USMLE STEP 2 CK PLATINUM NOTES

The Complete Preparatory Guide

Second Edition

Ashfaq Ul Hassan
MBBS MS
Consultant Anatomy
SKIMS Medical College
Bemina, Srinagar, Jammu and Kashmir, India

JAYPEE The Health Sciences Publisher
New Delhi | London | Panama | Philadelphia

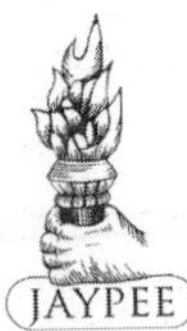

Jaypee Brothers Medical Publishers (P) Ltd

Headquarters

Jaypee Brothers Medical Publishers (P) Ltd.
4838/24, Ansari Road, Daryaganj
New Delhi 110 002, India
Phone: +91-11-43574357
Fax: +91-11-43574314
Email: jaypee@jaypeebrothers.com

Overseas Offices

J.P. Medical Ltd.
83, Victoria Street, London
SW1H 0HW (UK)
Phone: +44-20 3170 8910
Fax: +44-(0)20 3008 6180
Email: info@jpmedpub.com

JP Medical Inc.
325 Chestnut Street, Suite 412
Philadelphia, PA 19106, USA
Phone: +1215-713-7181
Email: jrusko@jpmedus.com

Jaypee Brothers Medical Publishers (P) Ltd.
Bhotahity, Kathmandu, Nepal
Phone: +977-9741283608
Email: Kathmandu@jaypeebrothers.com

Jaypee-Highlights Medical Publishers Inc.
City of Knowledge, Bld. 237, Clayton
Panama City, Panama
Phone: +1 507-301-0496
Fax: +1 507-301-0499
Email: cservice@jphmedical.com

Jaypee Brothers Medical Publishers (P) Ltd.
17/1-B, Babar Road, Block-B, Shaymali
Mohammadpur, Dhaka-1207, Bangladesh
Mobile: +08801912003485
Email: jaypeedhaka@gmail.com

Website: www.jaypeebrothers.com
Website: www.jaypeedigital.com

© 2016, Jaypee Brothers Medical Publishers

The views and opinions expressed in this book are solely those of the original contributor(s)/author(s) and do not necessarily represent those of editor(s) of the book.

All rights reserved. No part of this publication may be reproduced, stored or transmitted in any form or by any means, electronic, mechanical, photocopying, recording or otherwise, without the prior permission in writing of the publishers.

All brand names and product names used in this book are trade names, service marks, trademarks or registered trademarks of their respective owners. The publisher is not associated with any product or vendor mentioned in this book.

Medical knowledge and practice change constantly. This book is designed to provide accurate, authoritative information about the subject matter in question. However, readers are advised to check the most current information available on procedures included and check information from the manufacturer of each product to be administered, to verify the recommended dose, formula, method and duration of administration, adverse effects and contraindications. It is the responsibility of the practitioner to take all appropriate safety precautions. Neither the publisher nor the author(s)/editor(s) assume any liability for any injury and/or damage to persons or property arising from or related to use of material in this book.

This book is sold on the understanding that the publisher is not engaged in providing professional medical services. If such advice or services are required, the services of a competent medical professional should be sought.

Every effort has been made where necessary to contact holders of copyright to obtain permission to reproduce copyright material. If any have been inadvertently overlooked, the publisher will be pleased to make the necessary arrangements at the first opportunity.

Inquiries for bulk sales may be solicited at: jaypee@jaypeebrothers.com

USMLE Step 2 CK Platinum Notes

First Edition: 2013

Second Edition: **2016**

ISBN: 978-93-5250-172-4

Printed at Rajkamal Electric Press, Plot No. 2, Phase-IV, Kundli, Haryana.

Contributors

Ashfaq Ul Hassan
MBBS MS
Consultant–Anatomy
SKIMS Medical College
Bemina, Srinagar, Jammu and Kashmir, India

Prof. Showkat A Zargar
MD DM (Gastroenterology)
Director and Principal
Sher-i-Kashmir Institute of Medical Sciences (SKIMS)
Srinagar, Jammu and Kashmir, India

Prof. Naseer Mir
MS (Orthopedics)
Professor and Head – Orthopedics
Sher-i-Kashmir Institute of Medical Sciences (SKIMS)
Srinagar, Jammu and Kashmir, India

Dr Sheikh Manzoor Ahamed
MD (Dermatology)
Associate Professor and Head–Dermatology
Sher-i-Kashmir Institute of Medical Sciences (SKIMS)
Srinagar, Jammu and Kashmir, India

Preface to the Second Edition

I am extremely obliged to the Almighty Allah and no words would be enough to express my thanks to his holiness for guiding me.

This book *USMLE Step 2 CK Platinum Notes* consists of complete revision material for the preparation of the USMLE examinations with important latest questions asked in these examinations and most of the students do not fare well with these questions, thus significantly lowering their scores.

The book is for complete revision with special focus on the most common and most important cases asked. It covers special and important topics which are most frequently asked by the examiners.

The prime focus for the students to go through the most important points and recapitulating these at the end is important for any examination and special focus for the same has been given for their benefit.

Like the other series of books for the USMLE examinations being authored by me, which have had a tremendous success, I hope this effort of mine again would be helpful for the students throughout the world in their pursuit of academic excellence along with the important fact of getting a very good score in the examinations.

I hope the book proves to be useful for our students to the fullest.

I would encourage any aspiring student to join me for his/her contribution.

Ashfaq Ul Hassan
ashhassan@rediffmail.com

Preface to the First Edition

It gives me a great pleasure to introduce Platinum Notes for USMLE Step 1 and Step 2.

A need was felt by most of the students for a comprehensive book for USMLE for preparing extensively and simultaneously getting a very good score.

My efforts are directed to benefit the students to the maximum.

For a student preparing, revising, forgetting and consulting different books is a part of the game. In this journey some students tend to get nervous and anxious and I thought of putting all my best efforts into one book which would make the preparation simpler, interesting, more lucid and palatable.

High yield points, important topics, clinical correlations, in-depth focus on subjects, easy retention and quick revision are the points on which I have focused taking into account the latest trends of the examinations.

The matter in the book is highly concentrated, needs multiple revisions and deep concentration for retention.

The book has been framed to simulate the study pattern of USMLE examinations to its best.

The questions in the text and after every subject are almost similar to the questions put in the actual USMLE examination which gives a student a good chance to understand the standard of USMLE as well as to prepare for the examinations in a better way.

I feel that the students would be benefitted through my effort and a feedback from the students would be highly appreciated at ashhassan@rediffmail.com

I wish you good luck for your academic pursuits.

Ashfaq Ul Hassan
ashhassan@rediffmail.com

Acknowledgments

No words would be enough to express my regards to Prof. Showkat A Zargar, Director, Sher-i-Kashmir Institute of Medical Sciences (SKIMS), Srinagar, Jammu and Kashmir, India for his constant encouragement.

I am also thankful to my father Prof. Ghulam Hassan for his constant encouragement in all my academic pursuits and guiding me throughout the process of the completion of this book.

I convey my sincere thanks to Jaypee Brothers Medical Publishers (P) Ltd, New Delhi, India for their efforts and suggestions, especially Shri Jitendar P Vij (Group Chairman), Ms Chetna Vohra (Associate Director), and Ms Payal Bharti (Project Manager) for helping me through my idea.

Abbreviations

1°	Primary
2°	Secondary
#	Fracture
ACE	Angiotensin converting enzyme
ACE-I	Angiotensin converting enzyme inhibitor
ACTH	Adrenocorticotropic hormone
ACh	Acetylcholine
Adr	Adrenaline
AD	Autosomal dominant
ADH	Anti-diuretic hormone
AF	Atrial fibrillation
AFB	Acid-fast bacilli
AFP	Alpha-fetoprotein
A.k.a	Also known as
ALL	Acute lymphocytic leukemia
AML	Acute myelogenous leukemia
ANA	Antinuclear antibody
ANS	Autonomic nervous system
AP	Anteroposterior
AR	Autosomal recessive
ARDS	Acute respiratory distress syndrome
ARF	Acute renal failure
AS	Aortic stenosis
ATP	Adenosine triphosphate
ASD	Atrial septal defect
AV	Atrioventricular
A/E	All except
Acc/ to	According to
Ad/E, ad/e	Adverse effects
A/W or a/w	Associated with
BBB	Bundle branch block
bid	Twice a day
BMR	Basal metabolic rate
BP	Blood pressure
BPH	Benign prostatic hypertrophy
BUN	Blood urea nitrogen
B/L	Bilateral
BM	Bone marrow, basement membrane
b/n or b/w	Between
C/S	Culture and sensitivity
Ca^{2+}	Calcium
CABG	Coronary artery bypass graft
CAD	Coronary artery disease
CCF	Congestive cardiac failure
CT	Computerized tomography
CHF	Congestive heart failure
CHO	Carbohydrate
CML	Chronic myelogenous leukemia
CMV	Cytomegalovirus
CN	Cranial nerves
CNS	Central nervous system
CO	Cardiac output
C/O	Complaining of
COLD	Chronic obstructive lung disease
COPD	Chronic obstructive pulmonary disease
CPK	Creatine phosphokinase
CRF	Chronic renal failure
CRP	C-reactive protein
CSF	Cerebrospinal fluid
CVA	Cerebrovascular accident
CVP	Central venous pressure
CVS	Cardiovascular system

CXR	Chest X-ray
Ca	Carcinoma/Cancer
C/c	Complication
C_T	Chemotherapy
C/I	Contraindication
Cl/f	Clinical features
CTD	Connective tissue disease
Cont./L	Contralateral
Cx	Cervix
D and C	Dilation and curettage
DI	Diabetes insipidus
DIC	Disseminated intravascular coagulopathy
DIP	Distal interphalangeal joint
DKA	Diabetic ketoacidosis
dL	Deciliter
DM	Diabetes mellitus
DTR	Deep tendon reflexes
DVT	Deep venous thrombosis
d/to	Due to
D/g	Diagnosis
DOC	Drug of choice
Ds, d/s	Disease, disease
DM	Diabetes mellitus
ECG	Electrocardiogram
ECT	Electroconvulsive therapy
ECHO	Echocardiography
EMG	Electromyogram
EOM	Extraocular muscles
ESR	Erythrocyte sedimentation rate
ERCP	Endoscopic retrograde cholangio-Pancreatography
EUA	Examination under anesthesia
FBS	Fasting blood sugar
FEV	Forced expiratory volume
FFP	Fresh frozen plasma
FRC	Functional residual capacity
FTT	Failure to thrive
FVC	Forced vital capacity
FA	Fatty acid
FFA	Free fatty acid
GFR	Glomerular filtration rate
GH	Growth hormone
GIT	Gastrointestinal tract
GTT	Glucose tolerance test
GU	Genitourinary
HAV	Hepatitis A virus
HCG	Human chorionic gonadotropin
HDL	High density lipoprotein
Hb	Hemoglobin
HIV	Human immunodeficiency virus
HLA	Histocompatibility locus antigen
H/O	History of
HR	Heart rate
HSV	Herpes simplex virus
HTN	Hypertension
HS	Hereditary spherocytosis
HCC	Hepato cellular carcinoma
HD	Hodgkin's disease
I and D	Incision and drainage
IDDM	Insulin dependent diabetes mellitus
Ig	Immunoglobulin
IM	Intramuscular
INR	International normalized ratio
ITP	Idiopathic thrombocytopenic purpura
IV	Intravenous
IVP	Intravenous pyelogram
IVU	Intravenous urogram
ICT	Intracranial tension
IOC	Investigation of choice
ILD	Interstitial lung disease
IOT	Intraocular tension
Ipsi/L	Ipsilateral

JVP	Jugular venous pressure
K^+	Potassium
K/as	Known as
LAE	Left atrial enlargement
LBBB	Left bundle branch block
LDH	Lactate dehydrogenase
LMN	Lower motor neuron
LE	Lupus erythematosus
LP	Lumbar puncture
LV	Left ventricle
LVH	Left ventricular hypertrophy
LN	Lymph node
MAO	Monoamine oxidase
MEN	Multiple endocrine neoplasia
MI	Myocardial infarction or mitral insufficiency
mL	Milliliter
MMR	Measles, mumps, rubella
MRI	Magnetic resonance imaging
MRSA	Methicillin resistant staph aureus
MG	Myasthenia gravis
Mc or MC	Most common
MN	Malnutrition
M/m	Management
Ms, m/s	Muscle
Na	Sodium
NIDDM	Non-insulin dependent diabetes mellitus
NSAID	Non-steroidal anti-inflammatory drugs
n.or nv	Nerve
NHL	Non-Hodgkin's lymphoma
OCG	Oral cholecystogram
PA	Posteroanterior
PDA	Patent ductus arteriosus
PMN	Polymorphonuclear leukocyte (neutrophil)
PP	Patient profile
PT	Prothrombin time, or physical therapy
PTCA	Percutaenous transluminal coronary angioplasty
PTH	Parathyroid hormone
PTT	Partial thromboplastin time
P/g	Prognosis
P_x	Prophylaxis
PBC	Primary bilary cirrhosis
RA	Rheumatoid arthritis
RBBB	Right bundle branch block
RBC	Red blood cell
RIA	Radioimmunoassay
RNA	Ribonucleic acid
RTA	Renal tubular acidosis
RVH	Right ventricular hypertrophy
Rx	Treatment
R, or T/t	Treatment
R_T	Radiotherapy
SBE	Subacute bacterial endocarditis
SGOT	Serum glutamic-oxaloacetic transaminase
SGPT	Serum glutamic-pyruvic transaminase
SIADH	Syndrome of inappropriate antidiuretic hormone
SLE	Systemic lupus erythematous
SCLC	Small cell lung carcinoma
SM	Smooth muscle
Supf.	Superficial
SqCC	Squamous cell carcinoma
TIBC	Total iron binding capacity
tid	Three times a day
TSH	Thyroid stimulating hormone
TT	Thrombin time
TTP	Thrombotic thrombocytopenic purpura
TURP	Transurethral resection of prostate
TOC	Treatment of choice
UC	Ulcerative colitis

UMN	Upper motor neuron
URI	Upper respiratory infection
US, U/S	Ultrasound
UTI	Urinary tract infection
UVA	Ultraviolet A light
U/L	Unilateral
VF	Ventricular fibrillation
VDRL	Venereal disease research laboratory (test for syphilis)
V/Q	Ventrilation-perfusion
VT	Ventricular tachycardia
vWD	von Willebrand's virus
VZV	Varicella zoster virus
V/s	Vessel
Vs	Versus (= against)
WBC	White blood cell
WPW	Wolff-Parkinson-White
WG	Wegner's granulomatosis
WT	Wilm's tumor
XLR	X linked recessive
Yr	Year
Zn	Zinc
ZES	Zollinger Ellison Syndrome
—	Reaction block by, inhibited by
~	Denotes heading
!	Increase

Contents

1. Medicine 1
2. Pediatrics 217
3. Psychiatry 327
4. Dermatology 369
5. Surgery 421
6. Orthopedics 609
7. Ophthalmology 625
8. Obstetrics and Gynecology 675

Plate 1

Dermatological Diseases

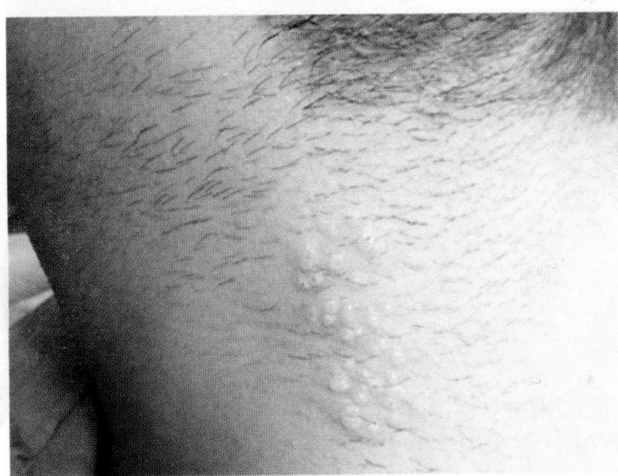

A young male presented with multiple grouped vesicular lesions of herpes zoster

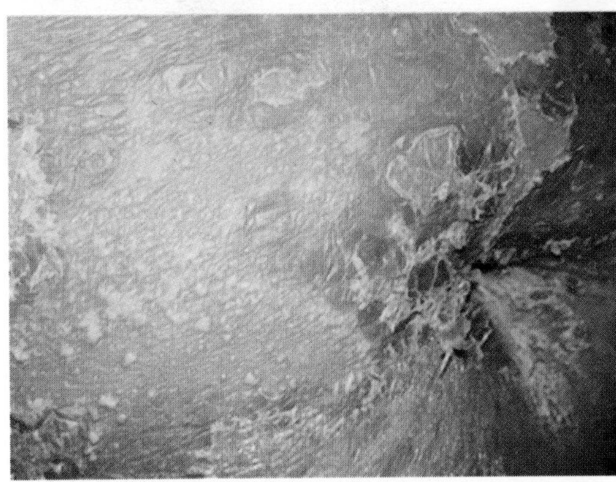

A young pregnant female patient developed annular lesions which spreaded in a ring form accompanied by fever and leucocytosis diagnosed as pustular psoriasis

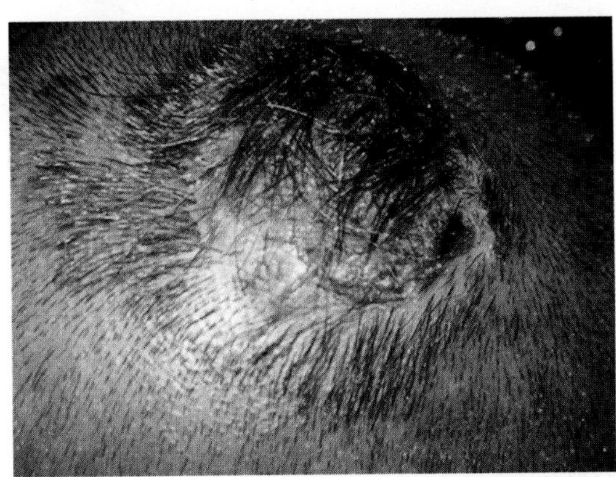

A young boy presented with a boggy inflammatory mass studded with broken hairs and follicular orifices oozing with pus suggestive of Kerion

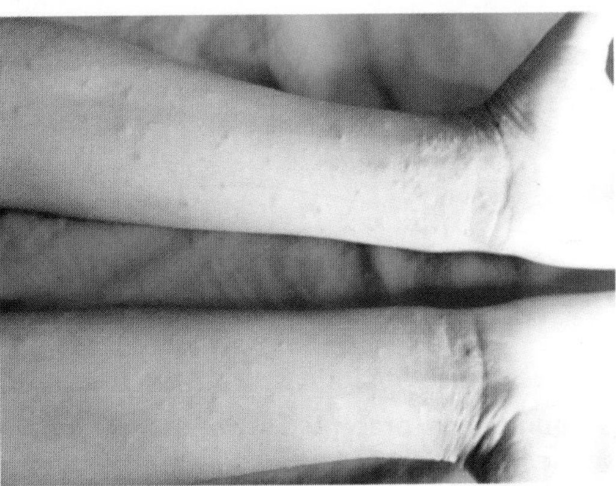

A child presented with multiple itchy papular lesions on the hands. Similar lesions were also seen in younger brother having scabies

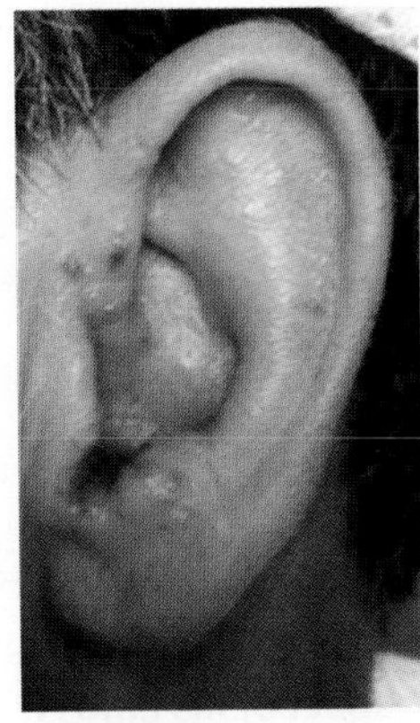

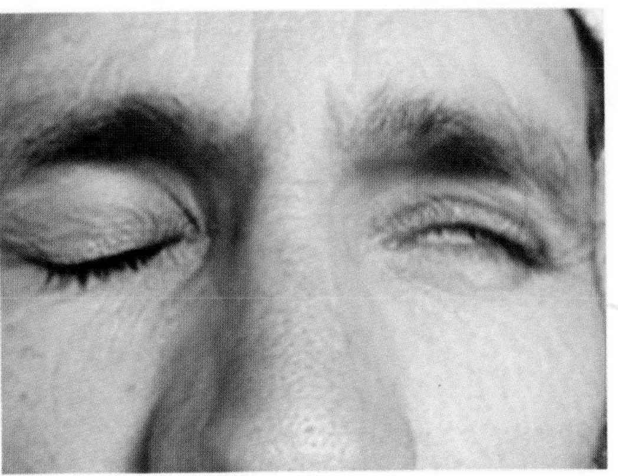

This patient presented with multiple vesicles on his pinna which was followed by palsy of facial nerve having Ramsay Hunt syndrome

Plate 2

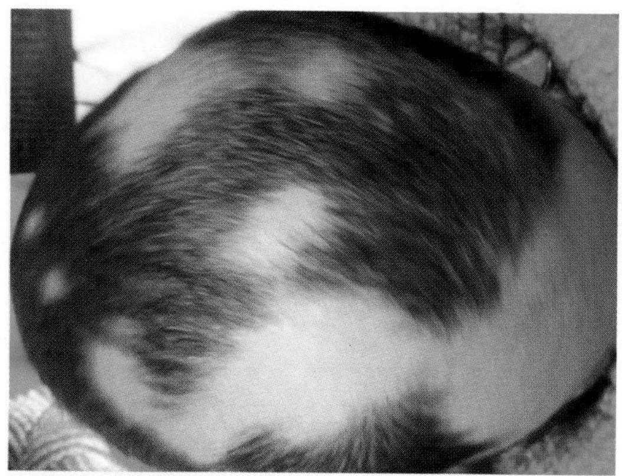

The patient has diffuse hair loss and having alopecia areata

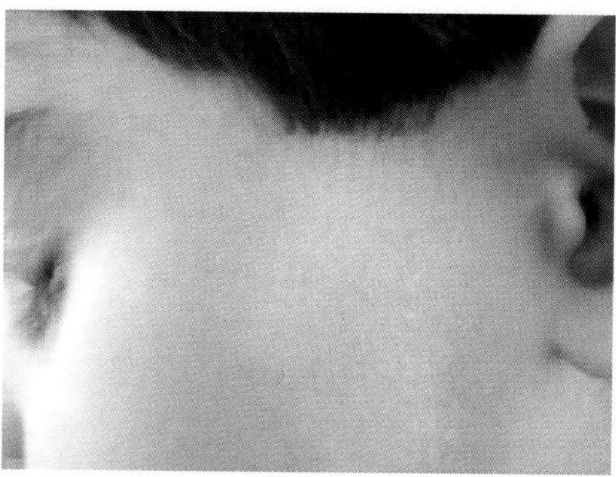

A young child presented with a pink patch which progressively developed into a hypopigmented macule having P. alba (Pityriasis alba)

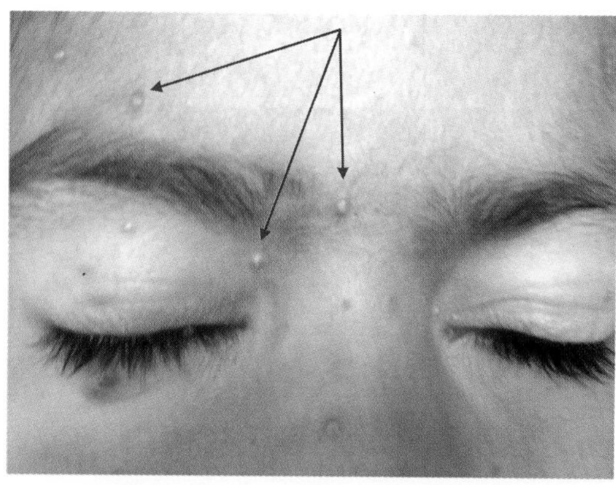

A young child presented with multiple dome shaped umbilicated lesions on the face which are molluscum contagiosum lesions

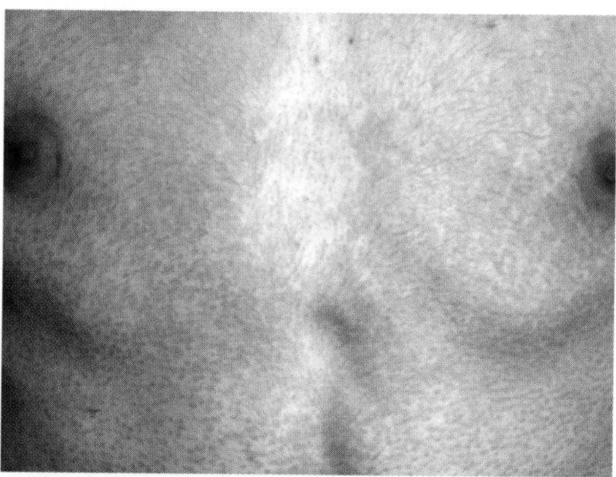

A young old adult presented with oval scaly hypopigmented macules over the chest having PV (pityriasis versicolor)

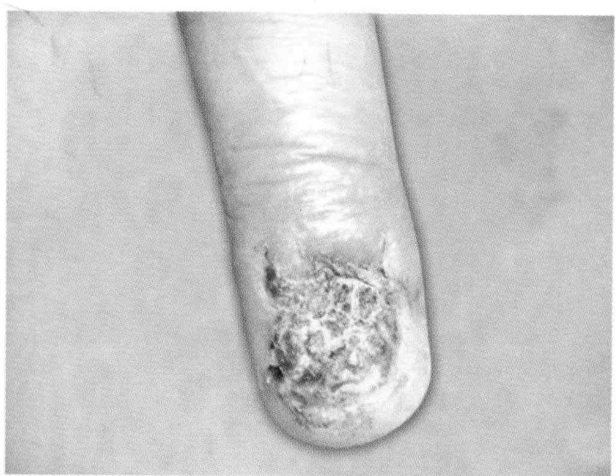

An elderly patient presented with a lesion as shown in figure which is dark in color with irregular borders there is periungual brownish black pigmentation there is longitudinal melanonychia suggestive of melanoma of nail

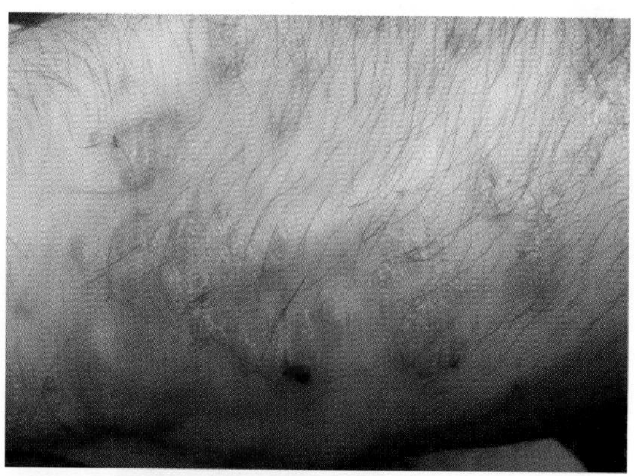

A 44-year-old developed scaly eruption on extensor aspect of his limbs having psoriasis

Plate 3

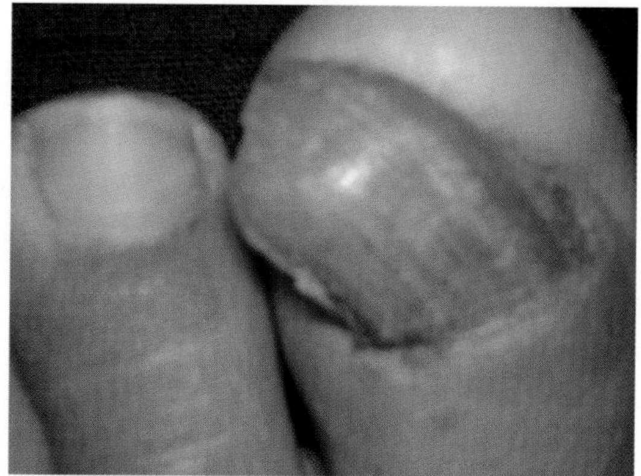

Nail pathology suggesting onchogryphosis

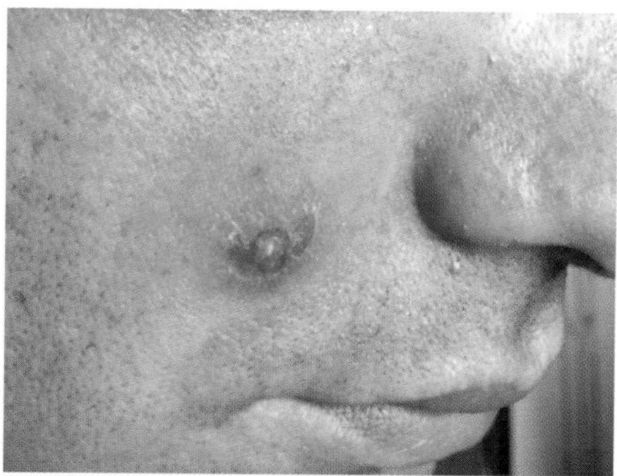

A 26-year-old man with diabetes mellitus presents with recurrent furunculosis caused mostly by staphylococci

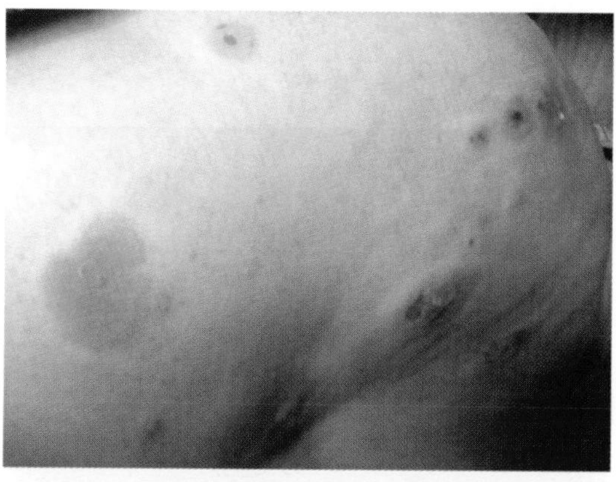

A patient after taking phenytoin present with targetoid lesion as erythema multiforme

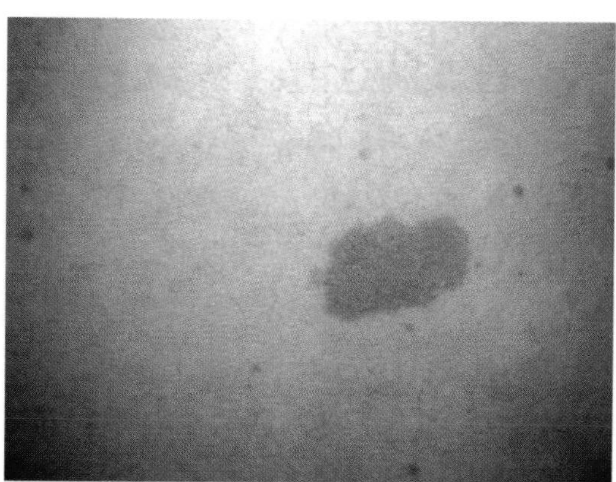

A typical café au lait spot on back

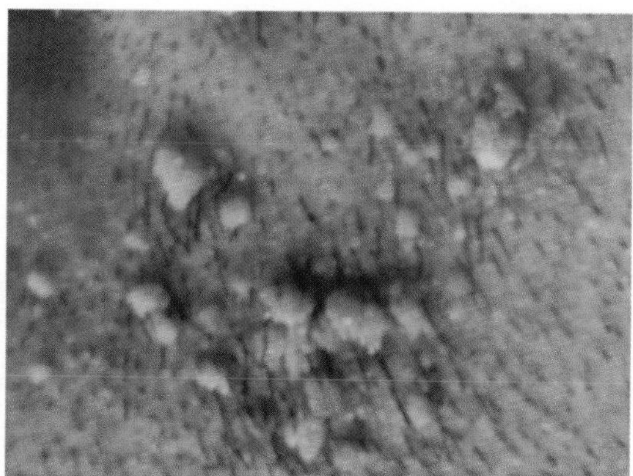

A patient has multiple, large exophytic filiform and cauliflower like masses suggestive of HPV warts

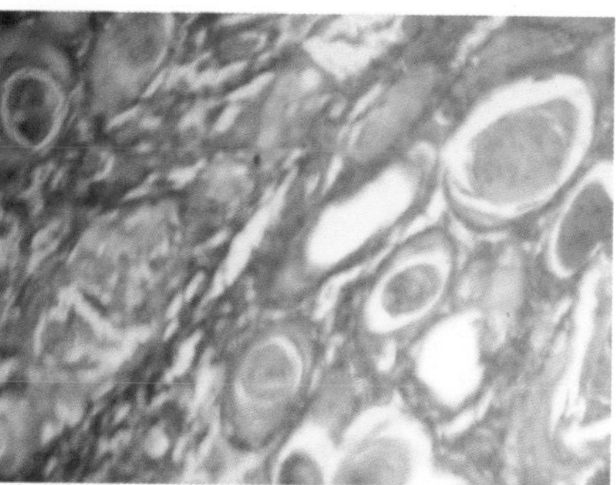

This 45-year-old female, who presented with a skin lesion which on histopathology showed characteristic keratin pearls is pathologically most commonly used in describing squamous cell carcinoma

Plate 4

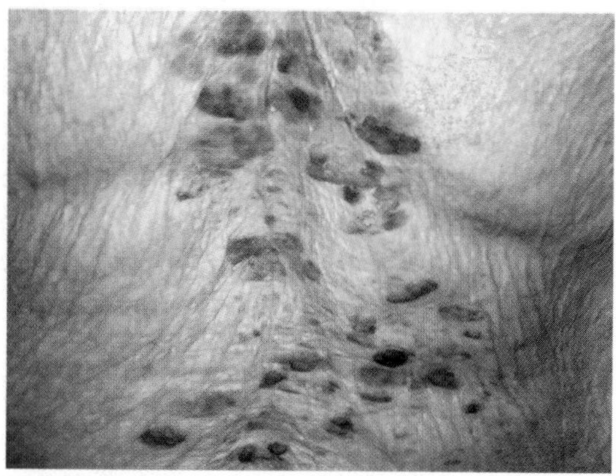

An elderly patient presented with appearance of multiple lesions diagnosed as multiple seborrheic keratoses. The patient was found to have an underlying cancer. The sign is called the leser-trelat sign

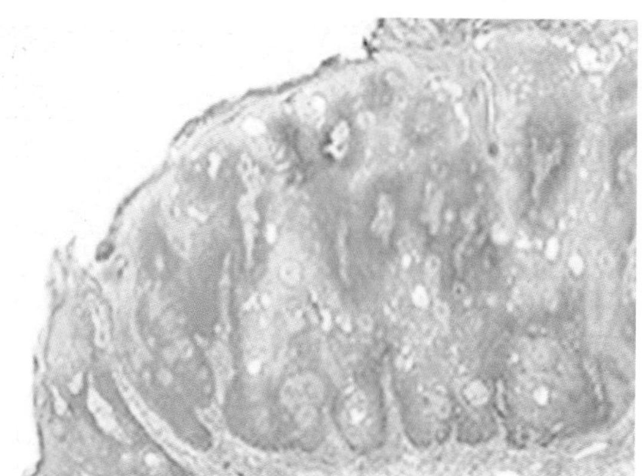

Histopathological slide revealing keratocanthoma skin

Orthopedic Images

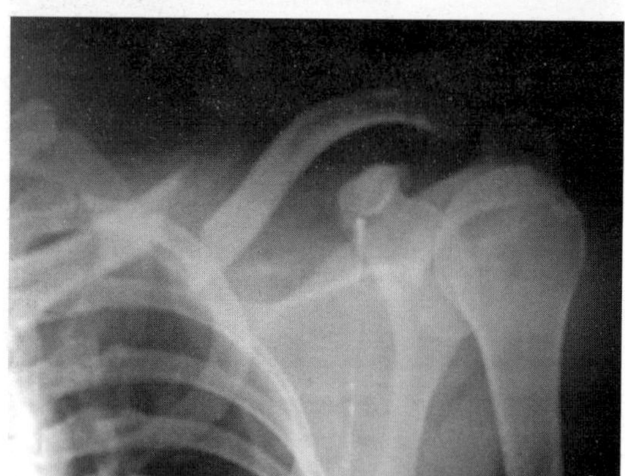

Well-defined mid shaft fracture clavicle

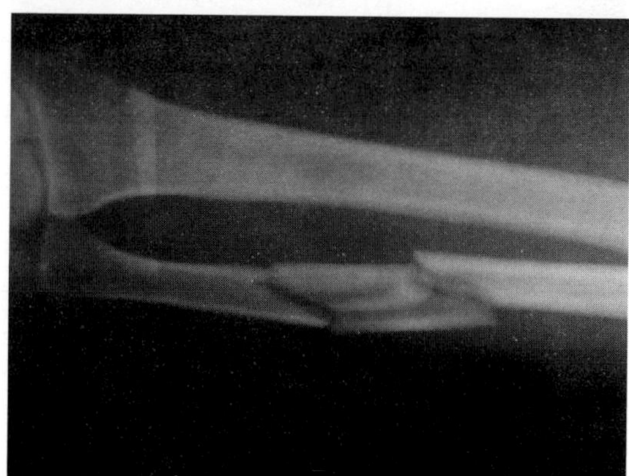

Fracture ulna

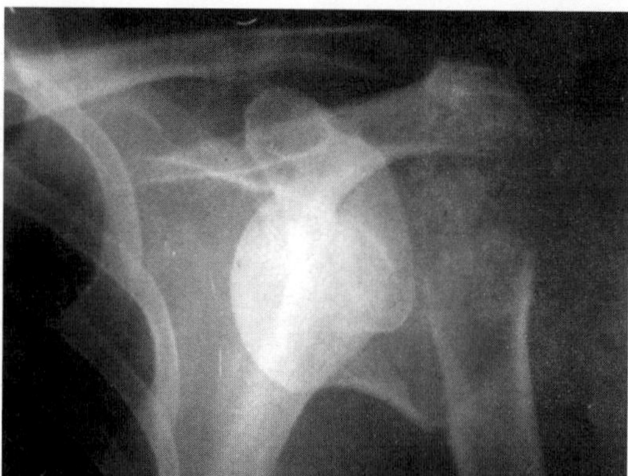

Fracture dislocation of shoulder joint

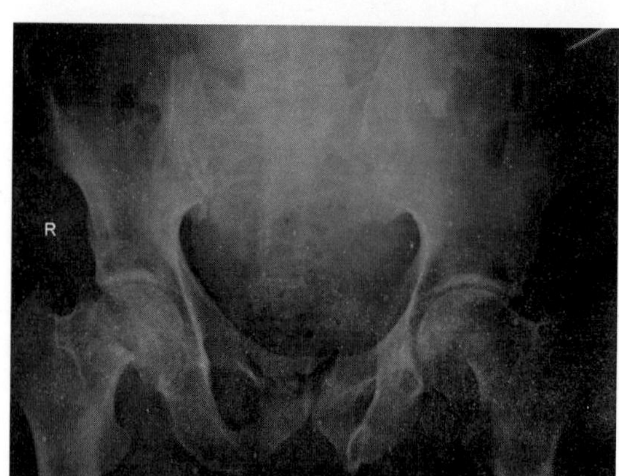

Bilateral subcapital fracture neck of femur

Plate 5

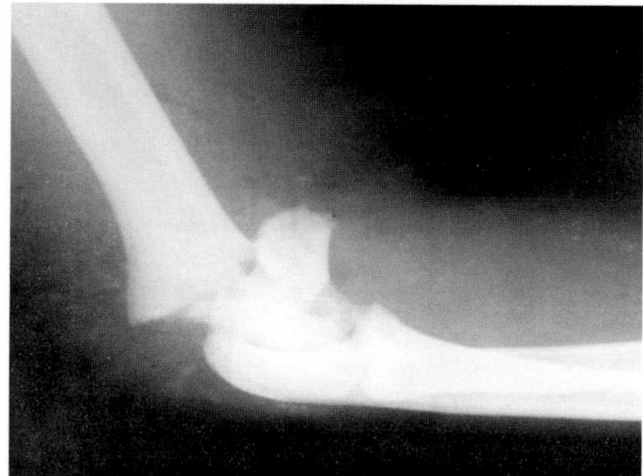
Lateral view intercondylar fracture elbow

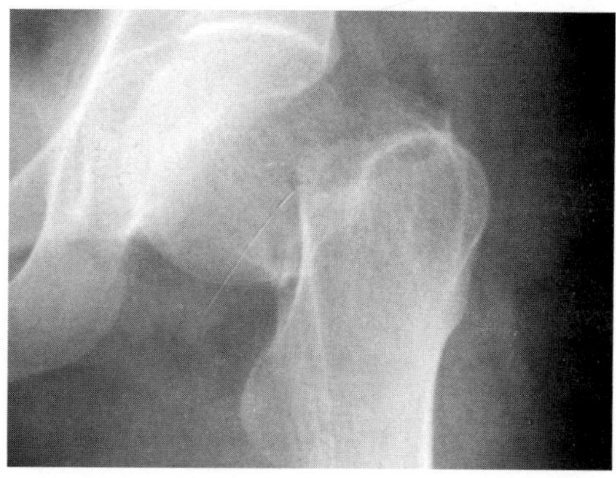
Fracture neck of femur

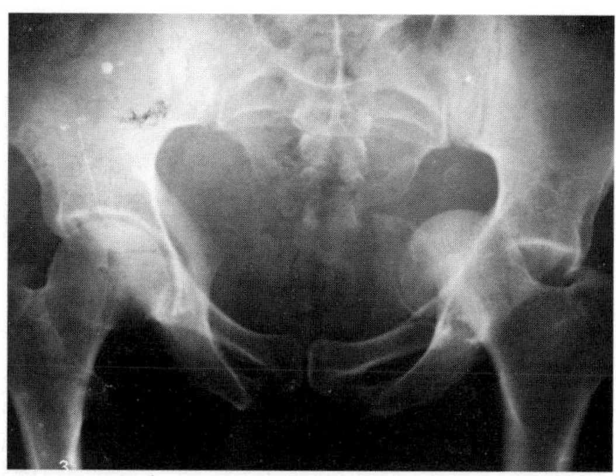
Central dislocation of left hip

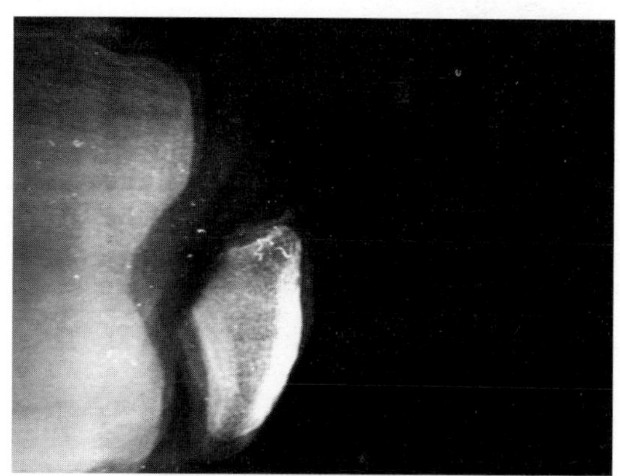
Fracture patella

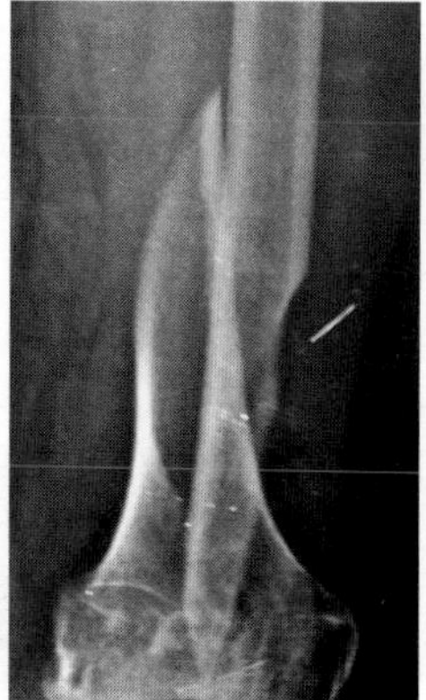
Intercondylar fracture femur

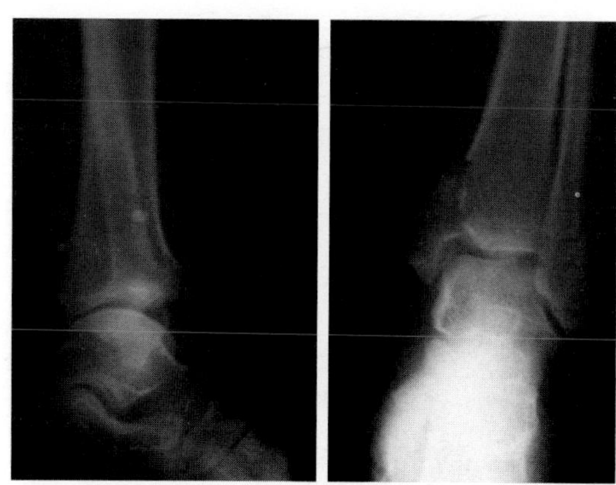
Well-defined bimalleolar fracture

Plate 6

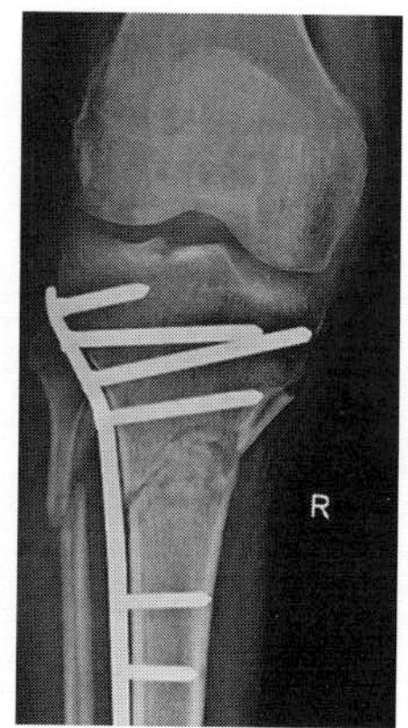

Upper tibial and fibula fracture

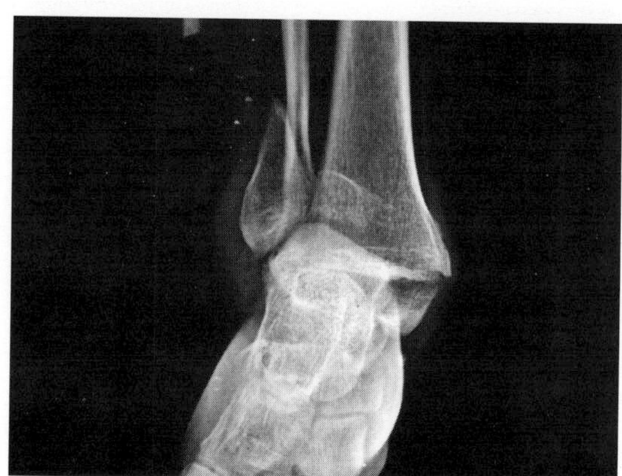

Well-defined trimalleolar fracture

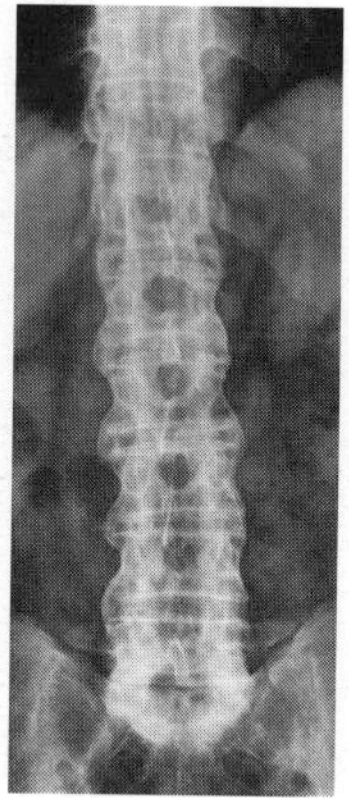

Bamboo spine characteristic of ankylosing spondylitis

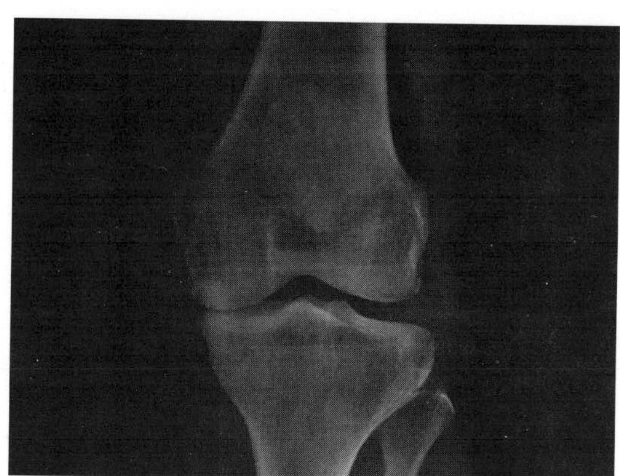

Medial compartment osteoarthritis knee

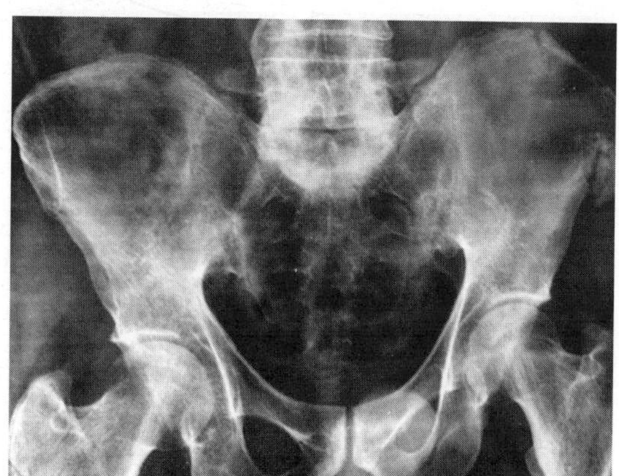

Sacroiliac ankylosis characteristic of ankylosing spondylitis

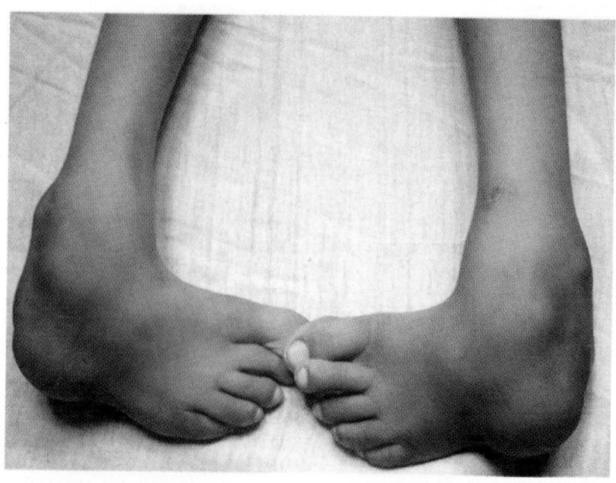

Congenital talipes equinovarus (CTEV)

Plate 7

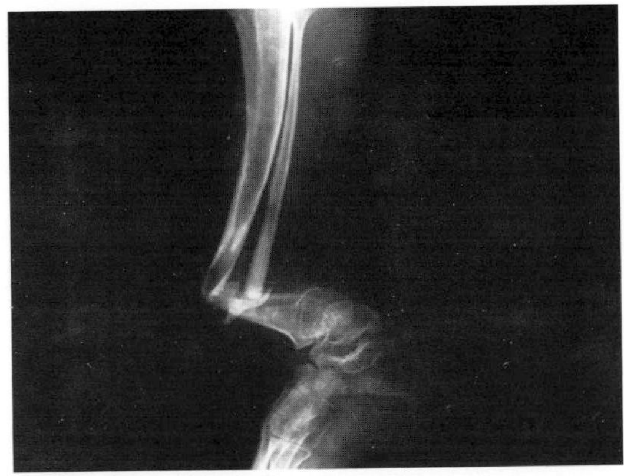

Congenital pseudarthrosis tibia

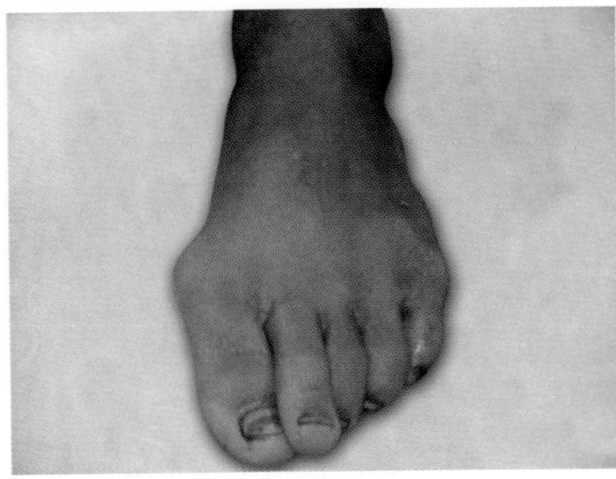

Hallux valgus

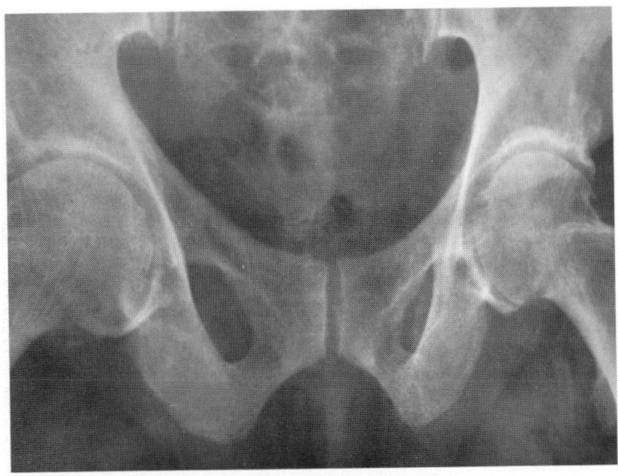

Severe bilateral osteoarthritis hip

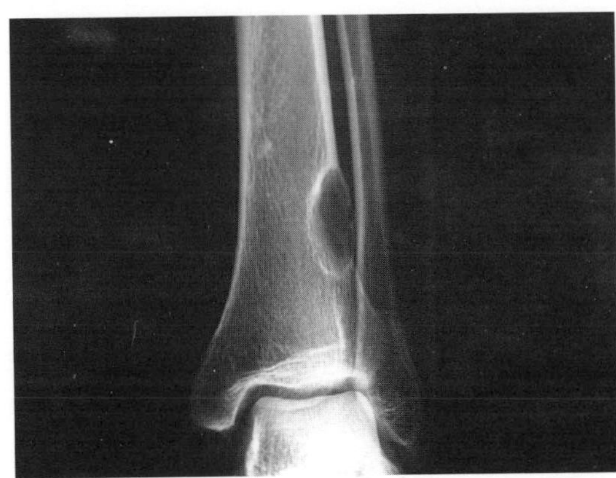

Fibrous dysplasia

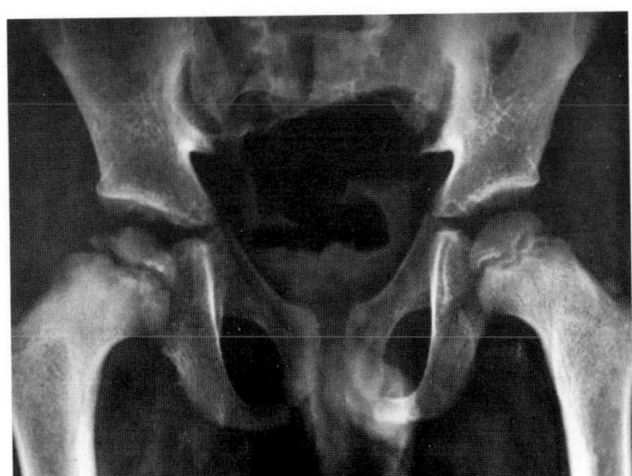

Severe Perthes disease

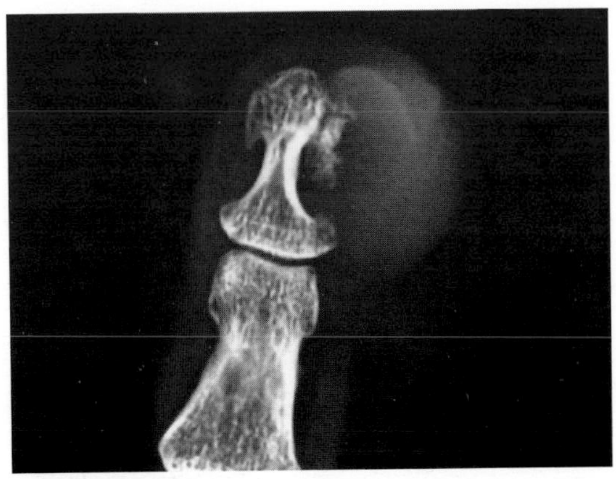

Exostosis terminal phalanx

Plate 8

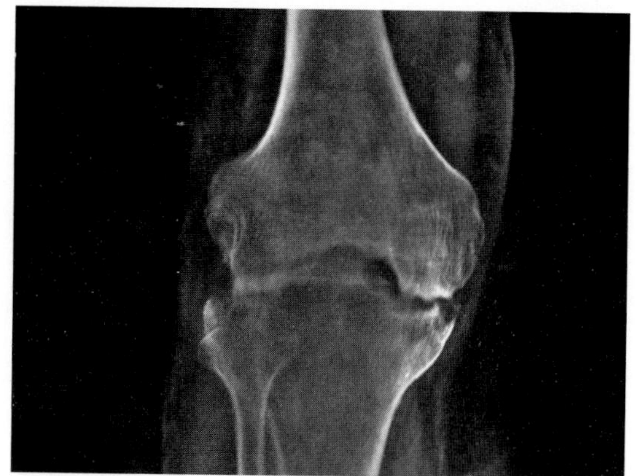
Tuberculosis knee joint

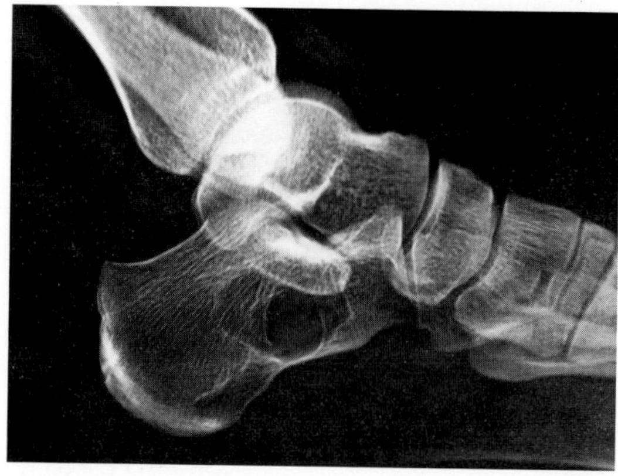
Bone cyst calcaneum

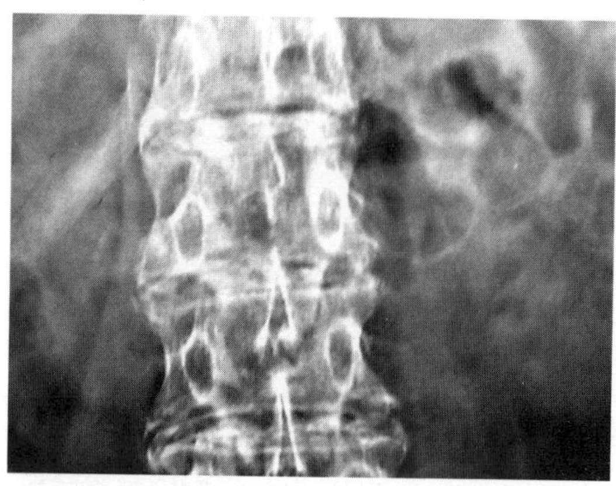
Intervertebral disk calcification in alkaptonuria

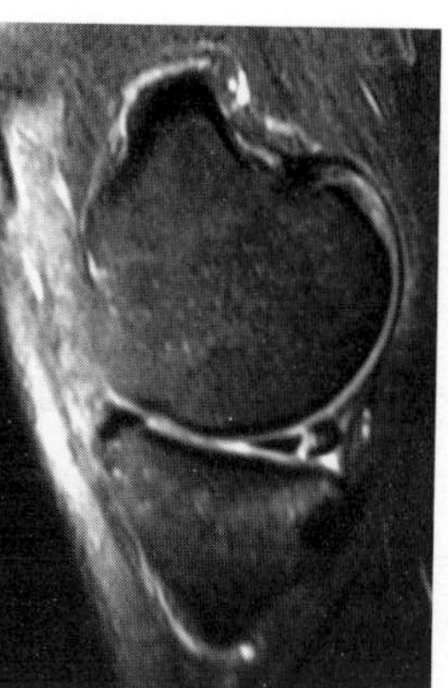
Medial meniscal tear

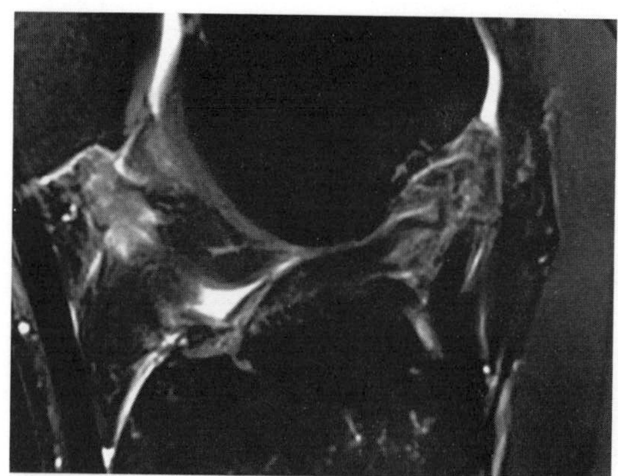
Avulsion of ACL (Anterior Cruciate Ligament)

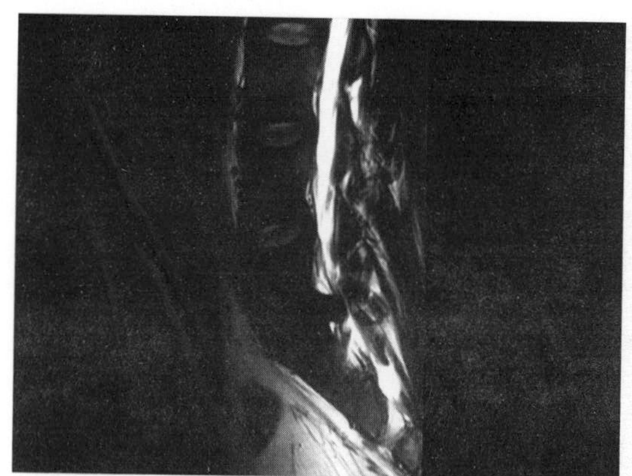
L5 S1 disk prolapse

All Orthopedic Figures Courtesy: Prof. Naseer Mir, Head Orthopedics, SKIMS Medical College, Bemina

Plate 9

Important Radiological Images

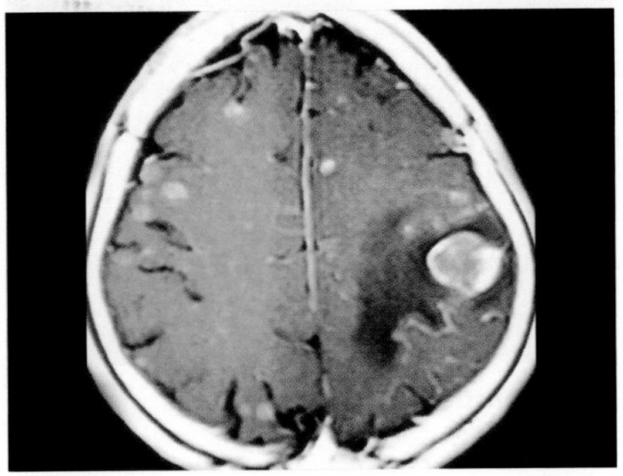

CT demonstrating tuberculomas brain

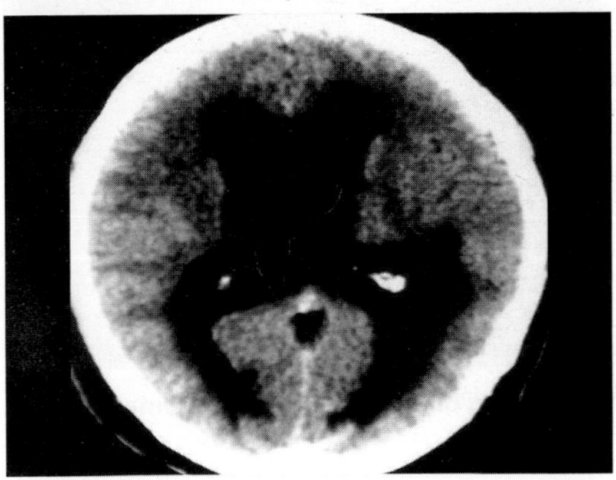

CT demonstrating enlarged ventricles brain (hydrocephalus)

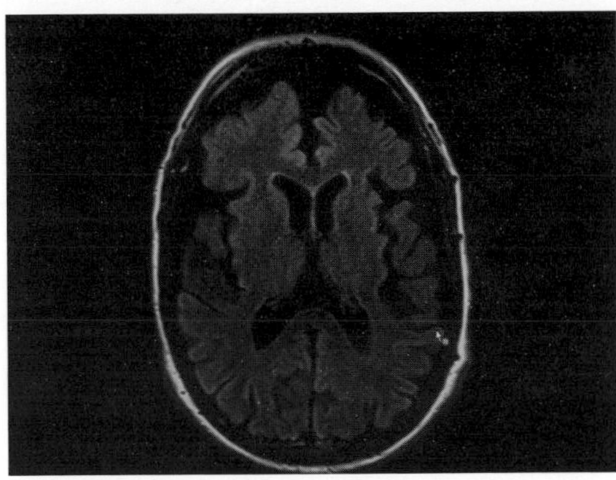

CT showing cortical atrophy

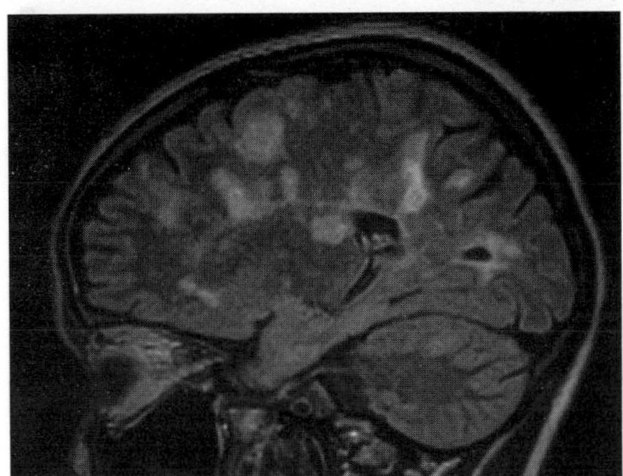

CT showing demyelinating plaques in multiple sclerosis

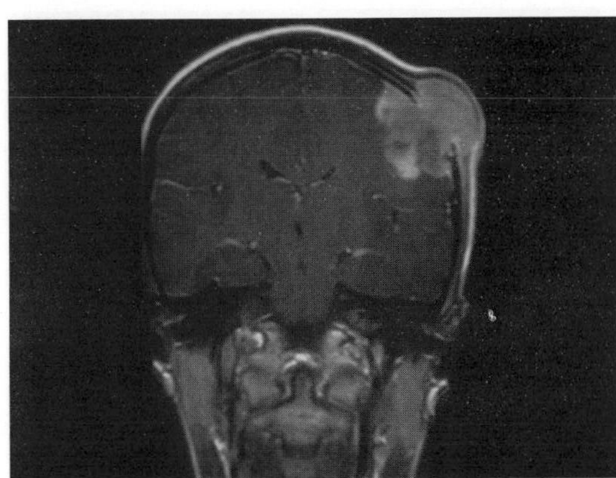

CT demonstrating metastasis skull

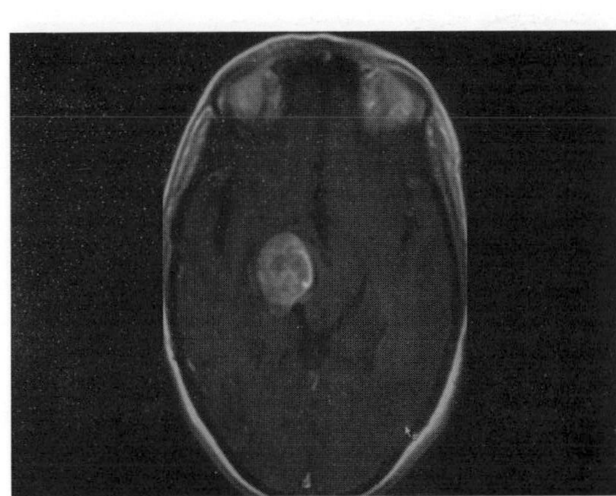

CT showing acoustic neuroma

Plate 10

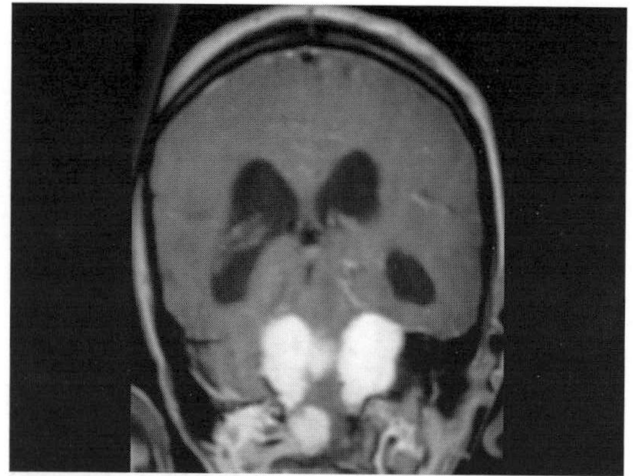
CT showing bilateral acoustic neuromas

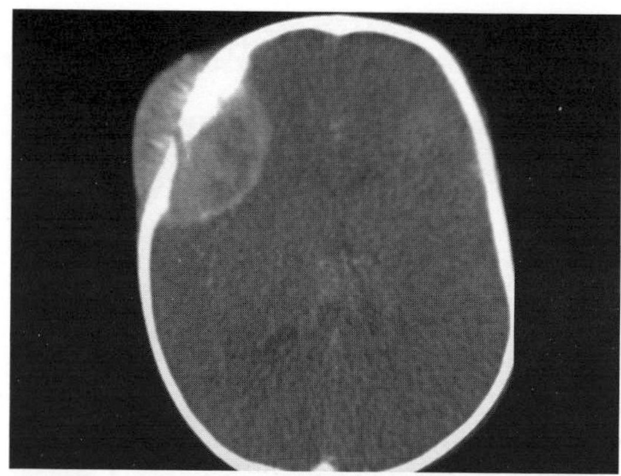
CT demonstrating a neuroblastoma

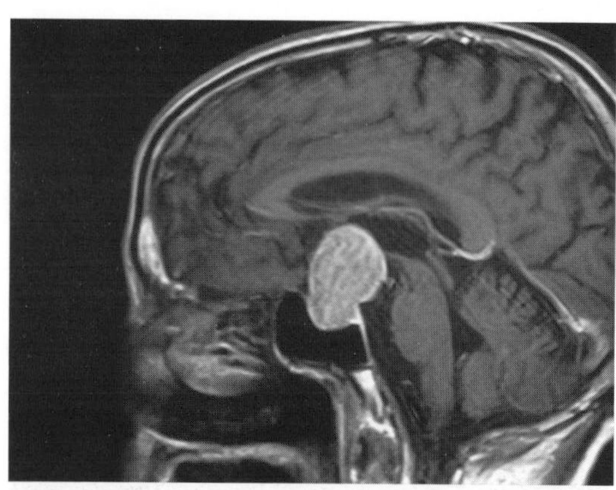
CT demonstrating pituitary tumor

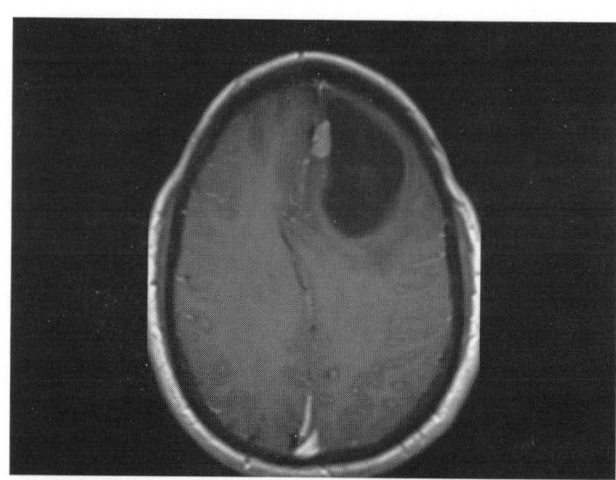
CT demonstrating pilocytic astrocytoma

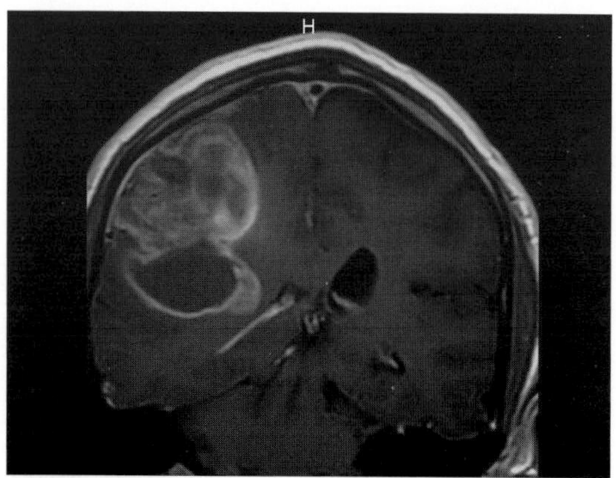

CT demonstrating a large ICSOL (oligodendroglioma)

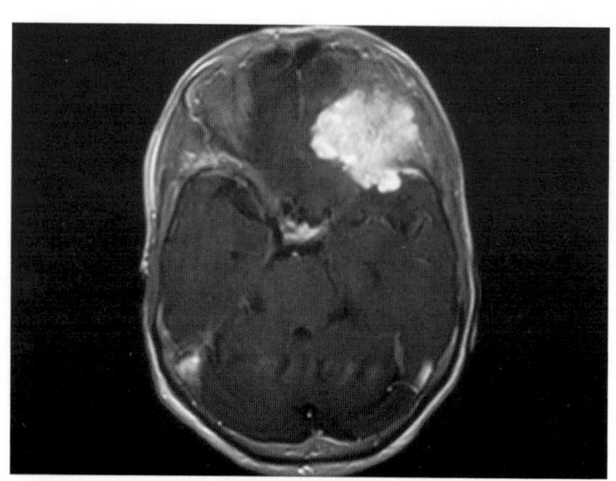
CT scan showing meningioma

Plate 11

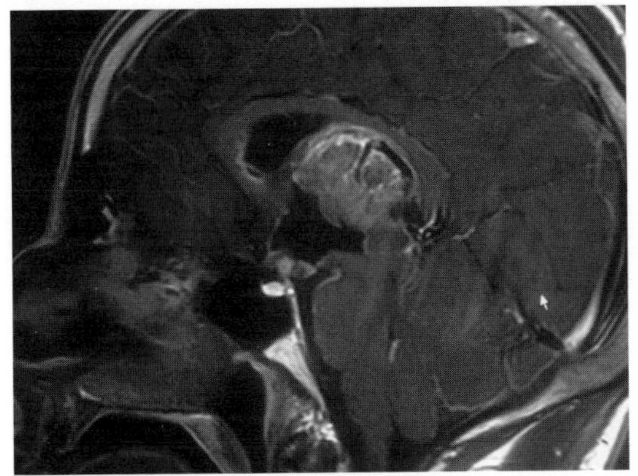

CT demonstrating pineal tumor

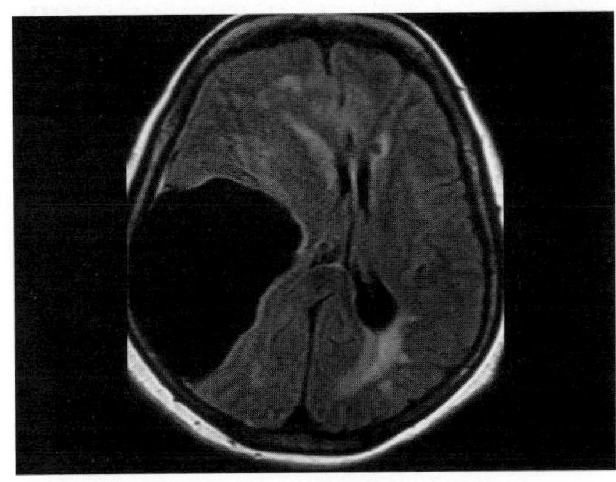

CT demonstrating porencephalic cyst

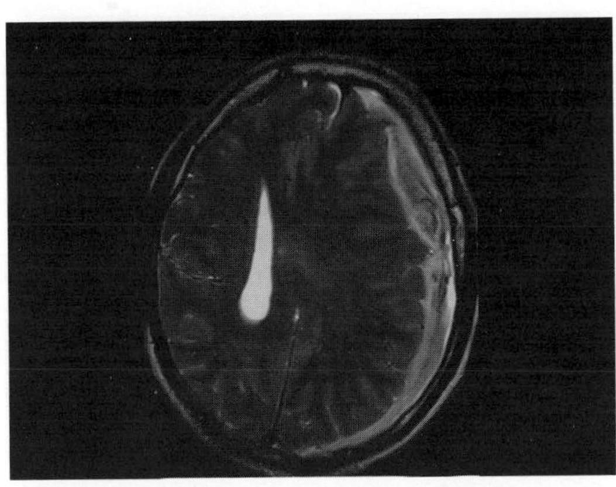

CT demonstrating subdural hemorrhage

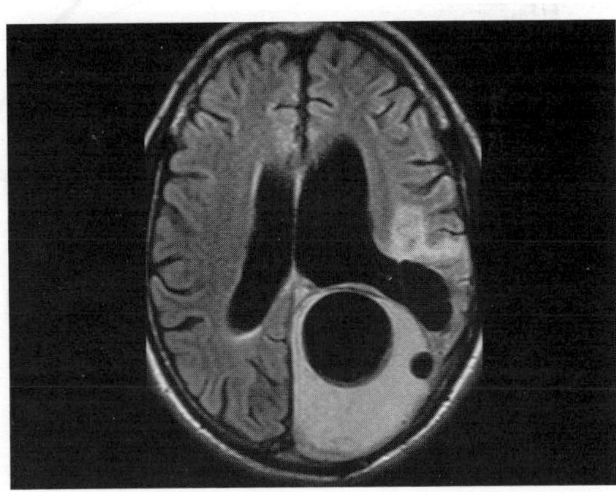

CT showing rare hydatid cyst in brain

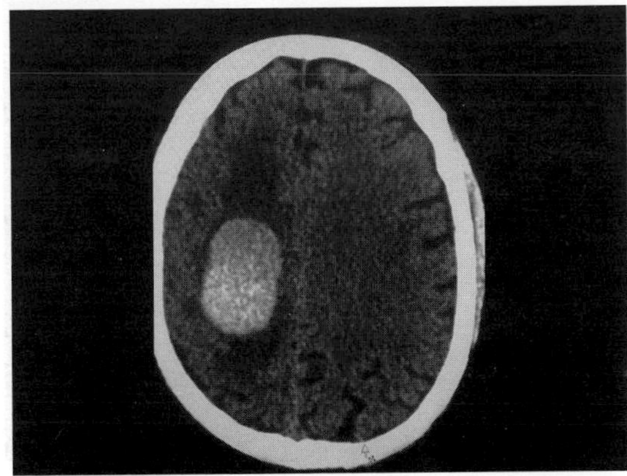

CT Scan showing intracranial hemorrhage

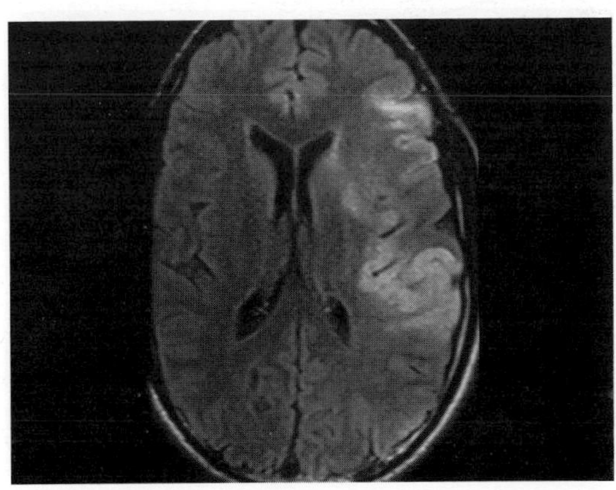

CT scan showing infarct in territory of right middle cerebral artery

Plate 12

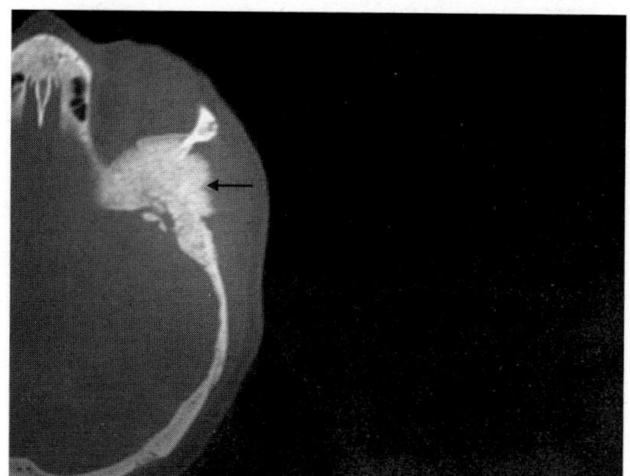

CT scan showing fibrous dysplasia

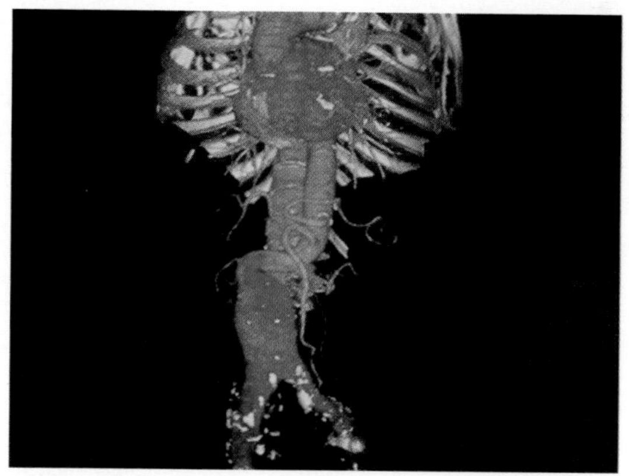

Angiogram revealing aortic aneurysm

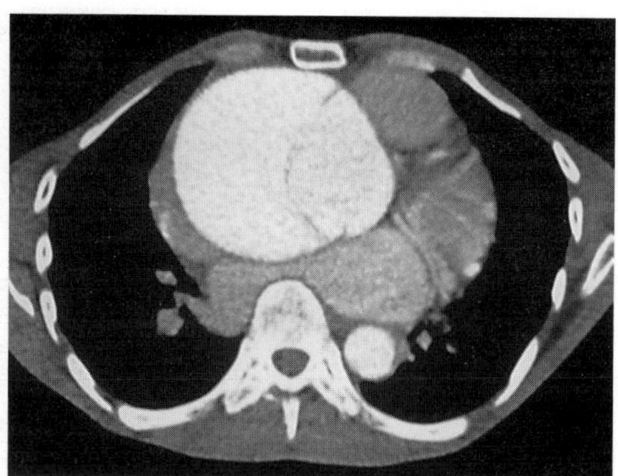

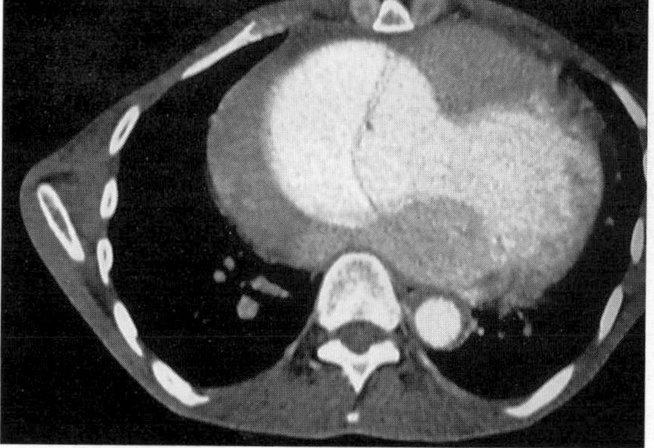

CT scan showing aortic dissection

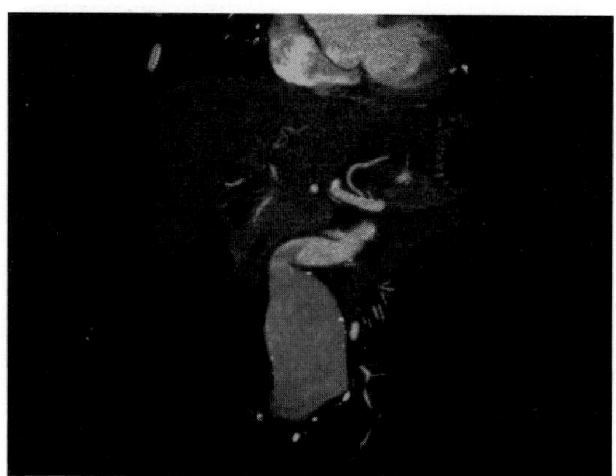

CT revealing aortic aneurysm

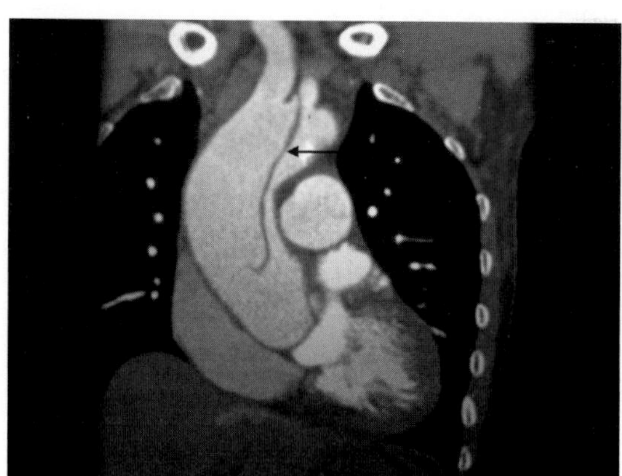

CT scan showing aortic dissection longitudinal tear

Plate 13

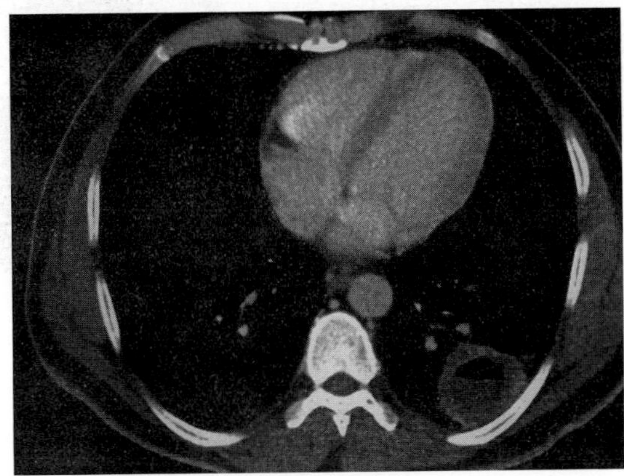

CT showing abscess in left lung

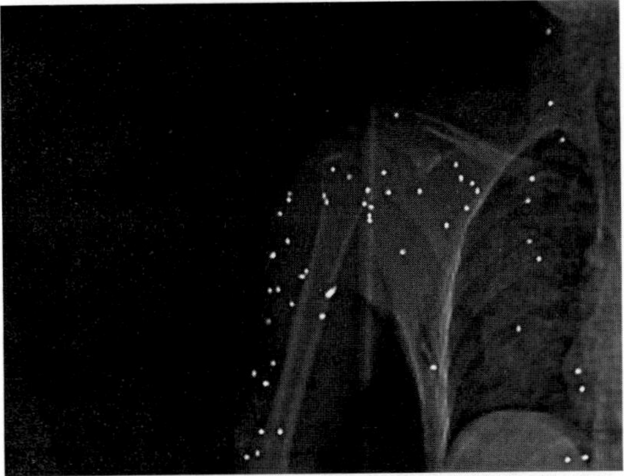

Radiograph demonstrating pellet Injuries in right lung and arm

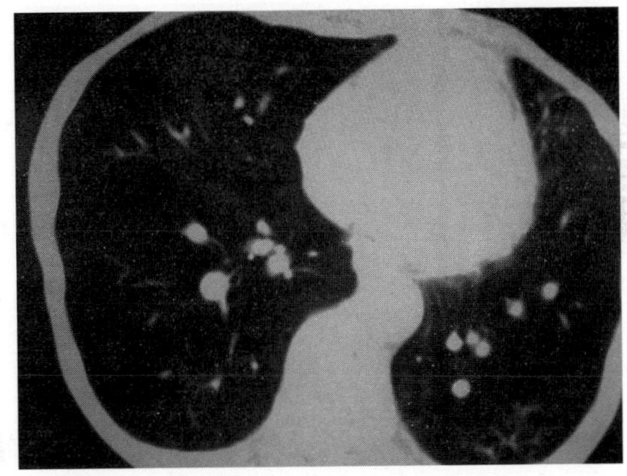

CT showing emphysematous lungs

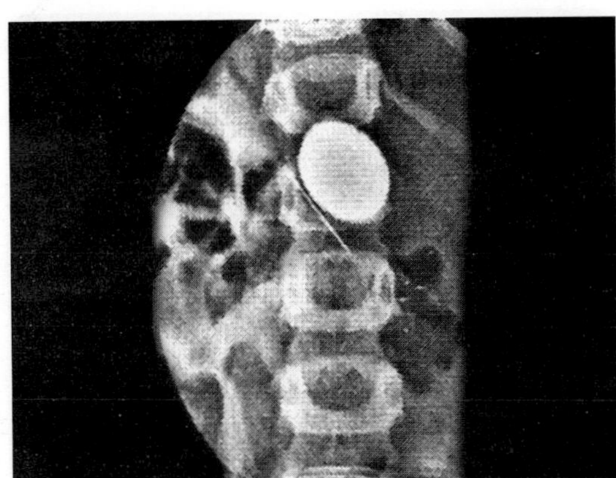

Plain radiograph demonstrating foreign body in esophagus

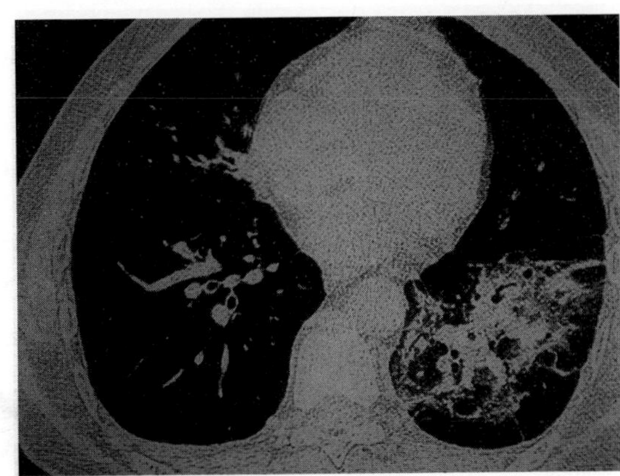

CT showing consolidation lung

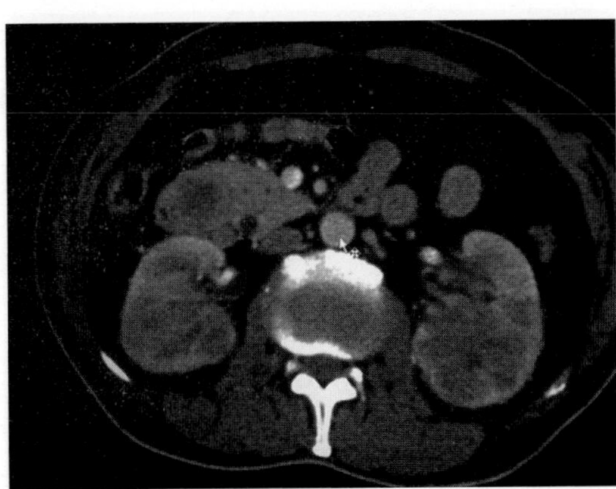

CT demonstrating multicentric renal cell cancers in VHL

Plate 14

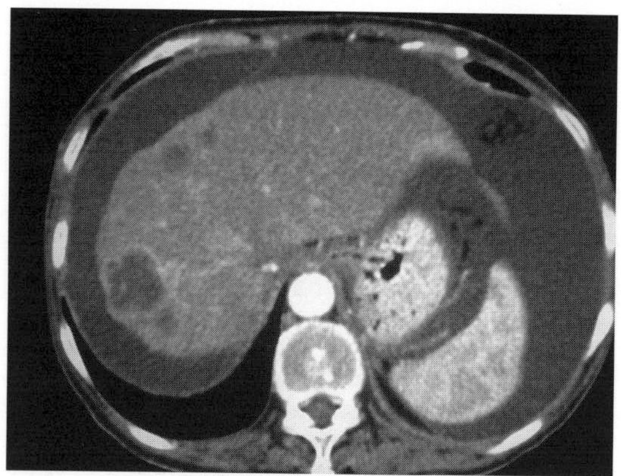

CT scan showing metastatsis liver

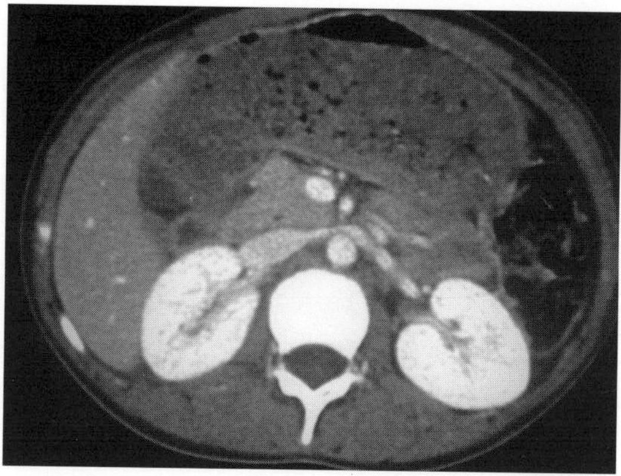

Liver laceration and renal injury in a case of trauma

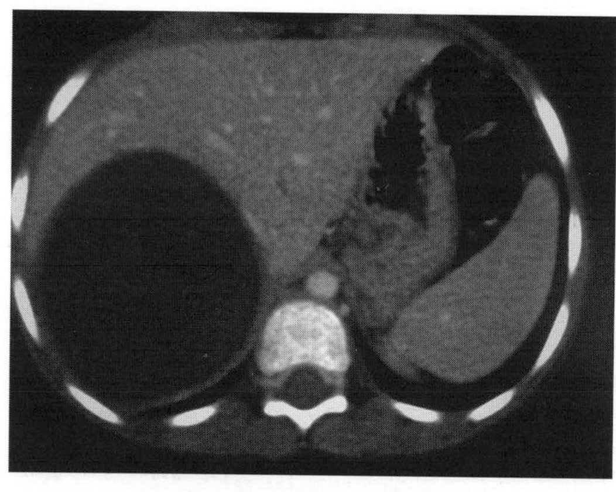

CT demonstrating hydatid cyst liver

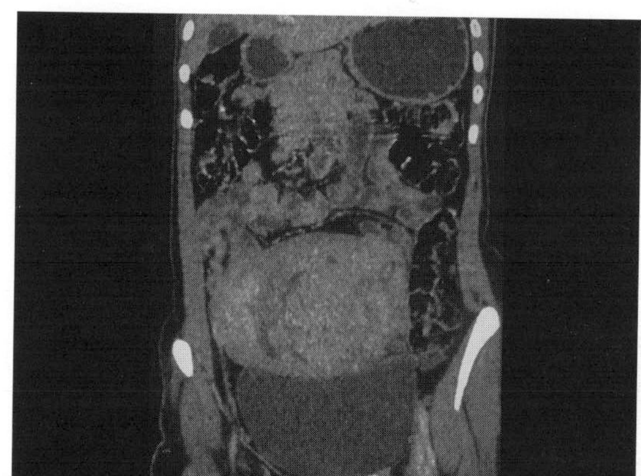

CT demonstrating a big fibroid

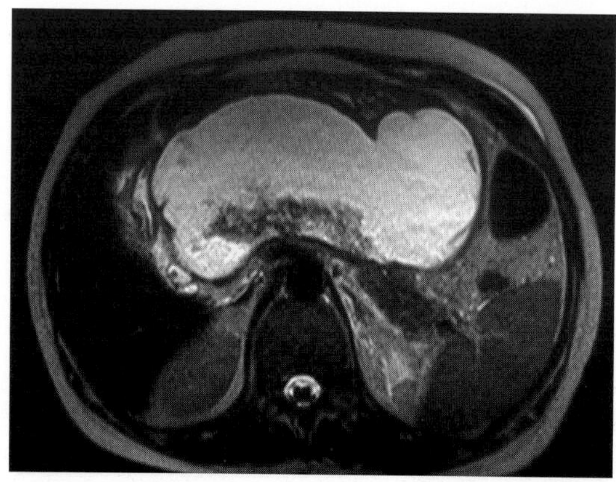

CT demonstrating a large pancreatic pseudocyst

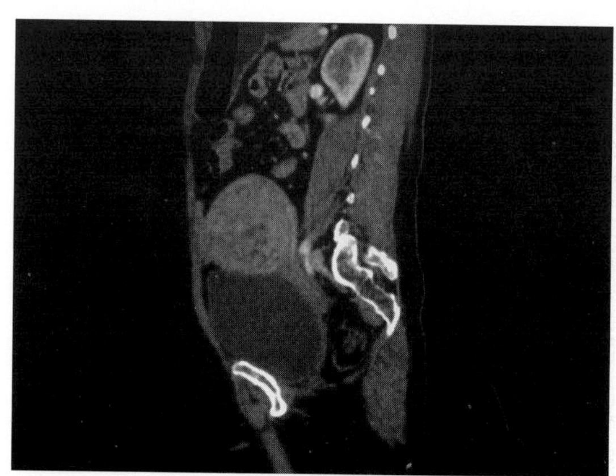

CT demonstrating a big uterine fibroid

Plate 15

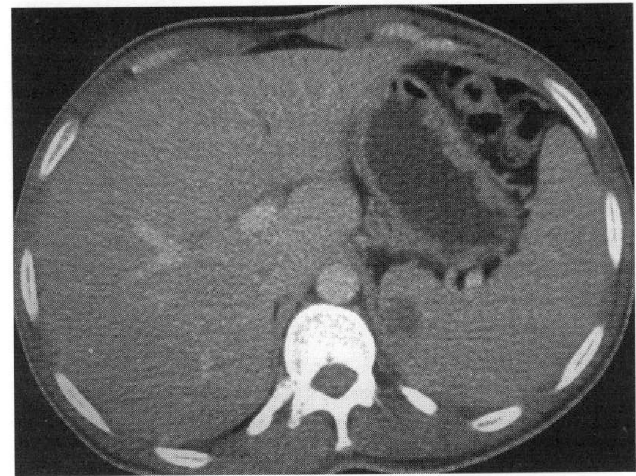

CT demonstrating an abscess in spleen

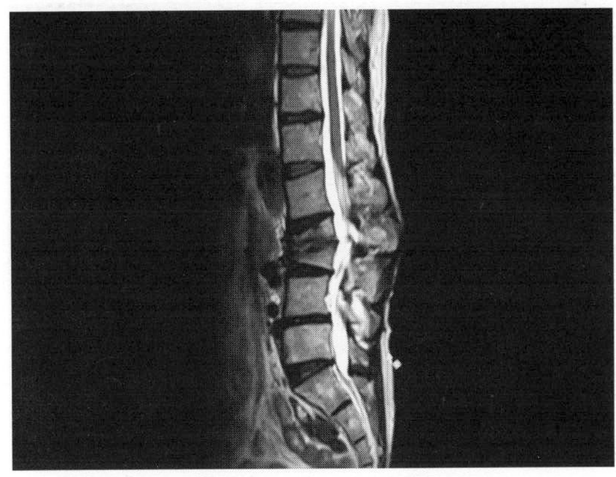

CT scan showing tuberculosis spine

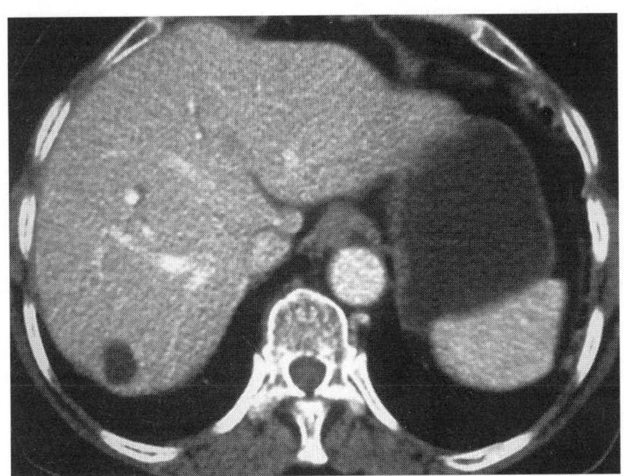

CT demonstrating cyst in liver

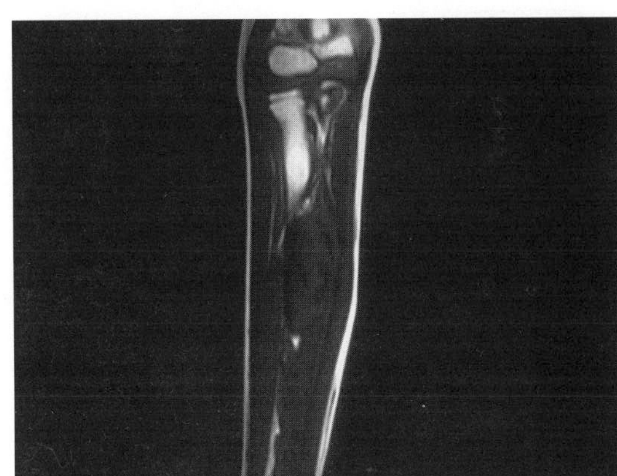

CT showing Ewing's sarcoma

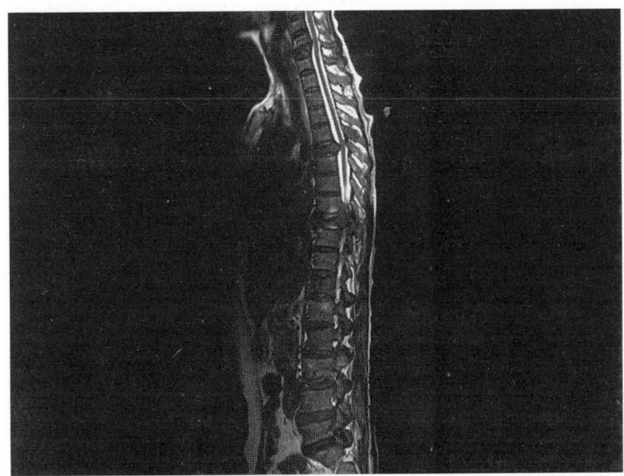

CT demonstrating spinal metastasis

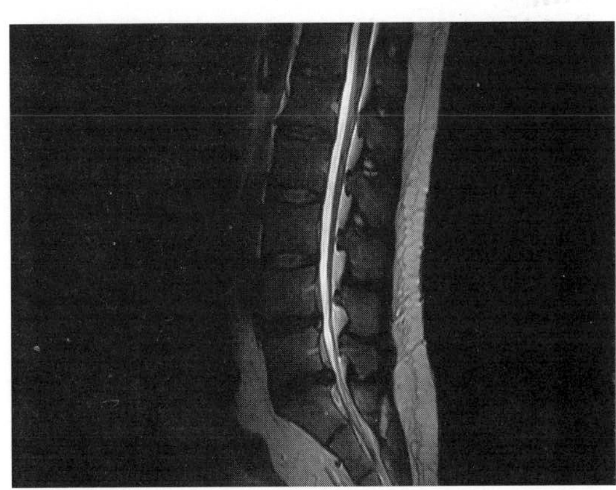

Disk protrusion at multiple sites

Plate 16

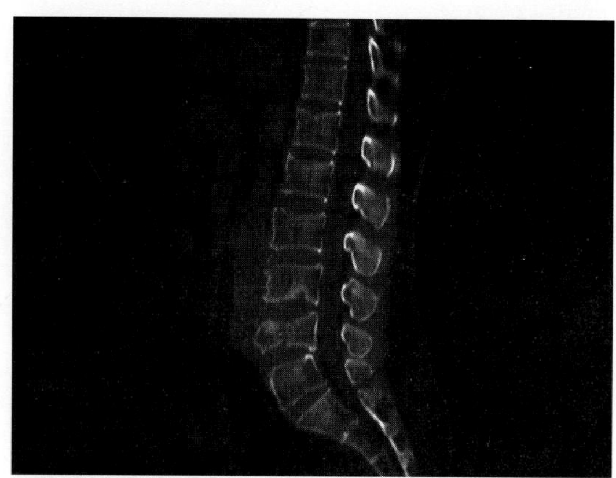

CT demonstrating vertebral fracture

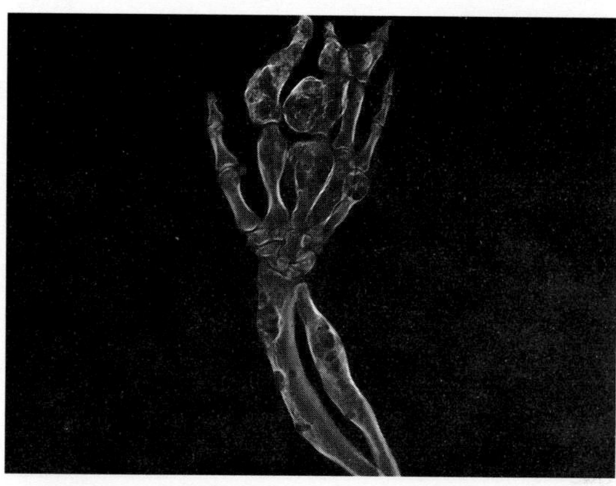

Radiograph demonstrating multiple enchondromas

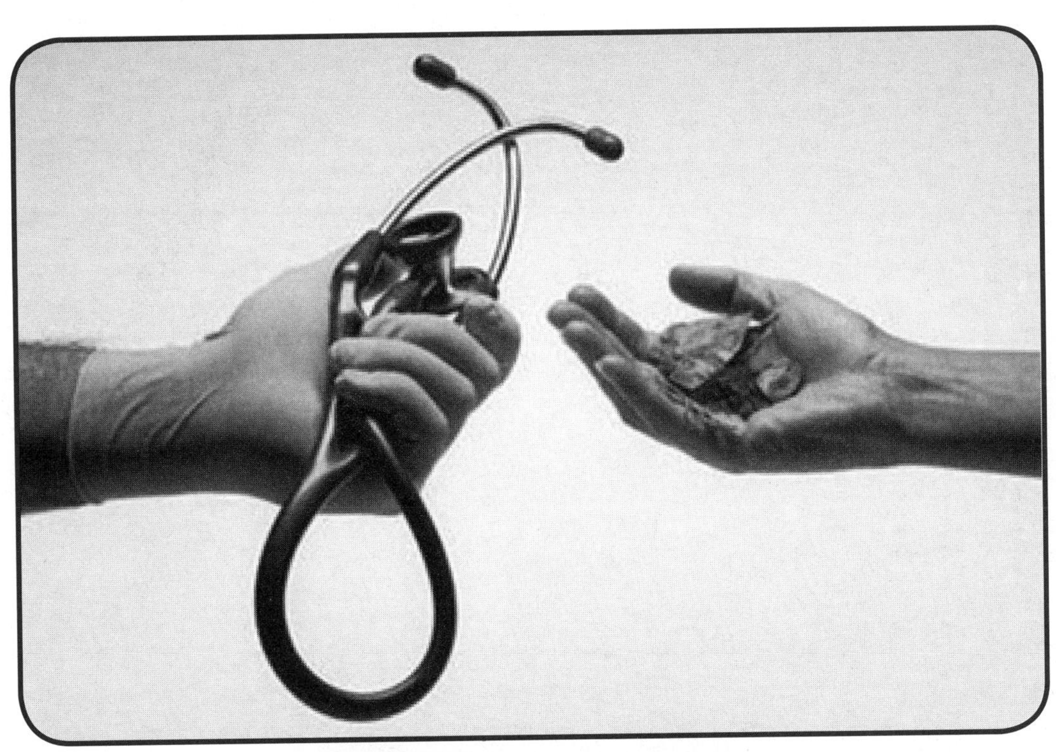

MEDICINE

Medicine 1

MINERAL-ASSOCIATED DISEASES

Zinc

- Zinc is an integral component of many metalloenzymes in the body
- It is involved in the **synthesis and stabilization of proteins, DNA, and RNA and plays a structural role in ribosomes and membranes**
- Zinc is necessary for the binding of steroid hormone receptors and several other transcription factors to DNA and thereby plays an important role in the regulation of gene transcription
- Zinc is absolutely required for normal **spermatogenesis, fetal growth, and embryonic development**
- **Deficiency:** Mild zinc deficiency has been described in many diseases including:
  - **Diabetes mellitus**
  - **AIDS**
  - **Cirrhosis**
  - **Alcoholism**
  - **Inflammatory bowel disease**
  - **Malabsorption syndromes and**
  - **Sickle-cell anemia**

Mild chronic zinc deficiency can cause **stunted growth in children, decreased taste sensation (hypogusia), impaired immune function, and night blindness** due to impaired conversion of retinol to retinaldehyde

Severe chronic zinc deficiency has been described as a cause of **hypogonadism and dwarfism** in several Middle-Eastern countries. In these children, **hypopigmented hair** is also part of the syndrome '**Acrodermatitis enteropathica**'

It is a rare autosomal recessive disorder characterized by abnormalities in zinc absorption. Clinical manifestations include **diarrhea, alopecia, muscle wasting, depression, irritability, and a rash involving the extremities, face, and perineum.** The rash is characterized **by vesicular and pustular crusting with scaling and erythema**. In addition, **hypopigmentation and corneal edema** have been described in these patients

- The diagnosis of **zinc deficiency is usually made by ↓serum zinc level**
- **Pregnancy and birth-control pills** may cause a slight depression in serum zinc levels, and **hypoalbuminemia** from any cause can result in hypozincemia

Copper

Copper is an integral part of numerous enzyme systems including:

- Amine oxidases
- Ferroxidase (ceruloplasmin)
- Cytochrome-c oxidase
- Superoxide dismutase and
- Dopamine hydroxylase
- Dietary copper deficiency is relatively rare, although it has been described in premature infants fed milk diets and in infants with malabsorption

- Signs and symptoms of copper deficiency include:
- **A hypochromic-normocytic anemia**
- Osteopenia
- Depigmentation
- Mental retardation
- Psychomotor abnormalities
- The diagnosis of copper deficiency is usually made on the basis of low serum levels of copper.

Selenium

- Selenium, in the form of selenocysteine, is a component of the enzyme **glutathione peroxidase**, which serves to protect proteins, cell membranes, lipids, and nucleic acids from oxidant molecules. Selenocysteine is also found in the **deiodinase enzymes**, which mediate the deiodination of thyroxine to the more active triiodothyronine
- **Keshan disease** is an endemic cardiomyopathy found in children and young women residing in regions of China where dietary intake of selenium is low. Low blood levels of selenium in various populations have been correlated with an increase in coronary artery disease and certain cancers, although the data are not consistent.

Chromium

- Chromium **potentiates the action of insulin in patients with impaired glucose tolerance**, presumably by increasing insulin receptor-mediated signaling
- Chromium deficiency has been reported to cause **glucose intolerance, peripheral neuropathy and confusion.**

Magnesium

Magnesium deficiency is a common clinical problem:

- Reduced renal reabsorption due to loop diuretics and alcohol use is a common cause of hypomagnesemia
- Vomiting and nasogastric suctioning, fluid loss from diarrhea
- Hypomagnesemia is prevalent in alcoholics

The clinical manifestations of hypomagnesemia are similar to those of severe hypocalcemia

The signs and symptoms of hypomagnesemia include:

- **Muscle weakness**
- **Prolonged PR and QT intervals**
- **Cardiac arrhythmias**
- **Positive Chvostek's and Trousseau's signs**
- **Carpopedal spasm can also occur with hypomagnesemia**
- **Remember:** Magnesium is important for effective PTH secretion as well as the renal and skeletal responsiveness to PTH; thus, hypomagnesemia is often associated with hypocalcemia due to impaired PTH secretion and function.

Ultratrace Elements

Are those for which the need is <1 mg/d

- **Molybdenum** is necessary for the activity of sulfite **and xanthine oxidase, and molybdenum deficiency may result in skeletal and brain lesions**
- **Arsenic (impaired growth, infertility)**
- **Boron (impaired energy metabolism, impaired brain function)**
- **Nickel (impaired growth and reproduction), silicon (impaired growth) and**
- **Vanadium (impaired skeletal formation) might also be essential.**

Cadmium

- Environmental exposure to cadmium can result from the **ingestion of basic foodstuffs, especially grains, cereals, and leafy vegetables, which readily absorb cadmium** occurring naturally or in soil contaminated by sewage sludge, fertilizers, and polluted groundwater
- Cigarette smoke contains cadmium
- **Occupational exposure** takes place in the metal-plating, pigment, battery, and plastics industries
- Most absorbed cadmium is concentrated in the liver and kidneys. In erythrocytes and soft tissues, cadmium is bound to metallothionein. The toxicity of cadmium may involve its binding to key **cellular sulfhydryl groups**, its competition with other metals (zinc and selenium) for inclusion in metalloenzymes, and its competition with calcium for binding sites on regulatory proteins such as calmodulin

Acute high-dose cadmium inhalation can cause **severe respiratory irritation with pleuritic chest pain, dyspnea, cyanosis, fever, tachycardia, nausea, and life-threatening noncardiogenic pulmonary edema**

Acute exposure through ingestion can cause **severe nausea, vomiting, salivation, abdominal cramps, and diarrhea**

Chronic effects of cadmium exposure are dose-dependent and include **anosmia, yellowing of the teeth, emphysema, minor changes in liver function, microcytic hypochromic anemia unresponsive to iron therapy, renal tubular dysfunction characterized by proteinuria and increased urinary excretion of β_2-microglobulin and (with prolonged poisoning) osteomalacia leading to bone lesions and pseudofractures. In follow-up studies of occupationally exposed workers, β_2-microglobulinuria was found to be irreversible**

Chelation therapy is not useful, and dimercaprol is contraindicated as this agent may exacerbate nephrotoxicity. Avoidance of further exposure and supportive therapy (including vitamin D if osteomalacia exists) are the mainstays of management.

Deficiency of Minerals

Iron deficiency	**Microcytic anemia**
Iodine	**Goiter**
Zinc	**Acrodermatitis enteropathica**
Copper	**Menkes disease**
Selenium	**Cardiomyopathy**
Chromium	**Impaired glucose tolerance**

Arsenic-related Diseases

Chronic arsenic (As) exposure has been linked to many cancers. Most common cancers associated are:

- **Basal cell carcinoma**
- **Squamous cell carcinoma**
- **Angiosarcoma of liver**
- **Lung Ca**
- **Kidney Ca**
- **Colon Ca**
- **Noncirrhotic portal fibrosis is a medical condition associated with As exposure**

ACID-BASE/ELECTROLYTE DISORDERS

Medically Important Electrolyte Imbalances

Potassium Deficit and Hypokalemia	Potassium Excess and Hyperkalemia
1. K depletion usually is due to **excessive losses of K in the urine or stool** 2. **Bartter's syndrome** is characterized by sodium wasting, excessive production of renin and aldosterone, and normotension	**Hyperkalemia (serum K > 5.5 mEq/L)** Must be distinguished from **pseudohyperkalemia due to hemolysis of the blood sample, or the release of K from erythrocytes, leukocytes, and platelets** during the clotting

Contd...

Contd...

Potassium Deficit and Hypokalemia	Potassium Excess and Hyperkalemia
3. **Cushing's syndrome** due to adrenal cancer or the ectopic ACTH syndrome and **hyperaldosteronism** 4. In association with diuretics **(e.g. thiazides, bumetanide, furosemide, ethacrynic acid,** but not spironolactone or triamterene) 5. **Hypomagnesemia** in osmotic diuresis **(e.g. diabetic ketoacidosis); in renal tubular disease, such as type I or type II renal tubular acidosis, Fanconi's syndrome** 6. **Excessive licorice ingestion and Liddle's syndrome** 7. **Amphotericin B** and with antipseudomonal penicillins (e.g. carbenicillin) or **high-dose penicillin** treatment 8. Gastrointestinal losses usually are due to **diarrhea, chronic laxative abuse or clay ingestion, vomiting or gastric suction** (renal K wasting with developing metabolic alkalosis is of primary importance) and bowel diversion 9. **Villous adenoma of the colon** is a rare cause of K loss from the GI tract 10. **Beta 2-Adrenergic agonists such as albuterol or terbutaline** may produce hypokalemia due to cellular K uptake 11. **Cystic fibrosis** 12. **Theophylline intoxication** 13. **Cortisol**	process in patients with marked leukocytosis (> 50,000/μL) or thrombocytosis (> 500,000/μL) Hyperkalemia may occur when: 1. **Acidosis** (due to accumulation of inorganic acids) 2. Hyperglycemia (in the presence of insulin deficiency) 3. **Moderately heavy exercise** (particularly in the presence of ß-blockade) 4. **Digitalis intoxication, Beta blockers** 5. **Acute tumor lysis** 6. **Acute intravascular hemolysis or** 7. **Hyperkalemic familial periodic paralysis** produces a shift of K out of cells into the ECF; or as a consequence of K excess 8. Since the kidneys normally excrete K loads rapidly, sustained hyperkalemia usually implies diminished renal K excretion 9. K excess is particularly common in acute oliguric states **(especially acute renal failure)** associated with **severe crush injuries, burns, bleeding into soft tissue or the GI tract, or adrenal insufficiency** **TREATMENT:** Acute emergency: Calcium gluconate, sodium bicarbonate, insulin, albuterol Nonemergency: Furosemide, resins, hemodialysis, peritoneal dialysis

Hypokalemia

- Severe hypokalemia (serum K < 3 mEq/L) may produce:
- **Muscular weakness and lead to paralysis and respiratory failure. Muscular malfunction may result in respiratory hypoventilation, paralytic ileus**
- **The characteristic ECG changes are**
  - ST segment depression
  - Increased U wave amplitude and
  - T wave amplitude <U wave amplitude
  - Severe hypokalemia may produce **premature ventricular and atrial contractions and ventricular and atrial tachyarrhythmias.**

Hyperkalemia

The ECG Changes are:

- **Shortening of the QT interval and**
- **Tall, peaked T waves (serum K > 5.5 mEq/L)**
- Progressive hyperkalemia produces **nodal and ventricular arrhythmias, widening of the QRS complex (serum K > 6.5 mEq/L)**
- **PR interval prolongation and disappearance of the P wave and finally**
- **Degeneration of the QRS** complex to a **sine wave pattern** and ventricular asystole or fibrillation.

USMLE Case Scenario

A 44-year-old Hypertensive, Diabetic man from Chicago with end-stage renal disease presents with syncope. An electrocardiogram reveals sinus bradycardia with a sine-wave pattern. Which of the following is the most appropriate initial step in management?

1. Oral calcium
2. Intravenous calcium
3. Intravenous lactate
4. Intravenous furosemide
5. Intravenous sodium bicarbonate

Ans. 2. Intravenous Calcium

It will work very rapidly to counteract the effect of the high potassium on the heart and muscle and should be given first.

Hypomagnesemia

- **Serum magnesium concentration < 1.6 mEq/L (< 1.9 mg/dL)**
- **Magnesium depletion usually results from:**
  - **Inadequate intake/alcoholism**
  - **Impairment of renal or gut absorption**
  - **Prolonged parenteral feeding, usually in combination with loss of body fluids via gastric suction or diarrhea**
  - **Lactation (increased requirement for Mg)**
  - **Conditions of abnormal renal conservation of Mg, such as hypersecretion of aldosterone, ADH, or thyroid hormone, hypercalcemia, diabetic acidosis, and cisplatin or diuretic therapy**
  - **It is often associated and presents with hypocalcemia and hypophosphatemia**
- Anorexia, nausea, vomiting, lethargy, weakness, personality change, **Tetany (e.g. positive Trousseau's or Chvostek's sign, or spontaneous carpopedal spasm), tremor, and muscle fasciculations may be present. The neurologic signs, particularly tetany, correlate with the development of hypocalcemia and hypokalemia**
- **Myopathic potentials are found on electromyography.**

Hypermagnesemia

Serum magnesium > 2.1 mEq/L (> 2.5 mg/dL)

- Symptomatic hypermagnesemia is common in **Renal failure** when patients are taking magnesium-containing antacids, laxatives, enemas, or infusions
- Acute rhabdomyolysis. Volume depletion
- Lithium
- Ketoacidosis without treatment
- Renal failure

Hypermagnesemia leads to generalized impairment of neuromuscular transmission, probably as the result of inhibition of acetylcholine release at the neuromuscular junction. ECG shows:

- **Prolongation of the PR interval,**
- **Widening of the QRS complex, and increased T wave amplitude**

Deep tendon reflexes disappear; hypotension, respiratory depression and narcosis develop with progression of the hypermagnesemia, cardiac arrest occurs

Treatment of Severe Mg Intoxication:

- Consists of circulatory and respiratory support, with IV administration of 10 to 20 mL of **10% calcium gluconate. The latter may reverse many of the Mg-induced changes, including the respiratory depression**
- **Administration of IV furosemide or ethacrynic acid** increases Mg excretion, if continuous and adequate hydration is maintained and renal function is adequate
- **Hemodialysis may be of value in severe hypermagnesemia**
- **When hemodialysis is impractical, peritoneal dialysis may be effective.**

Hypocalcemia

- **Hypoparathyroidism:** Characterized chemically by **low serum calcium and high serum phosphorus levels** usually follows **accidental removal of or damage to several parathyroid glands during thyroidectomy.**
  - **Idiopathic hypoparathyroidism**, in which the **parathyroids are absent or atrophied, is uncommon**. It may occur sporadically as an isolated or inherited condition, or in association with the **DiGeorge syndrome**
  - It also occurs as part of a **Genetic syndrome of hypoparathyroidism, Addison's disease and mucocutaneous candidiasis.**
  - **Pseudohypoparathyroidism (PHP)** differs from the postoperative and idiopathic forms and is characterized not by deficiency of PTH but by **target organ (bone and kidney) unresponsiveness to its action.**
- **Vitamin D deficiency**, due to **inadequate dietary intake, decreased exposure to sunlight, hepatobiliary disease, or intestinal malabsorption and associated with rickets or osteomalacia**. Functional vitamin D deficiency may occur during prolonged anticonvulsant therapy with **barbiturates and phenytoin**, presumably the result of increased catabolism of 25-(OH) D3.
- **Vitamin D-dependent rickets (VDDR),** in which the formation **of 1,25-DHCC is defective (Type I),** or there is **marked resistance of target organs to the effects of 1,25-DHCC and other vitamin D metabolites (Ttype II)** and **familial hypophosphatemic (Vitamin D-resistant) rickets.**
- **Renal tubular disease**, including **Fanconi's syndrome due to nephrotoxins** (e.g. heavy metals) and distal renal tubular acidosis.
- **Renal failure**, where diminished formation of 1, 25-DHCC coupled with hyperphosphatemia produces hypocalcemia.
- **Magnesium depletion** occurring with intestinal malabsorption or dietary deficiency, which causes hypocalcemia by relatively deficient secretion of PTH, as well as end-organ resistance to its action.
- **Acute pancreatitis**, which lowers serum Ca levels when Ca is chelated by lipolytic products.
- **Hypoproteinemia** of any cause with reduction in protein-bound Ca **(e.g. nephrotic syndrome, cirrhosis, protein-losing enteropathy)**. Hypocalcemia due to diminished protein-binding is asymptomatic, since the ionized Ca fraction is unaltered and the effects of Ca upon membrane excitability are produced by the ionized fraction.
- **During periods of increased Ca utilization** coupled with inadequate intake (e.g. after surgical correction of hyperparathyroidism with healing bone lesions), hypocalcemia can also develop. It may develop in oxalic acid poisoning and during sodium edetate therapy.
- **Septic shock** may be associated with hypocalcemia due to suppression of PTH release and 1, 25-DHCC formation.

Symptoms and Signs: The clinical manifestations of hypocalcemia are primarily neurologic

Slowly developing, insidious hypocalcemia may produce mild, diffuse encephalopathy and thus should be suspected in any patient with unexplained dementia, depression, or psychosis.

Severe hypocalcemia (Serum Ca < 7 mg/dL) may cause **<u>laryngospasm and generalized convulsions.</u>**

The most characteristic syndrome is tetany, resulting from severe hypocalcemia or a reduction in the serum ionized Ca fraction without marked hypocalcemia (e.g. in respiratory or metabolic alkalosis). **Tetany** is characterized by:

1. Sensory symptoms consisting of paresthesias of the lips, tongue, fingers and feet
2. Carpopedal spasm, which may be prolonged or painful
3. Generalized muscle aching
4. Spasm of facial musculature

- **Chvostek's sign** is contraction of the facial muscles, elicited by a light tapping of the facial nerve. It is occasionally present in normal individuals and is often absent in chronic hypocalcemia.
- **Trousseau's sign** is carpopedal spasm caused by reduction of the blood supply to the hand when a tourniquet or blood pressure cuff above systolic pressure is applied to the forearm for 3 min
- **Erbs's sign**: Muscle contraction can be produced by subthreshold electric stimulus
- **Peroneal sign:** Tapping of peroneal nerve will produce pedal spasm.

The ECG typically **shows 'prolongation' of the QT interval.**

Causes of Hypercalcemia

Total serum calcium>10.5 mg/dL.

- **Primary hyperparathyroidism** usually characterized by hypercalcemia, hypophosphatemia, and excessive bone resorption.
- **Sarcoidosis** is associated with hypercalcemia in up to. Hypercalcemia and/or hypercalciuria have also been described in **other granulomatous diseases (e.g. tuberculosis, leprosy, berylliosis, histoplasmosis, and coccidioidomycosis)**. Similarly, elevated serum levels of 1, 25-DHCC have been reported in hypercalcemic patients with **tuberculosis, silicosis, and Hodgkin's and non-Hodgkin's lymphoma.**
- **Milk-alkali syndrome**, excessive amounts of Ca and absorbable alkali are ingested, usually during peptic ulcer therapy, resulting in increased Ca absorption and hypercalcemia.
- **Idiopathic hypercalcemia of infancy** is recognized by the combination of suppressed levels of PTH, hypercalciuria, and in some severely affected patients, the somatic abnormalities of **'Williams' syndrome'** (e.g. supravalvular aortic stenosis, mental retardation, and an elfin facies).
- **Myeloma** should be suggested by the syndrome of anemia, azotemia, and hypercalcemia. This diagnosis is confirmed by bone marrow examination or finding a monoclonal gammopathy or free light chains in the serum or urine on immunoelectrophoresis
- **Lithium** causes hypercalcemia.

Endocrine causes of hypercalcemia **(e.g. Thyrotoxicosis, Addison's disease)**

- Polyuria
- Depression
- Abdominal pain, are features

Effective in treatment:

- **Furosemide**
- **Prednisolone**
- **Pamidronate are used for treatment**
- **Calcitonin**
- **Gallium nitrate**
- **Plicamycin**

Hypercalciuria is treated by: Thiazides

Hypercalcemia is not caused by tumor lysis but **HYPOCALCEMIA**

A 40-year-old male from California who presented with **polyuria, pain abdomen, nausea, vomiting,** and **altered sensorium** was found to have **Bronchogenic carcinoma.** The electrolyte abnormality seen in him would be **Hypercalcemia**

Simplest Explanation of Metabolic Disorders

	CO_2	pH	HCO_3
Respiratory Acidosis	↑	↓	↑
Respiratory Alkalosis	↓	↑	↓
Metabolic Acidosis	**No change**	↓	↓
Metabolic Alkalosis	**No change**	↑	↑

USMLE Case Scenario

A 45-year-old woman with glaucoma is treated by an ophthalmologist with acetazolamide. Three weeks later, the woman has an arterial pH of 7.34, an arterial PCO_2 of 29 mm Hg, and plasma HCO_3 of 15 mEq/L. Which of the following abnormalities has this woman most likely developed?

1. Metabolic acidosis
2. Metabolic alkalosis

3. Respiratory acidosis
4. Respiratory alkalosis

Ans. 1. Metabolic Acidosis

The laboratory results indicate that the arterial pH, arterial PCO_2, and plasma HCO_3^- concentrations are all low. These changes clearly demonstrate metabolic acidosis, which occurs commonly when a carbonic anhydrase inhibitor is administered.

USMLE Case Scenario

A 73-year-old male diabetic has a cardiopulmonary arrest, and is transported to the Texas Coronary Care unit by paramedics. The data shown below are derived from an arterial blood sample obtained upon admission. Plasma pH: 7.09, Plasma Bicarbonate: 15 mEq/L, Arterial Carbon Dioxide: 50 mm Hg. What type of acid-base abnormality is present in this man?

1. Respiratory acidosis
2. Respiratory alkalosis
3. Metabolic acidosis
4. Metabolic alkalosis
5. Mixed acidosis
6. Mixed alkalosis

Ans. 5. A mixed acidosis

It commonly occurs with cardiopulmonary arrest. Cardiac arrest victim experiences some degree of lactic acidosis (metabolic acidosis) as a result of poorly perfused tissues. A simultaneous respiratory acidosis due to ventilatory standstill also occurs. This combination of metabolic acidosis and respiratory acidosis is referred to as a 'mixed acidosis.'

Remember:

- **Respiratory Acidosis**: Any cause of hypoventilation causes Respiratory Acidosis (COAD, CNS Depression, Neuromuscular disease)
- **Respiratory Alkalosis**: Hyperventilation, Hypoxia, Hyperthyroidism, High Altitude (H4)
- **Metabolic Alkalosis**: Conditions causing Hypokalemia usually
- **Metabolic Acidosis**: Lactic acidosis, Ketoacidosis, Liver failure, Cardiac failure, Ethylene glycol, Renal tubular acidosis, Diarrhea.

Anion Gap (AG)

- It represents those **unmeasured anions in plasma**
- **(Normally** = 10 to 12 mmol/L) and
- Calculated as follows: AG = $\mathbf{Na^+ - (Cl^- + HCO_3^-)}$
- The **unmeasured anions** include anionic proteins, phosphate, sulfate, and organic anions
- When acid anions, such as acetoacetate and lactate, accumulate in extracellular fluid, the AG increases, causing a **high-AG acidosis**

Increased anion gap is seen in:

- Renal failure
- Lactic acidosis
- Diabetic ketoacidosis
- Starvation
- Salicylate poisoning

Hypoalbumenemia
Lithium toxicity
IgG myeloma
Hypercalcemia
Hypermagnesemia
Hyperkalemia

Conditions with decreased anion gap

Lactic Acidosis

An increase in plasma L-lactate may be secondary to:

Poor tissue perfusion (Type A):
- Circulatory insufficiency
- Shock, circulatory failure
- Severe anemia, mitochondrial enzyme defects
- Inhibitors (carbon monoxide, cyanide)

Aerobic disorders (Type B): Malignancies, diabetes mellitus, renal or hepatic failure, severe infections (cholera, malaria), seizures, AIDS, or drugs/toxins:
- **Biguanides**
- **Ethanol**
- **Methanol**
- **Isoniazid**
- **AZT analogues**
- **Fructose**

HYPOTHERMIA

Degrees of Hypothermia

- **Mild Hypothermia 95–90 °F**
- **Moderate Hypothermia 90–82.4 °F**
- **Severe Hypothermia less than 82.4 °F**

Accidental hypothermia occurs when there is an unintentional drop in the body's core temperature below 35 °C (95 °F)

Causes

- Primary accidental hypothermia is **geographically and seasonally pervasive**. Although most cases occur in the winter months and in colder climates, it is surprisingly common in warmer regions as well.
- Multiple variables make individuals at the **extremes of age, the elderly and neonates,** particularly vulnerable to hypothermia. **Dementia, psychiatric illness, and socioeconomic factors** often compound these problems by impeding adequate measures to prevent hypothermia.
- Individuals whose occupations or hobbies entail **extensive exposure to cold weather** are clearly at increased risk for hypothermia. Military history is replete with hypothermic tragedies. **Hunters, sailors, skiers, and climbers** are also at great risk of exposure, whether it involves injury, changes in weather, or lack of preparedness.
- **Ethanol, Amphetamine, chlorpromazine**
- **Wernicke's encephalopathy, phenothiazines, barbiturates, benzodiazepines, cyclic antidepressants**, and many other medications reduce centrally mediated vasoconstriction.
- Several types of endocrine dysfunction can lead to hypothermia. **Hypothyroidism, Adrenal insufficiency and hypopituitarism** can also increase susceptibility to hypothermia. **Hypoglycemia,** most commonly caused by insulin or oral hypoglycemic drugs, is associated with hypothermia, in part the result of neuroglycopenic effects on hypothalamic function.
- **Neurologic injury from trauma, cerebrovascular accident, subarachnoid hemorrhage, or hypothalamic lesions** increases susceptibility to hypothermia. **Agenesis of the corpus callosum, or Shapiro syndrome** is one cause of '**episodic hypothermia**', characterized by profuse perspiration followed by a rapid fall in temperature. Acute spinal cord injury disrupts the autonomic pathways that lead to shivering and prevents cold-induced reflex vasoconstrictive responses.
- Hypothermia is **confirmed by measuring the core temperature, preferably at two sites**. Rectal probes should be placed to a depth of 15 cm and not adjacent to cold feces.

Brain activities are slowed at temperatures below 35 °C.

Hypothermia provides protection against ischemia and hypoxia by reducing BMR.

Hypothermia is used in:

- **Neurosurgery**
- **Cardiac surgery**
- **Malignant hypoerthermia**
- **Prolonged surgeries**

Osborn waves (also known as **camel-hump sign, late delta wave or current of injury**) are usually observed on the electrocardiogram of people suffering from hypothermia, though they may also occur in people with high blood levels of calcium (hypercalcemia), brain injury, vasospastic angina, or ventricular fibrillation. **Osborn waves are positive deflections occurring at the junction between the QRS complex and the ST segment, where the S point, also known as the J joint, has a myocardial infarction-like elevation**

QT INTERVAL PROLONGED

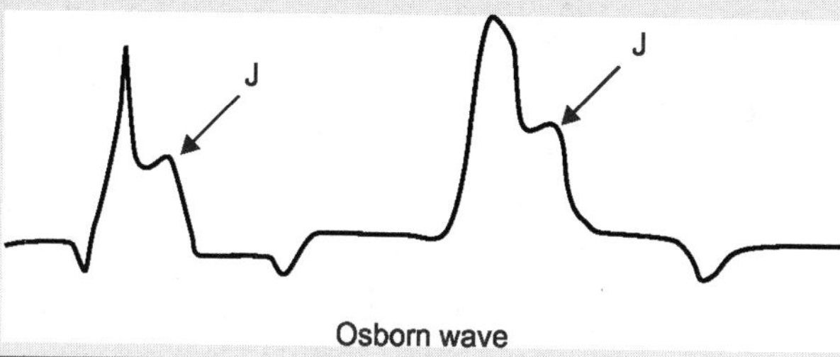

Osborn wave

'<u>Hyper Thermic</u>' Syndromes

- <u>**Hyperthermia:**</u> It is present when core body temperature > 37.2 °C. Heat injury syndromes may result in body temperatures in > 40 °C (104 °F) When temperatures are > 41 °C, enzymes are denatured, mitochondrial function is disturbed, cell membranes are destabilized, and oxygen-dependent metabolic pathways are disrupted
- <u>**Heat Cramps**</u>**: Painful spasm of major muscle groups** is the hallmark of heat cramps. Typically seen in **young, unacclimatized athletes or laborers** who exert themselves excessively in a hot climate, heat cramps are related to excessive losses of sodium, chloride, and water. Patients complain of nausea, vomiting, and fatigue in addition to muscle cramps, with onset of symptoms typically occurring several hours after they stop exercising
- <u>**Heat Exhaustion**</u>**:** The most common heat injury syndrome seen in athletes, may be preceded by heat cramps and is due to **severe dehydration and electrolyte loss**. In the young, heat exhaustion usually occurs following strenuous activity by unacclimatized individuals in a hot, humid environment. In the elderly, the problem is usually related to inadequate cardiovascular response to heat with disruption of normal compensatory mechanisms. Patients frequently complain of cramps, headache, fatigue, nausea, and vomiting. They appear listless, with pallor of the skin and profuse sweating. Other clinical findings include **orthostatic hypotension, core temperatures of 37.5 to 39 °C (99.5 to 102.2 °F), altered mental status, incoordination, and diffuse weakness**
- <u>**Heatstroke**</u>**:** Classified as exertional or nonexertional, is a syndrome **due to acute disruption of thermoregulatory mechanisms manifested by central nervous system depression, hypohidrosis, core temperatures {greater than or equal to} 41 °C**, and severe physiologic and biochemical abnormalities. Exertional heatstroke occurs in people working or exercising in a warm environment with an overwhelmed but unimpaired central thermoregulatory center. Nonexertional heatstroke occurs most frequently in elderly, debilitated, schizophrenic, intoxicated, or paralyzed individuals. <u>**These people have impaired central and/or peripheral thermoregulatory mechanisms (physiologic or drug-induced autonomic impairment), impaired awareness of or inability to leave a hot environment, poor acclimatization, and inadequate ability to increase cardiac output in response to heat.**</u>

Consequences of Heat-induced Cell Damage are:

- **Rhabdomyolysis**
- **Cardiac failure and arrhythmias**
- **Vasodilation**
- **Cytotoxic cerebral edema**
- **Hypotension**
- **Acute renal failure**

- **Adult respiratory distress syndrome (ARDS)**
- **Gastrointestinal hemorrhage and**
- **Acute hepatic failure**

Laboratory Abnormalities include:

- **Hyperkalemia**
- **Hypocalcemia**
- **Hyperphosphatemia or hypophosphatemia**
- **Rising creatinine**
- **Hemoconcentration**
- **Stress leukocytosis**
- **Thrombocytopenia**
- **Consumptive coagulopathy**
- **Lactic acidosis**
- **Hypoglycemia**
- **Proteinuria**

- **Neuroleptic malignant syndrome (NMS)** is a complex of extrapyramidal muscular rigidity, high-core temperature, altered level of consciousness, and elevated creatine kinase levels occurring as an acute or subacute reaction to therapy with neuroleptic medications
- **Malignant hyperthermia** is a hypermetabolic, myopathic syndrome, chemically or stress-induced, and is manifested by an abrupt rise in core temperature, vigorous muscle contractions, metabolic and respiratory acidosis, and ventricular arrhythmias, usually when inducing anesthesia.

RESPIRATORY MEDICINE

Importance of Different Presentations

- **Wheeze (Rhonci): Monophonic Obstruction in Airway**
- **Wheeze: Polyphonic Asthma**
- **Crepitations (Crackles): Fine and high-pitched: Pulmonary edema**
- **Persistent coarse crepitations: Bronchiectasis**
- **Pleural rub: Pleuritis, pulmonary infarction**
- **Silent chest: Severe bronchospasm**

- **Paradoxical breathing: Diaphragmatic palsy**
- **Tubular breathing: Consolidation, cavity**
- **Cavernous breathing: Cavity**
- **Amphoric breathing: Pneumothorax**

Sputum

- **Copious, pink, frothy: Pulmonary edema**
- **Copious, pungent, purulent: Bronchiectasis, lung abscess**
- **Black: Coal dust**

Differentiate between Obstructive and Restrictive Lung Disease

Obstructive lung disease	Restrictive lung disease
• TLC↑	• TLC↓
• RV↑	• RV↓

Obstructive lung disease	Restrictive lung disease
• TV↓	• TV↓
• VC↓	• VC↓
• FEV1↓	• FEV1↓
• FVC↓	• FVC↓
• FEV1/FVC↓	• FEV1/FVC↑
• $PaCO_2$↑	• $PaCO_2$ (N)or ↓

Carbon Monoxide Diffusion Capacity DLCO

Increased In	Decreased In
• Alveolar hemorrhage	• Interstitial lung disease
• Congestive heart failure	• Emphysema
	• Pulmonary embolism
	• Pulmonary hemorrhage

Respiratory Failure

Type I respiratory failure: PaO_2: ↓, $PaCO_2$: n or ↓, $PA–aO_2$↑Hypoxemia with decreased $PaCO_2$

Caused by:

- **Parenchymal diseases**
- **Pneumoniae**
- **ARDS**
- **Emphysema**
- **R-L shunts**

Type II respiratory failure: Pa O_2: ↓, $PaCO_2$: ↑, PA–a O_2 n. Hypoxemia with increased $PaCO_2$

Caused by:

- **COAD**
- **Interstitial lung diseases**
- **Musculoskeletal problems: Polymyositis, kyphoscoliosis**

Asthma

- **Category of COAD/COPD**
- **Hyperesponsiveness of airways with bronchoconstriction**
- **Incidence is increasing day by day**
- **Hypoxia is a common feature**
- **Leukotrienes ↑**
- **Hyperesponsiveness of airways**
- **Mast cell stabilizer used: Ketotifen**
- **Hypersensitive lung**
- **Constriction of small airways**
  - **Creola bodies seen**
  - **Charcot-Leyden crystals seen**
  - **Curschmann's spirals seen**
- **FEV1 is the parameter to improve maximum on bronchodilator therapy**
- **Mast cell stabilizers are used in treatment (chronic)**
- **Omalizumab is used now for treatment**

Speech difficulty Diaphoresis Altered sensation Cyanosis Silent chest	⟶	**Bad signs of asthma**

Severe asthma

Emphysema and Chronic Bronchitis

- **Emphysema** is defined anatomically as a permanent and destructive enlargement of **airspaces distal to the terminal bronchioles** without obvious fibrosis and with loss of normal architecture
- **Smoking is the commonest precipitant**
- **α_1 antitrypsin (α_1AT)** deficency is associated with **panacinar** emphysema
- Breathlessness is a characteristic feature
- Panacinar **emphysema** involves both the central and peripheral portions of the acinus, which results, if the process is extensive, in a reduction of the alveolar-capillary gas exchange surface and loss of elastic recoil properties
- Chronic bronchitis is defined clinically as the **presence of a cough productive of sputum not attributable to other causes on most days for at least 3 months over 2 consecutive years**
- **Diurnal variation in the peak expiratory flow rate is seen**
  - **Pink puffers** = emphysema
  - **Blue bloaters** = chronic bronchitis

Reid's index is used for chronic bronchitis

Bronchiectasis

Bronchiectasis describes a permanent dilatation of the airways secondary to chronic infection or inflammation.

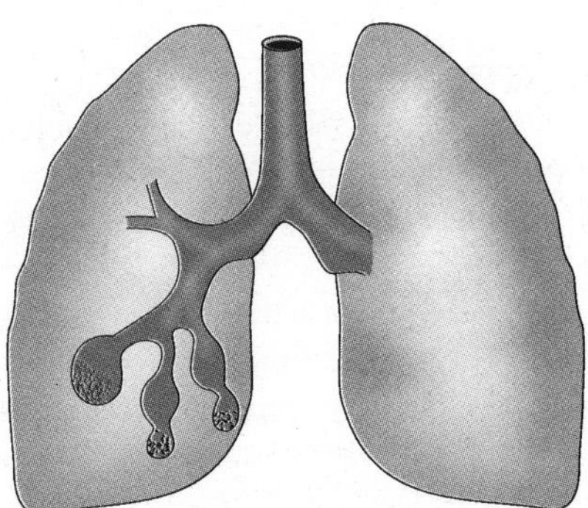

Bronchiectasis

- **Cylindrical bronchiectasis**—the bronchi appear as uniformly dilated tubes that end abruptly at the point that smaller airways are obstructed by secretions
- **Varicose bronchiectasis**—the affected bronchi have an irregular or beaded pattern of dilatation resembling varicose veins
- **Saccular (cystic) bronchiectasis**—the bronchi have a ballooned appearance at the periphery, ending in blind sacs without recognizable bronchial structures distal to the sacs
  - **Nodular bronchiectasis is seen in infection with mycobacterium avium**
  - **Feature of Kartagener's syndrome**
  - **Tram-track lines on CXR**
  - **Commonest in left lower lobe**
  - **Clubbing is a feature**
  - **Does not predispose to lung cancer**
  - **HRCT is the diagnostic technique of choice**

Causes

- **Postinfective: Tuberculosis, measles, pertussis, pneumonia**
- **Cystic fibrosis**
- **Bronchial obstruction, e.g. lung cancer/foreign body**
- **Immune deficiency: Selective IgA, hypogammaglobulinemia**
- **Allergic bronchopulmonary aspergillosis (ABPA)**
- **Ciliary dyskinetic syndromes: Kartagener's syndrome, Young's syndrome**
- **Yellow nail syndrome**

Primary Ciliary Dyskinesia

The primary disorders associated with ciliary dysfunction, **termed Primary Ciliary Dyskinesia**, are responsible for 5 to 10% of cases of bronchiectasis. The clinical effects include recurrent upper and lower respiratory tract infections, such as sinusitis, otitis media, and bronchiectasis

Approximately half of the patients with primary ciliary dyskinesia fall into the subgroup of **Kartagener's syndrome**:

- **Situs inversus**
- **Bronchiectasis and sinusitis**
- **Infertility**

Cystic Fibrosis (CF)

- Cystic fibrosis (CF) is a **monogenetic disorder** that presents as a multisystem disease
- This disease is characterized by chronic airways infection that ultimately leads to **bronchiectasis, exocrine pancreatic insufficiency and intestinal dysfunction, abnormal sweat gland function, and urogenital dysfunction**
- CF is an **autosomal recessive disease**
- Resulting from mutations in a gene located on **chromosome 7**
- The most common mutation in the CF gene results in an **absence of phenylalanine at amino acid position 508 (DF_{508}) of the CF** gene protein product, known as the CF transmembrane regulator **(CFTR)**
- The diagnostic biophysical hallmark of CF is **the raised transepithelial electric potential difference (PD) detected in airway epithelia**
- The transepithelial PD reflects components of both the rate of active ion transport and the resistance to ion flow of the superficial epithelium
- The unique predisposition of CF airways to chronic infection by ***Staphylococcus aureus and Pseudomonas aeruginosa*** raises the issue that other as yet undefined abnormalities in airway surface liquids may also contribute to the failure of lung defense
- **Cavitation is usually seen with staph infections.**

Interstitial Lung Diseases

The **interstitial lung diseases (ILDs)** represent a large number of conditions that involve the parenchyma of the **lung**, the alveoli, the alveolar epithelium, the capillary endothelium as well as the perivascular and lymphatic tissues

- Sarcoidosis
- Idiopathic pulmonary fibrosis (IPF) and
- **Pulmonary fibrosis associated with CTDs** are the most common ILDs of unknown etiology
  - Among the ILDs of known cause, the largest group comprises occupational and environmental exposures, especially the inhalation of inorganic dusts, organic dusts, and various fumes or gases
  - Patients with ILDs come to medical attention mainly because of the onset of progressive exertional dyspnea or a persistent, nonproductive cough. Hemoptysis, wheezing, and chest pain may be present. Often, the identification of **interstitial** opacities on chest X-ray focuses on the diagnostic approach toward one of the ILDs.

- Dyspnea is a common and prominent complaint in patients with ILD, especially the idiopathic **interstitial** pneumonias, hypersensitivity pneumonitis, COP, sarcoidosis, eosinophilic pneumonias, and PLCH
- **HRCT** is superior to the plain chest X-ray for early detection and confirmation of suspected ILD
- **Drug Therapy:** Glucocorticoids are the mainstay of therapy for suppression of the alveolitis present in ILD
- Many cases of ILD are chronic and irreversible despite the therapy discussed above and
- **Lung transplantation** may be considered.

Restrictive Lung Disease

- **TLC ↓**
- **RV ↓**
- **TV ↓**
- **VC ↓**
- **FEV1 ↓**
- **FVC ↓**
- **FEV1/FVC ↑**
- **$PaCO_2$ (N) or ↓**

Pleural Effusion

Transudate	Exudate
• Protein < 3 gm/100 ml • LDH < 200 IU • LDH Ratio < 0.6 • Pleural fluid/serum protein < 0.5 – **CHF** – **Cirrhosis** – **Nephrotic syndrome** – **Meig's syndrome** – **Pulmonary embolism**	• Protein > 3 gm/100 ml • LDH > 200 IU • LDH Ratio > 0.6 • Pleural fluid/serum protein > 0.5 – **Pneumoniae** – **Pulmonary infarction** – **Tuberculosis** – **Rheumatoid arthritis** – **Myxedema** – **Lupus erythematosus** – **Pulmonary embolism** – **Bronchogenic cancer**

QUESTIONS ASKED

Pleural Fluid Characteristics

- **Bloodstained:** Pulmonary infarction, metastatic carcinoma, tuberculosis
- **Low Glucose:** Rheumatoid arthritis, empyema
- **PH < 7.2:** Empyema
- **PH < 6.0:** Esophageal rupture
- **↑Amylase:** Esophageal perforation, pancreatitis
- **Chylous effusion:** Lymphomas, chest trauma
- **Cholesterol:** Hypothyroidism, TB, rheumatoid arthritis
- **Left sided effusion:** Pancreatitis, esophageal rupture

- **Tuberculous pleuritis:** The pleural fluid is an exudate with predominantly small lymphocytes. The diagnosis is established by demonstrating high levels of TB markers in the pleural fluid (**adenosine deaminase** > 45 IU/L, **gamma interferon** > 140 pg/mL, or **positive PCR for tuberculous DNA**).

- **Effusion secondary to malignancy** treat by: (1) tube thoracostomy with the instillation of a sclerosing agent such as talc; (2) outpatient insertion of a small indwelling catheter; or (3) thoracoscopy with pleural abrasion or the insufflation of talc
- **Parapneumonic effusion** parapneumonic effusions are associated with bacterial pneumonia, lung abscess, or bronchiectasis and are probably the most common exudative **pleural effusion**
  - **Loculated pleural fluid**
  - **Pleural fluid pH below 7.20**
  - **Pleural fluid glucose less than 60 mg/dL**
  - **Positive Gramstain or culture of the pleural fluid**
  - **The presence of gross pus in the pleural space.**

Pneumonias

'Typical' pneumonia syndrome is characterized by the **sudden onset of fever, cough productive of purulent sputum, shortness of breath, and (in some cases) pleuritic chest pain; signs of pulmonary consolidation**

- **Dullness**
- **Increased fremitus**
- **Egophony**
- **Bronchial breath sounds, and rales)** may be found on physical examination in areas of radiographic abnormality

The typical pneumonia syndrome is usually caused by the most common bacterial pathogen in community-acquired pneumonia, ***S pneumoniae***, but can also be due to other bacterial pathogens, such as ***H influenzae*** and mixed anaerobic and aerobic components of the oral flora.

'Atypical' pneumonia syndrome is characterized by a **more gradual onset, a dry cough, shortness of breath, a prominence of extrapulmonary symptoms (such as headache, myalgias, fatigue, sore throat, nausea, vomiting, and diarrhea),** and abnormalities on chest radiographs despite minimal signs of pulmonary involvement (other than rales) on physical examination

Atypical pneumonia is classically produced by:

- ***M pneumoniae***
- ***L pneumophila***
- ***C pneumoniae***
- **Oral anaerobes**
- ***P carinii***

Less frequently encountered pathogens. *C psittaci, Coxiella burnetii, Francisella tularensis, H capsulatum, and Coccidioides immitis.*

Remember

- **Mycoplasma pneumonia:** May be complicated by **erythema multiforme, hemolytic anemia, bullous myringitis, encephalitis, and transverse myelitis.**
- **Staph aureus:** Postinfluenza and pneumatocele formation
- **Klebsiella pneumonia:** It is characterized by **red current jelly sputum**
- **Legionella pneumonia:** It is frequently associated with **diarrhea, deterioration in mental status (delirium), renal and hepatic abnormalities, and marked hyponatremia; (walking pneumonia), failure to respond to beta lactam antibiotics**
- **Self-limiting form of legionella infection is called pontaic fever (Flu-like illness without pneumonia)**
- **C pneumonia:** Pneumonia, sore throat, hoarseness, and wheezing are relatively common.
- The atypical pneumonia syndrome in patients whose **HIV infection** suggests **Pneumocystis infection.**

USMLE Case Scenario

A highly encapsulated organism is found to cause bronchopneumonia with patchy infiltrates involving one or more lobes with red sputum in a debilitated alcoholic. Most likely disease is:
Klebsiella pneumonia

'Community-acquired 'Atypical Pneumonia'

- It is atypical in its gradual onset, absence of higher fevers and rigors, and nonproductive cough
- The results of the lung examination and the chest X-ray film reveal the typical findings of a bilateral interstitial infiltrate
- This clinical pattern can be caused by Mycoplasma pneumoniae or alternatively by viral agents
- Although the Mycoplasma can be cultured, this takes 7 to 10 days and requires special culture techniques that are not commonly available in hospital laboratories. Gram's stain of sputum usually shows sparse bacteria, clumps of desquamated respiratory epithelial cells, and a mixture of neutrophils and mononuclear cells (most helpful in practice in distinguishing from the more usual bacterial agents that tend to have a dense neutrophilic infiltrate)
- A single cold agglutinin reaction with titer greater than 1:64 is a helpful (but a little nonspecific) confirmatory test; sequential specimens with a fourfold increase in titer are also considered confirmatory. Common antibacterial agents used to treat M pneumoniae include tetracycline (not used for children) and erythromycin; clarithromycin and azithromycin are also effective.

High-yield Points in Pneumonia

- **Pnuemonia alba is due to treponnema palladium**
- **Bronchopneumonia in measles is due to immunosuppression**
- **Bulging fissure sign in pneumoniae is due to: Klebsiella pneumoniae**
- **Plasma cell pneumnoniae is caused by pneumocystis carnii**

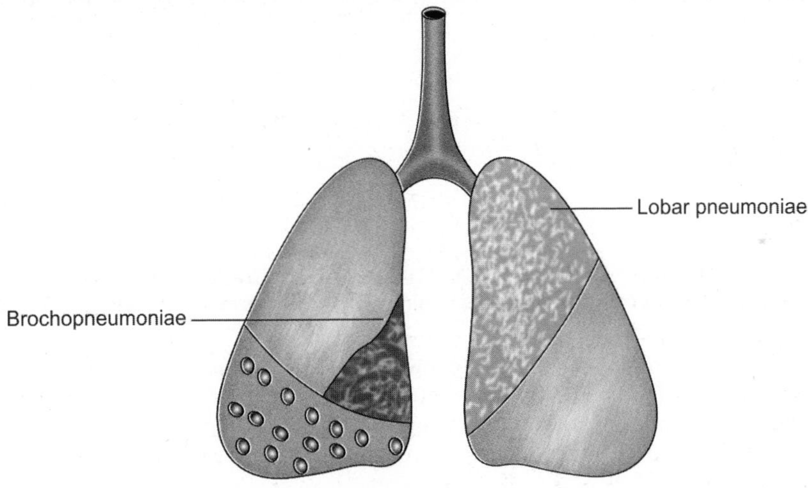

Mycoplasma Pneumonia

- Cause of **atypical pneumonia** which often affects younger patients
- It is associated with a number of complications such as **Erythema multiforme and Cold autoimmune hemolytic anemia**

Features

- **Flu-like symptoms** classically precede a dry cough
- **Bilateral** consolidation on X-ray
- **Serology useful in diagnosis**

Complications:

- **Cold agglutins (IgM) may cause hemolytic anemia, thrombocytopenia**
- **Erythema multiforme, erythema nodosum**
- **Meningoencephalitis, Guillain-Barre syndrome**
- **Bullous myringitis: painful vesicles on the tympanic membrane**
- **Pericarditis/myocarditis**

- **Gastrointestinal: Hepatitis, pancreatitis**
- **Renal: Acute glomerulonephritis**
- **Erythromycin is effective in treatment**

Nosocomial Pneumonia

The usual criteria for nosocomial pneumonia, which include **new or progressive pulmonary infiltrates, purulent tracheobronchial secretions, fever, and leukocytosis**, are frequently unreliable in those patients who often have **preexisting pulmonary disease, endotracheal tubes that irritate the tracheal mucosa** and may elicit an inflammatory exudate in respiratory secretions, or multiple other problems likely to produce fever and leukocytosis.

Aspiration Pneumonia and Anaerobic Lung Abscess

- Aspiration of a sufficient volume of gastric acid produces a **chemical pneumonitis** characterized by **acute dyspnea and wheezing** with hypoxemia and infiltrates on chest radiographs in one or both the lower lobes
- Clinical findings following aspiration of particulate matter depend on the extent of endobronchial obstruction and range from acute apnea to persistent cough with or without recurrent infection
- Although the aspiration of oral anaerobes can initially lead to an infiltrative process, it ultimately results in **putrid sputum, tissue necrosis,** and **pulmonary cavities**. In about three-quarters of cases, the clinical course of an abscess of **anaerobic polymicrobial etiology is indolent**
- Patients with anaerobic abscesses are usually prone to aspiration of oropharyngeal contents and have periodontal disease.

Aspiration of Solids

- Usually food. Obstruction of major airways typically results in atelectasis and moderate nonspecific inflammation. Therapy consists of **removal of the foreign body.**

Mendelson's Syndrome

- **Results from regurgitation of stomach contents and aspiration of chemical material, usually gastric juices. Pulmonary inflammation including the destruction of the alveolar lining, with transudation of fluid into the alveolar space, occurs with remarkable rapidity**
- **Typically this syndrome develops within hours, often following anesthesia when the gag reflex is depressed. The patient becomes tachypneic, hypoxic, and febrile.** The leukocyte count may rise, and the chest X-ray may evolve suddenly from normal to a complete bilateral 'whiteout' within 8 to 24 hours. Sputum production is minimal. The pulmonary signs and symptoms can resolve quickly with symptom-based therapy or can culminate in respiratory failure, with the subsequent development of bacterial superinfection over a period of days.

In contrast to these syndromes, **bacterial aspiration pneumonia:**
- Develops **more slowly**
- It is seen **in patients who are hospitalized**
- Have a **depressed gag reflex, impaired swallowing, or a tracheal or nasogastric tube**
- **Elderly patients**
- Those with transiently impaired consciousness in the wake of seizures, cerebrovascular accidents, or alcoholic blackouts
- **Tachypnea** is the mc sign.

Paroxysmal (Nocturnal) Dyspnea

Also known as **cardiac asthma**, this condition is characterized by attacks of severe shortness of breath that generally occur at night and usually awaken the patient from sleep. The attack is precipitated by stimuli that aggravate previously existing pulmonary congestion; frequently, the total blood volume is augmented at night because of the reabsorption of edema from dependent portions of the body during recumbency.

Necrotizing Pneumonitis

This form of **anaerobic pneumonitis** is characterized by numerous small abscesses that spread to involve several pulmonary segments. The process can be indolent or fulminating. This syndrome is less common than either aspiration pneumonia or lung abscess and includes features of both types of infection.

FREQUENTLY ASKED

Differentiate

Tropical eosinophilia

It is usually caused by **filarial infection**; however, eosinophilic pneumonias also occur with other parasites such as ***Ascaris, Ancyclostoma sp, Toxocara sp,*** *and* ***Strongyloides stercoralis, Wuchereria bancrofti or W malayi.***

Drug-induced eosinophilic pneumonias
Are exemplified by acute reactions to nitrofurantoin, which may begin 2 h to 10 days after nitrofurantoin is started, with symptoms of dry cough, fever, chills, and dyspnea; an eosinophilic pleural effusion accompanying patchy or diffuse pulmonary infiltrates may also occur. Other drugs associated with eosinophilic pneumonias include sulfonamides, penicillin, chlorpropamide, thiazides, tricyclic antidepressants, hydralazine, mephenesin, mecamylamine, nickel carbonyl vapor, gold salts, isoniazid and para-aminosalicylic acid.

Eosinophilia-myalgia syndrome

Caused by dietary supplements of **L-tryptophan**, is occasionally associated with pulmonary infiltrates.

Loeffler's syndrome

It is a benign, acute eosinophilic pneumonia of unknown cause characterized by migrating pulmonary infiltrates and minimal clinical manifestations

Acute eosinophilic pneumonia has been described recently as an idiopathic acute febrile illness **lasting less than 7 days** with severe hypoxemia, pulmonary infiltrates, and no history of asthma

Chronic eosinophilic pneumonia presents with significant systemic symptoms including fever, chills, night sweats, cough, anorexia, and weight loss lasting for **several weeks to months**. The chest X-ray classically shows peripheral infiltrates resembling a photographic negative of pulmonary edema. Some patients also have bronchial asthma of the intrinsic or nonallergic type. Dramatic clearing of symptoms and chest X-rays is often noted within 48 h after initiation of glucocorticoid therapy.

Allergic Angiitis and Granulomatosis of Churg and Strauss

- It is a **multisystem vasculitic disorder that frequently involves the skin, kidney, and nervous system in addition to the lung**
- The disorder may occur at any age and favors persons with a history of bronchial asthma. The asthma often is progressive until the onset of fever and exaggerated eosinophilia, at which time the symptoms of asthma may ease
- **Zafirlukast, zileuton,** and **montelukast** are recognized causes of Churg-Strauss syndrome.

The Hypereosinophilic Syndrome

- The presence of **more than 1500 eosinophils per microliter of peripheral blood for 6 months or longer**
- Lack of evidence for parasitic, allergic, or other known causes of eosinophilia; and signs or symptoms of multisystem organ dysfunction
- Consistent features are blood and bone marrow eosinophilia with tissue infiltration by relatively mature eosinophils
- The heart may be involved with tricuspid valve abnormalities or endomyocardial fibrosis and a restrictive, biventricular cardiomyopathy
- Other organs affected typically include the lungs, liver, spleen, skin, and nervous system. Treatment consists of **glucocorticoids and/or hydroxyurea**

Remember: Hypersensitive Pneumonitis

• Farmer's lung	Micropolyspora faeni	Moldy hay
• Humidifier lung	Thermophilic actinomyces	Air conditioners
• Bird Fancier's lung	Avian proteins	Bird excreta
• Baggassosis	Thermoactinomyces sacchri	Sugar cane dust
• Sequoisis	Graphium/aureobasidium	Sawdust
• Suberosis	Pencillium frequentans	Cork dust
• Mushroom Picker's Lung	Micropolysporafaeni	Moldy composite

ABPA (Allergic Bronchopulmonary Aspergillosis)

It is characterized by episodic airway obstruction, fever, eosinophilia, mucous plugs, positive sputum cultures, and the presence of grossly visible brown flecks in the sputum (hyphae), transient infiltrates and parallel 'tram-line' or ring markings on chest radiographs, proximal bronchiectasis, upper lobe contraction, and elevated levels of total IgA and immunoglobulin E (IgE).

- Bronchial asthma
- Pulmonary infiltrates
- Peripheral eosinophilia
- Immediate wheal and flare to aspergillus fumigates
- Serum precipitins to aspergillus fumigates
- Elevated IgE
- **'Central'** bronchiectasis

- **Noncontagious**
- **Upper lobe dominance**
- **Effusion is rare**

Nocardiosis

The clinical manifestations are nonspecific and include fever, cough, weight loss, and dyspnea. The range of pulmonary involvement extends from transient or inapparent infection to confluent bronchopneumonia with complete consolidation. Radiographic examination of the chest may reveal one or more of the following: fluffy infiltrates, multiple abscess formation with cavitation, bulging fissures, masses, nodules, and empyema.

Caused by:

- **Filamentous, aerobic Gram-positive Bacteria:**
- **Partially acid causes disseminated infections in immunocompromised**
- The risk of pulmonary or disseminated disease is greater than usual among people with deficient cell-mediated immunity especially that associated with lymphoma, transplantation, or AIDS
- In persons with AIDS, **Nocardiosis** usually presents at a $CD4^+$ lymphocyte concentration of <250/ul
- Prophylaxis with sulfamethoxazole and trimethoprim appears to reduce the risk of **nocardiosis** in persons with AIDS or transplanted organs
- **Nocardiosis** has also been associated with pulmonary alveolar proteinosis, tuberculosis and other mycobacterial diseases, and chronic granulomatous disease.

Pneumonia is by far the **most common respiratory tract nocardial disease.** Nocardial pneumonia is typically subacute; symptoms have usually been present for days or weeks at presentation. The onset may be more acute in immunosuppressed patients. Cough is prominent and produces small amounts of thick, purulent sputum that is not malodorous. Fever, anorexia, weight loss, and malaise are common; dyspnea, pleuritic pain, and hemoptysis are less common. Remissions and exacerbations over several weeks are frequent

The most common site of dissemination is the brain.

Pulmonary Tuberculosis

- **Ghon Complex:** Primary subpleural granuloma in the inferior upper lobe/superior lower lobe region (Ghon Focus) along with draining Hilar nodes
- **Puhl's lesion:** Isolated lesion of **chronic pulmonary TB in apex of lung**
- **Assmann's Focus: Infraclavicular** lesion of **chronic pulmonary TB**
- **Rancke Complex:** Combination of **calcified peripheral lesion (Ghon Complex) and calcified Hilar nodes seen in primary TB**

Obligate aerobe
Acid fast
Acid fastness is due to **mycolic acid and cell wall**
Lung is the mc organ involved
Koch's phenomenon is seen in Tuberculosis

Primary Pulmonary Tuberculosis

- Results from an initial infection with tubercle bacilli
- This form of disease is **often seen in children** and is frequently localized to the **middle and lower lung zones**
- The lesion forming after infection is usually **peripheral** and **accompanied by hilar or paratracheal lymphadenopathy**, which may not be detectable on chest radiography. In the majority of cases, the lesion heals spontaneously and may later be evident as a small calcified nodule **(Ghon lesion)**
- **Fibrocaseous lesion or phylenticular conjunctivitis can be a part of primary TB**
- **USUALLY unilateral lymphadenopathy is seen**
- In children and in persons with impaired immunity, such as those with malnutrition or HIV infection, primary pulmonary **tuberculosis** may progress rapidly to clinical illness.

Postprimary Disease

- Also called **adult-type**, **reactivation,** or **secondary tuberculosis**, postprimary disease results from **endogenous reactivation of latent infection** and is usually localized to the apical and posterior segments of the **upper lobes**, where the high oxygen concentration favors mycobacterial growth
- In addition, the superior segments of the lower lobes are frequently involved
- The extent of lung parenchymal involvement varies greatly, from small infiltrates to extensive cavitary disease
- Hemoptysis, however, may also result from rupture of a dilated vessel in a cavity **(Rasmussen's aneurysm)** or from aspergilloma formation in an old cavity
  - **Popcorn calcification** can occur
  - **Patients of atopic asthma are prone to develop TB**
  - **'Hemorrhagic' pleural effusions can ocuur in TB**
  - 'Cavitatory' lesions in lung can occur

Pleural Tuberculosis

- Involvement of the pleura is common in primary **tuberculosis** and results from penetration by a few tubercle bacilli into the pleural space
  - **The fluid is straw-colored and, at times, hemorrhagic**
  - **It is an exudate with a protein concentration > 50% of that in serum, a normal-to-low glucose concentration**
  - **A pH that is generally < 7.2**
  - **And detectable white blood cells** (usually 500 to 2500/ml). Neutrophils may predominate in the early stage, while mononuclear cells are the typical finding later
  - **Mesothelial cells are generally rare or absent**. AFB are very rarely seen on direct smear, but cultures may be positive for **M tuberculosis** in up to one-third of cases
- Necrotic Lymph nodes with peripheral rim enhancement is due to TB
- **PCR and BACTEC are now used for diagnosis.**

Tuberculous Empyema

It is a less common complication of **pulmonary tuberculosis**

It is usually the result of the rupture of a cavity, with delivery of a large number of organisms into the pleural space, or of a bronchopleural fistula from a pulmonary lesion

Tuberculous empyema may result in severe pleural fibrosis and restrictive lung disease.

Cryptic Miliary Tuberculosis

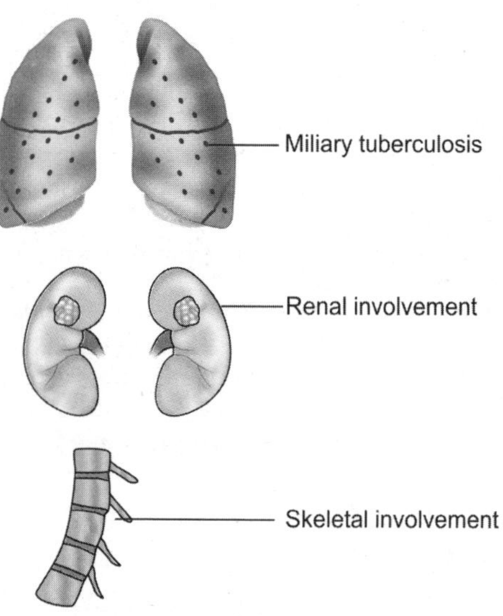

- A rare presentation which has a chronic course characterized by **mild intermittent fever, anemia, and ultimately meningeal involvement preceding death**
- An **acute septicemic form,** nonreactive miliary tuberculosis, occurs very rarely and is due to massive hematogenous dissemination of tubercle bacilli
- **Pancytopenia** is common in this form of disease, which is rapidly fatal
- At postmortem examination, multiple necrotic but **nongranulomatous (nonreactive)** lesions are detected

In miliary TB:

- **Large cavities are formed**
- **Radiologically diffuse consolidation**
- **Pleural effusions seen**

Tuberculo**cidal** drugs	Isoniazid, Rifampin, Pyrazinamide, Streptomycin
Tuberculo**static** drugs	Ethambutol, Thiacetazone, PAS, Ethionamide, Cycloserine

Important Points about TB in HIV-Positive Individuals

- Tuberculosis can appear at any stage of HIV infection
- In **early stages,** TB can present as typical pattern as upper lobe involvement with Cavitation without significant Lymphadenopathy or effusion
- In **late stages,** TB can present as diffuse interstitial or miliary pattern with little Cavitation with Lymphadenopathy
- Active TB can **accelerate** course of HIV infection
- **Extrapulmonary TB** is common in HIV patients
- **The diagnosis of TB in HIV patients is difficult because of:**
  - **Increased sputum negativity**
  - **Atypical radiography**

- Lack of classic granulomas
- Negative PDD skin tests

- Worldwide about **one-third** of all AIDS-related deaths are due to TB
- Clinical manifestations **'depend on CD4 CELL COUNTS'**
- In patients with **low CD4 CELL COUNTS**, disseminated disease is more common
- Pleural effusions, miliary spread, lymphadenopathy and bilateral reticulonodular pattern is seen
- In patients with **High CD4 CELL COUNTS**, typical pattern as upper lobe involvement with cavitation without significant lymphadenopathy or effusion is seen
- Heart disease is a common postmortem finding in HIV-infected patients
- **'Paradoxical reactions'** (Exacerbations in signs and symptoms) have been reported with administration of HAART.

MAC Mycobacterium Avium Complex

- Formerly known as MAI, it stands for Mycobacterium Avium Complex. MAC is a group of mycobacteria
- (The two most common being **M avium and M intracellulare)** that cause a serious disease in people with advanced AIDS. MAC most often causes a disseminated illness (bacteria is spread though the bloodstream) and can cause many symptoms throughout the body
- MAC bacteria are found in air, water, soil, foods, some tobacco products, and in many animals. It is impossible to avoid contact with MAC bacteria. A recent study showed that person-to-person transmission of MAC bacteria is unlikely
- **Risk factors** for developing MAC include having **fewer than 50 CD4 cells, a high viral load (greater than 90,000 copies per/ml) and having had another opportunistic infection such as CMV (cytomegalovirus)**

Signs and symptoms of MAC

- MAC can infect a person's entire body. The signs and symptoms of MAC can be the same signs of other diseases
- They include: high fever, drenching sweats, diarrhea, weight loss, abdominal pain, fatigue, weakness, anemia (low levels of red blood cells), neutropenia (low levels of white blood cells) or thrombocytopenia (low levels of platelets), and elevated liver function tests
- The liver or spleen may be enlarged. Blood infections, hepatitis, skin lesions, and pneumonia may also occur
- **Prophylaxis** is recommended for anyone who is HIV-positive and has 50 CD4 cells or less. While **rifabutin, clarithromycin, and azithromycin are all approved drugs for prophylaxis of MAC, clarithromycin and azithromycin** are the preferred choices
  - **Treatment for MAC** involves taking a combination of antibiotics. MAC treatment must include at least two drugs, one of which should be either **clarithromycin or azithromycin**
  - **Ethambutol** is the recommended second drug
  - **Rifabutin, ciprofloxacin, or amikacin** may be added for people with more severe MAC.

Pneumocystis Carinii

- Pneumocystis carinii, recently suggested to be a fungus rather than a parasite, is usually dormant in the host lung, causes disease when defenses are compromised
- **Fungus causing pneumonia in AIDS**
- **Damage of type I pneumocytes**
- **Hypertrophy of type II pneumocytes**
- **Interstitial pneumonitis**
- Nearly all patients have **immunologic deficiencies**
- The most common being **defects in cell-mediated immunity as with hematologic malignancies, lymphoproliferative diseases, cancer chemotherapy, and AIDS**
- Among patients with HIV infection, about 60% have *P. carinii* pneumonia as the initial AIDS-defining diagnosis, and >80% of AIDS patients have this infection at some time during their course
- Most patients have a history of **fever, dyspnea, and a 'dry, nonproductive cough'** that may evolve in a subacute fashion over several weeks or acutely over several days
- The chest X-ray characteristically shows **diffuse, bilateral, perihilar infiltrates**, but 10 to 20% of patients have normal X-rays.

- Arterial blood gases show '**hypoxemia, with a marked increase in the alveolar-arterial O_2 gradient**', and pulmonary function shows altered diffusing capacity
- Patients with HIV become vulnerable to *P. carinii* pneumonia when the **CD4 helper cell count is <200/µL**
- The diagnosis requires histopathologic demonstration of the organism with **methenamine silver, Giemsa, Wright-Giemsa, modified Grocott, Gram-Weigert, or monoclonal antibody stain,** with specimens obtained by transtracheal aspiration, transthoracic needle aspiration, open lung biopsy, induced sputum, or bronchoscopy
- The preferred diagnostic method is **induced** sputum when technical expertise is available
- Alternatively, the **preferred method is bronchoscopy with bronchioalveolar lavage and brush biopsy.**

- **'Pneumocystis carinii or Pneumocystis jerovici'** is an **opportunistic** pathogen
- It is **'yeast-like fungus'**
- Natural habitat is **lung**
- People at risk of PCP
- **Immunocompromised**
- **Patients undergone solid organ transplants**
- **Patients with HIV**
- **Children with primary immunodeficiency**
  - **Symptoms:** Dyspnea, fever, **nonproductive cough**
  - **Signs:** Tachypnea, Tacycardia, Cyanosis
  - **X-ray findings: Bilateral diffuse infiltrates in perihilar region**
  - **ABG:** Hypoxia, Increased Alveolar Arteriolar gradient, respiratory alkalosis
- Associated with **eosinophilic exudates**
- Damage of **type I pneumocytes** and hypertrophy of type II pneumocytes
- Adults present as **'alveolar predominant'** type disease
- **Infants present as predominant 'interstitial' type**
- **Bronchoalveolar lavage** is done for confirmation
- Risk of PCP increases when **CD4 count in children drops below 200 cells/micro liter** and it is the most common opportunistic infection in pediatric population with severly depressed cell counts.

Several Antimicrobials are Effective for PCP Infection

They are:

- TMP-SMZ (cotrimoxazole)
- TMP+Dapsone is also used
- **Dapsone alone** or along with Pyremethamine is also effective
- Combination therapy of Clindamycin + Primaquine
- Atavaquone
- **Pentamidine** is also used for the treatment of PCP
- **Glucocorticoids** are used in severe cases of PCP infection

Sarcoidosis

- **Sarcoidosis** is a **systemic disease**, and thus the clinical manifestations may be generalized or focused on one or more organs. However, because the **lung is almost always involved, most patients have symptoms referable to the respiratory system**
- The first manifestation of the disease is an accumulation of mononuclear inflammatory cells, mostly **CD4+ T_H1 lymphocytes and mononuclear phagocytes**, in affected organs. The giant cells within the granuloma can be of the Langhans' or foreign-body variety and often contain inclusions such as **noncaseating granulomas with bilateral hilar lymphadenopathy**
  - **Schaumann bodies** (conch-like structures)
  - **Asteroid bodies** (stellate-like structures) and
  - **Residual bodies** (refractile calcium-containing inclusions)

Two syndromes have been identified in the acute group:

- **Lofgren's syndrome** includes the complex of **erythema nodosum and X-ray findings of bilateral hilar adenopathy,** often accompanied by joint symptoms, including arthritis at the ankles, knees, wrists, or elbows
- **Heerfordt-Waldenstrom syndrome** describes individuals with **fever, parotid enlargement, anterioruveitis and facial nerve palsy**

- **Lupus pernio** is characterized by **indurated blue-purple, swollen, shiny lesions on the nose, cheeks, lips, ears, fingers, and knees**
- **Eye** involvement occurs in ~25% of patients with **sarcoidosis**, and it can cause blindness, **~75% have anterior uveitis and 25 to 35% have posterior uveitis**. There is blurred vision, tearing, and photophobia. When the lacrimal gland is involved, a **keratoconjunctivitis sicca syndrome**, with dry, sore eyes, can result
- **Parotid enlargement** is a classic feature of **sarcoidosis. Bilateral involvement is the rule**. The gland is usually nontender, firm, and smooth. Xerostomia can occur; other exocrine glands are affected only rarely

Common abnormalities in the blood include:

- **Lymphocytopenia**
- **Occasional mild eosinophilia**
- **↑erythrocyte sedimentation rate**
- **Hyperglobulinemia and**
- **↑Angiotensin-converting enzyme (ACE)**
- **False-positive tests for rheumatoid factor or antinuclear antibodies can be observed**
- **Hypercalcemia**
- **The Kveim-Siltzbach skin test**, the intradermal injection of a heat-treated suspension of a **sarcoidosis** spleen extract which is biopsied 4 to 6 weeks later, yields **sarcoidosis**-like lesions in 70 to 80% of individuals with sarcoidosis. Biopsy is **confirmatory test**
- Egg-shell calcification of hilar lymph nodes may be seen.

Typical USMLE Case Scenario

A 54-year-old engineer is having nonproductive cough and dyspnea. Chest radiograph shows bilateral hilar adenopathy. Over the next month, the patient undergoes a series of laboratory tests and, eventually, mediastinoscopy with a lymph node biopsy. Laboratory testing is remarkable for a (total) serum calcium level of 11.5 mg/dL and an elevated angiotensin-converting enzyme (ACE) level. Lymph node biopsy reveals nodular fibrotic lesions surrounded by histiocytes without necrosis (Noncaseous) (Noncaseating Granuloma).

Lymphangioleiomyomatosis (LAM)

- **Lymphangioleiomyomatosis (LAM)** is a rare lung disease that results in disorderly smooth muscle proliferation throughout the bronchioles, alveolar septa, perivascular spaces, and lymphatics, resulting in the obstruction of small airways (leading to pulmonary cyst formation and pneumothorax) and lymphatics (leading to chylous pleural effusion)
- LAM occurs in a sporadic form, which only affects females, who are usually of childbearing age. LAM also occurs in patients who have tuberous sclerosis
- Symptoms are dyspnea, cough, chest pain, and hemoptysis; spontaneous pneumothorax is common
- Diagnosis is suspected on the basis of symptoms and chest X-ray and is confirmed by high-resolution CT. Prognosis is uncertain, but the disorder is slowly progressive and over the years often leads to respiratory failure and death. Primary treatment is lung transplantation
- Lymphangioleiomyomatosis (LAM) is not an interstitial lung disease, but patients are occasionally misdiagnosed as having interstitial lung disease (and also asthma or COPD).

Pulmonary Hypertension PPH

GENE involved: Bone morphogenetic protein receptor II

Causes:

- Primary pulmonary hypertension

- COPD (mc cause for **chronic cor pulmonale**)
- Pulmonary thromboembolism (mc cause of **acute cor pulmonale**)
- Congenital heart disease (Eisenmenger's syndrome)
- Recurrent pulmonary embolism
- HIV
- Sarcoidosis
- Connective tissue disease
- Sickle cell anemia
- Obesity
- High altitude
- Fenfluamine

Features

- **Exertional dyspnea**
- **Chest pain, syncope**
- **Loud P2**

Guidelines for Treatment in PPH

- **Digoxin** may increase cardiac output and lower circulating levels of norepinephrine.
- **Diuretic therapy** relieves dyspnea and peripheral edema and may be useful in reducing right ventricular volume overload.
- Because pulmonary vascular resistance increases dramatically with exercise, patients should be cautioned against participating in activities demanding increased physical stress, **i.e. physical stress has got an effect on PPH.**
- In one study, it is recommended that **anticoagulant therapy be given to all patients** as it increases survival but does not cause regression of disease
- Other important points in treatment are:
  - Patients with substantial reductions in pulmonary vascular resistance from short-acting vasodilators may be candidates for **calcium channel blocker therapy**
  - **Prostacyclin** is an important modality in treatment
  - It causes improvement in symptoms, improves exercise tolerance and causes reduction in mortality
  - **Transplantation** may be considered in patients on prostacyclin who develop or continue to manifest heart failure. Heart lung, bilateral lung and single lung transplants are done.

Lung Cancer

Lung Cancer

- Lung Ca with worst prognosis **Small cell Ca**
- Lung Ca most responsive to radiotherapy **Small cell Ca**
- Lung Ca most responsive to chemotherapy **Small cell Ca**
  - Most common type of lung Ca **Adenocarcinoma**
  - Most commonly metastasizing to opposite lung **Adenocarcinoma**
  - Most common type in females **Adenocarcinoma**
  - Most common type in nonsmokers **Adenocarcinoma**
  - Most common in young **Adenocarcinoma**
  - Most common in peripheral location **Adenocarcinoma**
- Second most common lung Ca **Squamous cell carcinoma**
- Most common cavitating lung Ca **Squamous cell carcinoma**
- Best prognosis among lung Ca **Squamous cell carcinoma**
- Most common to produce hypercalcemia **Squamous cell carcinoma**

C associated with squamous cell carcinoma

- **C**entral in location
- **C**avitation
- **C**lubbing
- **C**alcium level↑

Small Cell Carcinoma of Lung: Oat Cell Carcinoma

- Highly malignant
- MC cancer causing SVC
- Metastasis occurs early especially to **brain**
- Usually associated with smoking
- Usually occurring in males
- Causes paraneoplastic syndrome: **Cushing's Syndrome, SIADH**
- Treated by **Chemotherapy**
- Surgical intervention not done usually

Lambert-Eaton Syndrome

Lambert-Eaton myasthenic syndrome is seen in association with small cell lung cancer, and to a lesser extent, breast and ovarian cancer. It may also occur independently as an autoimmune disorder. Lambert-Eaton myasthenic syndrome is caused by an antibody directed against presynaptic voltage-gated calcium channel in the peripheral nervous system.

Features:

- **Repeated muscle contractions lead to increased muscle strength *(in contrast to myasthenia gravis)**
- **Limb girdle weakness (affects lower limbs first)**
- **Hyporeflexia**
- **Autonomic symptoms: Dry mouth, impotence, difficultly micturating**
- **Ophthalmoplegia and ptosis not commonly a feature (unlike in myasthenia gravis)**

EMG

- **Incremental response** to repetitive electrical stimulation

Management

- Guanidine is sometimes used

Pulmonary Embolism

- Dyspnea **most common symptom and earliest manifestation**
- Tachypnea **most common sign**
- **Tachycardia, $S_3Q_3T_3$** (an S wave in lead I, a Q wave in lead III, and an inverted T wave in lead III Pattern in ECG) Abnormalities include sinus tachycardia; new-onset atrial fibrillation or flutter; and an inverted T wave in lead III. Often, the QRS axis is greater than 90. T wave inversion in leads V1 to V4 reflects right ventricular strain
  - **West Mark's Sign:** Focal oligemia on CXR
  - **Hamptons's Sign:** Wedge shaped density on CXR
  - **Palla's Sign:** Enlarged Right Descending Pulmonary Artery
- **Plasma D-dimer enzyme-linked immunosorbent assay (ELISA)** level is elevated in more than 90% of patients with PTE, reflecting plasmin's breakdown of fibrin
- **Pulmonary angiography:** Selective pulmonary angiography is the **most specific test** available for establishing the definitive diagnosis of PTE and can detect emboli as small as 1 to 2 mm
- A definitive diagnosis of PTE depends upon visualization of an **intraluminal filling defect** in more than one projection
- **Secondary signs of PTE include:**
  - **Abrupt occlusion (cut-off) of vessels**
  - **Segmental oligemia or avascularity**
  - A prolonged **arterial phase** with slow filling
  - Or tortuous, **tapering peripheral vessels**

A **Hypercoagulable state is characteristic of pregnancy**, and deep venous thrombosis (DVT) is a common complication. Indeed, **pulmonary embolism** is the most common cause of maternal death in the United States. Activated protein C resistance caused by the factor V Leiden mutation increases the risk for DVT and **pulmonary embolism** during pregnancy

- **Well's grading of pulmonary embolism is based on: clinical symptoms**
- **Definitive method of diagnosing pulmonary embolism is pulmonary angiography**
- **Most reliable method for diagnosis of PE is angiography**

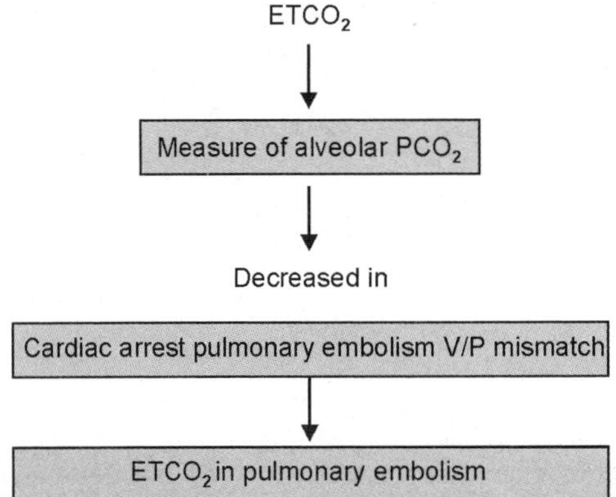
ETCO2
Measure of alveolar PCO2
Decreased in
Cardiac arrest pulmonary embolism V/P mismatch
ETCO2 in pulmonary embolism

USMLE Case Scenario

On 8th postoperative day after repair of a broken hip, a 68-year-old man from Texas suddenly develops pleuritic chest pain and shortness of breath. On examination by a physician, he is found to be anxious, diaphoretic, and tachycardic, with a blood pressure of 146/85 mm Hg. He has prominent distended veins in his neck and forehead. Blood gases show both hypoxemia and hypocapnia. His chest X-ray film is unremarkable. Which of the following is the most appropriate next step in management?

1. Aortogram
2. Cardiac enzymes
3. Hyperventilation and PEEP
4. Retinal examination
5. Ventilation-perfusion lung scan, or spiral CT scan of the chest
6. CXR

Ans. 5. Ventilation-perfusion lung scan, or spiral CT scan of the chest

The clinical picture is that of a pulmonary embolus. Although pulmonary angiogram is the 'gold standard' diagnostic test, confirmation is usually obtained with the less invasive ventilation-perfusion scan.

Pneumothorax

- **Pneumothorax** is the presence of gas in the pleural space
- Sudden dyspnea following cough and chest pain is seen
- **Spontaneous pneumothorax** occurs without antecedent trauma to thorax common in males/smokers
- **Rupture of subpleural bleb is a common cause**
- **Primary spontaneous pneumothorax** occurs in the absence of underlying lung disease, while
- **Secondary spontaneous pneumothorax** occurs in its presence. A traumatic **pneumothorax** results from penetrating or nonpenetrating chest injuries
  - **Tension pneumothorax** is a **pneumothorax** in which the pressure in the pleural space is positive throughout the respiratory cycle
  - **Primary Spontaneous Pneumothorax:** Primary spontaneous pneumothoraces are usually due to rupture of apical pleural blebs, small cystic spaces that lie within or immediately under the visceral pleura. Primary spontaneous pneumothoraces **occur almost exclusively in smokers**
  - **Secondary Spontaneous Pneumothorax:** Most secondary spontaneous pneumothoraces are due to **chronic obstructive pulmonary disease**
  - **Traumatic Pneumothorax:** Traumatic pneumothoraces can result from both penetrating and nonpenetrating chest trauma. Traumatic pneumothoraces should be treated with tube thoracostomy unless they are very small.

- **Tension Pneumothorax:** This condition usually occurs during mechanical ventilation or resuscitative efforts. The positive pleural pressure is life-threatening both because ventilation is severely compromised and because the positive pressure is transmitted to the mediastinum, which results in decreased venous return to the heart and reduced cardiac output

- **Decreased breath sounds**
- **Hyper-resonant percussion note**
- **Intrapleural pressure is equal to atmospheric pressure in Open Pneumothorax.**

Tension Pneumothorax

This is a life-threatening emergency that needs to be managed immediately with either chest tube thoracostomy or needle thoracocentesis to relieve the tension on the affected side of the thorax. Physical examination reveals tachycardia, tachypnea, decreased or absent breath sounds over the involved hemithorax, increased resonance to percussion, subcutaneous emphysema, and deviation of the trachea to the opposite side. Tension pneumothorax develops when air leaking into the chest increases intrathoracic pressure, completely collapsing the lung on that side. It results in displacement of the mediastinum and trachea to the opposite side of the chest and impedes venous return.

Remember

- **Shrinking lung syndrome** is seen in SLE
- **Bovine cough** is a feature of laryngeal palsy
- **White lung** is a feature of asbestosis
- **Sequestration lung** is best diagnosed by angiography
- **Shock lung/DAD (Diffuse Alveolar Damage) is ARDS**

USMLE High Yield

The risk of a smoker with asbestos exposure developing lung cancer is about greater than the regular population. The patient has an increased risk for lung cancer and would greatly benefit from smoking cessation. Asbestosis can lead to an interstitial lung disease in patients with or without a smoking history. Even nonsmokers may present with dyspnea on exertion, cough, chest wall pain, and ultimately, end-stage lung disease. Patients with asbestosis are at increased risk for pleural or peritoneal mesotheliomas.

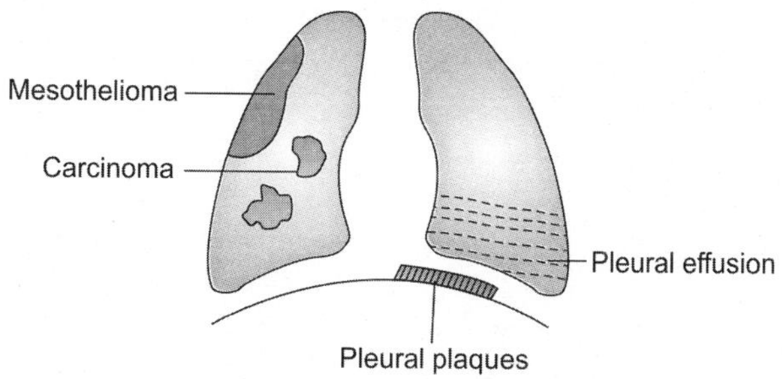

X-ray presentations of asbestosis

ARDS Shock Lung/DAD (Diffuse Alveolar Damage)

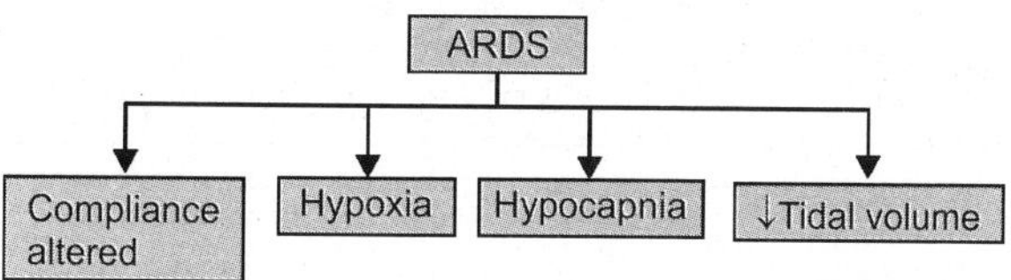

Features of ARDS

- **Stiff lungs**
- **Hypoxemia**
- **Hypercapnia**
- **Pulmonary edema**
- **Normal PCWP**
- ↑Pulmonary artery pressure
- No response to oxygen
- Ground glass appearance
- Acute onset of respiratory failure
- Air bronchogram sign is positive
- Associated with
- Pancreatitis
- Trauma
- Septicemia
- Embolism
- Multiple blood transfusions

Respiratory Causes of Clubbing

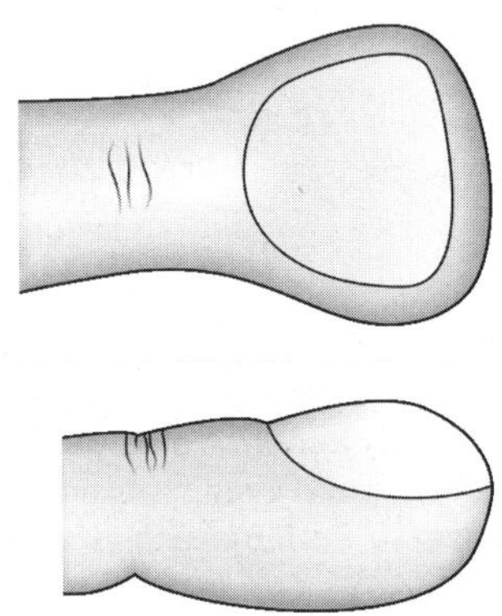

Clubbing of nails

- **Bronchogenic cancer**
- **COLD**
- **Bronchiectasis**
- **Lung abscess**
- **Empyema**
- **Pulmonary fibrosis**
- **Mediastinal tumors**
- **Pleural tumors**
- **Cryptogenic organizing pneumonia**

- **Opacification with no mediastinal shift: consolidation**
- **Opacification with ipsilateral mediastinal shift: collapse**
- **Opacification with contralateral mediastinal shift**
- **Haemothorax, hydrothorax**

Most common cause of **hemoptysis**	Bronchitis
Most common cause of **hemoptysis in india**	Tuberculosis
Most common cause of **massive hemoptysis**	Bronchiectasis

• Most common cause of **massive hemoptysis in India**	• Tuberculosis
• Most common **presenting symptom of lung cancer**	• Cough
• Most common site for **bronchogenic cysts**	• Middle mediastinum
• Most common cause of **stridor in children**	• Foreign body

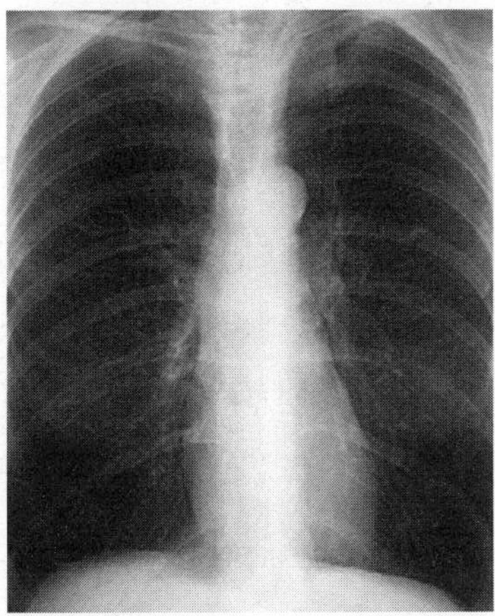

CXR demonstrating COPD (Emphysematous Lung)

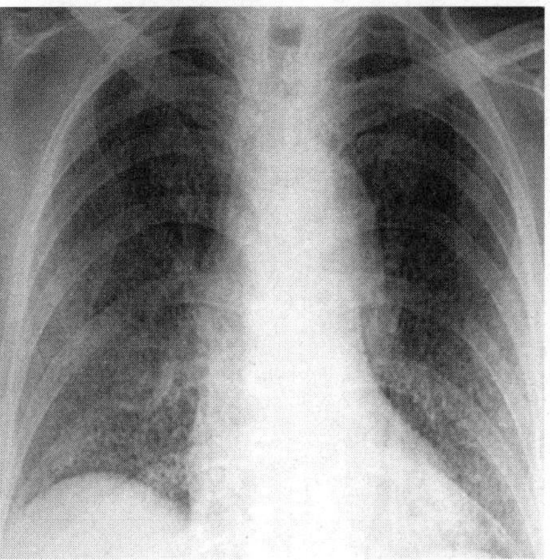

CXR demonstrating miliary tuberculosis

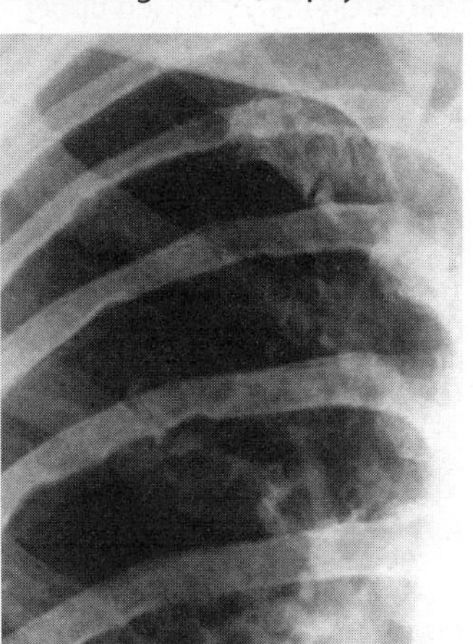

Rib-notching in coarctation of aorta

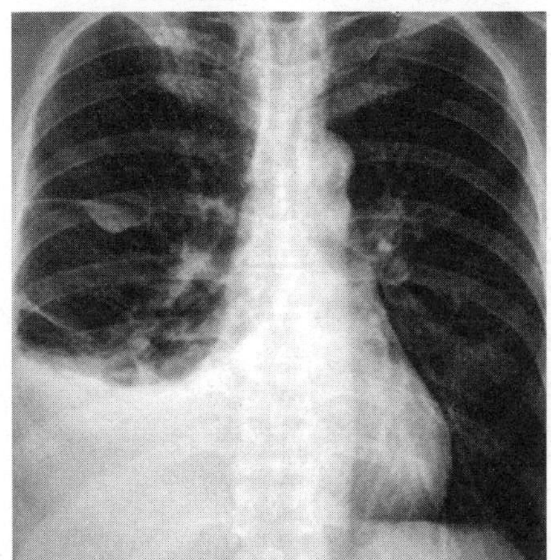

CXR demonstrating a big right-sided pleural effusion

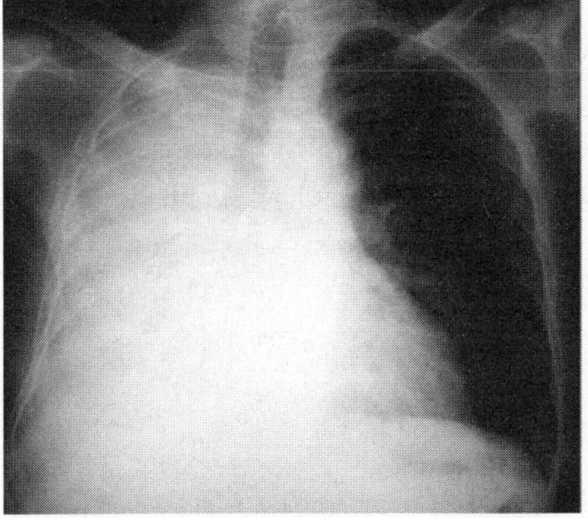

CXR demonstrating atelectasis of right lung

(i) Homogenous density right hemithorax, (ii) Mediastinal shift to right, (iii) Right hemithorax smaller, (iv) Right heart and diaphragmatic silhouette are not identifiable

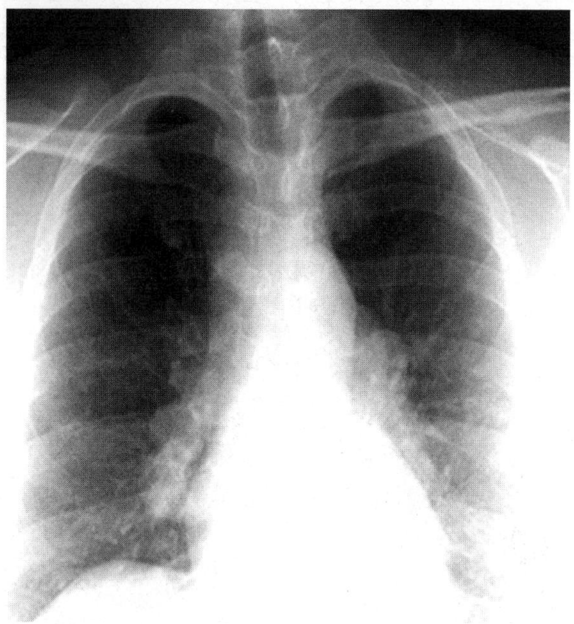

CXR demonstrating bihilar adenopathy

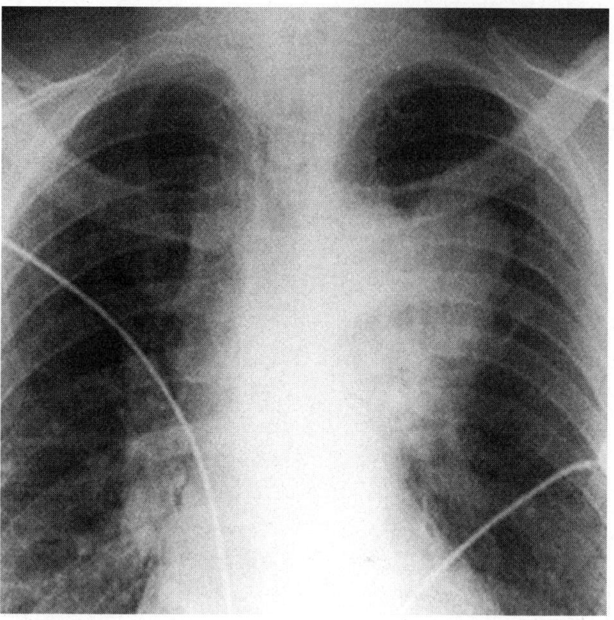

CXR of a squamous cell carcinoma of the left upper lobe of lung

CARDIOVASCULAR MEDICINE

Different Types of Pulse

- **Small volume, slow rising pulse: (Anacrotic):** Aortic Stenosis
- **Collapsing and slow rising (Bisferiens):** AS with AR
- **Collapsing Pulse:** Hyperdynamic circulation, AR, Thyrotoxicosis, PDA, AR
- **Pulsus alternans.** LVF
- **Jerky pulse:** HOCM
- **Pulsus paradoxus:** Asthma, cardiac tamponade, pericarditis

Waves in JVP

- **'a'** wave – 1st positive wave and it is due to **atrial systole.** Absent in AF
- **'x'** wave – fall of pressure in atrium, coincides with **atrial diastole**
- **'c'** wave – it is due to rise in atrial pressure during **isometric contraction** during which the **AV valves bulge into atrium**
- **'x_1'** wave – occurs during ejection period, when AV ring is pulled towards ventricles causing distension of atria
- **'v'** wave – occurs during **isometric relaxation** period or during atrial diastole
- **'Y'** wave – due to **opening of AV valve** and emptying of blood into ventricle.

Jugular venous distension suggests:

- **Right heart failure**
- **Pulmonary hypertensin**
- **Tricuspid regurgitation**
- **Volume overload**
- **Pericardial disease**

<u>Hepatojugular reflux:</u> seen in fluid overload, impaired right ventricular compliance

<u>Kussmaul's sign</u> is an increase in JVP with inspiration.

Heart Sounds

Heart sounds	Cause
First	Closure of AV valves (Mitral Tricuspid) **High-pitched** duration: 14 seconds **SOFT S1** is seen in: – **MS (long-standing, calcified)** – Obesity – MR – Pleural effusion – **Loud S1** is heard in: anemia, anxiety, fever, Thyrotoxicosis ASD, PDA **MS (Polonged flow through AV valve)**
Second	Closure of semilunar valves (aortic, pulmonary) **Wide split of S2** is seen in: **ASD, MR, PS** **Reverse splitting of S2 is seen in:** **LBBB, HTN, AS**

- **AS: Aortic stenosis**
- **AR: Aortic regurgitation**
- **MS: Mitral stenosis**
- **MR: Mitral regurgitation**
- **HTN: Hypertension**
- **LBBB: Left bundle branch block**
- **RBBB: Right bundle branch block**

S_3

- **S_3 is low-pitched and because of ventricular filling**
- **Diastolic occurring after S_2**
- **Best heard at apex**
- **Best heard with bell of stethoscope**

Causes of S_3:

- **In children, hyperdynamic states**
- **LVF, RVF**
- **Regurgitant lesions**

S_4

- **S_4 is low-pitched**
- **Presystolic, produced during second rapid filling phase (before S_1)**
- **Best heard with bell of stethoscope**

Seen in:

- **Hypertension**
- **AS**

- **HOCM**
- **Ischemic heart diseases**
- **Acute MR**

Differentiating Different Types of Shock		
• **Cardiogenic shock**	↑PCWP	↓CO
• **Volume overload**	↑PCWP	↑CO
• **Hypovolemic shock**	↓PCWP	
• **Noncardiogenic shock (ARDS)**	n PCWP	

Hypovolemic shock

↓PCWP
↓CO
↑SVR

Cardiogenic shock

↑PCWP
↓CO
↑SVR

Neurogenic shock

↓PCWP
↓CO
↓SVR

Parameters in shock

Recognizing Certain ECG Rhythms

ECG Identification:

- Identify the atrial rhythm and measure its rate. Establishing the rate allows the atrial rhythm to be characterized as bradycardia (rate < 60 per minute), normal (rate between 60 and 100 per minute), and tachycardia (rate >100 per minute)
- If atrial and ventricular rates are different from each other, their rates must be determined separately
- Determine the regularity or irregularity of the rate. Irregular rhythms should be further described as totally irregular ('irregularly' irregular as, for example, in atrial fibrillation) or regular with periods of irregularity ('regularly' irregular as, for example, in atrial bigeminy)
- Determine the P wave axis, duration, and morphology to provide information about the focus or origin of the atrial rhythm and whether the atria are being depolarized antegradely or retrogradely
- If the atrial rhythm is sinus, the P wave morphology and duration can suggest the presence of atrial enlargement or hypertrophy
- Identify the ventricular rate and whether it is regular or irregular. Ascertain whether it is associated with the atrial rhythm and what their relationships are: Is there one P wave for each QRS complex? Do the P waves precede or follow the QRS complexes? What is the PR interval? Is it constant or does it change?
- Determine the QRS axis and duration, and describe the QRS morphology. The duration, morphology, and axis of the QRS complexes can help define the origin of the ventricular rhythm
- Rhythms originating above the ventricles usually use the normal His-Purkinje system to active ventricular muscle, and the QRS complexes are narrow and normal-appearing unless bundle branch block is present. QRS complexes originating from ventricular tissue, on the other hand, are broad and bizarre. If the ventricles are depolarized using the normal His-Purkinje pathways, the QRS morphology (including voltage), duration, and axis can suggest the presence of left and/or right ventricular hypertrophy
- Finally, compare the present ECG with previous records.

Conduction Abnormalities

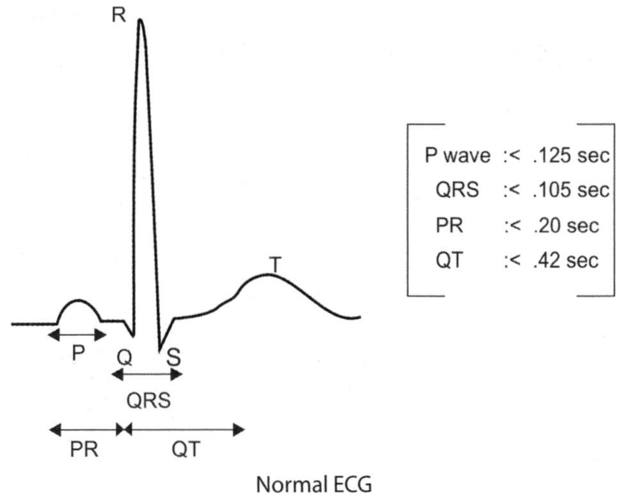

Normal ECG

Waves of Normal ECG

Wave/Segment	From – To	Cause	Duration (second)
P wave	–	**Atrial depolarization**	**0.1**
QRS complex	–	**Ventricular depolarization**	**0.08 – 0.10**
T wave	–	**Ventricular repolarization**	**0.2**
P–R interval	**Onset of P wave to onset of Q wave**		**(0.12 to 0.2)**
Q–T interval	**Onset of Q wave and end of T wave**		**0.4 – 0.42**

Prolonged

- **Lev's disease**: There is **calcification and sclerosis of the fibrous cardiac skeleton**, which frequently involves the aortic and mitral valves, the central fibrous body, and the summit of the ventricular septum
- **Lenegre's disease** appears to be a **primary sclerodegenerative disease within the conducting system** itself with no involvement of the myocardium or the fibrous skeleton of the heart
- **First-degree AV block**, more properly termed **prolonged AV conduction**, is classically characterized by a PR interval > 0.20 s
- **Second-degree heart block** (intermittent AV block) is present when some atrial impulses fail to conduct to the ventricles
- **Mobitz type I second-degree AV block (AV Wenckebach block)** is characterized by progressive PR interval prolongation prior to block of an atrial impulse. This type of block is almost always localized to the AV node and associated with a normal QRS duration, although bundle branch block may be present
- **There is progressive lengthening of the PR interval and a drop beat occurs**
- **Mobitz type II second-degree AV block**, conduction fails suddenly and unexpectedly without a preceding change in PR intervals. It is generally due to disease of the His-Purkinje system and is most often associated with a prolonged QRS duration
- **Third-degree AV block** is present when no atrial impulse propagates to the ventricles. If the QRS complex of the escape rhythm is of normal duration, occurs at a rate of 40 to 55 beats per minute, and increases with atropine or exercise, AV nodal block is probable. Congenital complete AV block is usually localized to the AV node. If the block is within the His bundle, the escape pacemaker is usually less responsive to these perturbations. If the escape rhythm of the QRS is wide and associated with rates 40 beats per minute, block is usually localized in, or distal to, the His bundle and mandates a pacemaker, since the escape rhythm in this setting is unreliable
- Some patients with infra-His bundle block are capable of retrograde conduction. In such patients, a **'pacemaker syndrome'** may develop if a simple ventricular pacemaker is used. Dual-chamber pacemakers eliminate this potential problem.

Important Points to Note in ECG

- **LBBB: QRS duration greater than 120 msec. W pattern of QRS in V1-V2 and M pattern of QRS in V3-V6**
- **RBBB: QRS duration greater than 120 msec. M pattern of QRS in V1-V2 and W pattern of QRS in V3-V6**
- **Long QT syndrome: QT_c greater than 440 msec**
- **LVH: S in V1+R in V6 > 35 mm**
- **RVH: Right axis deviation and wave in V1 > 7 mm**
- **Ischemia/Infarction: Inverted T waves, Poor R wave Progression in precordial chest leads. ST segment elevation/depression**
- **Transmural infarction: Significant Q waves**

'Pacemaker' Syndrome

The pacemaker syndrome consists of fatigue, dizziness, syncope, and distressing pulsations in the neck and chest and can be associated with adverse hemodynamic effects. The pathophysiologic contributors to the pacemaker syndrome include:

- Loss of atrial contribution to ventricular systole
- Vasodepressor reflex initiated by cannon A waves, which are caused by atrial contractions against a closed tricuspid valve and observed in the jugular venous pulse and
- Systemic and pulmonary venous regurgitation due to atrial contraction against a closed AV valve

The symptoms associated with the pacemaker syndrome can be **prevented by maintaining AV synchrony by dual-chamber pacing** or, in the case of a ventricular demand pacemaker, by programming an escape rate of 15 to 20 beats per minute below that of the paced rate.

Relative Bradycardia

- **Typhoid fever**
- **Brucellosis**
- **Leptospirosis**
- **Drug-induced fever**
- **Factitious fever**

ECG: Axis Deviation

Causes of left axis deviation (LAD)

- **Left anterior hemiblock**
- **LBBB**
- **Wolff-Parkinson-White syndrome**
- **Hyperkalemia**
- **Congenital: ostium primum ASD, tricuspid atresia**
- **Minor LAD in obese people**

Causes of Right Axis Deviation (RAD)

- **Right ventricular hypertrophy**
- **Left posterior hemiblock**
- **RBBB**
- **Chronic lung disease**
- **Pulmonary embolism**
- **Ostium secundum ASD**
- **Normal in infant < 1 year old**
- **Minor RAD in tall people**

ST Elevation is seen in

- **Acute MI**
- **Prinzmetal's angina**
- **Acute pericarditis**
- **Ventricular aneurysm**
- **Early repolarization variant**

Torsades De Pointes

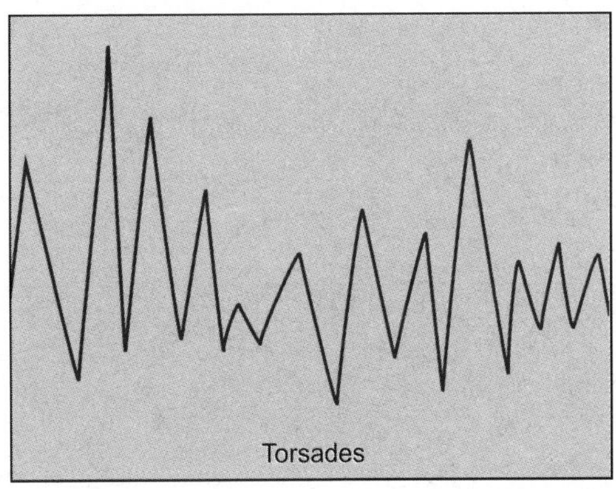
Torsades

Causes: Prolonged QT Syndrome

- **Quinidine**
- **Procanamide**
- **Disopyramide**
- **Terfenadine, astemizole**
- **Cisapride**
- **Gatifloxacin**
- **Sparfloxacin**
- **Halofantrine**
- **Mefloquine**
- **TCA**
- **Hypomagnesemia**

Wolff-Parkinson-White Syndrome

- The term Wolff-Parkinson-White syndrome is applied to patients with both pre-excitation on the ECG and paroxysmal tachycardias. AV bypass tracts can be associated with certain congenital abnormalities, the most important of which is Ebstein's anomaly
- AV bypass tracts that conduct in an antegrade direction produce a typical ECG pattern of a:
  - Short PR interval (< 0.12 s)
  - A slurred upstroke of the QRS complex (delta wave) and
  - A wide QRS complex
- During PSVT in **WPW**, the impulse is usually conducted antegradely over the normal AV system and retrogradely through the bypass tract
- **Procainamide** is helpful
- **Radiofrequency ablation** is done.

Drugs and Arrhythmias

• DOC for ventricular arrhythmias	Lidocaine
• DOC for AF without heart failure	Beta blockers
• DOC for Atrial flutter without heart failure	Beta blockers
• DOC for AF with heart failure	Digoxin
• DOC for Atrial flutter with heart failure	Digoxin
• DOC for PSVT	Adenosine
• DOC for WPWS	Procainamide
• DOC for ventricular ectopics	Beta blockers
• DOC for sinus bradycardia	Atropine

Sinus Bradycardia

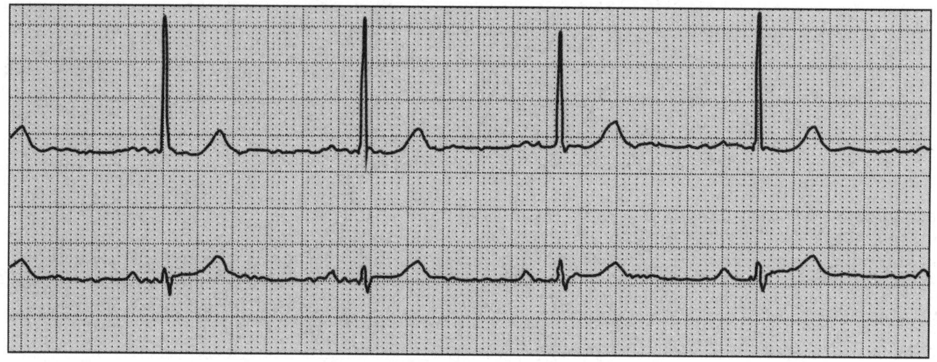

Heart rate: < 60 bpm, regular rhythm

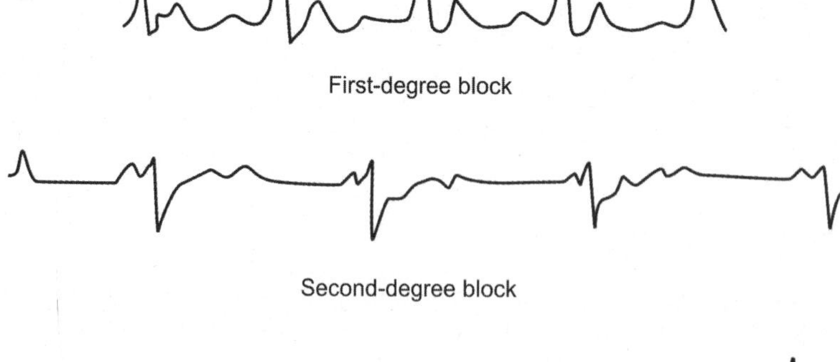

First-degree block

Second-degree block

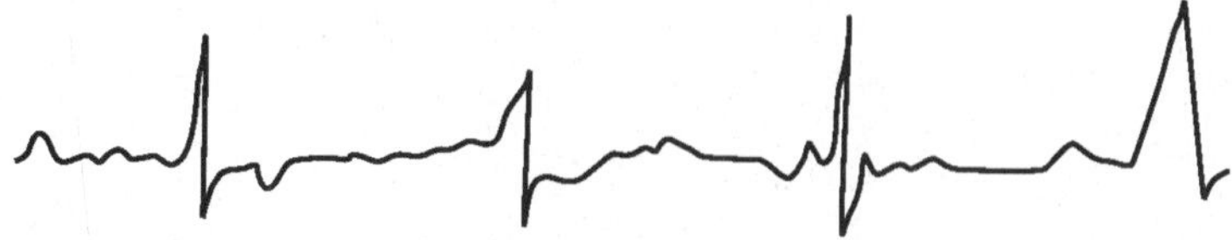

Complete heart block

Atrial Fibrillation

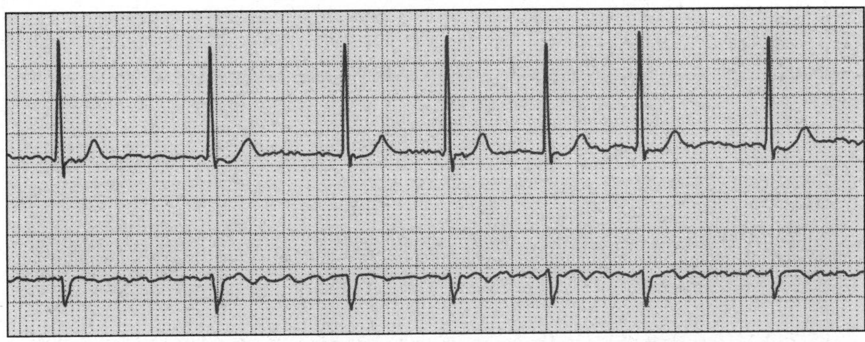

Heart rate greater than 350, irregular rhythm, fibrillatory p wave

PVC

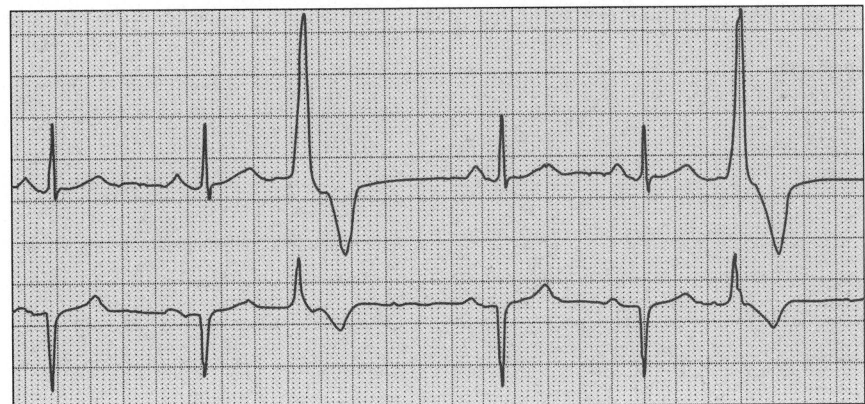

Every third beat is a PVC

Ventricular Tachycardia

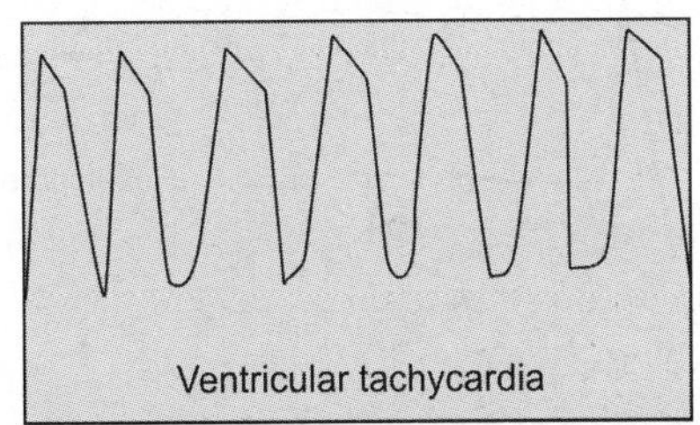

Ventricular tachycardia

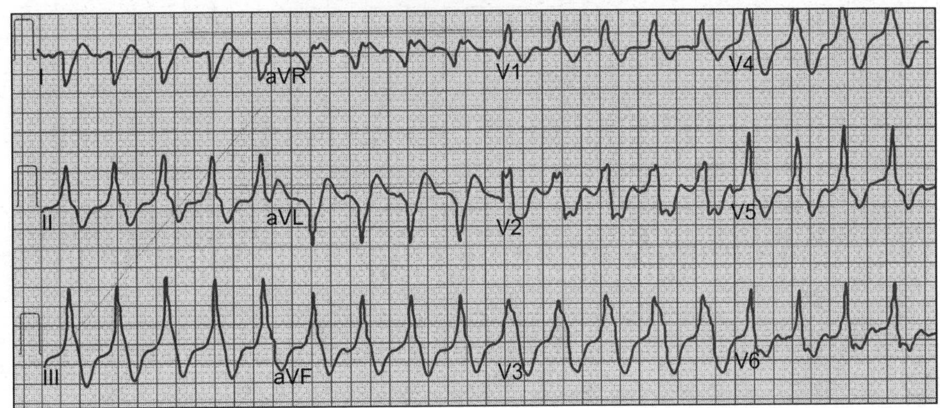

Ventricular Fibrillation

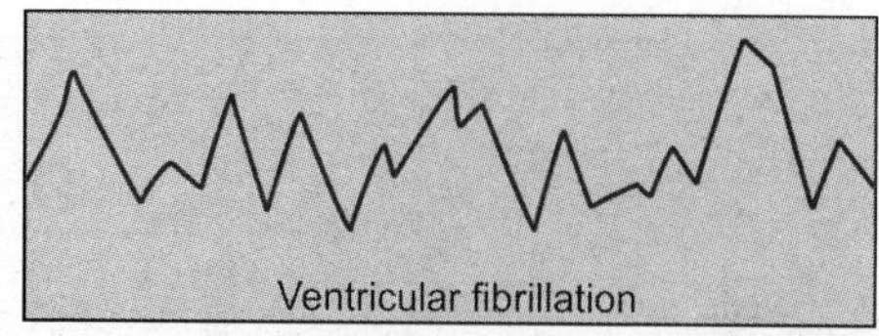

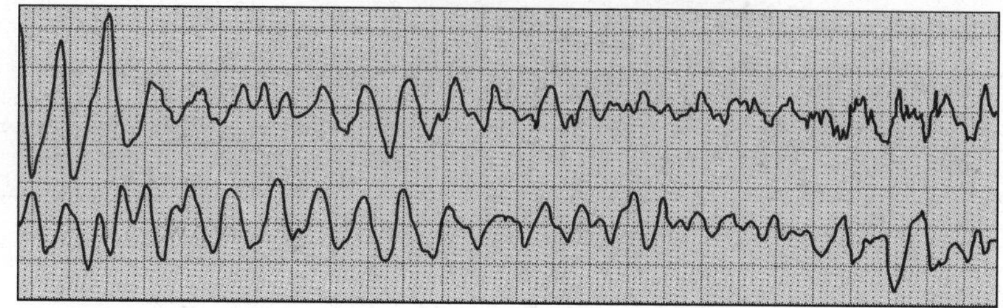

VF: Here heart rate is greater than 300, irregular rhythm, absent P wave, fibrillatory base line

Myocardial Infarction

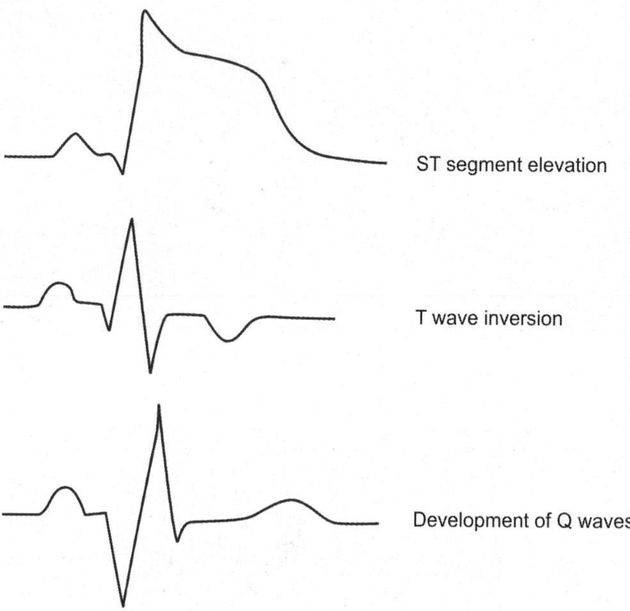

Anteroseptal MI

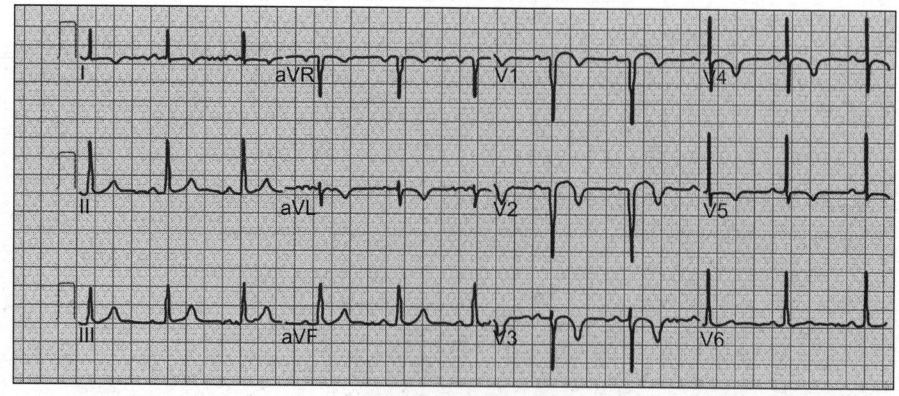

The QS complexes, resolving ST segment elevation and T wave inversions in V1-2 are evidence for a fully evolved anteroseptal MI

Old Inferior MI

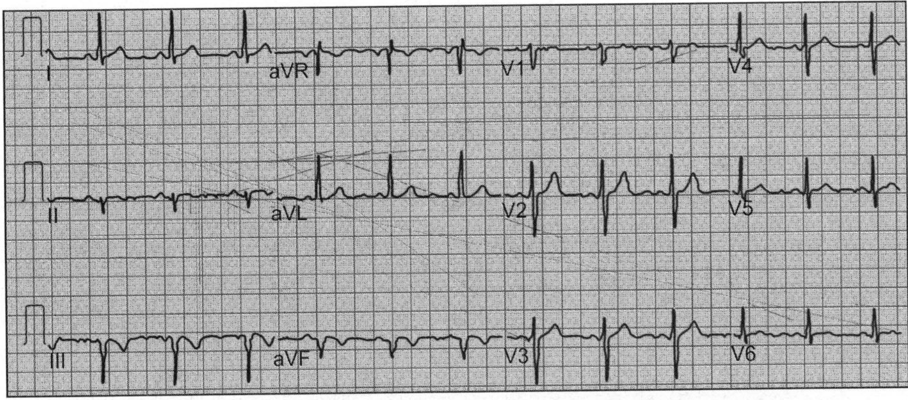

Anteroseptal MI

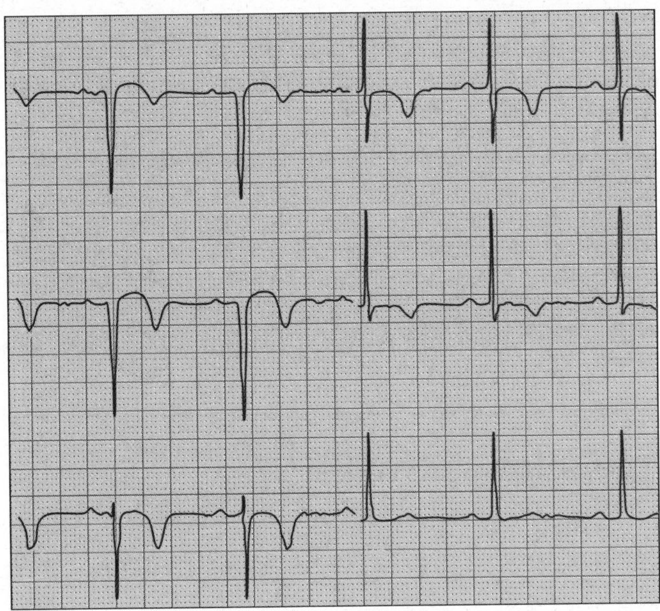

LVH with 'Strain'

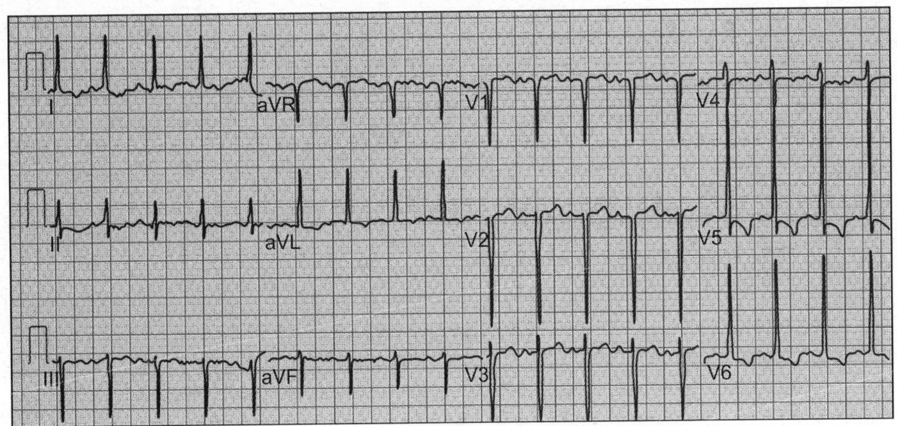

Left Atrial Enlargement

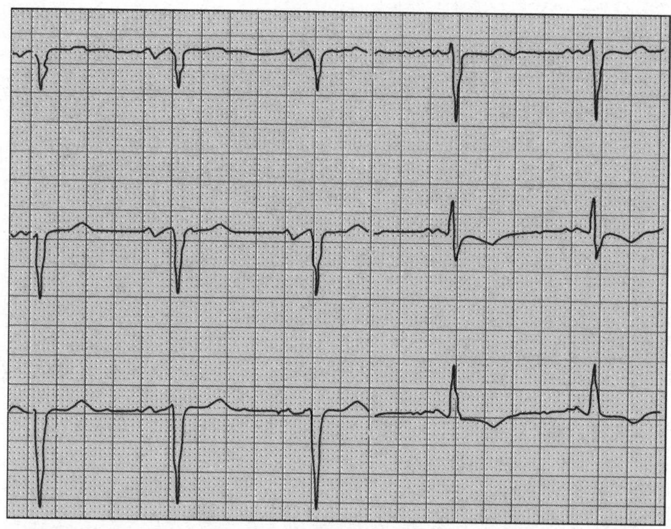

LAE is best seen in V1 with a prominent negative (posterior) component measuring 1 mm wide and 1 mm deep hypothermia: J-waves or Osborn waves

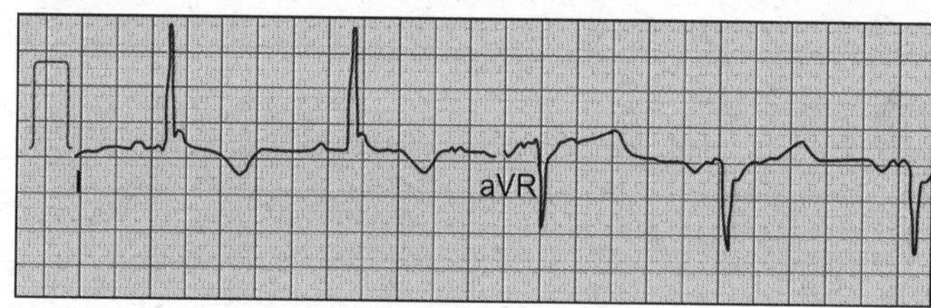

In hypothermia, a small extra wave is seen immediately after the QRS complex (best seen in Lead I in this example) This wave is called a J-wave, or Osborn wave. This wave disappears with the warming of body temperature

MURMURS: INNOCENT MURMUR FEATURES

7 Ss

- **Soft**
- **Systolic**
- **Short**
- **Sounds (S1 and S2) normal**
- **Symptomless**
- **Special tests normal (X-ray, EKCG)**
- **Standing/Sitting (vary with position)**

Murmurs

Ejection systolic	Pan-systolic	Late systolic	Early diastolic	Mid-diastolic
• Aortic stenosis • Pulmonary stenosis • HOCM • ASD • Fallot's	• Mitral regurgitation • Tricuspid regurgitation • Mitral prolapse • VSD	• HOCM • Mitral valve prolapse • Coarctation of aorta	• Aortic regurgitation	• Mitral stenosis • Austin-Flint murmur (severe aortic regurgitation)

Continous murmur is seen in

- **PDA**
- **AV fistula**
- **Rupture of sinuses of valsalva**
- **Coarctation of aorta**
- **Venous hum**
- **VSD with AR**

REMEMBER
Coarctation of the aorta

Coarctation of the aorta occurs in two patterns:

In the infantile type, the stenosis is proximal to the insertion of the ductus arteriosus (preductal); this pattern is associated with Turner's syndrome

In the adult form, the stenosis is distal to the ductus arteriosus (postductal) and is associated with notching of the ribs (secondary to continued pressure from the aorta on them), hypertension in the upper extremities, and weak pulses in the lower extremities. Headache, cold extremities, and lower extremity claudication with exercise are typical if the patient is symptomatic (many adults with mild distal coarctation may remain asymptomatic for years). Upper extremity hypertension with weak pulses in the lower extremities, and a midsystolic (or continuous) murmur over the chest or back may be the only obvious signs in some.

Cyanotic Congenital Heart Diseases

5 Ts:

- **Truncus arteriosus**
- **Transposition of the great arteries**
- **Tricuspid atresia**
- **Tetralogy of Fallot**
- **Total anomalous pulmonary venous return**

MS is a female title (Ms) and it is female-predominant
MR is a male title (Mr) and it is male-predominant

Rheumatic Heart Disease

JONES CRITERION

- According to revised Jones criteria, the diagnosis of rheumatic fever can be made when **two of the major criteria, or one major criterion plus two minor criteria are present along with evidence of streptococcal infection**
- Exceptions are chorea and indolent carditis, each of which by itself can indicate rheumatic fever

Major criteria

- **Migratory polyarthritis:** A temporary migrating inflammation of the large joints, usually starting in the legs and migrating upwards
- **Carditis:** Inflammation of the heart muscle which can manifest as congestive heart failure with shortness of breath, pericarditis with a rub, or a new heart murmur
- **Subcutaneous nodules:** Painless, firm collections of collagen fibers over bones or tendons. They commonly appear on the back of the wrist the outside elbow, and the front of the knees
- **Erythema marginatum:** A long-lasting rash that begins on the trunk or arms as macules and spreads outward to form a snake-like ring
- While clearing in the middle, this rash never starts on the face and it is made worse with heat.

- **Sydenham's chorea (St. Vitus' dance):** A characteristic series of rapid movements without purpose of the face and arms
- This can occur very late in the disease

Minor Criteria

- **Fever**
- **Arthralgia: Joints pain without swelling**
- **Raised erythrocyte sedimentation rate or C-reactive protein**
- **Leukocytosis**

Rheumatic Heart Disease

- **Preceded by streptococcal pharyngitis**
- **Aschoff bodies are a feature**
- **Anitschkow cells/caterpillar cells are seen**
- **Pancarditis is a feature**
- **Bread and butter pericarditis**
- **Vegitations along the line of closure of valves**
- **Subendocardial MacCallum's patches present**
- **Most common cause of mitral stenosis**

Mitral Stenosis

Mitral stenosis: It is said that the causes of mitral stenosis are **rheumatic fever, calcium deposits** and **narrowing of motral valve in Newborn babies.** Rarer causes that may be seen include mucopolysaccharidoses, carcinoid and endocardial fibroelastosis

Features:

- **Mid-diastolic murmur (Best heard in expiration)**
- **Loud S1, opening snap**
- **Low volume pulse**
- **Malar flush**
- **Atrial fibrillation**
- **Hemoptysis seen**
- **Hoarseness of voice is seen in MS**
- **Left atrial myxoma is an important differential diagnosis**
- **Pulmonary hypertension occurs**

Features of severe MS:

Length of murmur increases, opening snap becomes closer to S2

Echocardiography:

Most useful in MS is echocardiography

- The normal cross-sectional area of the mitral valve is 4–6 sq cm
- A 'tight' mitral stenosis implies a cross-sectional area of < 1 sq cm
- < 0.6 cms of mitral vavle area is incompatible with life.

USMLE Case Scenario

A 68-year-old woman who is normotensive presents to her cardiac physician after several episodes of syncope. Physical examination is remarkable for a low-pitched 'plopping' sound during mid-systole. Two-dimensional echocardiography demonstrates a ball-valve type obstruction of the mitral valve. Most likely diagnosis would be:
Myxoma

Aortic Stenosis

Aortic stenosis:

Features

- **Ejection systolic murmur**
- **Slow rising pulse**
- **Narrow pulse pressure**
- **Sustained heaving apex is seen**
- **Angina is a feature**
- **Sudden death is a feature**
- **Exercise testing is contraindicated in AS**

Causes of Aortic Stenosis:

- Degenerative calcification
- Bicuspid aortic valve
- William's syndrome (supravalvular aortic stenosis)
- Postrheumatic disease
- Subvalvular: HOCM

Management:

- If asymptomatic, then observe the patient as a general rule
- If symptomatic, then valve replacement
- If asymptomatic but valvular gradient > 50 mm Hg and with features such as left ventricular systolic dysfunction, then consider surgery
- Balloon valvuloplasty is limited to patients with critical aortic stenosis who are not fit for valve replacement.

Aortic Regurgitation

Aortic regurgitation:

Features

- **Early diastolic murmur**
- **Collapsing pulse**
- **Wide pulse pressure**
- **Mid-diastolic Austin-Flint murmur in severe AR—due to partial closure of the anterior mitral valve cusps caused by the regurgitation streams**

Causes (due to valve disease)

- Rheumatic fever
- Infective endocarditis
- Connective tissue diseases e.g. RA/SLE
- Bicuspid aortic valve

Causes (due to aortic root disease)

- Aortic dissection
- Spondylarthropathies (e.g. ankylosing spondylitis)
- Hypertension
- Syphilis
- Marfan's, Ehler-Danlos syndrome

Signs seen in AR	
• Corrigan's sign	Dancing carotids
• De Musset's sign	Head movements with cardiac pulse
• Quincke's sign	↑Capillary pulsations
• Traube's sign	Pistol shot sounds over femorals

• **Duroziez's murmur**	**Diastolic murmur over femorals**
• **Hill's sign**	**Femoral-Brachial pulse gradient**
• **Lighthouse sign**	**Blanching/flushing of forehead**
• **Landolfi's sign**	**Alternate constriction/dilation of pupil**
• **Muller's sign**	**Uvual pulsations**
• **Rosenbach's sign**	**Liver pulsations**
• **Gerhard's sign**	**Splenic pulsations**
• **Lincoln's sign**	**Pulsating popliteals**
• **Mayer's sign**	**Diastolic drop on raising arm**

AR

An 20-year-old male comes to the physician for a routine physical examination. His height is 198 cm. He has long fingers and toes. Blood pressure is 150/65 mm Hg, and pulse is 66/min. On auscultation, there is a grade 2/6, long, high-frequency diastolic murmur at the second right intercostal space.

MVP: Floppy Valve Syndrome/Mitral Valve Prolapse

- Systolic click-murmur syndrome, **Barlow's syndrome, floppy-valve syndrome, and billowing mitral leaflet syndrome**
- **Myxomatous degeneration**
- Frequent finding in patients with heritable disorders of connective tissue, including the:
  - **Marfan syndrome**
  - **Osteogenesis imperfecta** and the
  - **Ehlers-Danlos syndrome**
- MVP is **more common in females**
- Most patients are asymptomatic and remain so for their entire lives
- Chest pain is seen
- Midsystolic murmur with myxomatous degeneration
- **Sudden death has been noted but is a very rare complication**
- The most important finding is the **mid- or late (nonejection) systolic click.**

CARDIOMYOPATHIES

HOCM

Hypertrophic cardiomyopathy is a common cause of sudden cardiac death in young patients. It usually causes problems during exertion. Clues to the diagnosis include: dyspnea, palpitations, bifid apical impulse, coarse systolic murmur at the left sternal border, and ventricular hypertrophy with asymmetric septal thickening on echocardiogram. Left ventricular outflow obstruction typically plays an important role in the pathophysiology of this condition. Maneuvers that decrease preload, such as the Valsalva maneuver, will accentuate the heart murmur because they result in less ventricular filling, contributing to greater outflow obstruction.

HOCM: Hypertrophic obstructive cardiomyopathy (HOCM) is an autosomal dominant disorder of muscle tissue caused by defects in the genes encoding contractile proteins

Features:

- **Dyspnea, angina, syncope**
- **Sudden death (most commonly due to ventricular arrhythmias), arrhythmias, heart failure**
- **Jerky pulse**
- **Large 'A' waves**
- **Double apex beat**
- **Ejection systolic murmur: Increases with Valsalva maneuver and decreases on squatting**

Associations: Friedreich's ataxia, WPWS

ECHO:

- Systolic anterior motion **(SAM)** of the anterior mitral valve leaflet
- Asymmetric hypertrophy **(ASH)**
- Mitral regurgitation

- Hypertrophic obstructive cardiomyopathy (HOCM) caused by mutations in the **myosin heavy chain b gene**
- Udually follows **AD inheritance**
- **Sudden death** is a feature
- **Ejection systolic murmur of HOCM ↑STANDING, ↓Lying down, supine**
- **Avoid digoxin**
- Cardiac catheterization shows **Banana shaped left biventricular cavity** in systole
- **Usual Premature closure of Aortic cusps**
- **Predominantly Left ventricular outflow tract gradient.**

Dilated Cardiomyopathy

Dilated cardiomyopathy

Basics:

- Dilated heart leading to systolic (+/– diastolic) dysfunction
- All 4 chambers affected but LV more so than RV
- Features include arrhythmias, emboli, mitral regurgitation
- Absence of congenital, valvular or ischemic heart disease

Causes:

- Infections, e.g. coxsackie A and B, HIV, diphtheria, parasitic
- Endocrine, e.g. hyperthyroidism
- Infiltrative*, e.g. hemochromatosis, sarcoidosis
- Neuromuscular, e.g. Duchenne muscular dystrophy, Friedreich's ataxia
- Nutritional, e.g. kwashiorkor, pellagra, thiamine/selenium deficiency

Restrictive Cardiomyopathy

Restrictive cardiomyopathy is the least prevalent form of cardiomyopathy

- Amyloidosis
- Hemochromatosis
- Sarcoidosis and
- Fabry's disease

The main hemodynamic consequence of these pathologic states is a rigid, noncompliant chamber with a high-filling pressure

- Systolic function may deteriorate if compensatory hypertrophy is inadequate to compensate for infiltrated or fibrosed chambers
- Mural thrombosis and systemic emboli can complicate either the restrictive or obliterative variety

Echocardiography shows normal systolic function

- The atria are often dilated
- **Myocardial hypertrophy** is often seen in restrictive myopathy
- High atrial pressure with a prominent **'y' descent**
- **Kussmaul's sign is seen**
- **Normal-sized ventricular cavities** with normal or decreased systolic shortening
- Biopsy can demonstrate endocardial fibrosis and thickening, myocardial infiltration with iron or amyloid or chronic myocardial fibrosis.

Infective Endocarditis

Infective Endocarditis

- Patients affected by endocarditis
- Previously normal valves (50%, typically acute presentation)
- Rheumatic valve disease (30%)
- Prosthetic valves
- Congenital heart defects
- Intravenous drug users (IVDUs, e.g. typically causing tricuspid lesion)

Causes:

- **Streptococcus viridans (most common cause – 40–50%)**
- **Staphylococcus epidermidis (especially prosthetic valves)**
- **Janeway's lesions, (nontender maculopapular lesions in palms/soles)**
- **Splinter hemorrhages (NAILS)**
- **Roth's spots seen (RETINA)**

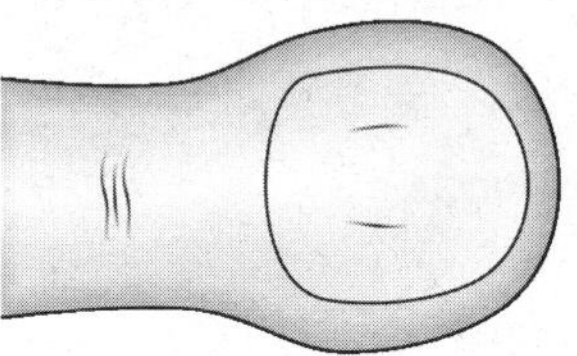

Splinter hemorrhages

LOW RISK:

- **ASD**
- **MVP without MR**

Atherosclerosis

Risk factors for atherosclerosis:

- Smoking
- Hypertension
- Low HDL, raised apolipoprotein A
- Familial hypercholesterolemia
- Familial hypertriglyceridemia
- Familial dysbetalipoproteinemia
- Diabetes mellitus
- Family history
- Obesity
- Physical inactivity

Associated with coronary atherosclerosis:

- **CMV**
- **Chlamydiae**
- ***H. pylori***

Amino acid associated with atherosclerosis: homocysteine

ECG Changes seen in Acute Myocardial Infarction

Hyperacute phase:

- ST elevation
- Tall T wave
- Increased ventricular activation time

Fully evolved phase:

- Pathological Q wave
- Elevated ST segment
- Inverted T waves

Old infarct:

- Pathological Q waves

ECG: Coronary Territories (Infarct areas)

Anteroseptal

- V1-V4
- Left anterior descending

Inferior

- II, III, aVF
- Right coronary

Anterolateral

- V4 – 6, I, aVL
- Left mainstem

Lateral

- I, aVL +/ – V5 – 6
- Left circumflex

Posterior

- Tall R waves V1 – 2

Key Points for the Exam

- In **stable angina** enzyme levels are normal
- **Myoglobin** is the first to rise
- CK-MB is useful to look for reinfarction as it returns to normal after 2-3 days (troponin T remains elevated for up to 10 days)
- CK-MB is raised earlier than other enzymes
- Troponin is a marker of cardiac infarction
- **Sensitive marker for myocardial infarction is Troponin T**

	Begins to rise	Peak value	Returns to normal
Myoglobin	1–2 hours	6–8 hours	1–2 days
CK-MB	2–6 hours	16–20 hours	1–2 days
CK	4–8 hours	16–24 hours	3–4 days
Trop T	4–6 hours	12–24 hours	7–10 days
AST	12–24 hours	36–48 hours	3–4 days
LDH	24–48 hours	72 hours	8–10 days

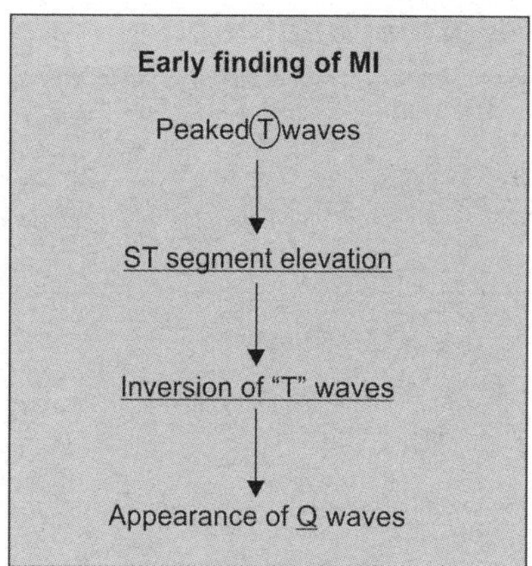

Sequence of MI

Wolff-Parkinson-White (WPW) Syndrome (ADDITIONAL)

Wolff-Parkinson-White (WPW) syndrome: It is caused by a congenital accessory conducting pathway between the atria and ventricles leading to an atrioventricular re-entry tachycardia (AVRT). As the accessory pathway does not slow conduction, AF can degenerate rapidly to VF. Possible ECG features include:

- **Short PR interval**
- **Wide QRS complexes with a slurred upstroke—'delta wave'**
- **Left axis deviation**

Differentiating between type A and type B

- **Type A** (left-sided pathway): dominant R wave in V1
- **Type B** (right-sided pathway): no dominant R wave in V1

<u>**Associations of WPW**</u>

- **HOCM**
- **Mitral valve prolapse**
- **Ebstein's anomaly**
- **Thyrotoxicosis**
- **Secundum ASD**

Management

- Definitive treatment: radiofrequency ablation of the accessory pathway
- Medical therapy: Procainamide flecainide.

- **Eisenmenger's syndrome**
  Describes the **reversal of a left to right shunt** in a congenital heart defect due to pulmonary hypertension associated with:
  - **VSD**
  - **ASD**
  - **PDA**

Features

- **Original murmur may disappear**
- **Cyanosis**
- **Clubbing**
- **Right ventricular failure**
- **Hemoptysis, embolism**

- **Carey Coombs Murmur**: Transient soft **mid-diastolic murmur** of acute rheumatic fever due to mitral valvulitis
- **Graham Steel Murmur**: Early diastolic murmur of Pulmonary Regurgitation
- **Means Murmur**: Pulmonary systolic murmur in Thyrotoxicosis
- **Seagull's Murmur**: Aortic regurgitation murmur.

Mitral Valve Prolapse: (ADDITIONAL)

Usually idiopathic but may be associated with a wide variety of cardiovascular disease. Associations:

- **Congenital heart disease: PDA, ASD**
- **Cardiomyopathy**
- **Turner's syndrome**
- **Marfan's syndrome, Fragile X syndrome**
- **Osteogenesis imperfecta**
- **Pseudoxanthoma elasticum**
- **Wolff-Parkinson-White syndrome**
- **Long-QT syndrome**

Features

- Patients may complain of atypical chest pain or palpitations
- **Mid-systolic click (occurs later if patient squatting)**
- **Late systolic murmur (longer if patient standing)**
- Complications: mitral regurgitation, arrhythmias (including long QT), emboli, sudden death

Management: Antibiotic prophylaxis against infective endocarditis is only required if mitral regurgitation is present.

Digoxin Toxicity

- **Digoxin toxicity**
  Features: Generally unwell, lethargy, N/V, confusion, **yellow-green vision**, arrhythmias (e.g. AV block, bradycardia, VF, VT)
  Idioventricular rhythm is a feature:

Precipitating factors

- **Classically: hypokalemia***
- **Myocardial ischemia**
- **Hypomagnesemia, hypercalcemia, hypernatremia, acidosis**
- **Hypoalbuminemia**
- **Hypothermia**
- **Hypothyroidism**
- **Drugs: amiodarone, quinidine, verapamil, spironolactone (compete for secretion in distal convoluted tubule, therefore, reduce excretion)**

Management

- Withdrawal of digitalis, potassium supplements
- Correct arrhythmias, phenytoin used, digitalis antibody (fab fragments)
- Monitor K^+

Long QT Syndrome (ADDITIONAL)

Long QT syndrome:

Important as it may lead to ventricular tachycardia and can, therefore, cause collapse/sudden death. A normal corrected QT is less than 440 ms

Congenital

- **Jervell-Lange-Nielsen syndrome (includes deafness and is due to an abnormal potassium channel)**
- **Romano-Ward syndrome (no deafness)**

Drugs

- **Amiodarone**
- **Sotalol**
- **Class 1a antiarrhythmic drugs**

- **Tricyclic antidepressants**
- **Chloroquine**
- **Terfenadine:** A nonsedating antihistamine and classic cause of prolonged QT in a patient, especially if also taking P450 enzyme inhibitor, e.g. patient with cold takes terfenadine and erythromycin at the same time

Other causes

- Electrolyte: Hypocalcemia
- Hypokalemia
- Hypomagnesemia
- Hypothermia
- Acute MI
- Myocarditis
- Subarachnoid hemorrhage

Management

- Beta-blockers
- Implantable cardioverter defibrillators in high-risk cases.

Acute Pericarditis

Pain, a pericardial friction rub, electrocardiographic changes, and pericardial effusion with **cardiac tamponade** and paradoxic pulse are cardinal manifestations:

- **Chest pain is an important but not invariable symptom in various forms of acute pericarditis**
- **The pericardial friction rub is the most important physical sign of acute pericarditis; it may have up to three components per cardiac cycle and is high-pitched, scratching, and grating**
- **The electrocardiogram: Widespread elevation of the ST segments, often with upward concavity.**

Cardiac Tamponade

The accumulation of fluid in the pericardium in an amount sufficient to cause serious obstruction to the inflow of blood to the ventricles results in **cardiac tamponade**

The three most common causes of **tamponade** are neoplastic disease, idiopathic pericarditis, and uremia. **Tamponade** may also result from bleeding into the pericardial space either following **cardiac** operations and trauma (including **cardiac** perforation during diagnostic procedures) or from tuberculosis and hemopericardium. The latter may occur when a patient with any form of acute pericarditis is treated with anticoagulants

The three principal features of **tamponade** are:

- **Elevation of intracardiac pressures**
- **Limitation of ventricular filling and**
- **Reduction of cardiac output**

Look for

- **Electrical alternans**
- **Pulsus paradoxus**
- **JVP↑**
- **Prominent x descent**
- **Absent y descent**
- **Beck's triad: hypotension, silent heart, ↑JVP**
- **Absent Kussmaul's sign**

Constrictive Pericarditis

- **Right heart failure occurs**
- **Raised JVP seen**
- **Ascites precox seen**
- **Prominent x descent**
- **Prominent y descent**
- **Thickened pericardium**
- **Kussmaul's sign +**
- **Square root sign+**

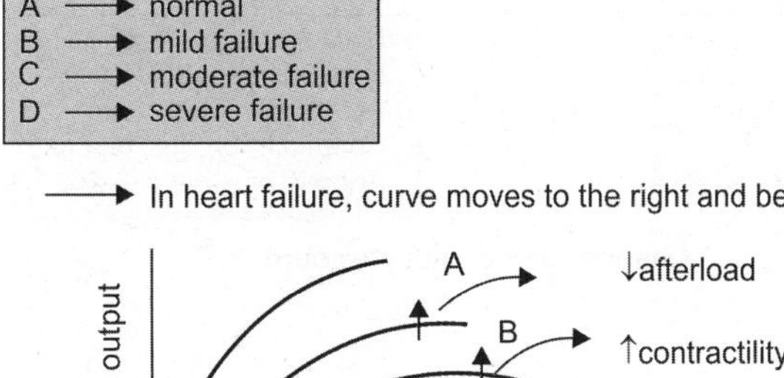

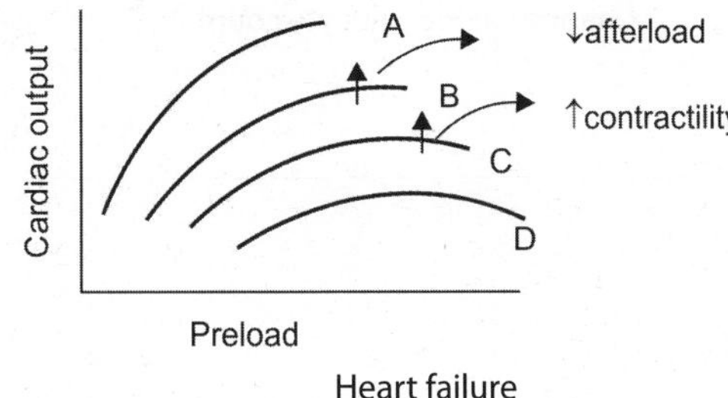

Heart failure

Pericardial Effusion

Pericardial effusion nearly always has the physical characteristics of **an exudate:**

Bloody fluid is commonly due to:

- **Tuberculosis**
- **Tumor**
- **Effusion of rheumatic fever**
- **Postcardiac injury**
- **Postmyocardial infarction (especially following the administration of anticoagulant) and in uremic pericarditis**
- **Transmural myocardial infarction**
- **Aortic aneurysm dissection**
- **Metastasis to pericardium.**

A man with fever, dull-aching retrosternal chest pain reported to the emergency. On examination, he was found to show pulsus paradoxus, Kussmaul's sign and increased jugular venous pressure. His apex beat was impalpable and heart sounds were muffled. Probable diagnosis is: Pericardial effusion.

HEMATOLOGY

Iron deficiency anemia of long duration is characterized by:

- Erythroid hyperplasia in bone marrow
- Normal reticulocyte count
- Normal WBC count

- Normal platelet count
- Microcytosis, hypochromasia, anisocytosis, poikilocytosis in PBF
- Normoblastic hyperplasia in bone marrow
- **Raised free erythrocyte protoporphyrin**
- **Raised transferring receptor levels**

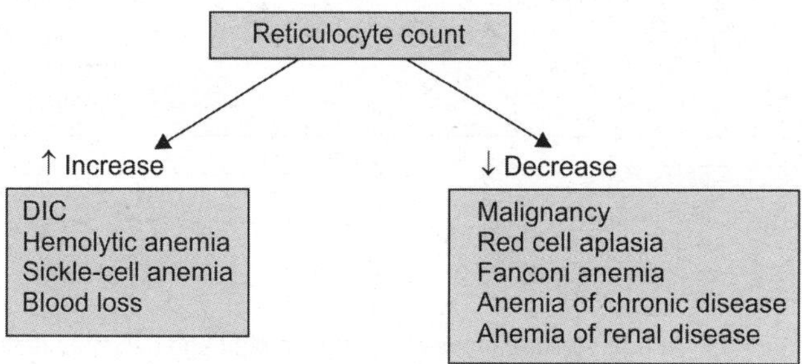

Changes in reticulocyte count

Microcytic Anemia

Causes:

- **Iron deficiency**
- **Thalassemia**
- **Sideroblastic anemia**
- **Anemia of chronic disease**
- **Lead poisoning**

Blood Changes:

- **Hypochromia**
- **Microcytosis**
- **Poikilocytosis**
- **Bone marrow with ↑ normoblasts**
- **Microcytic hypochromic anemia not responding to iron is thalassemia usually.**

	Iron deficency	Thalassemia	Sideroblastic anemia	Chronic anemia
Sr Fe	↓	n	n	↓
TIBC	↑	n	n	↓
% Saturation	↓	↑	↑	↓
Ferritin	↓	↑	↑	↑

- **Hypochromic microcytic anemia with ↓Sr, Fe, ↑TIBC: Iron deficiency anemia**
- **Hypochromic microcytic anemia with ↓Sr, Fe, ↓TIBC: Anemia of chronic disease**
- **↓ Sr Ferritin is the early indicator of iron deficiency**

Paterson-Kelly Syndrome is Characterized

- **Koilonychia**
- **Microcytic hypochromic anemia**
- **Iron-deficiency anemia**

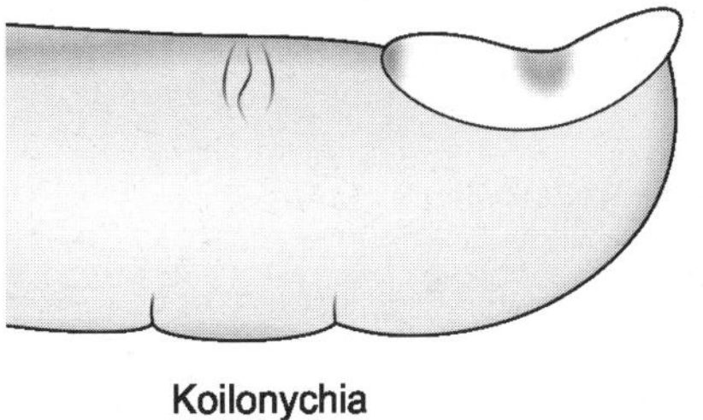

Koilonychia

Megaloblastic Anemia

<u>Causes:</u>

- **Liver diseases**
- **Hypothyroidism**
- **Orotic aciduria**
- **Thiamine deficiency**
- **B12 deficiency**
- **Folic acid deficiency**
- **Hemodialysis**
- **Fish tapeworm infestation**
- **Drugs: Phenytoin, primidone, nitrous oxide, phenobarbitone, folate antagonists.**

<u>Hematological findings</u>

- **Decreased red blood cell (RBC) count and hemoglobin levels**
- **Increased mean corpuscular volume** (MCV, >95 fl) **and mean corpuscular hemoglobin (MCH)**
- **<u>Normal mean corpuscular hemoglobin concentration</u>** (MCHC, 32–36 g/dL)
- The reticulocyte count is decreased due to destruction of fragile and abnormal megaloblastic erythroid precursor
- The platelet count may be reduced
- Neutrophil granulocytes may show **multisegmented nuclei** (senile neutrophil). This is thought to be due to decreased production and a compensatory prolonged lifespan for circulating neutrophils, which increase number of nuclear segments with age
- **Anisocytosis** (increased variation in RBC size) and **poikilocytosis** (abnormally shaped RBCs)
- **Macrocytes** (larger than normal RBCs) are present
- **Howell-Jolly bodies** (chromosomal remnant) also present
- **Pancytopenia can also occur.**

Blood chemistries will also show:

- **Increased homocysteine and methylmalonic acid in B12 deficiency**
- **Increased homocysteine in folate deficiency**
- **Normal levels of both methylmalonic acid and total homocysteine rule out clinically significant cobalamin deficiency with virtual certainty**

Bone marrow shows

- (Not normally checked in a patient suspected of megaloblastic anemia) **megaloblastic hyperplasia**
- Increased stainable iron
- Megaloblastic erythropoiesis
- Large megakaryocytes

Possible associated neurological findings: **Subacute combined degeneration of spinal cord** and its symptoms may be present due to demyelination secondary to deficiency of vitamin B12.

Tongue in Megaloblastic Anemia

- **Large (macroglossia)**
- **Atrophic glossitis (loss of papillae)**
- **Red patches and red lines on ventral surface (Moeller's glossitis)**
- **Sore**
- **Angular cheilitis and ulcers**

Folate Deficiency

It is commonly seen in alcoholics (poor intake) and pregnant women (increased need). All women of reproductive age should take folate supplements to prevent neural tube defects in their offspring. Rare causes of folate deficiency include poor diet (e.g. tea and toast), methotrexate, prolonged therapy with trimethoprim-sulfamethoxazole, anticonvulsant therapy (especially phenytoin), and malabsorption. Look for macrocytes and hypersegmented neutrophils (either one should make you think of the diagnosis) with no neurologic symptoms or signs and low folate levels in serum or red blood cells. Treat with oral folate.

USMLE Case Scenario

A 53-year-old woman from New York is being treated for long-standing severe rheumatoid arthritis. Screening blood studies demonstrate anemia with a hemoglobin level of 9 g/dL. The patient's nutritional status is good, and the clinician suspects she has anemia of chronic disease. Which of the following erythrocyte findings would be most likely to be seen on peripheral blood smear?

1. All normal morphology
2. Macrocytes
3. Numerous spherocytes
4. Target cells
5. Tear drop forms
6. Siderroblasts
7. Spherocytes

Ans. 1. All normal morphology

The anemia of chronic disease is seen in patients with underlying severe chronic disorders, such as infections, inflammatory diseases (such as this patient's rheumatoid arthritis), and cancers. The anemia is usually initially normocytic but may, with time, become microcytic.

Hemolytic Anemias: By Site

In intravascular hemolysis, free hemoglobin is released which binds to haptoglobin. As haptoglobin becomes saturated, hemoglobin binds to albumin forming methemalbumin (detected by Schumm's test). Free hemoglobin is excreted in the urine as hemoglobinuria, hemosiderinuria.

Intravascular Hemolysis: Causes

- **Mismatched blood transfusion**
- **G6PD deficiency**
- **Red-cell fragmentation: Heart valves, TTP, DIC, HUS**
- **Paroxysmal nocturnal hemoglobinuria**
- **Cold autoimmune hemolytic anemia**

Extravascular Hemolysis: Causes

- **Hemoglobinopathies: Sickle-cell, Thalassemia**
- **Hereditary spherocytosis**
- **Hemolytic disease of newborn**
- **Warm autoimmune hemolytic anemia**

Features of Hemolytic Anemia

- **Increased reticulocyte count**
- **Increased serum lactate dehydrogenase level**
- **Decreased serum haptoglobin level**
- **Increased serum unconjugated bilirubin**
- **Autoimmune hemolytic anemia is seen in SLE**

Features of Hemolysis

- **Elevated lactate dehydrogenase (LDH)**
- **Elevated bilirubin (unconjugated as well as conjugated if the liver is functioning)**
- **Jaundice**
- **Low or absent haptoglobin (intravascular hemolysis only)**
- **Urobilinogen, bilirubin, and hemoglobin in urine (only conjugated bilirubin shows up in the urine, and hemoglobin shows up in the urine only when haptoglobin has been saturated, as in brisk intravascular hemolysis).**

Sickle-cell Crises

- **AR condition**
- **Glutamine-valine change**

TO BE EXACT: Replacement of glutamate by valine at position 6 beta chain of Hb A

<u>Features:</u>

- **Bone pain commonest. (acute presentation)**
- Pulmonary HTN
- Cardiomegaly
- Fish mouth vertebrae
- Osteomyelitis, priaprism, renal pappilary necrosis
  - **Hemosidenuria**
  - **↑LDH**
  - **↑unconjugated bilirubin**
  - **↓haptoglobin**
  - **Leucocytosis**
  - **Target cells seen**
- Autosplenectomy
- **Crewcut hair skull** along with thalassemia
- **Improved with Hb F**

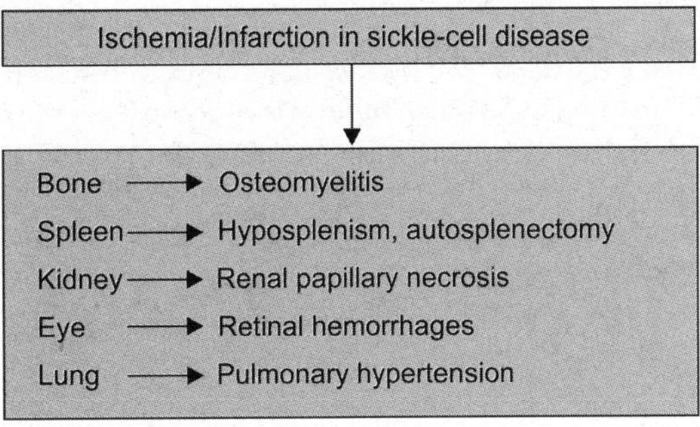

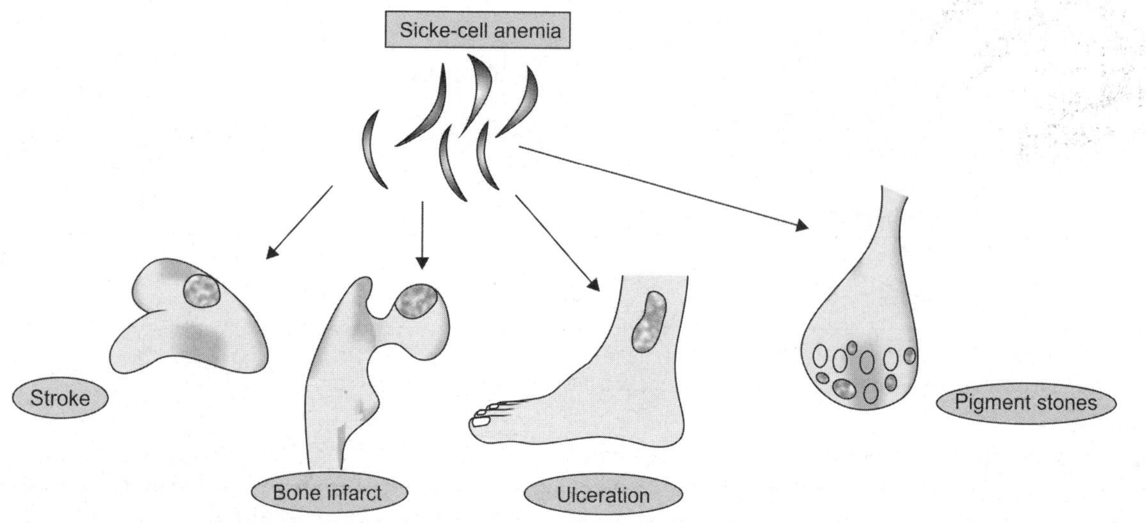

Four Main Types of Crises are recognized

- **Thrombotic 'painful crises'**
- **Sequestration**
- **Aplastic**
- **Hemolytic**

Thrombotic crises

- Also known as **'painful crises'** or **'vaso-occlusive crises'**
- Precipitated by infection, dehydration, deoxygenation
- Infarcts occur in various organs including the bones (e.g. avascular necrosis of hip, hand-foot syndrome in children, lungs, spleen and brain

Sequestration crises

- **Sickling within organs** such as the spleen or lungs causes pooling of blood with worsening of the anemia
- **Acute chest syndrome:** Dyspnea, chest pain, pulmonary infiltrates, low pO_2—the most common cause of death after childhood

Aplastic crises

- Caused by infection with **parvovirus**
- Sudden fall in hemoglobin

Hemolytic crises

- Rare
- Fall in hemoglobin due an **increased rate of hemolysis**

USMLE Case Scenario

An 18-year-old African-American woman with sickle-cell disease is brought to the Medical OPD because she is having some respiratory problems. About 8 days before the visit, she developed a low-grade fever of 101.6 °F with complaints of generalized body aches, loss of appetite. Her mother noticed development of a rash that has since disappeared. Laboratory studies show: A peripheral blood smear shows no evidence of any erythroid precursor. Which of the following is the most likely pathogen?

1. Chlamydia
2. EBV
3. CMV
4. Neisseria
5. Parvovirus
6. Streptococcus
7. Staphylococcus

Ans. 5. Parvovirus
This patient is presenting with aplastic crisis, organism is parvovirus B19, a virus implicated in erythema infectiosum (fifth disease). The virus causes a transient red cell aplasia; bone marrow often shows lack of erythroid precursors.

USMLE Case Scenario

A 26-year-old black man comes to the New York Emergency complaining of a few hour's history of bilateral knee pain and a severe painful erection. He had a similar episode two-and-a-half years ago. He has no nausea, vomiting or fever and his vital signs are within normal limits. After receiving treatment with oxygen and intravenous fluids, his symptoms resolve and he is discharged home. What is the most likely diagnosis?

1. Osteoarthritis
2. Gonococcal infection
3. Leukemia
4. Sickle-cell disease
5. Traumatic injury

Ans. 4. Sickle-cell disease
It is the likely cause of this patient's unusual combination of symptoms

USMLE High Yield

Patients with sickle-cell anemia are at risk for pain crises when they are exposed to cold, have infection, become dehydrated or are under severe stress resulting in oxygen deprivation. Pain occurs due to occlusion of small vessels by the sickle-shaped cells. Although pain may be felt anywhere, more common sites include the bones, joints, and abdomen. Men may present with priapism (a persistent, painful erection unrelated to sexual activity or excitement). Treatment is largely symptomatic and supportive.

Applications of Gene Therapy

- Cystic fibrosis
- SCID
- GH deficiency
- Familial hypercholesterolemia
- Lesch-Nyhan syndrome
- Parkinsonism, Alzheimer's disease, Huntington's chorea, Gaucher's disease
- Stroke, head injury, multiple sclerosis
- Anemia, **sickle-cell anemia**
- Hemophilia, HIV
- Cancers

Glucose 6 Phosphate Dehydrogenase Deficiency G6PD

- It is **X-linked recessive**
- Causes **episodic hemolytic anemia because of decreased ability of RBCs to withstand oxidative stress**
- **G6PD is the first and rate-limiting step of HMP shunt responsible for NADPH production**
- **NADPH is the cofactor for production for glutathione reductase forming reduced glutathione which is a potent antioxidant**
- **In its absence, H_2O_2 accumulates in RBC causing cell membrane damage leading to hemolysis**
- Pallor, hemoglobinuria, jaundice, **Heinz bodies, bite cells** are seen
- **Oxidized hemoglobin denatures** and precipitates in the form of Heinz bodies
- **Agents implicated:**
  - **Primaquine**

- **Chloroquine**
- **Dapsone**
- **Nitrofurantoin**
- **Nalidixic acid**

Hereditary Spherocytosis

- **Primary abnormality in the cytoskeletal proteins that form RBC membrane**
- **Cytoskeletal proteins: maintain RBC shape, strength and flexibility**

Structure of RBC Membrane

- **Lipid bilayer**
- **Proteins: Stabilize lipid bilayer**
- **Spectrin: Major protein, inner surface of cell membrane**
- **Ankyrin: 'Anchors' spectrin to transmembrane proteins**

- **Spherical RBC** due to a molecular defect in one of the proteins in the cytoskeleton of the RBC membrane, leading to a loss of membrane
- Decreased ratio of surface area to volume
- Usually has an **autosomal dominant** inheritance pattern
- The major clinical features of hereditary **spherocytosis** are anemia, splenomegaly, and jaundice
- Assessed by measurement of the osmotic fragility of the RBC (↑)
- Aplastic crisis is triggered by parvovirus
- **About 50% of patients have a defect in ankyrin, the protein that forms a bridge between protein 3 and spectrin**
- **A mutation of protein 3, resulting in a deficiency of that protein and mild anemia with dominant inheritance**
- **Mutations of spectrin, leading to impaired synthesis or self-association**
- **Paladin defect**
- **Splenectomy is curative**

Hereditary pyropoikilocytosis: This condition results from a deficiency of spectrin and an abnormality of spectrin self-assembly. Hemolysis is usually severe, is recognized in childhood, and is partially responsive to splenectomy

Hereditary stomatocytosis: Stomatocytes are cup-shaped RBCs (concave on one face and convex on the other).

Paroxysmal Nocturnal Hemoglobinuria (PNH)

Paroxysmal nocturnal hemoglobinuria (PNH) is an **acquired disorder** leading to hemolysis (mainly intravascular) of hematological cells (STEM CELL DEFECT).

- It is thought to be caused by **increased sensitivity of cell membranes to complement** due to a lack of glycoprotein glycosylphosphatidylinositol **(GPI)**.
- Patients are more prone to venous thrombosis. GPI can be thought of as an anchor which attaches surface proteins to the cell membrane complement-regulating surface proteins, e.g. **decay-accelerating factor (DAF)** are not properly bound to the cell membrane due a lack of GPI.

Features

- **Hemolytic anemia**
- **Red blood cells, white blood cells, platelets or stem cells may be affected: Therefore, pancytopenia may be present**
- **Hemoglobinuria: Classically dark-colored urine in the morning (although has been shown to occur throughout the day)**
- **Thrombosis, e.g. Budd-Chiari syndrome/Thrombocytopenia**
- **Aplastic anemia may develop in some patients**

- ↓LAP score
- **Hypercellular marrow**

Diagnosis: Ham test: Acid-induced hemolysis (normal red cells wouldn't)

Management: Blood product replacement, anticoagulation, stem cell transplantation

HAM test is a complement-based test

Analysis of GPI-linked proteins is used as a diagnostic test.

The LAP Score

It is a semiquantitative cytochemical assessment of alkaline phosphatase in neutrophils. The LAP score is based on staining intensity, with a possible score of 0-400. It differentiates **chronic myeloid leukemia (low)** from **reactive leucocytosis (high)**, e.g. bacterial infection. It may assist in the differentiation of **polycythemia rubra vera (high)** from other causes of **erythrocytosis (normal)**

Sideroblastic Anemia

- Red cells contain **abnormal iron granules in the mitochondria** around the nucleus: ring sideroblasts
- Peripheral blood cells are **hypochromic whilst increased marrow iron**
- **High or normal transferrin saturation, ↑Serum ferritin, ↑Sr iron**
- May be congenital or acquired
- **Congenital cause: Delta-aminolevulinate synthase-2 deficiency**

Acquired causes

- **Myelodysplasia**
- **Alcohol**
- **Lead**
- **Anti-TB medications**

Investigations

- Hypochromic microcytic anemia (more so in congenital)
- Bone marrow: Sideroblasts and increased iron store
- Management: Supportive, pyridoxine may help.

Pyridoxine-responsive conditions
Homocystinuria Oxaluria Xanthinuria Convulsions

Pyridoxine response +ve

Pernicious Anemia

Deficiency of **intrinsic factor of Castle:**

- **Antigastric parietal cell antibodies** in 90%
- **Anti-intrinsic factor antibodies** in 50%
- **Macrocytic anemia:** Low WCC and platelets
- LDH may be raised due to ineffective erythropoiesis
- Also low-serum B12, hypersegmented polymorphs on film, megaloblasts in marrow
- Schilling test

Remember

• **Uremia** • **G6PD deficiency** • **Helmet cells**	• **Burr cells** are seen • Bite cells • **Hemolytic Uremic Syndrome**
• **Cirrhosis**	• **Spur cells** are seen
• **Iron depletion**	• Seen in iron-deficiency anemia, polycythemia vera
• **Thalassemia minor**	• Decreased osmolysis, microcytic hypochromic anemia, increased HbA2.
• **Sickle-cell anemia**	• **Tactoids and sickling** seen
• **Acquired spherocytosis**	• **Schistocytes present**, Coombs positive
• **Hereditary spherocytosis**	• Coombs negative
• **Aplastic anemia**	• Platelets maximum affected and last to recover, pancytopenia present
• **Pernicious anemia and folate deficiency anemia**	• Anisocytosis, poikilocytosis, fragmented RBCs, neutrophil lobes increased, platelets normal. Absolute reticulocyte count low.
• **Sideroblastic anemia**	• Ring sideroblasts present (These are iron granules in mitochondria around the nucleus), microcytic, hypochromic RBCs, macrocytic hypo- or normochromic RBCs

Autoimmune gastritis causes a lack of the intrinsic factor needed to absorb vitamin B12. Autoantibodies that are often present include those directed against the microsomal fraction of parietal cells and those capable of neutralizing intrinsic factor.

USMLE Case Scenario

A 77-year-old woman has a four-month history of weight loss, burning sensation of the tongue, fatigue, anorexia, and poorly localized abdominal pain. The woman appears pale to the physician. Intraoffice hematocrit is 25% with peripheral smear showing large erythrocytes and hypersegmented neutrophils. Serum folate is 2.6 ng/ml (normal greater that 1.9 ng/ml) and serum vitamin B12 is 111 pg/ml (normal 200–800 pg/ml). Stomach biopsy demonstrates chronic gastritis.

Pan Cytopenia is seen in

- **Hypoplastic anemia**
- **Megaloblastic anemia**
- **PNH**

Polycythemia Rubra Vera

Polycythemia rubra vera is a **myeloproliferative disorder** caused by clonal proliferation of a marrow stem cell leading to an **increase in red cell volume**, often accompanied by overproduction of neutrophils and platelets. It has peak incidence in the sixth decade, with typical features including:

- **Hyperviscosity (thrombosis)**
- **Even bleeding as well**
- **Pruritus**
- **Splenomegaly**
- **Normal erythropoietin levels**
  - **↑LAP score**
  - **↑Vitamin B12 levels**
- Management

- **Venesection—first-line treatment**
- **Hydroxyurea-slight increased risk of secondary leukemia**
- **Phosphorus-32 therapy**
- Prognosis
- Progress to **myelofibrosis**
- Progress to **acute leukemia**

USMLE Case Scenario

A 66-year-old lady from Texas is investigated for recurrent episodes of gouty arthritis. On examination, she looked plethoric and has a 6 cm splenomegaly. She has the following results:

Hb 19.45 gm/dl
Hct 0.632
Platelet count 466 x 109/l
ESR 2 mm/1st hour
Coagulation screen normal
AST normal
ALT normal
BUN normal
Creatinine normal

Most likely diagnosis is: Polycythemia

Myelophthisic Anemia

It is due to a space-occupying lesion in the bone marrow. The common causes are malignant invasion that destroys bone marrow (most common) and myelodysplasia or myelofibrosis. On the peripheral smear, look for marked anisocytosis (different size), poikilocytosis (different shape), nucleated red blood cells, giant and/or bizarre-looking platelets, and teardrop-shaped red blood cells. A bone marrow biopsy may reveal no cells ('dry tap' if the marrow is fibrotic) or malignant-looking cells.

Tumors Associated with Polycythemia

- **Hypernephroma**
- **Cerebellar hemangioblastoma**
- **Hepatoma**
- **Fibroid (uterine)**
- **Pheochromocytoma**
- **Meningioma**
- **Adrenal adenoma**

Thrombocytopenia

Causes of 'severe' thrombocytopenia:

- ITP
- DIC
- TTP
- Hematological malignancy

Causes of 'moderate' thrombocytopenia:

- Heparin-induced thrombocytopenia (HIT)
- Drug-induced, (e.g. quinine, diuretics, sulphonamides, aspirin, thiazides)
- Alcohol
- Liver disease

- Hypersplenism
- Viral infection (EBV, HIV, hepatitis)
- Pregnancy
- SLE/antiphospholipid syndrome
- B12 deficiency
- **Hess' (tourniquet) test** is used for ITP

Hemophilia

- **Decreased VIII level**
- **Increased PTT**
- **Bleeding into soft tissue**
- **Anti-factor VIII antibodies are seen in hemophilia who have received infusion of plasma concentrates**

Coagulation Defects

• **Hemophilia A**	Deficiency of factor **VIII C**
• **Hemophilia B (Christmas disease)**	Deficiency of factor **IX** (X-linked)
• **Hemophilia C**	Deficiency of factor **XI** (autosomal inherited defect)
• **Parahemophilia**	Deficiency of factor **V**
• **von Willebrand's disease**	Deficiency of **v WF** along with VIII C

von Willebrand's Disease

- von Willebrand's disease is the **most common inherited bleeding disorder**
- It is inherited in an **autosomal dominant fashion** and
- Characteristically behaves like a platelet disorder, i.e. epistaxis and menorrhagia are common whilst hemoarthroses and muscle hematomas are rare

Role of von Willebrand Factor:

- Large glycoprotein which forms massive multimers up to 1,000,000 Da in size
- Promotes platelet adhesion to damaged endothelium
- Carrier molecule for factor VIII

Types

- Type 1: partial reduction in vW
- Type 2: abnormal form of vW
- Type 3: total lack of vWF

Investigation

- Prolonged bleeding time
- APTT may be prolonged
- Factor VIII levels may be moderately reduced
- Defective platelet aggregation with ristocetin
- Normal PT

Management

- Tranexamic acid for mild bleeding
- DDAVP: raises levels of vWF by inducing release of vWF from Weibel-Palade bodies in endothelial cells
- Factor VIII concentrate
- **Cryoprecipitate** is used to treat.

Ristocetin-induced platelet aggregation—Ristocetin-induced platelet aggregation (RIPA) measures the affinity with which vWF binds to the platelet receptor GP Ib by limiting the concentration of ristocetin in the assay. It is used primarily to look for the type 2B variant of vWF which has mutations in the binding site for GP Ib such that the type 2B vWF binds to GP Ib more readily than normal.

USMLE Case Scenario

An 18-month-old fell from a staircase while learning to walk. The toddler has an enlarging, swollen bruise on his forehead, which is now over 5 cm across and increasing in size. A blood sample is drawn, and the child oozes blood at the puncture site for 25 minutes. Clotting studies on the blood sample show a prolonged PTT and a normal PT. Follow-up studies show very low levels of factor VIII. Which of the following is the most likely diagnosis?

1. Disseminated intravascular coagulation
2. Hemophilia B
3. Hyperhomocysteinemia
4. von Willebrand disease

Ans. 2 Hemophilia B

Hemophilia

- **It is an X-linked clotting disorder that occurs in two forms:**
  - **Hemophilia A due to deficient factor VIII and**
  - **Hemophilia B due to deficient factor IX**
- **Some individuals with hemophilia have levels of these factors that are 5% of normalor even higher, and have relatively mild disease, only requiring replacement therapy during surgical procedures or other situations in which significant bleeding might occur**
- **In contrast, individuals with factor levels less than 1% of normal have severe bleeding problems throughout life that usually become apparent by 18 months of age. In these individuals, excessive bleeding into joints and tissues may cause crippling musculoskeletal disorders.**

von Willebrand's Disease (NUTSHELL)

- von Willebrand's disease is an **autosomal dominant** disease
- von Willebrand's disease is the **commonest hereditary** bleeding disorder
- von Willebrand's disease is characterized by platelet adhesion defect
- **Postoperative traumatic or mucosal bleeding,** epistaxis, menorrhagia common
- Hemarthosis or muscle hematomas are rare
- **Increased BT and increased PTT** are findings
- **A vWF (von** Willebrand's **factor) level** which is synthesized in platelets is **low**
- Treatment: **Factor VIII cryoprecipitate, vasopressin**

Factor V Leiden Mutation

In the normal person, factor V functions as a cofactor to allow factor X to activate an enzyme called thrombin. Thrombin in turn cleaves fibrinogen to fibrin, which polymerizes to form the dense meshwork that makes up the majority of a clot. Activated protein C (aPC) is a natural anticoagulant that acts to limit the extent of clotting by cleaving and degrading factor V

- **Factor V Leiden mutation is an autosomal dominant condition**
- The gene that codes the protein is referred to as **F5**
- As a missense substitution, it changes a protein's amino acid from **arginine to glutamine**
- When factor V remains active, it facilitates overproduction of thrombin leading to excess fibrin generation and **excess clotting**

- The excessive clotting that occurs in this disorder is almost always **restricted to the veins**, where the clotting may cause a deep vein thrombosis (DVT). If the venous clots break off, these clots can travel through the heart to the lung, where they block a pulmonary blood vessel and cause a pulmonary embolism
- Women with the disorder have an **increased risk of miscarriage and stillbirth.** It is extremely rare for this disorder to cause the formation of clots in arteries that can lead to stroke or heart attack, though a 'mini-stroke', known as a transient ischemic attack, is more common.

Genetical Hypercoagulable States

- **Factor V Leiden Mutation (Most Common)**
- Antithrombin III Deficiency
- Protein C and Protein S Deficiency
- Homocysteinemia
- Defects in fibrinolysis

Parameters in Different Disorders (Bleeding)

• **von Willebrand's disease**	**↑BT**	**↑PTT**
• **Liver failure**	**↑PT**	**↑PTT**
• **Heparin**	**↑PTT**	
• **Warfarin**	**↑PT**	
• **Scurvy**	**↑N**	
• **ITP**	**↑BT**	**↓Platelets**
• **TTP**	**↑BT**	**↓Platelets**

Antiphospholipid Syndrome

Antiphospholipid syndrome is an acquired disorder characterized by a predisposition to **both venous and arterial thromboses, recurrent fetal loss and thrombocytopenia.** It may occur as primary disorder or secondary to other conditions, most commonly systemic lupus erythematosus (SLE)

A key point for the exam is to appreciate that antiphospholipid syndrome causes a **paradoxical rise in the APTT.** This is due to an ex-vivo reaction of the lupus anticoagulant autoantibodies with phospholipids involved in the coagulation cascade

<u>Features:</u> Can be asymptomatic

- **Venous/arterial thrombosis NOT BLEEDING**
- **Recurrent fetal loss (2nd trimester abortions)**
- **Livedo reticularis**
- **Thrombocytopenia**
- **Prolonged APTT**
- **Other features: preeclampsia, pulmonary hypertension**
- **Not Bleeding Disorder**

Leukemoid Reaction

The leukemoid reaction describes the presence **<u>of immature cells,</u>** such as myeloblasts, promyelocytes and nucleated red cells in the peripheral blood. This may be due to infiltration of the bone marrow causing the immature cells to be 'pushed out' or sudden demand for new cells

<u>Causes:</u>

- **Severe infection**
- **Severe hemolysis**
- **Massive hemorrhage**
- **Metastatic cancer with bone marrow infiltration**

A relatively common clinical problem is differentiating chronic myeloid leukemia from a leukemoid reaction. The following differences may help:

Leukemoid reaction:

- **High leucocyte alkaline phosphatase score**
- **Toxic granulation (Döhle bodies) in the white cells**
- **'Left shift' of neutrophils, i.e. three or less segments of the nucleus**

Chronic myeloid leukemia

- **Low leucocyte alkaline phosphatase score.**

USMLE Case Scenario

A 70-year-old retired male from Washington complains of chronic fatigue. On examination, the patient is noted to have Lymphadenopathy and an enlarged liver and spleen. Laboratory examination reveals a white blood cell count of 29,000/µl with 96% lymphocytes; the lymphocytes appear small and mature. Both the hematocrit and platelet counts are within normal limits. The likely diagnosis is:
Chronic lymphocytic leukemia (CLL) is typically a disease of the elderly.

Chronic Lymphocytic Leukemia (CLL)

It is typically a disease of the elderly, with most of the cases occurring after the age of 50; the median age is 65. Patients will typically present with a complaint of chronic fatigue and/or lymphadenopathy. Approximately, half of all the patients with CLL present with an enlarged liver and/or spleen. CLL typically pursues an indolent course but can occasionally present as a rapidly progressive disease. The hallmark of CLL is the isolated lymphocytosis in which the white blood cell count is usually greater than 20,000/ml and between 75% and 98% of the circulating cells are small 'mature' lymphocytes.

Blood Transfusion Complications

Hemolytic: Immediate or delayed

- Febrile reactions
- Transmission of viruses, bacteria, parasites
- **Hyperkalemia, citrate toxicity**
- Iron overload
- ARDS
- Clotting abnormalities

Immediate hemolytic reaction

- For example, ABO mismatch
- Massive intravascular hemolysis

Febrile reactions

- **Due to white blood cell HLA antibodies**
- Often the result of sensitization by previous pregnancies or transfusions

Causes a degree of immunosuppression

- Patients with colorectal cancer who have blood transfusions have a worse outcome than those who do not.

Others:

- **ARDS**
- **Hypothermia**
- **In nonmismatch blood transfusion reaction, direct Coombs test should be done.**

Viruses Transmitted by Blood Transfusion

- **Hepatitis B**
- **Hepatitis C**
- **Hepatitis G**
- **HIV type I**
- **HTLV type I**
- **CMV**
- **Parvovirus B19**

Thrombophilia

Inherited

- Activated protein C resistance (Factor V Leiden)
- Antithrombin III deficiency
- Protein C deficiency
- Protein S deficiency

Acquired

- Antiphospholipid syndrome
- OCP

ITP (Idiopathic Thrombocytopenic Purpura)

In many cases, the cause is not actually idiopathic but **autoimmune**, with antibodies against platelets being detected in approximately 60 percent of patients

Most often these **antibodies are against platelet membrane glycoproteins IIb-IIIa or Ib-IX,** and are of the **IgG type**

- The diagnosis of ITP is a **process of exclusion**
- In approximately one percent of the cases, autoimmune hemolytic anemia and immune thrombocytopenic purpura coexist, a condition called **'Evans syndrome'**
- **Bleeding time is prolonged** in ITP patients
- On examination of the **bone marrow, an increase in the production of megakaryocytes** may be observed and may help in establishing a diagnosis of ITP.

DIFFERENTIATE ITP FROM TTP AND HUS

TTP (Thrombotic Thrombocytopenic Purpura)

There is widespread formation of platelet thrombi

'Pentad of signs' is:

- **Fever**
- **Thrombocytopenia**
- **Microangiopathic hemolytic anemia**
- **Neurological symptoms**
- **Renal failure**

Lab features:

- **Decreased platelet count and increased bleeding time**
- **Normal PT and PTT**
- **Normal complement.**

HUS: (Hemolytic Uremic Syndrome)

It is a complication of the Shiga toxin or Shiga-like toxin: exotoxins released by Shigella species and the enterohemorrhagic *E. coli*. HUS in children usually develops after a gastrointestinal or flu-like illness, and is characterized by bleeding, oliguria and hematuria, and microangiopathic hemolytic anemia. Presumably the Shiga toxin is toxic to the microvasculature, producing microthrombi that consume platelets and RBCs, and may fragment the red cell membrane.

- Occurs most commonly in **children**
- Follows gastroenteritis
- Pentad similar to TTP seen
- Verocytotoxin producing ***E. coli*** **0157: H7** is most commonly encountered

Some Specific Splenomegalic Syndromes

- **Myeloproliferative disorders** include:
  - **Polycythemia vera**
  - **Myelofibrosis with myeloid metaplasia**
  - **Chronic myelogenous leukemia and**
  - **Essential thrombocythemia**
- **Lymphoproliferative disorders:** The spleen is enlarged in **chronic lymphocytic leukemia** and the **lymphomas** (including Hodgkin's disease)
- **Lipid storage diseases:** Glucocerebroside **(in Gaucher's disease)** or sphingomyelin (**in Niemann-Pick disease)** may accumulate in the spleen
- **Collagen vascular disorders:** In both SLE and RA, splenomegaly and leukopenia may coexist. In the latter, often termed **Felty's syndrome,** neutropenia may be severe and associated with frequent infections.

Congestive splenomegaly (Banti's syndrome): Chronically increased splenic venous pressure may result from hepatic cirrhosis, portal or splenic vein thrombosis, or certain malformations of the portal venous vasculature. Associated bleeding from esophageal varices may be worsened by the superimposed thrombocytopenia induced by splenomegaly.

Common Translocations associated with Hematological Malignancies

t(9;22) Philadelphia chromosome

- Present in > 95% of patients with **CML**
- This results in part of the Abelson proto-oncogene being moved to the BCR gene on chromosome 22
- The resulting BCR-ABL gene codes for a fusion protein which has tyrosine kinase activity in excess of normal
- Poor prognostic indicator in ALL

t(15;17)

- Seen in **acute promyelocytic leukemia (M3)**
- Fusion of PML and RAR-alpha genes

t(8;14)

- Seen in **Burkitt's lymphoma**
- MYC oncogene is translocated to an immunoglobulin gene

t(11;14)

- **Mantle cell lymphoma**
- Deregulation of the cyclin D1 (BCL-1) gene

Hodgkin's Disease

- **Bi modal age distribution** (late 20 years and after 50 years)
- The commonest presentation of Hodgkin's Lymphoma is **painless enlargement of lymph nodes**
- Prognosis is **directly proportional to number of RS** cells and **inversely proportional to number of lymphocytes**
- Spread is to be contigious to **adjacent lymph nodes**
- Extranodal spread **is uncommon**
- EBV is causative in some cases
- Malignant cell is **Reed-Sternberg Cell**. (Owl-eyed, bilobed nucleus with prominent nucleoli)
- RS cells are positive for **CD 15 and CD 30**. (Except lymphocyte predominant)
- CNS involvement is uncommon
- **Cerebellar degeneration** is seen in HD (anti-Tr antibodies)

Hodgkin's lymphoma is a malignant proliferation of lymphocytes characterized by the presence of the Reed-Sternberg cells. It has a bimodal age distributions being most common in the third and seventh decades

Ann-Arbor Staging of Hodgkin's Lymphoma

- **I: Single lymph node**
- **II: 2 or more lymph nodes/regions on same side of diaphragm**
- **III: Nodes on both sides of diaphragm**

Each Stage May be Subdivided into A or B

- **A = No systemic symptoms other than pruritus**
- **B = Weight loss > 10% in last 6 months, fever > 38 °C, night sweats (poor prognosis)**

Nodular sclerosing CHL

It is the most common subtype and is composed of large tumor nodules showing scattered lacunar classical RS cells set in a background of reactive lymphocytes, eosinophils and plasma cells with varying degrees of collagen fibrosis/sclerosis

- **Most common type in females**
- **Mediastinal involvement common**
- **Lacunar cell present**

Mixed-cellularity subtype

It is a common subtype and is composed of numerous classic RS cells admixed with numerous inflammatory cells including lymphocytes, histiocytes, eosinophils, and plasma cells without sclerosis. This type is most often associated with EBV infection and may be confused with the early, so-called 'cellular' phase of nodular sclerosing CHL

MC type in India

Lymphocyte-rich

It is a rare subtype, shows many features which may cause diagnostic confusion with nodular lymphocyte predominant B-cell

Non-Hodgkin's Lymphoma (B-NHL)

'Popcorn cells' are a feature of this type

Lymphocyte-depleted

It is a rare subtype, composed of large number of often pleomorphic RS cells with only few reactive lymphocytes which may easily be confused with diffuse large cell lymphoma. Many cases previously classified within this category would now be reclassified under anaplastic large cell lymphoma.

Lymphocyte predominant is considered a histogenetically different subtype. CD 15 –, CD 30 –, CD 45+

Popcorn cells are seen in this variety

Best prognosis

Burkitt's lymphoma

This type of lymphoma is a high-grade B-cell lymphoma that occurs in endemic form in and sporadically in the United States and Europe. The sporadic form is often in an abdominal site and occurs in young adults. The African form of Burkitt's lymphoma has been strongly associated with antibodies directed against Epstein-Barr virus; the association is weaker in sporadic cases. A characteristic translocation, t(8;14) (q24.l3;q32.33) has been described.

Hairy Cell Leukemia

Hairy cell leukemia is a rare malignant proliferation disorder of **B cells**

- Express CD 19, 20, CD 11, CD 25
- CD 103 is exclusive
- It is more common in **males** (4:1)

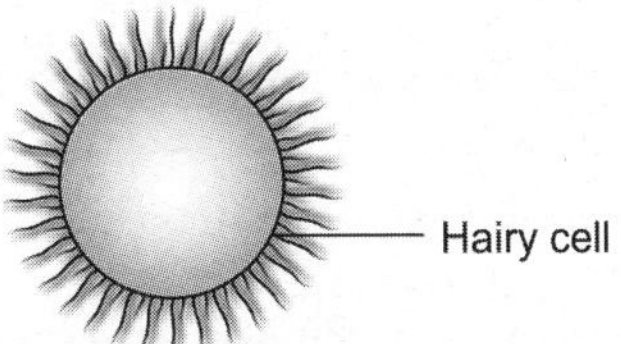

Features:

- **Pancytopenia**
- **Splenomegaly**
- **Skin vasculitis in 1/3rd patients**
- **'Dry tap' despite bone marrow hypercellularity**
- **Tartrate-resistant acid phosphotase (TRAP) stain positive**
- **Cladribine is DOC**
- **Pentostatin and interferon alpha are also used**

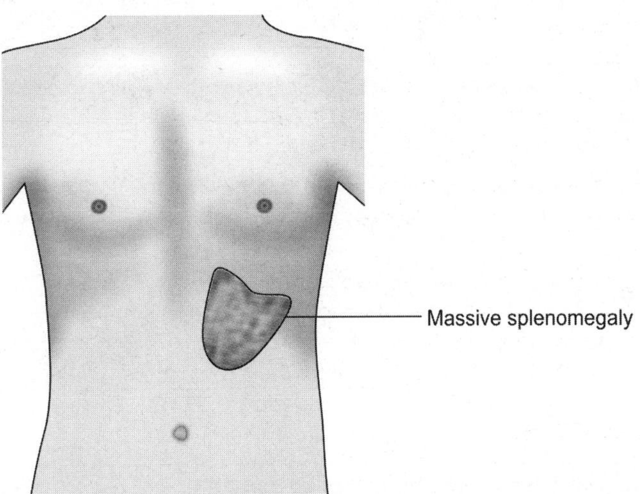

- **Hairy cell leukemia: CD 103+**
- **Mantle cell lymphoma: CD5+, CD103–**
- **CLL: CD 23+**
- **Apoptosis: CD95+**

Mantle Cell Lymphoma

- **Painless lymphadenopathy**
- **Splenomegaly**
- **Occasional GI involvement**
- **CD5+, CD23 –. CD10 –, CD 19+, CD 79 b+**
- **t (11 – 14) translocation**

- **Popcorn type of Reed Sternberg cell is seen in: Lymphocyte-predominant type of Hodgkin's lymphoma**
- **ABVD and MOPP Regimes are used in Hodgkin's lymphoma**
- **B-cell lymphomas are hairy cell leukemia, mantle cell lymphoma, Burkitt's Lymphoma**
- **HTLV 1 is associated with Adult T cell lymphoma**
- **IgA lymphoma involves stomach**

Blood Films: Typical Pictures

Hyposplenism, e.g. postsplenectomy	Iron-deficiency anemia	Myelofibrosis	Megaloblastic anemia
• Target cells • Howell-Jolly bodies	• Target cells • 'Pencil' poikilocytes	• 'Tear-drop' poikilocytes	• Hypersegmented neutrophils
• Cabot's rings • Siderotic granules • Acanthocytes • Schizocytes	• If combined with B12/folate deficiency, a **'Dimorphic' film** occurs with mixed microcytic and macrocytic cells		

Leucocyte Alkaline Phosphatase (LAP)

Raised In	Low In
• Myelofibrosis • **Leukemoid reactions** • **Polycythemia rubra vera** • Infections • Steroids, Cushing's syndrome • Pregnancy, oral contraceptive pill	• **Chronic myeloid leukemia** • Pernicious anemia • **Paroxysmal nocturnal hemoglobinuria** • Infectious mononucleosis

Castleman's disease, which can present with **localized or disseminated lymphadenopathy**; some patients have systemic symptoms. The disseminated form is often accompanied by **anemia and polyclonal hypergammaglobulinemia**, and the condition seems to be related to an **overproduction of interleukin 6**, possibly produced by human herpesvirus 8.

Sinus histiocytosis with massive lymphadenopathy (Rosai-Dorfman's disease) usually presents with **bulky lymphadenopathy in children or young adults.** The disease is usually nonprogressive and self-limited, but patients can manifest **autoimmune hemolytic anemia.**

Lymphomatoid papulosis is a **cutaneous lymphoproliferative disorder** that is often confused with anaplastic large-cell **lymphoma** involving the skin. The cells of lymphomatoid papulosis are similar to those seen in **lymphoma** and stain for CD30, and T cell receptor gene rearrangements are sometimes seen. However, the condition is characterized by waxing and waning skin lesions that usually heal, leaving small scars.

Cat Scratch Disease

Typical Cat Scratch Disease presents with **Painful Regional Lymphadenopathy** persisting for weeks to months after a cat scratch
Only occasionally a generalized lymphadenopathy may occur
Tender Regional Lymphadenopathy occurs in 1–2 weeks after inoculation
Epitrochlear, axillary, pectoral and cervical lymph nodes may be affected
Lymph nodes become suppurative occasionally
Lymphadenopathy persists for weeks.

Takayasu's Arteritis

- Also called **'Pulseless Disease' or 'Aortic Arch Syndrome'**
- It is a **vasculitis** common in **Asia,** especially in **young and middle-aged females**, affecting medium to large size arteries including aorta and its branches.
- Characterized by **granulomatous inflammation leading to arterial thrombosis, stenosis or aneurysm.**
- Clinical features are:
  - Aortic involvement with palpable purpura and panarteritis
  - Loss of pulse in upper extremities, (radial pulse not felt)
  - Systemic features: fever, weight loss, arthalgias, fatigue
  - Anemia and increased ESR
  - Visual loss or field defects, retinal hemorrhages
  - Neurological abnormalities like headache, pulsating chest pain, hypertension

Treatment is by **steroids (Drug of choice)**

Polyarteritis Nodosa and Microscopic Polyangiitis

- **'Necrotizing vasculitis' of small- and medium-sized muscular arteries** in which involvement of the renal and visceral arteries is characteristic
- **Intimal proliferation is a feature**
- **Classic PAN does not involve pulmonary arteries**
- **Preceded by history of asthma**
- The **microscopic polyangiitis (microscopic polyarteritis)** connot a **necrotizing vasculitis with few or no immune complexes (pauci-immune) affecting small vessels (capillaries, venules, or arterioles).** Since necrotizing arteritis involving small- and medium-sized arteries may also be present, it shares features with classic PAN except that **glomerulonephritis is very common (90%) in microscopic polyangiitis, and pulmonary capillaritis often occurs**
- **Multiple organ systems are involved**
- **Skin involvement: livedo reticularis, hyperpigmentation**
- The pathology in the kidney in **classic PAN is predominantly that of arteritis without glomerulonephritis**
- The presence **of hepatitis B antigenemia** in approximately 20 to 30% of patients with systemic vasculitis
- **Hypergammaglobulinemia may be present,** and up to 30% of patients have a positive test for hepatitis B surface antigen
- **Positive ANCA titers (usually of the p-ANCA type) are found in a low percentage (< 20%) of patients with classic PAN**
- **Microscopic polyangiitis is strongly associated with ANCA that are usually of the p-ANCA type**, but c-ANCA have also been reported
- The diagnosis of classic PAN is based on the demonstration of characteristic findings of **vasculitis on biopsy**

Kawasaki Disease

- **Kawasaki disease (also known as 'lymph node syndrome', 'mucocutaneous node disease', 'infantile polyarteritis')**
- **Kawasaki disease** is an inflammation (vasculitis) of the middle-sized arteries
- **Kawasaki disease** affects **many organs**, including the skin, mucous membranes, lymph nodes, and blood vessel walls, but the **'most serious'** 'effect is on the **heart** where it can cause **'severe aneurysmal dilations'**

Classically, five days of fever plus four of five **'diagnostic criteria'** must be met in order to establish the diagnosis

The criteria are:

- Erythema of the lips or oral cavity or cracking of the lips
- Rash
- Swelling or erythema of the hands or feet
- Red eyes (conjunctival injection)
- **Swollen lymph node in the neck of at least 15 millimeters**

Strawberry tongue seen

Intravenous immunoglobulin (IVIg) is the **standard treatment for Kawasaki disease** and is administered in high doses with marked improvement usually noted within 24 hours. If the fever does not respond, an additional dose may have to be considered. IVIg by itself is most useful within the first 7 days of onset of fever, in terms of preventing coronary artery aneurysm

Salicylate therapy, particularly aspirin, remains an important part of the treatment. '**Aspirin therapy**' is started at high doses until the fever subsides, and then is continued at a low dose when the patient returns home, usually for 2 months, to prevent blood clots from forming. **'Except for Kawasaki disease, aspirin is otherwise normally not recommended for children due to its association with Reye's syndrome.'**

Corticosteroids have also been used especially when other treatments fail or symptoms recur.

Polymyositis/Dermatomyositis

- A systemic connective tissue disease characterized by inflammatory and degenerative changes in the muscles **(polymyositis)** and frequently also in **the skin (dermatomyositis)**, leading to symmetric weakness and some degree of muscle atrophy, principally of the limb girdles
- **Dermato + Myositis:** Involves skin and muscles usually
- **Females** are more commonly affected. Features are **'rash and muscle weakness'**
- **'Proximal'** muscle weakness with loss of fine motor movements is seen
- Dermatomyositis **can be associated with malignancy in 10–20% cases**
- **Rash involves:**
  - **Eyelids with edema (Heliotrope rash)**
  - **Erythema of knuckles with scaly eruption (Gottron's rash)**
  - **Neck and anterior chest (V sign)**
  - **Back and shoulder (Shawl sign)**

Creatine kinase is increased especially in damage to muscles and in conditions like:

- Myocardial infarction
- Trauma to muscles (Rhabdomyolysis)
- Muscular dystrophies
- Dermatomyositis
- Polymyositis
- Hypothyroidism and
- Cerebral infarction
  - It has been reliably suggested that Creatine kinase is a **reliable biochemical marker of myositis in dermatomyositis.** Serum muscle enzymes, especially the **transaminases, creatine kinase (CK), and aldolase, are usually elevated**; the **'most sensitive and useful'** is **CK**
  - **Periodic enzyme determinations are helpful in monitoring treatment**
  - **Elevated levels decrease with effective therapy.**

Reiter's Syndrome (RS)

- Arthritis associated with **nonbacterial urethritis or cervicitis, conjunctivitis, and mucocutaneous lesions.**
- RS is classified with the **seronegative spondyloarthropathies.**
- Arthritis usually is the 2nd or 3rd feature of RS and may be mild or severe.
- Joint involvement generally is **asymmetric and polyarticular,** occurring in the large joints of the lower extremities as well as the toes. Back pain may occur, usually with more severe disease
- **Enthesopathy** (inflammation at tendinous insertion into bone) is common in RS and other seronegative arthritides, e.g. **plantar fasciitis, digital periostitis, Achilles tendinitis.**

- Mucocutaneous lesions, small, painless superficial ulcers are commonly seen on the oral mucosa, tongue, and glans penis **(balanitis circinata)**. Patients may also develop hyperkeratotic skin lesions of the palms and soles, and around the nails **(keratoderma blennorrhagica)**
- Cardiovascular involvement with **aortitis, aortic insufficiency, and conduction defects** occurs rarely

Temporal Arteritis

Temporal Arteritis (Giant Cell Arteritis; Cranial Arteritis)

- A **chronic inflammatory disease** of large blood vessels, particularly those with a **prominent elastica**, occurring primarily in the elderly
- More common in females
- Giant cell arteritis most often involves **arteries of the carotid system**, particularly the cranial arteries
- Segments of the aorta, its branches, the coronary arteries, and the peripheral arteries may also be affected
- The disease has a predilection for arteries containing elastic tissue; it is rarely seen in veins
- The histologic reaction is a **granulomatous inflammation** of the intima and inner part of the media
- Presentations are diverse, depending on the distribution of the arteritis, but typically include:
  - **Severe headache (MC)**
  - **(Especially temporal and occipital), scalp tenderness, and visual disturbances (amaurosis fugax, diplopia, scotoma, ptosis, and vision blurring)**
  - **Claudication of the masseter, temporalis, and tongue muscles** are characteristic
  - **Blindness due to ischemic optic neuropathy**
  - On physical examination, there may be **swelling and tenderness with nodularity over the temporal arteries** and
  - **Bruits** over the large vessels

- **ESR is usually markedly elevated** (often >100 mm/h, Westergren) during the active phase, but is normal in about 1% of patients
- **Normochromic and normocytic anemia** are often present and, at times, profound. Alkaline phosphatase may be elevated
- Other nonspecific findings include **'polyclonal hyperglobulinemia and leukocytosis.'**
- Diagnosis can be made clinically but should be verified by temporal artery biopsy because of the need for prolonged corticosteroid treatment
- Even a temporal artery that is normal to palpation and without tenderness or swelling may be abnormal on biopsy

USMLE Case Scenario

A 75-year-old African resident started to complain of occasional jaw pain 4 months ago. She also began complaining of headache 3 weeks ago, which is throbbing, rated as 5/10 on 0–10 scale, worse in the afternoon, and radiating down the neck.

Raynaud's Phenomenon and Disease

Spasm of arterioles, usually in the digits (and occasionally other acral parts such as the nose and tongue), with **intermittent pallor or cyanosis of the skin**

More common in females

Raynaud's phenomenon may be idiopathic (Raynaud's disease)

Or secondary to other conditions:

- Connective tissue disorders (e.g. scleroderma, RA, SLE)
- Obstructive arterial diseases (arteriosclerosis obliterans, thromboangiitis obliterans, thoracic outlet syndrome), neurogenic lesions
- **Drug intoxications (ergot and methysergide)**
- **Dysproteinemias, myxedema**
- **Primary pulmonary hypertension and trauma**
- Idiopathic Raynaud's disease is most common in young women (60 to 90% of reported cases)

Primary Raynaud syndrome commonly affects upper limb arteries

Hos good prognosis

Attacks of vasospasm of the digital arteries and arterioles may last from minutes to hours but are rarely severe enough to cause gross tissue loss. With long-standing Raynaud's disease, the skin of the digits may become smooth, shiny, and tight, with loss of subcutaneous tissue (sclerodactyly)

Small painful ulcers may appear on the tips of the digits

Vessels are histologically normal in early stages, but in advanced cases, the arterial intima may thicken and thromboses may form in small arteries

In secondary Raynaud's phenomenon, pathologic changes of the underlying disease are apparent.

Erythromelalgia

A rare syndrome of **paroxysmal vasodilation** with **burning pain, increased skin temperature, and redness of the feet and, less often, the hands**

Causes of secondary erythromelalgia:

- Myeloproliferative disorders
- Hypertension
- Venous insufficiency
- Diabetes mellitus, SLE, RA
- Lichen sclerosus et atrophicus, gout
- Spinal cord disease, or multiple sclerosis

Acrocyanosis

Persistent, painless, symmetric cyanosis of the hands and, less commonly, the feet, caused by vasospasm of the small vessels of the skin

The etiology is unknown but may be related to increased tone of the arterioles associated with dilation of capillaries and venules

The disorder usually occurs in women and is not associated with occlusive arterial disease

The digits and hands or feet are persistently cold and bluish, and sweat profusely; they may swell

Cyanosis is usually **intensified by cold and lessened by warming.**

Systemic Lupus Erythematosus (SLE)

- Ninety percent of cases are in women, usually of child-bearing age

Clinical Manifestations

Musculoskeletal Manifestations

- Almost all the patients experience **arthralgias and myalgias**; most develop intermittent arthritis
- **Erosions are rare. Differentiating point is nonerosive arthritis**
- Myopathy can be **inflammatory** (during periods of active disease), or secondary to treatment (hypokalemia, glucocorticoid myopathy, hydroxychloroquine myopathy)
- **Ischemic necrosis of bone** is a common cause of hip, knee, or shoulder pain in patients receiving glucocorticoids

Cutaneous Manifestations

- **The malar 'butterfly' rash** is a photosensitive, fixed erythematous rash, flat or raised over the cheeks and bridge of the nose, often involving the chin and ears
- **Scarring is absent; telangiectasia** may develop
- A more diffuse **maculopapular rash**, predominant in sun-exposed areas, is also common and usually indicates disease flare
- **Loss of scalp hair** is usually patchy but can be extensive
- Less frequent SLE skin lesions include **urticaria, bullae, erythema multiforme, lichen planus-like lesions,** and **panniculitis ('lupus profundus')**
- Patients with SLE can develop **vasculitic skin lesions.** These include purpura, subcutaneous nodules, nailfold infarcts, ulcers, vasculitic urticaria, panniculitis, and gangrene of digits. Shallow, slightly painful ulcers in the mouth and nose are frequent in patients with SLE.

Renal Manifestations

- Most patients with SLE have **immunoglobulins deposited in glomeruli**, but only one-half have clinical nephritis, defined by proteinuria
- Early in the disease, most are asymptomatic, although some develop the edema of nephrotic syndrome. Urinalysis shows hematuria, cylindruria, and proteinuria
- Papillary necrosis seen
- Most patients with **mesangial or mild focal proliferative nephritis** maintain good renal function. Patients with diffuse proliferative nephritis develop renal failure if untreated
- **Wire loop lesions** seen
- **Renal involvement** is the most common cause of death

Nervous System Manifestations

- **Mild cognitive dysfunction** is the **most frequent manifestation**
- **Headaches** are common and may be migraine-like or nonspecific
- **Seizures** of any type may occur
- Less frequent manifestations include psychosis, acute confusional states, demyelinating disorders, cerebrovascular disease, movement disorders, aseptic meningitis, myelopathy, mononeuropathy or polyneuropathy of cranial or peripheral nerves, autonomic dysfunction, acute demyelinating polyneuropathy (Guillain-Barre), mood disorders, optic neuritis, subarachnoid hemorrhage, pseudotumor cerebri, and hypothalamic dysfunction with inappropriate secretion of vasopressin. Depression and anxiety are frequent.

Vascular System

- **Thrombosis** in vessels of any size can be a major problem
- Although vasculitis may underlie thrombosis, there is increasing evidence that antibodies against phospholipids lupus anticoagulant (LA), anticardiolipin (ACL) are associated with clotting without inflammation.

Hematologic Manifestation

- **Anemia of chronic disease** occurs in most patients when lupus is active
- **Autoimmune hemolytic anemia seen**
- **Coombs' positive hemolysis occurs**
- **Cold antibodies**
- **Leukopenia (usually lymphopenia)**
- **Mild thrombocytopenia is common**
- **Pancytopenia can occur**
- **Clinical manifestations of lupus anticoagulant and anticardiolipin** include thrombocytopenia, **recurrent venous or arterial clotting, recurrent fetal loss, and valvular heart disease** usually respond to glucocorticoids; clotting syndromes do not

Cardiopulmonary System

- **Pericarditis is the most frequent manifestation** of cardiac lupus
- **Effusions** can occur and occasionally lead to tamponade; constrictive pericarditis is rare
- **Myocarditis** can cause arrhythmias, sudden death, and/or heart failure
- **Valvular insufficiency** (usually aortic or mitral) can occur, with or without **Libman-Sacks endocarditis**
- **Myocardial infarcts** usually result from degenerative disease, although they can result from vasculitis
- **Cavitation in lung**
- **Pulmonary fibrosis**
- **Pleurisy and pleural effusions** are common manifestations of SLE
- **Shrinking lung syndrome**
- **Lupus pneumonitis** causes fever, dyspnea, and cough; X-rays show fleeting infiltrates and/or areas of plate-like atelectasis; this syndrome responds to glucocorticoids. However, the most common cause of pulmonary infiltrates in patients with SLE is infection
- **Polyserositis**

Pregnancy and SLE

- Most patients **complete pregnancy safely** and deliver normal infants
- **Fertility rates are normal in patients with SLE**, but spontaneous abortion and stillbirths are frequent (10–30%), especially in women with lupus anticoagulant and/or anticardiolipin
- **NO strelity**
- **Neonatal lupus**, caused by transmission of maternal **anti-Ro** across the placenta, consists of **transient skin rash and (rarely) permanent heart block**. Transient thrombocytopenia from maternal antiplatelet antibodies also occurs.

Lab Tests

- **ANAs** are the **best screening test**
- Antibodies **to double-stranded DNA (dsDNA) and to CM are relatively specific for SLE**. High serum levels of ANAs and anti-dsDNA and low levels of complement usually reflect **disease activity**, especially in patients with nephritis.
- **Very low levels of CH_{50}** with **normal levels of C3** seen
- Hematologic abnormalities include **anemia** (usually normochromic normocytic but occasionally hemolytic), leukopenia, lymphopenia, and thrombocytopenia
- The Westergren **erythrocyte sedimentation rate** correlates with disease activity in some patients
- Urinalysis should be performed and serum creatinine levels should be measured periodically in patients with **SLE**
- With active nephritis, the urinalysis usually shows proteinuria, hematuria, and cellular or granular casts.

Drug-induced Lupus

- **Several drugs can cause a syndrome resembling SLE, including:**
  - **Procainamide**
  - **Hydralazine**
  - **Isoniazid**
  - **Chlorpromazine**
  - **D-penicillamine, practolol**
  - **Methyldopa, quinidine**
  - **Interferon A and**
  - **Possibly hydantoin, ethosuximide, and oral contraceptives**
- The syndrome is rare with all but procainamide, the most frequent offender, and hydralazine. There is genetic predisposition to drug-induced lupus, partly determined by **drug acetylation rates**
- Most common are systemic complaints and **arthralgias; polyarthritis and pleuropericarditis**
- **Renal and CNS involvement are rare**
- All patients have ANA and most have **antibodies to histones**
- **'Best marker' is antibodies to histones.**

Progressive Systemic Sclerosis (PSS) (Scleroderma)

A chronic disease of unknown cause, characterized by diffuse fibrosis; degenerative changes; and vascular abnormalities in the skin (scleroderma), articular structures, and internal organs (especially the esophagus, intestinal tract, lung, heart, and kidney).

PSS is about 4 times **more common in women** than men and is comparatively rare in children

- The disease varies in severity and progression, ranging from generalized cutaneous thickening (PSS with diffuse scleroderma) with rapidly progressive and often fatal visceral involvement, to a form distinguished by restricted skin involvement (often just the fingers and face) and prolonged passage of time, often several decades, before full manifestation of characteristic internal manifestations **(CREST syndrome: Calcinosis, Raynaud's phenomenon, Esophageal dysfunction, Sclerodactyly, Telangiectasia).**

- Raynaud's phenomenon is an important component of scleroderma.
- Anticentromere antibody seen
- The most common are **Raynaud's phenomenon** and insidious swelling of the acral portions of the extremities with gradual thickening of the skin of the fingers. **Polyarthralgia** also is a prominent early symptom.
- **The skin:** Induration is symmetric and may be confined to the fingers **(sclerodactyly)** and distal portions of the upper extremities, or it may affect most or all of the body. As the disease progresses, the skin becomes taut, shiny, and hyperpigmented; the face becomes mask-like; **telangiectases** appear on the fingers, chest, face, lips, and tongue. Subcutaneous calcifications develop **(calcinosis circumscripta),** usually on the fingertips and over bony eminences.
- **Musculoskeletal system**: **Friction rubs** develop over the joints (particularly the knees), tendon sheaths (**tendinitis**), and large bursae because of fibrin deposition on synovial surfaces. Flexion contractures of the fingers, wrists, and elbows result from fibrosis of the synovium and periarticular structures. **Trophic ulcers** are common, especially on the fingertips and overlying the finger joints
- **GI tract:**
- **Esophageal dysfunction** is the **most frequent visceral disturbance and eventually occurs in most patients**
- **Dysphagia, acid reflux** due to lower esophageal sphincter incompetence, and **peptic esophagitis** with possible **ulceration and stricture** are common
- **Barrett's metaplasia** of the esophagus occurs in 1/3rd of all patients with scleroderma; these patients have an increased risk of complications such as stricture or **adenocarcinoma**
- **Hypomotility** of the small intestine may be associated with malabsorption resulting from anaerobic bacterial overgrowth.
- **Pneumatosis cystoides intestinalis, biliary cirrhosis** has occurred in persons with CREST syndrome.

- **Cardiorespiratory system: Lung fibrosis**, with exertional dyspnea, its most prominent symptom, is associated early with an impairment in gas exchange. **Pleurisy and pericarditis** with effusion may occur. Recent studies indicate generally indolent progression of lung involvement, with substantial individual variability. **Pulmonary hypertension** may develop as a result of long-standing interstitial and peribronchial fibrosis or intimal hyperplasia of small pulmonary arteries; the latter is associated with the CREST syndrome. **Cardiac arrhythmias, conduction disturbances, and other ECG abnormalities** are common
- **The kidneys:** Severe renal disease may occur as a consequence of intimal hyperplasia of interlobular and arcuate arteries, and usually is heralded by the abrupt onset of **accelerated or malignant hypertension**
- An antibody that reacts with centromeric protein **(anticentromere antibody)** is found in the serum of a high proportion of patients with the CREST syndrome
- **Localized forms** of scleroderma occur as circumscribed patches **(morphea)** or linear sclerosis of the integument and immediately subjacent tissues without systemic involvement.

Sjogren's Syndrome

- Occurs as primary form/isolated disorder
- Secondary form with other CT disorders
- Sjogren's syndrome is a chronic, slowly progressive autoimmune disease characterized by **lymphocytic infiltration of the exocrine glands** resulting in **xerostomia and dry eyes**
- A small but significant number of the patients may develop **malignant lymphoma**
- The disease affects predominantly **middle-aged women** (female-to-male ratio 9:1)
- Sera of patients with Sjogren's syndrome often contain a number of autoantibodies directed against non-organ-specific antigens, such as immunoglobulins (rheumatoid factors) and extractable nuclear and cytoplasmic antigens **(Ro/SS-A, La/SS-B)**

Lymphoma is a well-known manifestation of Sjogren's syndrome that usually presents later in the illness. Persistent parotid gland enlargement, lymphadenopathy, cutaneous vasculitis, peripheral neuropathy, lymphopenia, and cryoglobulinemia are manifestations suggesting the development of lymphoma. Most lymphomas are extranodal, marginal zone B cell, and low grade. Salivary glands are the most common site of involvement.

- **Dry eye** or **Keratitis Sicca** or **Aqueous deficiency dry eye** occurs in **Sjogrens syndrome**
- **Dry mouth**
- **Dry nose**

- **Dry eyes**
- **Dry skin**
- **Dry throat**
- **Dry sex (vaginal involvement)**
- **Involvement of other exocrine glands** occurs less frequently and includes a decrease in mucous gland secretions of the upper and lower respiratory tree, resulting in dry nose, throat, and trachea **(xerotrachea),** and diminished secretion of the exocrine glands of the gastrointestinal tract, leading to **esophageal mucosal atrophy, atrophic gastritis, and subclinical pancreatitis. Dyspareunia due to dryness of the external genitalia and dry skin also may occur.**

Behçet's Syndrome: Oro-oculo-genital Syndrome

- **Recurrent oral and genital ocular involvement**
- **Associated with HLA B5**
- The **ulcers are usually painful**, shallow or deep with a central yellowish necrotic base, appear singly or in crops, and are located anywhere in the oral cavity. The ulcers persist for 1 to 2 weeks and subside without leaving scars
- The **genital ulcers resemble the oral ones**
- Skin involvement includes **folliculitis, erythema nodosum, an acne-like exanthem, and, infrequently, vasculitis**. Nonspecific skin inflammatory reactivity to any scratches or intradermal saline injection (pathergy test) is a common and specific manifestation
- Eye involvement is the most dreaded complication, since it occasionally progresses rapidly to blindness. **Iritis, posterior uveitis, retinal vessel occlusions, and optic neuritis** are seen in some patients with the **syndrome. Hypopyon, uveitis** is a feature
- Recurrent DVT is seen
- The arthritis of **Behçet**'s syndrome is **not deforming** and affects the knees and ankles.

USMLE Case Scenario

A 38-year-old lady from Mexico presents with myalgia and lethargy. Her blood tests show a positive ANA and rheumatoid factor is negative. The CK is raised at 360 U/l. Extranuclear antigen tests show a negative Ro and negative La, negative Scl 70 and positive ribonuclear protein antibody. Most likely diagnosis is:
Mixed connective tissue disease.

Henoch Schönlein Purpura

- Henoch-Schönlein Purpura (HSP): Abdominal pain with guaiac-positive stools, plus a prominent rash, mostly on his lower extremities. Other characteristic findings of HSP include hematuria and joint pains. The illness may follow an upper respiratory infection or strep throat
- Also referred to as **anaphylactoid purpura**, is a distinct **systemic vasculitis syndrome** that is characterized by:
  - **Palpable purpura** (most commonly distributed over the buttocks and lower extremities)
  - **Arthralgias**
  - **Abdominal pain**
  - **Glomerulonephritis**
- It is a **small vessel vasculitis**
- Henoch-Schönlein purpura is **usually seen in children;** most patients range in age from 4 to 7 years
- A seasonal variation with a **peak incidence in spring** has been noted
- **IgA** is the antibody class most often seen in the immune complexes and has been demonstrated in the renal biopsies of these patients
- Gastrointestinal involvement, which is seen in almost 70% of pediatric patients, is characterized by **colicky abdominal pain** usually associated with **nausea, vomiting, diarrhea, or constipation** and is frequently accompanied by the passage of blood and mucus per rectum; **bowel intussusception** may occur rarely
- It usually **resolves spontaneously** without therapy. Rarely, a progressive glomerulonephritis will develop.

- **Renal failure is the most common cause of death** in the rare patient who dies of Henoch-Schönlein purpura
- Routine laboratory studies generally show a **mild leukocytosis, a normal platelet count, and occasionally eosinophilia. Serum complement components are normal, and IgA levels are elevated** in about one-half of patients
- **Treatment:** The prognosis of Henoch-Schönlein purpura is **excellent. Most patients recover completely, and some do not require therapy**.

Differentiate

USMLE Case Scenario

A 7-year-old boy is brought to the emergency department. His parents assert that over the past 3 days, he has become progressively ill with generalized fatigue and mid-abdominal pain that have become steadily worse. On examination, he has a maculopapular rash on his thighs and feet with some spread of the rash to his buttocks. The rash does not blanch and some lesions near the ankles look petechial. His temperature is 103.4 °F He has dark stool, which is positive for occult blood.

Rocky Mountain Spotted Fever

It is a rickettsial disease associated with fever, headache, and a rash caused by Rickettsia rickettsii, the vector, a tick, and the reservoir rodents and mammals. Clinically, the onset is nonspecific. The patient may complain of fever, myalgias, nausea, and vomiting. The typical triad of the illness is headache, fever, and a rose-colored blanching, maculopapular rash that begins on the extremities and spreads centripetally to the entire body. The erythematous macules soon turn into petechiae as a result of vasculitis.

USMLE Case Scenario

A 22-year-old boy is brought to the emergency department because of sudden onset of headache, fever, vomiting, and a skin rash. He spent vacation camping in North Carolina. During his stay, he had experienced multiple insect bites and removed several ticks from all family members. The boy had started complaining of a headache and developed fever by noon. He vomited several times. He noticed that a rose-colored rash had developed around his ankles. He has multiple erythematous macules on his lower legs and hands, and rare petechiae interspersed between them.

Paraneoplastic Syndromes (Endocrine Syndromes)

• **Hypercalcemia of malignancy**	Hypercalcemia with cancer is classified as **humoral hypercalcemia of malignancy (HHM)**, which is caused by circulating hormones, or **local osteolytic hypercalcemia (LOH)**, which is caused by local paracrine factors secreted by cancers within the bone **Parathyroid hormone-related peptide (PTHrP) causes nearly all cases of HHM**, while the mediators of LOH in bone are heterogenous
• **Hyponatremia of malignancy**	Due to the inappropriate secretion of arginine vasopressin (AVP) and is termed as the **syndrome of inappropriate antidiuretic hormone secretion (SIADH)** **Small cell lung cancer** is the malignancy chiefly responsible for producing ectopic AVP
• **Ectopic acth syndrome**	Responsible for ~15% of all cases of **Cushing's syndrome** and for most cases of Cushing's syndrome that occur in cancer patients Ectopic ACTH syndrome is most commonly due to **small cell lung cancer (50% of cases), bronchial carcinoid tumors (10%), thymic carcinoid tumors or thymomas (10%), pancreatic islet cell tumors (10%), pheochromocytoma or other neural crest tumors (5%), or medullary carcinoma of the thyroid (5%).**
• **Ectopic acromegaly**	**Ectopic production of growth hormone-releasing hormone (GHRH)** is the predominant cause of ectopic acromegaly The cancers associated with **ectopic acromegaly include carcinoid tumors of the bronchus, pancreatic islet cell tumors, and cancers of the lung, breast, colon and adrenal glands.**

• **Gynecomastia**	**Ectopic production of hCG** is the most common cause of paraneoplastic gynecomastia; **hepatoma or a germ cell tumor with choriocarcinoma** elements contains aromatase enzyme activity that converts circulating androgens to estrogen. Other tumors rarely associated with ectopic gynecomastia include **carcinoid tumors of the bronchus, intestine, and small cell lung cancer** About 5% of men with **testicular choriocarcinoma** present with an enlarging breast mass.
• **Non-islet cell tumor hypoglycemia**	Can occur with large, slow-growing **sarcomas, mesotheliomas, and hepatomas.**

USMLE Case Scenario

A 55-year-old man visits his family doctor after his friend from New York, who has not seen him for 15 years, notices a change in his appearance. Overgrowth of his frontal bones and enlargement of his hands and feet have occurred. The patient complains of a tingling sensation in the 1st, 2nd, and 3rd digits of the right hand and loss of coordination and strength of the right thumb. He is most likely having Acromegaly.

Hematologic Syndromes

• **Erythrocytosis**	Renal cell cancer, 10% of patients with hepatoma, and 15% of patients with cerebellar hemangioblastomas have erythrocytosis
• **Granulocytosis**	Tumors and tumor cell lines from patients with lung, ovarian, and bladder cancers have been documented to produce granulocyte colony-stimulating factor (G-CSF), granulocyte-macrophage colony-stimulating factor (GM-CSF)
• **Thrombocytosis**	Lung and gastrointestinal cancers, 20% of patients with breast, endometrial, and ovarian cancers, and 10% of patients with lymphoma
• **Eosinophilia**	Eosinophilia is present in 10% of patients with lymphoma, 3% of patients with lung cancer, and occasional patients with cervical, gastrointestinal, renal, and breast cancer
• **Thrombophlebitis**	Lung, pancreatic, gastrointestinal, breast, ovarian, and genitourinary cancers, lymphomas, and brain tumors

Medical Oncology

Cytotoxic	Mechanism of action	Adverse effects
• **Vincristine**	**Inhibits formation of microtubules**	**Peripheral neuropathy (reversible)**
• **Cisplatin**	**Causes cross-linking in DNA**	**Ototoxicity, peripheral neuropathy**
• **Bleomycin**	**Degrades preformed DNA**	**Lung fibrosis**
• **Doxorubicin**	**Stabilizes DNA—topoisomerase II complex inhibits DNA and RNA synthesis**	**Cardiomyopathy**
• **Methotrexate**	**Inhibits purine synthesis**	**Myelosuppression, mucositis**
• **Cyclophosphamide**	**Alkylating agent—causes cross-linking in DNA**	**Hemorrhagic cystitis, myelosuppression**

TREATMENT-RELATED ONCOLOGICAL EMERGENCIES

Tumor Lysis Syndrome

Tumor lysis syndrome is a well-recognized clinical entity that is characterized by various combinations of:

- **Hyperuricemia**
- **Hyperkalemia**
- **Hyperphosphatemia**
- **Lactic acidosis and**
- **Hypocalcemia**

Frequently, acute renal failure develops as a result of the syndrome.

Human Antibody Infusion Reactions

The initial infusion of human or humanized antibodies **(rituximab)** is associated with fever, chills, nausea, asthenia, and headache in up to half of treated patients. Bronchospasm and hypotension occur in 1% of patients. The pathogenesis is thought to be activation of immune effector processes (cells and complement).

Hemolytic Uremic Syndrome

Hemolytic uremic syndrome (HUS) and, less commonly, thrombotic thrombocytopenic purpura (TTP) occurring after treatment with antineoplastic drugs have been described. **Mitomycin** is by far the most common agent causing this peculiar syndrome. Other chemotherapeutic agents, including **cisplatin, bleomycin, and gemcitabine,** have also been reported to be associated with this syndrome.

Neutropenia and Infection

These remain the **most common serious complications** of cancer therapy.

Pulmonary Infiltrates

Patients with cancer may present with **dyspnea associated with diffuse interstitial infiltrates on chest radiographs**. Such infiltrates may be due to progression of the underlying malignancy, treatment-related toxicities, infection, and/or unrelated diseases. The cause may be **multifactorial.**

Typhlitis

Neutropenic enterocolitis (Typhlitis) is a **necrosis of the cecum and adjacent colon** that may complicate the treatment of acute leukemia. The patient develops **right lower quadrant abdominal pain**, often with **rebound tenderness and a tense, distended abdomen, in a setting of fever and neutropenia**

Watery diarrhea (often containing sloughed mucosa) and bacteremia are common, and bleeding may occur).

Hemorrhagic Cystitis

Hemorrhagic cystitis can develop in patients receiving **cyclophosphamide and ifosfamide**. Both drugs are metabolized to **'Acrolein'** which is a strong chemical irritant that is excreted in the urine. Prolonged contact or high concentrations may lead to **bladder irritation and hemorrhage**. Symptoms include **gross hematuria, frequency, dysuria, burning, urgency, incontinence, and nocturia**. Maintaining a high rate of urine flow minimizes exposure. In addition, **'2-Mercaptoethane sulfonate' (Mesna)** detoxifies the metabolites and can be coadministered with the instigating drugs.

MUSCLE DISORDERS

Toxic Myopathies

Drugs and chemicals may produce focal or generalized damage to skeletal muscle

- The most common cause of focal damage is the injection of narcotic analgesics. Three agents in particular: **pentazocine, meperidine, and heroin**
- **D-Penicillamine** induces a condition simulating the clinical and pathologic picture of polymyositis. A similar condition has been reported with cimetidine
- **Procainamide** may cause myositis as part of a systemic lupus erythematosus-like reaction
- **Chloroquine** administration may cause a vacuolar myopathy
- **Zidovudine**, used in the treatment of AIDS, produces proximal weakness and pain
- Fibric acid derivatives **(clofibrate, gemfibrozil)**, 3-hydroxy-methyl-glutaryl-coenzyme A reductase inhibitors **(lovastatin, simivastatin, pravastatin)**, and **niacin** have all been implicated in myopathies, **occasionally**
- **Emetine hydrochloride** (used for treatment of amebiasis).

- **E-aminocaproic acid** (an antifibrinolytic agent) and
- **Perhexiline** (used for angina pectoris) have all been observed to cause muscle weakness and muscle fiber necrosis after several weeks of therapy
- Drug-induced myopathy accompanied by proximal weakness occurs with **glucocorticoid therapy**
- **Excess alcohol** intake causes acute muscle weakness with rhabdomyolysis and ↑CPK
- **Steroid myopathy mainly involves pelvis**
- A very serious drug-induced condition, **malignant hyperthermia** occurs in susceptible individuals after exposure to certain general anesthetic and depolarizing muscle relaxants.

Polymyositis

PM is a subacute inflammatory myopathy affecting adults, and rarely children, who do not have any of the following:

- **No rash**
- **No involvement of the extraocular and facial muscles**
- **No family history of a neuromuscular disease**
- **No cutaneous manifestations**
- **No history of exposure to myotoxic drugs or toxins**
- **No endocrinopathy**
- **No neurogenic disease**
- **No muscular dystrophy**

No biochemical muscle disorder (deficiency of a muscle enzyme), or PM may occur either in isolation, in association with a systemic autoimmune or connective tissue disease, or with known viral or bacterial infection

Proximal limb muscles are involved

Pharyngeal muscles are involved

Pain is a feature

Focal necrosis on biopsy is seen

CPK is increased

Inclusion Body Myositis

- **Weakness and atrophy of distal muscles**, especially foot extensors and deep finger flexors, occur
- Patients present with falls because their knees collapse due to early quadriceps weakness
- The diagnosis is always made by the characteristic findings on the muscle biopsy
- Disease progression is slow but steady, and most patients require an assistive device such as cane, walker, or wheelchair within several years of onset.

USMLE Case Scenario

A 69-year-old man from Ohio presents with muscle weakness and difficulty swallowing. On neurological examination, he has proximal and distal upper and lower limb weakness. Antibody profile is normal. There is wasting of the intrinsic muscles of the fingers and thigh muscles. CK is elevated and EMG findings are consistent with a myopathic process. Most likely diagnosis is: Inclusion Body Myositis

Duchenne's Muscular Dystrophy

- In Duchenne's muscular dystrophy, inheritance **is X-linked Recessive**
- Defect lies in **Dystrophin gene** and results in absence of dystrophin protein
- Onset is typically below **5 years of age**

- **Sarcolemal protein** defect
- Proximal limb muscles are involved and **pseudohypertrophy** of these muscles occurs
- Patient on standing tries to climb on himself **(Gowers' sign)**
- Characteristic pathological features are:
  - **Necrosis of muscle fibers**
  - **Muscle fibers of varying size**
  - **Fibrosis**
  - **Fatty infiltration**

The **less severe** form is the **Becker's dystrophy**

Features are:

- **Less common**
- **Less severe**
- **Not absence but decreased and altered dystrophin protein**
- **Later onset**
- **Cardiac involvement is rare**
- **May have normal lifespan**

Other Muscular Dystrophies

Facioscapulohumeral (Landouzy-Dejerine) muscular dystrophy:

- It is an **autosomal dominant** form characterized by weakness of the facial muscles and shoulder girdles, usually beginning at age 7 to 20 years
- Difficulty with whistling, eye closure, and elevation of the arms are early symptoms
- Anterior tibial and peroneal weakness develops in some kindreds and although foot drop develops, ambulation is rarely lost. Life expectancy is normal.

Limb-girdle Muscular Dystrophy: Describes patients with weakness of:

- Pelvis **(Leyden-Möbius [pelvifemoral] type)** and
- Shoulder **(Erb [scapulohumeral] type)** girdles

Mitochondrial myopathies are inherited through **maternal, non-Mendelian inheritance**

Some mitochondrial myopathies cause only progressive external ophthalmoplegia (ocular myopathy); others also cause patients to develop limb weakness and multisystem disorders, predominantly involving brain and muscle

Diagnosis is made either by finding biochemical abnormalities of mitochondria or **'ragged red fibers'** in muscle biopsy specimens stained with modified Gomori's trichrome stain.

Congenital myopathies have been named by their characteristic findings on muscle biopsy:

Central core disease

Centronuclear myopathy

Nemaline myopathy

These children present with delayed walking and mild proximal muscle weakness that is not progressive

The biochemical defect is unknown

Myotonic dystrophy (Steinert's disease)

- It is an **autosomal dominant** disorder that combines dystrophic muscular weakness with myotonia
- The gene for this disorder has been **localized to Chromosome 19q.** It occurs at any age and is variable in severity
- Myotonia is prominent in the hand muscles, and ptosis is common even in mildly affected individuals

- Severe cases show marked peripheral muscular weakness associated with:
- **High incidence of cataracts**
- **Testicular atrophy NOT ENLARGEMENT**
- **Premature balding**
- **Cardiac muscle conduction defects**
- **Hatchet facies, and endocrine abnormalities, i.e. diabetes mellitus**
- **Mental retardation** occurs frequently
- It is a **trinucleotide repeat disorder**
- Mostly affects **type 1 Fibers**
- Typically involves **Distal Muscles**

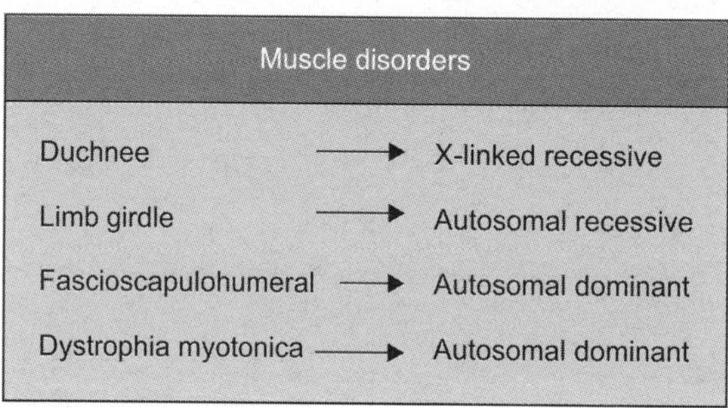

Pattern of inheritance

Calcium Channel Disorders of Muscle

- **Hypokalemic periodic paralysis**
- **Familial hemiplegic migrane**
- **Spinocerebellar ataxia-6**

Hypokalemic Periodic Paralysis (hypoKPP)

- Causes episodic weakness, which usually affects proximal limb muscles more than distal ones
- Rarely ocular, bulbar, or respiratory muscles are affected
- Respiratory muscle weakness may prove fatal
- Meals high in carbohydrate or sodium can provoke attacks
- Reflexes become hypoactive, and cardiac arrhythmias may occur during attacks owing to low serum potassium. Onset is at adolescence
- Men are more often affected because of decreased penetrance in women. Some women have only infrequent attacks
- Diagnosis is established by demonstrating a low serum potassium level during a paralytic attack and by excluding secondary causes of hypokalemia
- The molecular defect in the calcium channel can be defined in many patients
- The acute paralysis improves after the administration of potassium salts. Oral KCl (0.2 to 0.4 mmol/kg) should be given to patients with severe weakness and repeated at 15- to 30-min intervals depending on the response of the ECG, serum potassium level, and muscle strength.

Sodium Channel Disorders of Muscle

Hyperkalemic Periodic Paralysis (hyperKPP)

- Causes episodic weakness of limb muscles; cranial and respiratory muscles are rarely involved
- The term 'hyperkalemic' is misleading, since patients are often normokalemic during attacks
- Paresthesias and muscle pain are present during many attacks.

- Diagnosis is suggested by a modest elevation of the serum potassium level during attacks in nearly half of patients; at times, however, the serum potassium level is normal or even low. The so-called hyperkalemic and normokalemic forms of this disorder are not separate entities
- **Paramyotonia Congenita** Paramyotonia congenita (PC) causes attacks of paralysis either spontaneously or with cold provocation. PC with periodic paralysis is similar to hyperKPP, except that paradoxical myotonia (i.e. myotonia worsening with activity) and objective cold sensitivity are more prominent in PC
- **Potassium-aggravated Myotonia** Some patients with muscle sodium channel defects have severe muscle stiffness but no paralytic episodes. The stiffness is accentuated by elevations in serum potassium levels.

CHLORIDE CHANNEL DISORDERS OF MUSCLE

Myotonia Congenita

Myotonia congenita (Thomsen's disease):

It is a rare, **autosomal dominant** myotonia that begins usually in infancy. The myotonia produces symptoms most troublesome in the hands, legs, and eyelids

Weakness is usually minimal

Muscles may become hypertrophied, but muscle stiffness is the most important problem

Diagnosis usually is established by the characteristic physical appearance, by **inability to relax the handgrip rapidly after opening and closing the hand, and by sustained muscle contraction after direct muscle percussion**

The myotonic phenomenon causes a typical **dive-bomber sound** in electromyography studies

Family pedigrees are important.

Myasthenia Gravis (MG)

- A disease characterized by **episodic muscle weakness, chiefly in muscles innervated by cranial nerves, and characteristically improved by cholinesterase-inhibiting drugs**
- The disease is caused by an **autoimmune attack on the acetylcholine receptor of the postsynaptic neuromuscular junction**, resulting in loss or dysfunction of acetylcholine receptors and jeopardizing normal neuromuscular transmission
- Dercreased myoneural junction transmission
- The disease **predominates in women**, most commonly presents between 20 and 40 years of age, but may occur at any age
- **Neonatal myasthenia** is a syndrome of generalized muscle weakness seen in 12% of infants born to MG mothers because of passive transfer of Abs through the placenta. Symptoms resolve as the Ab titer declines in days to weeks
- **Congenital myasthenia** is a rare autosomal recessive disorder of neuromuscular transmission beginning in childhood, usually with ophthalmoplegia. Since acetylcholine-receptor Abs are absent, the disease is not regarded as autoimmune
- **The most common symptoms are ptosis, diplopia, and muscle fatigability after exercise.** Ocular muscles are affected first in 40% of patients and eventually in 85%
- **Dysarthria, dysphagia, and proximal limb weakness** are common
- **Sensory modalities and deep tendon reflexes are normal**
- **Pyridostigmine** or **neostigmine** are the most commonly used cholinergic drugs
- **Thymectomy** is indicated in most patients with generalized MG; 80% will subsequently remit or require less maintenance drug. If a thymoma is found, excision is adviced to prevent spread within the mediastinum

Should be done in all cases

- **Plasmapheresis** may be useful to prepare refractory patients for thymectomy and during respiratory crisis. During severe crisis, ventilating support should be given along with IV feeding and withdrawal of anticholinesterase therapy

REMEMBER

- It is done for myasthenia crisis and not cholinergic crisis
- Myasthenia gravis is one condition in **which biopsy is not specific for diagnosis**
- **ENMG is more diagnostic**. Decremental response is seen to repetitive nerve stimuli
- Role of muscle biopsy is limited. Inflammatory lymphorrhages and nonspecific atrophy are seen.

GIT

• **Migratory glossitis**	**Geographic tongue**
• **Atrophic glossitis**	**Iron deficiency**
• **Leutic glossitis**	**Syphilis**

Esophagitis

Most common causes are:
- **Reflux esophagitis (mc)**
- Infectious esophagitis
- Eosinophilic esophagitis
- Drug-induced esophagitis
- Radiation esophagitis
- Corrosive esophagitis

Plummer-Vinson Syndrome

- **Also called the Paterson-Brown-Kelly syndrome or sideropenic dysphagia**
- Describes young women with **koilonychias, iron-deficiency anemia and dysphagia** referred high in the neck
  - Commonest type of esophageal carcinoma: Squamous cell carcinoma
  - Commonest site of squamous cell carcinoma: Lower end of esophagus
  - Commonest feature of achalasia cardia: Dysphagia
  - Commonest feature of cancer esophagus: Progressive dysphagia
  - Difficulty in swallowing: Dysphagia
  - Pain during swallowing: Odynophagia

The metaplasia of esophageal squamous epithelium to columnar epithelium (Barrett's esophagus) is a complication of severe reflux esophagitis, and it is a risk factor for esophageal adenocarcinoma

Barrett's epithelium progresses through a dysplastic stage before developing into adenocarcinoma.

- Multiple sacculations and diverticulae with **corckscrew esophagus**: **diffuse esophageal spasm**
- **Rat tail esophagus** with dilated proximal and narrow distal end: **achalasia**
- **Narrow and irregular** esophageal lume: **esophageal cancer**
- **Stricture/ulcer in esophagus**: esophageal reflux—**GERD**

- **Initial investigation for dysphagia for solid food is barium swallow**
- **Best investigation for dysphagia for solid food is endoscopy**
- **Best investigation for dysphagia for solid and liquid food is manometry.**

Gastritis

The term **gastritis** should be reserved for histologically documented inflammation of the gastric mucosa

- **Acute Gastritis:** The most common causes of acute gastritis are infectious. Acute infection with ***H. pylori*** induces gastritis
- **Chronic Gastritis** is identified histologically by an inflammatory cell infiltrate consisting primarily of lymphocytes and plasma cells, with very scant neutrophil involvement. Chronic gastritis is also classified according to the predominant site of involvement
- **Type A** refers to the body-predominant form (**autoimmune**) and
- **Type B** is the central-predominant form **(*H. pylori*-related)**
- **The AB gastritis** has been used to refer to a **mixed antral/body picture**

- **Lymphocytic gastritis** is characterized histologically by intense infiltration of the surface epithelium with lymphocytes. The infiltrative process is primarily in the body of the stomach and consists of mature T cells and plasmacytes
- A subgroup of patients has thickened folds noted on endoscopy. These folds are often capped by small nodules that contain a central depression or erosion; this form of the disease is called **Varioliform gastritis**
- Marked eosinophilic infiltration involving any layer of the stomach (mucosa, muscularis propria, and serosa) is characteristic of **Eosinophilic gastritis**
- Several systemic disorders may be associated with **Granulomatous gastritis.** Gastric involvement has been observed in **Crohn's disease**. Involvement may range from granulomatous infiltrates noted only on gastric biopsies to frank ulceration and stricture formation. Gastric Crohn's disease usually occurs in the presence of small intestinal disease. Several rare infectious processes can lead to granulomatous gastritis, including histoplasmosis, candidiasis, syphilis, and tuberculosis.

Menetrier's Disease

- Menetrier's disease characterized by **large, tortuous gastric mucosal folds**
- The mucosal folds in Menetrier's disease are often most **prominent in the body and fundus**
- Histologically, massive foveolar hyperplasia (hyperplasia of surface and glandular mucous cells) is noted, which **replaces most of the chief and parietal cells**
- **Protein-losing enteropathy is common**
- **Gastric acid secretion is not increased**
- **Premalignant: Increased risk of adenocarcinoma**
- Hyperplasia and hypertrophy produce the prominent folds observed
- The pits of the gastric glands elongate and may become extremely tortuous
- Although the lamina propria may contain a mild chronic inflammatory infiltrate, Menetrier's disease is **not considered a form of gastritis.**

Schindler's Disease

- **Acid hypersecretion**
- **Giant rugae**
- **Normal protein balance**

H. pylori

H. pylori accounts for most of the peptic ulcer cases

More **prevalent in developing countries**

- It is a gram-negative bacillus
- **Microaerophilic**
- **Urease-producing**
- pH-gated urea channel in *H. pylori* bacterium is called **Urel**

Causes

- Gastritis
- Gastric Ca
- Gastric lymphoma
- Peptic ulcer disease

Extragastric diseases in which *H. pylori* is believed to play a role:

- Ischemic heart diseases
- Coronary atherosclerosis
- Idiopathic thrombocytopenic purpura

- Iron-deficiency anemia
- Hepatocellular carcinoma
- Cholangiocarcinoma
- Inflammatory Bowel diseases
- Raynaud's Phenomenon

Tests for *H. pylori:* Endoscopy-based biopsy urease test
- **Histology**
- **Culture**
- **Urea breath test (Documenting eradication)**
- **Serological test (Epidemiological)**
- **Stool antigen test**

Treatments to of *Helicobacter pylori are*:
- **Clarithromycin**
- **Bismuth subsalicylate**
- **Metronidazole**

Duodenal Ulcer	Gastric Ulcer
• **More** common • More associated with ***H. pylori*** • **Early age** of onset • Occur most often in the **first portion of duodenum**), with ~90% located within 3 cm of the pylorus • **Usually < 1 cm in diameter** • **Less chances of malignancy** • **No loss** of weight • Tenderness usually **in R Hypochondrium** • Night pain **common**	• Less common • Associated with *H. pylori* • Later age of onset • Occur most often in the lesser curvature • More chances of malignancy • Loss of weight • Tenderness usually midline • Night pain uncommon

- Gastric ulcers associated with **normal or ↓ acid output**
- *H. pylori* is more important as a cause of **duodenal ulcer**
- **Family history** is more important in duodenal ulcer
- Stress ulcers after head trauma: **Cushings ulcer**
- Commonest site for Cushings ulcer: distal duodenum
- Commonest site of peptic ulcer: first part of duodenum
- Stress ulcers after burns: **Curling's ulcer**
- **Most common complication of peptic ulcer—Hemorrhage**

GI BLEEDING: CAUSES
ABCDEFGHI

- **Angiodysplasia**
- **Bowel cancer**
- **Colitis**
- **Diverticulitis/Duodenal ulcer**
- **Epistaxis/Esophageal (cancer, esophagitis, varices)**
- **Fistula (anal, aortoenteric)**
- **Gastric (cancer, ulcer, gastritis)**
- **Hemorrhoids**
- **Infectious diarrhea/IBD/Ischemic bowel**

- **Hematemesis indicates an upper GI source of bleeding** (above the ligament of Treitz). Melena indicates that blood has been present in the GI tract for at least 14 h. Thus, the more proximal the bleeding site, the more likely melena will occur
- **Hematochezia usually represents a lower GI source of bleeding**, although an upper GI lesion may **bleed** so rapidly that blood does not remain in the bowel long enough for melena to develop
- **GIB of obscure origin.** Obscure GIB is defined as recurrent acute or chronic bleeding for which no source has been identified by routine endoscopic and contrast studies. Push enteroscopy, with a specially designed enteroscope or a pediatric colonoscope to inspect the entire duodenum and part of the jejunum, is generally the next step. Push enteroscopy may identify probable bleeding sites in 20 to 40% of patients with obscure GIB. If enteroscopy is negative or unavailable, a specialized radiographic examination of the small bowel (e.g. enteroclysis) should be performed
- **Occult GIB** is manifested by either a **positive test for fecal occult blood or iron-deficiency anemia**
- **Peptic ulcers are the most common cause of UGIB**, accounting for about 50% of cases. **Mallory-Weiss tears** account for 5 to 15% of cases. **Hemorrhagic or erosive gastropathy** [e.g. due to nonsteroidal anti-inflammatory drugs (NSAIDs) or alcohol] and erosive esophagitis often cause mild UGIB, but major bleeding is rare.

MALABSORPTION

Tropical Sprue

Tropical sprue: Malabsorptive disease in tropical regions with unknown etiology
Similar features to celiac sprue and responds to antibiotics, Vitamin B12, Folate.

Whipple's Disease

Whipple's disease: Malabsorptive disease caused by Tropheryma whippeli

- PAS positive, rod-shaped bacilli fill lamina propria, **Tropheryma whipelli**
- Biopsy is specific test
- **Malabsorption, fever, lymphadenopathy, arthralgia**
- **CNS involvement with dementia, seizures, coma, myoclonus**
- Treatment is with antibiotics
- **Trimethoprim sulfamethaxozole**

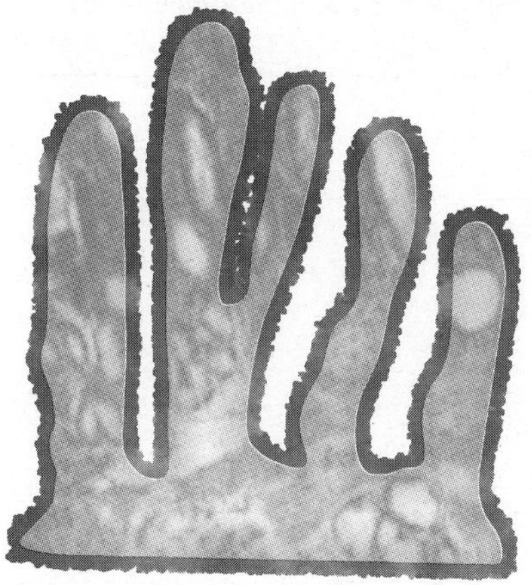

Normal jujenum

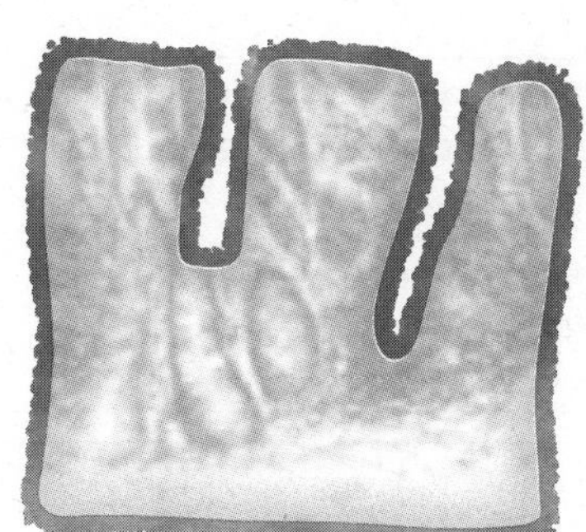

Villous atrophy

- Treatment is with antibiotics
- **Trimethoprim sulfamethoxazole**

Celiac Disease

Celiac disease: It is caused by **sensitivity to the protein gluten**. Repeated exposure leads to villous atrophy which, in turn, causes malabsorption. Conditions associated with celiac disease include dermatitis herpetiformis (a vesicular, pruritic skin eruption) and autoimmune disorders

- **Type 1 diabetes mellitus**
- **Autoimmune hepatitis**
- **Myasthenia gravis**
- **Sjogren's syndrome**
- **Lymphomas, Addison's, Grave's disease**
- **Diagnosis is made by a combination of immunology and jejunal biopsy. Villous atrophy and immunology should reverse on a gluten-free diet. Immunology:**
  - **Anti-endomyseal antibody**
  - **Alpha-gliadin antibody**
  - **TTG (tissue transglutinamise) antibodies**
  - **Anti-casein antibodies are also found in some patients**
- **Jejunal biopsy shows:**
  - **Villous atrophy**
  - Crypt **hyperplasia**
  - Increase in intraepithelial **lymphocytes**
  - Lamina propria infiltration with **lymphocytes**
  - Thickness of mucosa **unaltered.**

In Nutshell

- **Celiac sprue** is gluten-sensitive enteropathy or **nontropical sprue**
- Hypersensitivity to gluten/gliadin occurs with loss of villi and malabsorption
- **RICE is safe to use**
- Genetic predisposition: **HLA B8, DR 3 and DQ**
- **Pathology:** Loss of villi, increased intraepithelial lymphocytes
- Increased plasma cells in lamina propria
- **Presentation: Malabsorption, abdominal distension, bloating, diarrhea, steatorrhea, weight loss**
- Association with **dermatitis herpetiformis.**

Tests for GIT

- **Gastric analysis with pentagastrin stimulation: Zollinger-Ellison Syndrome**
- **Serum level of Vitamin B12: Pernicious anemia**
- **Lactose tolerance test: Milk intolerance**
- **Bile acid breath Test: Blind loop syndrome**
- **Urea breath test: *H. pylori* infection**
- **Secretin test: Pancreatic exocrine insufficiency**

Bloody diarrhea

- Salmonella
- Shigella
- Yersinia
- EIEC
- Campylobacter jejuni

Ulcerative Colitis	Crohn's disease
Involves rectum always	Involves ileum mostly
May cause **'pancolitis'** **Diffuse involvement**	Nondiffuse involvement Called **'regional enteritis'**
Retrograde spread to ileum is **backwash ileitis**	
Disease of continuity	Skip lesions
Pseudopolyps present	Pseudopolyps absent
Limited to mucosa and submucosa	**Transmural** inflammation
Noncaseating granulomas not seen	**Noncaseating granulomas** seen
Creeping fat not seen	Creeping fat seen
Strictures, ulcerations, fistula less frequent	Strictures, ulcerations, fistula frequent
Toxic megacolon occurs	Rare
Malignant transformation +++	Malignant transformation +

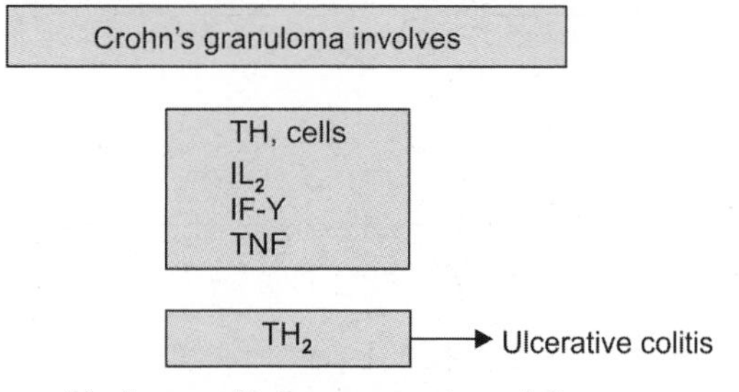

Mediators of inflammatory bowel diseases

- **Antisachromycies cereviase antibody: Crohn's disease**
- **p ANCA: more in favor of ulcerative colitis**
- **Antiendomyseal antibody: Celiac sprue**

Mainstay of therapy for inflammatory bowel diseases: 5 aminosalicylic acid

- **Sulfasalazine, olsalazine, mesolaminate also used**

Other drugs used:

- **Methotrexate**
- **Azathioprine**
- **Cyclosporine**
- **Cyclophosphamide**

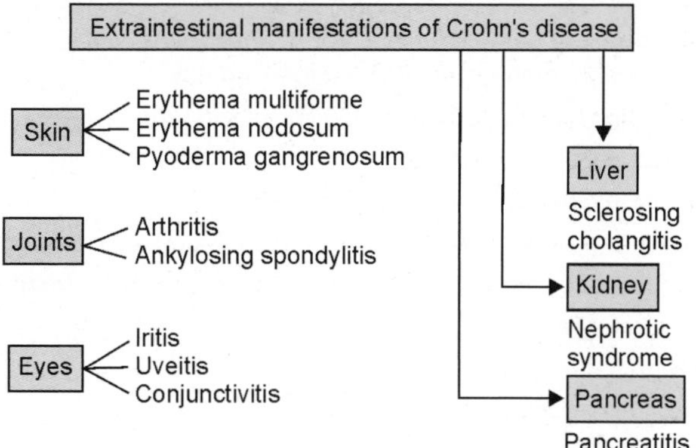

Extraintestinal manifestations of Crohn's disease

- **Multiple, longitudinal, oval ulcers, along antimesenteric border:** typhoid ulcers
- **Ulcers that heal; without scarring:** typhoid ulcers
- **Classical flask-shaped ulcers:** amebic ulcer

Verner-Morrison Syndrome

WDHA Syndrome

Pancreatic cholera is due to **increased secretion of VIP, GIP**

Delta cell tumor causes pancreatic cholera which is not an infective condition but simulates cholera due to increased secretion of water and salt

Diarrhea, weight loss and flushing occur

Electrolyte abnormalities include:

- **Hypokalemia**
- **Hypochlorrhydia**
- **Hyperglycemia**
- **'Hypercalcemia' and not Hypocalcemia**

VIRAL HEPATITIS

Incubation period

- Hepatitis A – incubation period 2–6 weeks
- Hepatitis B4 – 8 weeks
- Hepatitis C2 – 22 weeks
- Hepatitis D4 – 8 weeks
- Hepatitis E2 – 9 weeks

- Hepatitis B is a **DNA virus**; all others are RNA virus
- **P GENE** codes reverse transcriptase of Hepatitis B virus
- Spreads by feco-oral route—**Hepatitis A and E**
- Spreads by percutaneous route—**Hepatitis B, C and D**
- Hepatitis B also spreads by vertical and sexual route—most common
- Oncogenicity present in Hepatitis B especially after neonatal infection
- **Carrier state** present in Hepatitis B
- Hepatitis B virus may present in blood and other body fluids and excretions, such as saliva, breast milk, semen, vaginal secretions, urine, bile, etc
- Feces not known to be infectious
- **HBsAg** is the **first viral marker to appear in blood** after infection; it remains in circulation throughout icteric course of disease. In a typical case, it disappear within roughly 2 months but may last for 6 months
- HBcAg is not demonstrable in circulation but antibody, anti-HBe appears in serum a week or two after appearance of HbSAg
- **Anti-HbeAg** is the **antibody marker** to be seen in blood
- HBeAg (HB envelop antigen) appears in blood concurrently with HBsAg
- **HbeAg** is an indicator of intrahepatic viral replication and its presence in blood indicates **high infectivity**
- For diagnosis of HBV infection, simultaneous presence of IgM, HBC indicates **recent infection**
- And presence of **IgG; anti H-Be** indicates **remote** infection
- Hepatitis B is associated with **PAN**
- **Interferon, lamuvidine, adefovir** are used in treatment of Hepatitis B
- **Type E hepatitis:** enterically transmitted.

- **MC cause of sporadiac cases of hepatitis in adults: Hepatitis E**
- **Worst prognosis in pregnancy: Hepatitis E**
- **Most common route of spread of Hepatitis E is feco-oral**
- Non A–non B hepatitis caused by **Hepatitis C virus**
- **Interferon + ribavarin combinations are used for hepatitis C**
- Hepatitis most prone to chronicity: hepatitis C
- Hepatitis C is associated with:
- **Cryoglobinemia**
- **PAN**
- **Sjögren's syndrome**
- **Diabetes mellitus**
- **Throioditis**
- **Non-Hodgkin's lymphoma**
- **Glomerulonephritis**
- **Lichenoid eruption**
- **Arthritis**

HDV

- HDV is **'defective'** because it **does not have genes for its proteins**
- HDV **can replicate in cells only infected with HBV**
- HDV **uses surface antigen of HBV (HBsAg) as its envelop protein**
- HBV is a **helper virus for HDV**

- **HDV is an enveloped virus**
- **HDV is an RNA virus**
- **Genome of HDV is small and encodes only one protein—the delta antigen**
- **HDV genome is a ribozyme, i.e. has ability to self-cleave and self-ligate**
- **Infection with Hepatitis D can be prevented by vaccinating susceptible persons with Hepatitis B vaccine.**

Fitz-Hugh-Curtis Syndrome

- Fitz-Hugh-Curtis syndrome is a condition in which **bacteria, usually from a pelvic infection, spread through the abdomen and cause inflammation of the tissue surrounding the liver.** It occurs in 15–30% of women with pelvic inflammatory disease (PID), but may also occur in women without PID, and in men
- In Fitz-Hugh-Curtis syndrome, the inflammation of the liver tissue leads to the (adhesions) between the outside of the liver and the inside of the abdomen. In some individuals, these adhesions cause no symptoms. Others have severe pain in the **upper right part of the abdomen**, over the gallbladder. The pain may move to the right shoulder. Sometimes the pain increases with coughing, sneezing, or movement. Since the source of Fitz-Hugh-Curtis syndrome is most often a pelvic infection, symptoms such as nausea, vomiting, chills, fever, and headaches may be present
- **Diagnosis:** The presence of a pelvic infection would also provide a clue to the diagnosis, but without PID, the diagnosis may be difficult, since many conditions can cause abdominal pain. **In women, cervical cultures for two particular pelvic infections need to be done. Chlamydia and gonorrhea** are the most common causes of Fitz-Hugh-Curtis syndrome. If infection is present, the white blood cell (WBC) count in the blood will be high, as will the erythrocyte sedimentation rate (ESR)
- **Laparoscopy confirms diagnosis:** The physician can see the adhesions on the outside of the liver, which have a typical stringy look **(called 'violin-string' adhesions).**

Budd-Chiari Syndrome: (5 Ps)

- **Polycythemia vera**
- **Pregnancy**
- **Postpartum**
- **Pills (OCP)**
- **PNH**
- **Hepatocellular cancer**

- **Caplan's syndrome: Pneumoconiosis+rheumatiod arthritis**
- **Felty's syndrome: Rheumatiod arthritis+splenomegaly+**

Cholestasis is reflected by:

- **↑Alkaline phosphatase**
- **↑5 nucleotidase**
- **↑GGT**

Wilson's Disease

- It is an **AR** disorder
- Chromosome **13** is involved
- The diagnosis is confirmed by the demonstration of either:
  - A serum ceruloplasmin level < 20 mg/dl and Kayser-Fleischer rings or
  - A serum ceruloplasmin level < 20 mg/dl and a concentration of copper in a liver biopsy sample > 250 μg/g dry weight or
  - Most symptomatic patients excrete >100 μg copper per day in urine and have histologic abnormalities on liver biopsy

Pathognomonic features are:

- **Hepatic dysfunction:** Jaundice, Hepatomegaly, Cirrhosis, Portal hypertension, Hepatitis occur
- **Eye Changes:** Brownish or grayish **Kayser-Fleisher ring in Descement's membrane in cornea**
- These golden deposits of copper in Descemet's membrane of the cornea do not interfere with vision but indicate that copper has been released from the liver and has probably caused brain damage
- If a patient with frank neurologic or psychiatric disease does not have Kayser-Fleischer rings when examined by a trained observer using a slit lamp, the diagnosis of Wilson's disease can be excluded
- Rarely, Kayser-Fleischer rings may be accompanied by **sunflower cataracts**
- **The neurologic manifestations** include resting and intention tremors, spasticity, rigidity, chorea, drooling, dysphagia, and dysarthria. Babinski responses may be present, and abdominal reflexes are often absent. **Sensory changes never occur, except for headache**
- **Psychiatric disturbances** are present in most patients with neurologic symptoms. Schizophrenia, manic-depressive psychoses, and classic neuroses may occur, but the commonest disturbances are bizarre behavioral patterns that defy classification

Treatment consists of removing and detoxifying the deposits of copper as rapidly as possible and must be instituted once the diagnosis is secure, whether the patient is ill or asymptomatic

- **Zinc is the DOC**
- **Penicillamine** is administered orally in an initial dose of 1 g daily in single or divided doses at least 30 min before and 2 h after eating
- The dose of **Trientine** is 1 g/d on an empty stomach is more potent than pencillamine and used in patients not tolerating pencillamine

Zinc acetate or gluconate are effective as maintenance therapy, at doses of 150 mg/d of elemental zinc, for patients who are asymptomatic or have improved maximally on penicillamine or trientine.

Disease of C (Wilson's Disease)

- Ceruloplasmin ↓
- Chromosomal involvement
- Copper deposition in hepatocytes
- Chronic active hepatitis
- Cirrhosis
- Changes (Sensory) absent
- Cataract (Sunflower)
- Chorea is a feature
- Corneal Involvement (Kayser-Fleischer Ring)

Hemochromatosis

- It is a common disorder of iron storage
- In which there is an appropriate increase in intestinal iron absorption
- Results in deposition of excessive amounts of iron in parenchymal cells with eventual tissue damage and
- Impaired function of organs, especially the **liver, pancreas, heart, joints, and pituitary**
  - **Hereditary or genetic hemochromatosis:** This disorder is most often caused by inheritance of a **mutant HFE gene**, which is tightly linked to the HLA-A locus on **chromosome 6p**
  - Autosomal dominant
  - **Secondary iron overload:** Tissue injury usually occurs secondary to an **iron-loading anemia** such as thalassemia or **sideroblastic anemia,** in which increased erythropoiesis is ineffective. In the acquired iron-loading disorders, massive iron deposits in parenchymal tissues can lead to the same clinical and pathologic features as in hemochromatosis

In hemochromatosis, **mucosal absorption is inappropriate to body needs and amounts to 4 mg/d or more**. The progressive accumulation of iron causes an:

- **Early elevation in plasma iron**
- **An increased saturation of transferrin, and**
- **Progressive elevation of plasma ferritin level.**

Clinical Manifestations

Initial symptoms include weakness, lassitude, weight loss, change in skin color, abdominal pain, loss of libido, and symptoms of diabetes mellitus

The liver is usually the **first organ to be affected**, and **hepatomegaly** is present in more than 95% of symptomatic patients. **Hepatocellular carcinoma develops in about 30% of patients with cirrhosis, and it is the most common cause of death in treated patients**; hence the importance of early diagnosis and therapy. Its incidence increases with age, is more common in men, and occurs almost exclusively in cirrhotic patients. **Splenomegaly** occurs in approximately half of symptomatic cases

Excessive skin pigmentation is present in over 90% of symptomatic patients at the time of diagnosis. The characteristic **metallic or slate gray** hue is sometimes referred to as bronzing and results from increased melanin and iron in the dermis. Pigmentation usually is diffuse and generalized, but it may be more pronounced on the face, neck, extensor aspects of the lower forearms, dorsa of the hands, lower legs, genital regions, and in scars

Bronze color

Diabetes mellitus is more likely to develop in those with a family history of diabetes, suggesting that direct damage to the pancreatic islets by iron deposition occurs in combination with a genetic predisposition

Bronze Diabetes

Arthropathy develops in 25 to 50% of patients. It usually occurs after age 50, but may occur as a first manifestation, or long after therapy. The joints of the hands, especially **the second and third metacarpophalangeal joints,** which are usually the first joints involved may ensue

Acute brief attacks of synovitis may be associated with deposition of calcium pyrophosphate (chondrocalcinosis or pseudogout), mainly in the knees.

Cardiac involvement is the presenting manifestation in about 15% of patients. The most common manifestation is **congestive heart failure**, which occurs in about 10% of young adults with the disease, especially those with juvenile hemochromatosis

Hypogonadism occurs in both sexes and may antedate other clinical features. Manifestations include **loss of libido, impotence, amenorrhea, testicular atrophy, gynecomastia, and sparse body hair.** These changes are primarily the result of decreased production of gonadotropins due to impairment of hypothalamic-pituitary function by iron deposition; however, primary testicular dysfunction may be seen in some cases. Adrenal insufficiency, hypothyroidism, and hypoparathyroidism may also occur.

Diagnosis

The association of:

1. **Hepatomegaly**
2. **Skin pigmentation**
3. **Diabetes mellitus**
4. **Heart disease**
5. **Arthritis and**
6. **Hypogonadism should suggest the diagnosis**

Transferrin saturation and iron-binding capacity are used as initial screening tests

Treatment: Venesection, Phlebotomy (TOC) and desferroxamine.

Primary Biliary Cirrhosis

- PBC is associated with a variety of disorders, such as **CREST, the sicca syndrome (dry eyes and dry mouth); autoimmune thyroiditis; type 1 diabetes mellitus; and IgA deficiency**
- **IgG antimitochondrial antibody (AMA)** is detected in more than 90% of patients with PBC
- Many patients with PBC are **asymptomatic**, and the disease is initially detected on the basis of ↑ **serum alkaline phosphatase**
- 90% are **women** aged 35 to 60
- **Earliest symptom is pruritus,** which may be either generalized or limited initially to the palms and soles
- Steatorrhea and the malabsorption of lipid-soluble vitamins
- Protracted elevation of serum lipids, especially cholesterol, leads to subcutaneous lipid deposition around the eyes **(xanthelasmas)** and over joints and tendons **(xanthomas)**
- Over a period of months to years, the **itching, jaundice, and hyperpigmentation** slowly worsen. Eventually, signs of **hepatocellular failure and portal hypertension develop** and ascites appears

Laboratory Findings:

- **↑Serum alkaline phosphatase**
- **↑Serum 5-nucleotidase activity and**
- **↑γ-glutamyl transpeptidase levels**
- **Serum bilirubin is usually normal and aminotransferase levels minimally increased**
- The diagnosis is supported by a **positive AMA test**

Treatment: Ursodiol has been shown to improve biochemical and histologic features and might improve survival, particularly liver transplantation-free survival (although this remains unproven)

Secondary Biliary Cirrhosis

- SBC results from **prolonged partial or total obstruction of the common bile duct or its major branches** caused by **postoperative strictures or gallstones.** Chronic pancreatitis may lead to **biliary** stricture and secondary **cirrhosis**
- SBC is also an important complication of **primary sclerosing cholangitis**
- Patients with **malignant tumors of the common bile duct or pancreas** rarely survive long enough to develop SBC
- In children, **congenital biliary atresia and cystic fibrosis** are common causes of SBC.

- **Anti-smooth muscle antibody: Autoimmune hepatitis I**
- **Anti-liver/kidney microsomal antibody: Autoimmune hepatitis II**
- **Anti-mitochondrial antibody: Primary biliary cirrhosis**

- **Angiosarcoma liver:** Vinyl chloride, Aflatoxin, Thorotrast
- **Peliosis hepatitis:** Steroids, Danazol
- **Hepatic vein thrombosis:** OCP, cytotoxic drugs
- **Veno occlusive disease:** Pyrozziline alkaloids, cytotoxic drugs

Spontaneous Bacterial Peritonitis (SBP)

- Patients with ascites and cirrhosis may develop acute bacterial peritonitis without an obvious primary source of infection
- Patients with very advanced **liver** disease are particularly susceptible to SBP
- The ascitic fluid in these patients typically has especially **low concentrations of albumin and other so-called opsonic proteins,** which normally may provide some protection against bacteria
- An ascitic fluid leukocyte count of **500 cells/L (with a proportion of polymorphonuclear leukocytes of 50%) or more than 250 polymorphonuclear leukocytes** should suggest the possibility of bacterial peritonitis while results of bacterial cultures of ascitic fluid are pending
- The presence of **more than 10,000 leukocytes per liter, multiple organisms, or failure to improve after standard therapy for 48 h suggest** that the peritonitis may be secondary to an infection elsewhere in the body.

Carcinoid Syndrome

- **Kulchitsky Type I (typical carcinoid)**
- **Kulchitsky Type II (atypical carcinoid)**
- **Kulchitsky Type III (small cell lung cancer)**
- **'Carcinoid syndrome'** occurs in **less than 10% of patients with carcinoid tumors**

The carcinoid syndrome is encountered **when venous drainage from the tumor gains access to the systemic circulation so that vasoactive secretory substances escape hepatic degradation**

This situation obtains in three circumstances:

1. **When hepatic metastases are present**
2. **When venous blood from extensive retroperitoneal metastases drains into paravertebral veins, and**
3. **When the primary carcinoid tumor is outside the gastrointestinal tract, e.g. a bronchial, ovarian, or testicular tumor**

Hepatorenal Syndrome

Definition and Pathogenesis Hepatorenal syndrome is a serious complication in the patient with cirrhosis and ascites and is characterized by **worsening azotemia with avid sodium retention and oliguria in the absence of identifiable specific causes of renal dysfunction**

- **The kidneys are structurally intact**
- **Urinalysis and pyelography are usually normal**
- **Renal biopsy is also normal, and**
- **Kidneys from** such patients have been used successfully for renal transplantation

Clinical features and diagnosis:

- Worsening azotemia
- Hyponatremia
- Progressive oliguria
- Hypotensions are the hallmarks of the hepatorenal syndrome

This syndrome, which is distinct from prerenal azotemia, may be precipitated by severe gastrointestinal bleeding, sepsis, or overly vigorous attempts at diuresis or paracentesis; it may also occur without an obvious cause.

Hypoxemia and Hepatopulmonary Syndrome

Mild hypoxemia occurs in approximately one-third of patients with chronic **liver** disease

The hepatopulmonary syndrome is typically manifest by **hypoxemia, platypnea, and orthodeoxia**

Hypoxemia usually results from right to left intrapulmonary shunts through dilatations in intrapulmonary vessels that can be detected by **contrast-enhanced echocardiography or a macroaggregated albumin lung perfusion scan.**

Remember

- Commonest cause of lower GI bleed is: Hemorrhoid
- BUT commonest cause of massive bleed per rectum in elderly is diverticulosis
- Hypergastrenemia with hypochlorrydia is a feature of pernicious anemia
- **Clostridium difficile has been associated with Crohn's disease.**

RENAL SYSTEM

Significance of Casts

RBC Casts: Glomerulonephritis
Dysmorphic RBC: Glomerular pathology
WBC Casts: Pyelonephritis
Hyaline Casts: Normal, ARF
Coarse granular casts: ATN
Waxy casts: CRF
Tom Harsfall protein: normal, tubular in origin

Recurrent Gross Hematuria is seen in

- **IgA nephropathy**
- **Alport's syndrome**
- **Thin glomerular basement membrane disease**
- **Hypercalciuria**
- **Urolithiasis**

Prerenal Uremia-Kidneys hold on to sodium to preserve volume

	Prerenal uremia	**Acute tubular necrosis**
Urine sodium	< 20 mmol/L	> 30 mmol/L
Fractional sodium excretion*	< 1%	> 1%
Fractional urea excretion**	< 35%	>35%
Urine: plasma osmolality	> 1.5	< 1.1
Urine: plasma urea	> 10:1	< 8:1
Specific gravity	> 1020	< 1010
Urine	'bland' sediment	brown granular casts
Response to fluid challenge	Yes	No

Seen in CRF are

- **Broad casts in urine**
- **Restless legs**
- **Impotence**
- **Isothenuria**
- **Hypernatremia/hyponatremia**
- **Hypokalemia/hyperkalemia**
- **Hypocalcemia**
- **Hyperurecemia**

Causes of CRF:
- **Membranous GN**
- **Membranoproliferative GN**
- **FSGN**

- Azotemia (High levels of BUN and creatinine)
- Metabolic acidosis
- Hyperkalemia
- Fluid retention **(may cause hypertension, edema, congestive heart failure, and pulmonary edema)**
- Hypocalcemia and hyperphosphatemia **(impaired vitamin D production; bone loss leads to renal osteodystrophy)**
- Anemia (due to lack of erythropoietin; give synthetic erythropoietin to correct)
- Anorexia, nausea, vomiting (from build-up of toxins)
- Central nervous system disturbances **(mental status changes and even convulsions or coma from toxin build-up)**
- Bleeding **(due to disordered platelet function)**
- Uremic pericarditis (friction rub may be heard)
- Skin pigmentation and pruritus **(skin turns yellowish-brown and itches because of metabolic byproducts)**
- Increased susceptibility to infection (due to decreased cellular immunity).

Diabetes Mellitus

Epidemiology	IDDM	NIDDM
Age at onset	Younger, lean patients	Older, obese patients
Heredity	Usually < 25 years	Usually > 40 years
	HLA-DR 3 and/or DR 4 (95%)	No HLA links
	30–50% concordance in identical twins	90% concordance in identical twins
Autoimmunity	Presence of islet cell antibody, Insulin autoantibody. Association with other organ-specific autoimmune diseases	None
	Insulin deficiency	
	May develop ketoacidosis	
	Insulin	
Clinical		Partial insulin deficiency, Insulin resistance
treatment		May develop nonketotic hyperosmolar state
		Weight loss, drugs, insulin sometimes

Remember

- Glucose levels rise in the early morning **(Dawn phenomenon)**
- **Rebound hyperglycemia** may appear from 1/2 to 24 hours after moderate to severe hypoglycemia **(Somogyi phenomenon)**
- **Syndrome X** is a term used to describe a constellation of metabolic derangements that includes insulin resistance, hypertension, dyslipidemia, central or visceral obesity, endothelial dysfunction, and accelerated cardiovascular disease
- Chronic complications can be divided into vascular and nonvascular complications. The vascular complications of DM are further subdivided into:
  - **Microvascular (retinopathy, neuropathy, nephropathy)** and
  - **Macrovascular complications (coronary artery disease, peripheral vascular disease, cerebrovascular disease)**
  - **Nonvascular complications** include problems such as gastroparesis, sexual dysfunction, and skin changes.

RENAL COMPLICATIONS OF DIABETES MELLITUS

- **Diabetic nephropathy is the leading cause of ESRD** and a leading cause of DM-related morbidity and mortality
- Proteinuria in individuals with DM is associated with markedly reduced survival and increased risk of cardiovascular disease
- Individuals with diabetic nephropathy almost always have diabetic retinopathy also

OPHTHALMOLOGIC COMPLICATIONS OF DIABETES MELLITUS

- DM is the leading cause of blindness
- Blindness is primarily the result of progressive diabetic retinopathy and clinically significant macular edema
- Diabetic retinopathy is classified into two stages: nonproliferative and proliferative

NEUROPATHY AND DIABETES MELLITUS

- Diabetic neuropathy occurs in approximately 50% of individuals with long-standing type 1 and type 2 DM
- It may manifest as polyneuropathy, mononeuropathy, and/or autonomic neuropathy
- Development of neuropathy correlates with the duration of diabetes and glycemic control
- The absence of chest pain **(silent ischemia)** is common in individuals with diabetes.

DRUGS IN DIABETES

- **A-Adrenergic blockers** slightly improve insulin **resistance** and positively impact the lipid profile, whereas beta blockers and thiazide diuretics can increase insulin **resistance**
- **Beta blockers** cause masking of hypoglycemic symptoms
- **Central adrenergic antagonists** and vasodilators are lipid- and glucose-neutral

NONALCOHOLIC STEATOHEPATITIS

Nonalcoholic steatohepatitis (NASH) is a term used to describe liver changes similar to those seen in alcoholic hepatitis in the **absence of a history of alcohol abuse**. Associated factors:

- **Obesity**
- **Hyperlipidemia**
- **Type 2 diabetes mellitus**
- **Jejunoileal bypass**
- **Sudden weight loss/starvation**

Features: Usually asymptomatic, hepatomegaly, AST > ALT

MODY

Maturity-onset diabetes of the young (MODY) is characterized by the development of type 2 diabetes mellitus in patients <25 years old. It is typically inherited as an autosomal dominant condition. Over six different genetic mutations have so far been identified as leading to MODY. Ketosis is not a feature at presentation

MODY 2: 20% of cases, due to a defect in the **glucokinase gene**

MODY 3: 60% of cases, due to a defect in the **HNF-1 alpha gene**

Diabetic Nephropathy

Diabetic nephropathy is a clinical syndrome characterized by:

- **Persistent albuminuria (> 300 mg/d or > 200 mcg/min) that is confirmed on at least 2 occasions 3–6 months apart (early test)**
- **A relentless decline in the glomerular filtration rate (GFR)**
- **Elevated arterial blood pressure**
- **HbA1C is used to monitor diabetic control**

Diabetic Nephropathy: Stages

Diabetic nephropathy: Stages

Diabetic nephropathy may be classified as occurring in five stages*:

Stage 1

- Hyperfiltration: increase in GFR
- May be reversible

Stage 2 (silent or latent phase)
- Most patients do not develop microalbuminuria for 10 years
- GFR remains elevated

Stage 3 (incipient nephropathy)
- Microalbuminuria (albumin excretion of 30–300 mg/day, dipstick negative)

Stage 4 (overt nephropathy)
- Persistent proteinuria (albumin excretion > 300 mg/day, dipstick positive)
- Hypertension is present in most patients
- Histology shows diffuse glomerulosclerosis and focal glomerulosclerosis (Kimmelstiel-Wilson nodules)

Stage 5
- End-stage renal disease, GFR typically < 10 ml/min
- Renal replacement therapy needed.

- It is the leading cause of End-stage Renal disease, (ESRD)
- It is more common in blacks with type 2 DM
- Microalbuminuria is the first manifestation of injury to glomerular filtration barrier and predicts nephropathy
- Kidney size is normal or increased
- ACE inhibitors are the drugs of choice as they control both systemic and intraglomerular hypertension
- The determination of microalbuminuria in diabetes mellitus is important as it is the earliest indication of diabetic nephropathy which, left untreated, will eventually lead to end-stage renal disease.
- The pathological changes are identical in Type 1 and 2
- The main changes occur in the glomeruli. Rarely, changes may occur in the renal tubules
- Aggressive and sustained treatment of nephropathy would slow the progression of the condition
- Microalbuminuria is best determined on a 24-hour urine sample
- For convenience, a random sample can also be used and the test done with the Micral Test Strip.

Kimmelstiel-Wilson nodules are characteristic of diabetic nephropathy. 'Nodules of pink hyaline material form in regions of glomerular capillary loops in the glomerulus. This is due to a marked increase in mesangial matrix from damage as a result of non-enzymatic glycosylation of proteins.'

Differences between Nephritic and Nephrotic Syndromes

Nephritic Syndrome	Nephrotic Syndrome
1. Hematuria	1. Severe proteinuria
2. Hypertension	2. Hypoalbuminemia
3. Oliguria	3. Hyperlipidemia
4. Proteinuria	4. Fibrinogen increased
	5. Lipoproteins increased
	6. Low serum calcium
	7. Platelet activation
	8. Decreased HDL

Acute Nephritic Syndrome

- It is characterized by sudden onset (i.e. over days to weeks) of acute renal failure and **oliguria** (< 400 ml of urine per day)
- Renal blood flow and glomerular filtration rate (GFR) fall
- Extracellular fluid volume expansion, **edema**
- **Hypertension develops** because of impaired GFR and enhanced tubular reabsorption of salt and water

- As a result of injury to the glomerular capillary wall, urinalysis typically reveals **red blood cell casts, dysmorphic red blood cells, leukocytes, and subnephrotic proteinuria of < 3.5 g per 24 h (nephritic urinary sediment)**
- Hematuria is often macroscopic.

Glomerulonephritides: Membranous glomerulonephritis

- Presentation: proteinuria/nephrotic syndrome/CRF
- Cause: infections, rheumatoid drugs, malignancy
- Gold, pencillamine
- 1/3 resolve, 1/3 respond to cytotoxics, 1/3 develop CRF

IgA nephropathy aka Berger's disease mesangioproliferative GN

- Typically young adult with hematuria following an URTI
- Patient presents with gross hematuria often **'24 to 48 hrs' after a pharyngeal or GIT infection as compared to poststreptococcal glomerulonephritis which develops '10 days' after pharyngitis and '2 weeks' after skin infection**

Diffuse proliferative glomerulonephritis

- Classical poststreptococcal glomerulonephritis in a child
- Presents as nephritic syndrome/ARF

Minimal change disease (MCD)

- Typically a child with nephrotic syndrome (accounts for 80%)
- Causes: Idiopathic, HIV, Hodgkin's, NSAIDs, rifampicin,interferon alpha
- Good response to steroids
- IgA deposits
- **Fusion of foot processes on EM**
- **No change on light microscopy**
- **Polyanions** contribute to damage
- **Hypertension is not common in MCD**

Focal segmental glomerulosclerosis

- **May be** idiopathic or secondary to HIV, heroin
- **Presentation:** proteinuria/nephrotic syndrome/CRF

Rapidly progressive glomerulonephritis aka crescentic glomerulonephritis

- Rapid onset, often presenting as ARF, crescent formation, nonselective proteinuria

Causes include:

- Poststreptococcal GN
- Goodpasture's
- ANCA positive vasculitis
- SLE
- Infective endocarditis
- HS purpura
- Burger's disease

Mesangiocapillary glomerulonephritis (Membranoproliferative)

- **Type 1:** cryoglobulinemia, hepatitis C
- **Type 2:** partial lipodystrophy

Kidney in HIV

Aggressive form of 'focal segmental glomerulosclerosis' (FSGS) characterizes HIV infection along with microcystic tubular dilatation and interstitial fibrosis.

Viral genome has been detected in glomerular and tubular cells

1. HIV infection is associated with **focal segmental glomerulosclerosis, acute diffuse proliferative glomerulonephritis, and mesangioproliferative glomerulonephritis, including IgA nephropathy, MPGN, and membranous glomerulopathy**
2. The **'classic and most common' HIV-associated glomerulopathy** is an **'aggressive form of focal segmental glomerulosclerosis'**, an entity that is termed as HIV-associated nephropathy (HIVAN)
3. This disease may be the **first manifestation of infection** in otherwise asymptomatic patients. HIVAN is **more common in blacks** than in other ethnic groups and is **more frequent in intravenous drug abusers** with HIV infection than in homosexuals
4. The disease has been **described in all high-risk groups,** however, including infants of HIV-positive mothers
5. **Renal biopsy** typically reveals visceral epithelial cell swelling, collapse of the glomerular capillary tuft, severe tubulointerstitial inflammation, and microcystic dilatation of renal tubules
6. **Electron microscopy** characteristically reveals severe visceral epithelial cell injury and tubuloreticular inclusions in glomerular endothelial cells, tubular cells and infiltrating leukocytes. This constellation of findings has been termed as collapsing glomerulopathy, but it should be emphasized that a similar picture can be seen in the absence of HIV infection
7. The presence of **tubuloreticular inclusions** and the **aggressive clinical course** distinguish HIVAN from idiopathic focal segmental glomerulosclerosis
8. The typical clinical correlates of HIVAN are **severe nephrotic syndrome and rapid progression to ESRD**, occurring in weeks to months.

Wegner's Granulomatosis

- **Necrotizing vasculitis of small arteries and veins** together with **granuloma formation** that can be either intravascular or extravascular
- **Lung** involvement: Bilateral **nodular cavitary infiltrates** demonstrate **necrotizing granulomatous vasculitis**
- The renal biopsy lesion is that of a **pauci-immune necrotizing and crescentic GN.**

Goodpasture's Syndrome

- Autoimmune disease in which **autoantibodies are directed against type IV collagen**
- The clinical complex of **anti-GBM** nephritis and lung hemorrhage is referred to as **Goodpasture's syndrome**. Patients with **Goodpasture's syndrome** are typically young males (5 to 40 years; male-female ratio of 6:1)
- The target antigen is a component of the noncollagenous (NCI) domain of **the α3 chain of type IV collagen**, the α3 chain being preferentially expressed in glomerular and pulmonary alveolar basement membrane

Anti-GBM disease commonly presents with:

- **Hematuria**
- **Nephritic urinary sediment, subnephrotic proteinuria and**
- **Rapidly progressive renal failure over weeks, with or without pulmonary hemorrhage**
- About 20% of patients have **low titers of ANCA**, usually a perinuclear **(p ANCA)**
- **Renal biopsy is the gold standard** for diagnosis of anti-GBM nephritis
- The typical morphologic pattern on light microscopy is diffuse proliferative glomerulonephritis, with focal necrotizing lesions and crescents in >50% of glomeruli **(crescentic glomerulonephritis)**
- Immunofluorescence microscopy reveals **linear ribbon-like deposition of IgG along the GBM**
- C3 is present in the same distribution in 70% of patients. Prominent IgG deposition along the tubule basement membrane and tubulointerstitial inflammation is found occasionally
- Electron microscopy reveals nonspecific inflammatory changes without immune deposits. Typical features on **lung biopsy include alveolar hemorrhage.**

Alport's Syndrome (Hereditary Nephritis)

- Nephritis
- Nerve deafness
- Eye disorders (Lens dislocation, corneal dystrophy, posterior cataracts)

- Foamy cells in interstitium
- **Mutation in alpha 5 chain of collagen type IV**
- **Electron microscopy is used for diagnosis**

Rhabdomyolysis

Causes:
- Crush injury
- Burns
- Heroin, barbiturates
- Cocaine, amphetamines
- Hypokalemia
- Hypophosphatemia
- Hypothyroidism
- Diabetic ketoacidosis
- Clostridium, streptococcus

Liddle's Syndrome

Liddle's syndrome is a rare familial disease with a clinical presentation of **'hyperaldosteronism'**, consisting of:
- **Hypertension**
- **Hypokalemia and**
- **Metabolic alkalosis**

However, **aldosterone levels are undetectable** in these patients, and a nonaldosterone mineralocorticoid has not been isolated

Increased distal tubule sodium reabsorption, due to activating mutations in the amiloride-sensitive sodium channel, has been described in multiple families

Pharmacologic agents that block distal tubule sodium uptake, such as **amiloride and triamterene, are effective in treating the hypertension and electrolyte abnormalities**.

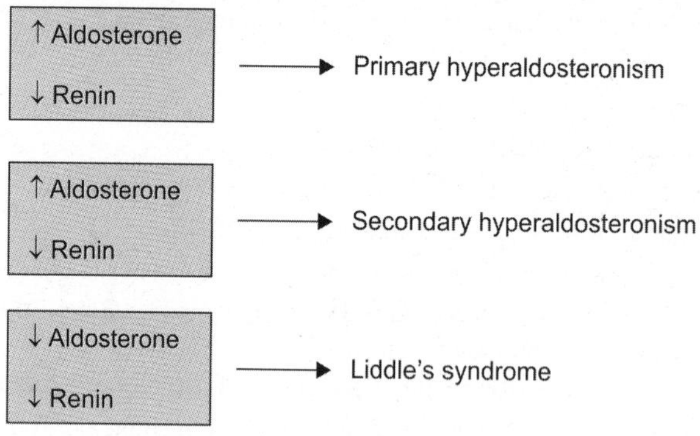

Differentiating features

Bartter's Syndrome

Antenatal Bartter's syndrome is characterized by **polyhydramnios and premature delivery**

The infants also have a characteristic facies consisting of a triangular face with prominent eyes and ears. **Prostaglandin E production is very high**

Characteristic of Bartter's syndrome:
- **Hypokalemia**

- **Metabolic alkalosis and**
- **Normal to low blood pressure 'Not Elevated'**

The 'Gitelman's variant' of Bartter's syndrome presents during **adolescence or adulthood** and generally has a **milder course** than Bartter's syndrome. The dominant features are fatigue and weakness. It is distinguished from Bartter's Syndrome by:

- **Hypocalciuria**
- **Hypomagnesemia with hypermagnesuria and**
- **Normal prostaglandin production.**

Renal Tubular Acidosis

All three types of renal tubular acidosis (RTA) are associated with hyperchloremic metabolic acidosis (normal anion gap):

Type 1 RTA (distal)

- Inability to generate acid urine (secrete H+) in distal tubule
- Causes hypokalemia
- Complications include nephrocalcinosis and renal stones
- Causes include idiopathic, RA, SLE, Sjogren's

Type 2 RTA (proximal)

- Decreased HCO_3– reabsorption in proximal tubule
- Causes hypokalemia
- Complications include osteomalacia
- Causes include idiopathic, as part of Fanconi syndrome, Wilson's disease, cystinosis, outdated tetracyclines

Type 4 RTA (hyperkalemic)

- Causes hyperkalemia
- Causes include hypoaldosteronism, diabetes.

- **Benign hypertension:** Hyaline arteriosclerosis
- **Malignant hypertension:** Fibrinoid necrosis
- **Renin-dependent hypertension:** Renovascular hypertension

Pheochromocytomas

Rule of '10' in pheochromocytomas:

- 10% malignant*
- 10% bilateral*
- 10% extra-adrenal*
- 10% extra-abdominal*
- 10% occur in children
- 10% familial
- 10% **not** associated with hypertension*

- Most common sign in pheochromocytoma = **Hypertension***
- Commonest cause of paroxysmal hypertension

Syndromes associated with pheochromocytoma:

- **MEN type I (Sipple's syndrome)**
- **MEN type II (Mucosal neuroma syndrome)**
- **von Hippel–Lindau's syndrome**
- **von Recklinghausen's neurofibromatosis**

Polycystic Kidney Disease

- APKD is **autosomal dominant**
- Type I involves **Chromosome 16**
- Type II involves **Chromosome 4**
- APKD has got other manifestations such as:

Colonic diverticuli (most common)
- Hepatic cysts
- Splenic cysts
- Aneurysms
- Mitral valve prolapse
- Hypertension is seen in 20–30% cases of children and 70% cases of adults
- Acute renal colic is due to hemorrhage into cyst
- Both gross and microscopic hematuria are seen along with UTI, pyelonephritis, pyocyst, ESRD.

Remember APKD: 11 B's

Bloody urine
Bilateral pain [vs stones, which are usually unilateral pain]
Blood pressure ↑
Bigger kidneys
Bumps palpable
Complications:
Berry aneurysm
Biliary cysts
Bicuspid valve [prolapse and other problems]
Accelerators:
Boys
Blacks
Blood pressure high

Tuberous Sclerosis

Patients with this multisystem disease most commonly present with skin lesions and benign tumors of the central nervous system

Renal involvement is common

Angiomyolipomas are the most frequent abnormality and are usually bilateral

Renal cysts may be present as well and can give an appearance similar to that of ADPKD

Histologically, the cysts are unique. **The cyst-lining cells are large with an eosinophilic-staining cytoplasm and may form hyperplastic nodules that can fill the cyst space.**

von Hippel-Lindau Disease

This autosomal dominant disease is characterized by:
- **Hemangioblastomas of the retina and the central nervous system**
- **Renal cysts** occur in the majority of cases and are usually bilateral
- The VHL gene is a tumor-suppressor gene and has been localized to chromosome 3. It is the same gene that is mutated in **sporadic renal cell carcinoma,** which may be found in up to 25% of patients with von Hippel-Lindau disease and is frequently multifocal.

Causes of Enlarged Kidneys: SHAPE

Scleroderma
HIV nephropathy
Amyloidosis
Polycystic kidney disease
Endocrinopathy (diabetes)

Diabetes Insipidus

Causes of cranial DI:

- **Idiopathic**
- **Post-head injury**
- **Pituitary surgery**
- **Craniopharyngiomas**
- **Histiocytosis X**

DIDMOAD is the association of cranial Diabetes Insipidus, Diabetes Mellitus, Optic Atrophy and Deafness **(also known as Wolfram's syndrome)**

Causes of nephrogenic DI:

- Genetic (primary)
- Electrolytes: hypercalcemia, hypokalemia
- Drugs: demeclocycline, lithium
- Tubulointerstitial disease: obstruction, sickle-cell, pyelonephritis

Investigation

- High-plasma osmolarity, low-urine osmolarity, water deprivation test

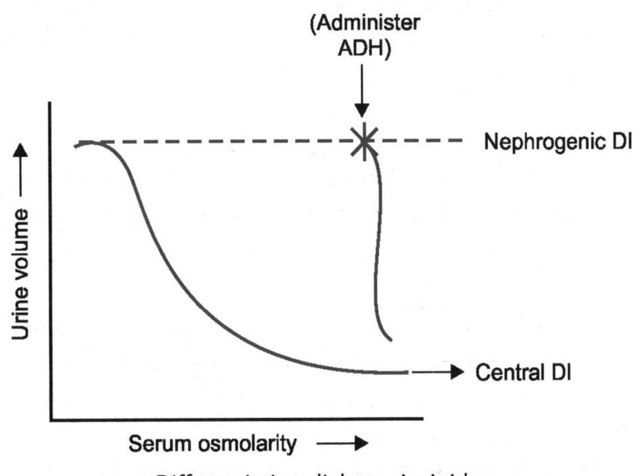

Differentiating diabetes insipidus

USMLE Case Scenario

A 66-year-old man from Toledo has severe polyuria and polydipsia, drinking 6 to 7 glasses of water and producing over one liter of urine each hour. An internal medicine resident places the patient on overnight water restriction for further analysis. The test results shown below were obtained the following morning. Plasma sodium concentration: 153 mEq/L, Urine osmolarity: 86 mosmol/L, Urine glucose concentration: 0 mg/d. There is no glucose in urine. The following is the most likely diagnosis:

1. Conn's Syndrome
2. Bartter's Syndrome

3. Liddle's Syndrome
4. Addison's disease
5. Diabetes insipidus
6. Diabetes mellitus
7. Fanconi syndrome

Ans. 5. Diabetes Insipidus

It is characterized by the excretion of abnormally large volumes of dilute urine (polyuria) with a commensurate increase in fluid intake (polydipsia). The most common type is due to inadequate secretion of antidiuretic hormone (also called vasopressin) and is usually referred to as 'neurogenic' diabetes insipidus. This condition rarely causes severe problems as long as the person has plenty of water to drink. Placing the patient on overnight water restriction caused severe dehydration and a greatly elevated plasma sodium concentration. The possibility of diabetes mellitus which can also be associated with polyuria and polydipsia is easily excluded by the lack of glucosuria.

Renal Vein Thrombosis (RVT)

- **Thrombosis** of one or both main **renal** veins occurs in a variety of settings (hypercoagulable states such as may develop in pregnant women, users of oral contraceptives, subjects with nephrotic syndrome, or dehydrated infants. Nephrotic syndrome accompanying **membranous glomerulopathy** and certain carcinomas predispose to the development of RVT
- **Acute cases** occur typically in children and are characterized by sudden loss of **renal** function, often accompanied by fever, chills, lumbar tenderness (with kidney enlargement), leukocytosis, and hematuria. Hemorrhagic infarction and **renal** rupture may lead to hypovolemic shock
- **In cases of gradual thrombosis**, usually occurring in the elderly, the only manifestation may be recurrent pulmonary emboli or development of hypertension. A Fanconi-like syndrome and proximal **renal** tubular acidosis have been described
- **The definitive diagnosis** can only be established through **selective renal venography** with visualization of the occluding thrombus. Short of angiography, magnetic resonance imaging (MRI) often provides definitive evidence of thrombus
- Treatment consists of anticoagulation, the main purpose of which is prevention of pulmonary embolization, although some authors have also claimed improvement in **renal** function and proteinuria. Thrombectomy is effective in some cases.

Renal Artery Stenosis

- Stenosis of the main **renal** artery and/or its major branches accounts for **2 to 5% of hypertension**
- The common cause in the **middle-aged and elderly is an atheromatous plaque at the origin of the renal artery**
- In **younger women, stenosis is due to intrinsic structural abnormalities** of the arterial wall caused by a heterogenous group of lesions termed as **fibromuscular dysplasia**
- **Renal** artery stenosis should be suspected when hypertension develops in a previously normotensive individual over 50 years of age or in the young (under 30 years) with suggestive features: symptoms of vascular insufficiency to other organs, high-pitched epigastric bruit on physical examination, symptoms of hypokalemia secondary to hyperaldosteronism (muscle weakness, tetany, polyuria), and metabolic alkalosis
- **The best initial screening test is a renal ultrasound**, which may reveal unilateral **renal** hypotrophy (but normal cortical echogenicity). Absence of compensatory hypertrophy in the contralateral kidney should raise the suspicion of bilateral stenosis or superimposed intrinsic (structural) **renal** disease, most commonly hypertensive or diabetic nephropathy
- **A positive captopril test, which has a sensitivity and specificity of greater than 95%, constitutes an excellent follow-up procedure** to assess the need for more invasive radiographic evaluation
- **Magnetic resonance angiography (MRA) has replaced previous modalities as the most sensitive (100%) and specific (95%) test for the diagnosis of renal arterial stenosis**
- The **most definitive diagnostic procedure** is **bilateral arteriography with repeated bilateral renal vein and systemic renin determinations.**

Dialysis

Commonly accepted criteria for putting patients on dialysis include:

- The presence of **uremic syndrome**
- The **presence of hyperkalemia unresponsive** to conservative measures
- **Extracellular volume expansion**
- **Acidosis refractory** to medical therapy
- A bleeding diathesis; and a creatinine clearance of < 10 cc/min per 1.73 m^2
- In chronic renal failure (ESRD), the options include:
  - Hemodialysis (in center or at home)
  - Peritoneal **dialysis**, either as continuous ambulatory peritoneal **dialysis** (CAPD) or
  - Continuous cyclic peritoneal **dialysis** (CCPD)
- **Hemodialysis** is the most common therapeutic modality
- Peritoneal **dialysis** is favored in younger patients.

Complications during Hemodialysis:

- Hypotension is the most common acute complication of hemodialysis
- Muscle cramps
- Anaphylactoid reactions to the dialyzer
- The major cause of death in patients with ESRD receiving chronic **dialysis** is cardiovascular disease.

Hemodialysis is done for Poisoning in Blood From

- Barbiturates
- Aspirin
- Methanol (Alcohol)
- Boric acid
- Thiocyanates
- Lithium
- Theophylline
- Atenolol

For Dialysis, Properties Should be

- Low molecular weight
- High water solubility
- Low protein binding
- Small volume of distribution
- Long half life
- High dialysis clearance

Cushing's Syndrome

ACTH-dependent causes

- Cushing's disease (80%): pituitary tumor secreting ACTH producing adrenal hyperplasia
- Ectopic ACTH production (5–10%): e.g. small cell lung cancer

ACTH-Independent causes

- Iatrogenic: steroids
- Adrenal adenoma (5–10%)

- Adrenal carcinoma (rare)
- Carney complex: Syndrome including cardiac myxoma
- Micronodular adrenal dysplasia (very rare)

Pseudo-Cushing's

- Mimics Cushing's
- Often due to alcohol excess or severe depression
- Causes false positive dexamethasone suppression test or 24-hr urinary free cortisol
- Insulin stress test may be used to differentiate.

Tests

- **The first test to perform is the dexamethasone suppression,** which consists of administering 1 mg of dexamethasone at 11 PM, and then measuring serum cortisol levels in a blood sample drawn at 8 AM the next day. Abnormally high cortisol levels after this test confirm hypercortisolism
- The next step is to find the source of excessive cortisol or ACTH

Baseline plasma ACTH measurement should be performed after a diagnosis:

- If hypercortisolism has been confirmed by dexamethasone suppression test. This test is used to determine whether excessive cortisol production is secondary to increased ACTH levels
- **CT scans of the chest and abdomen** are performed to look for ectopic
- Sources of ACTH. These radiologic studies are especially useful in finding neoplasms that may manifest with inappropriate ACTH secretion, the most frequent of which is small cell carcinoma of the lungs.

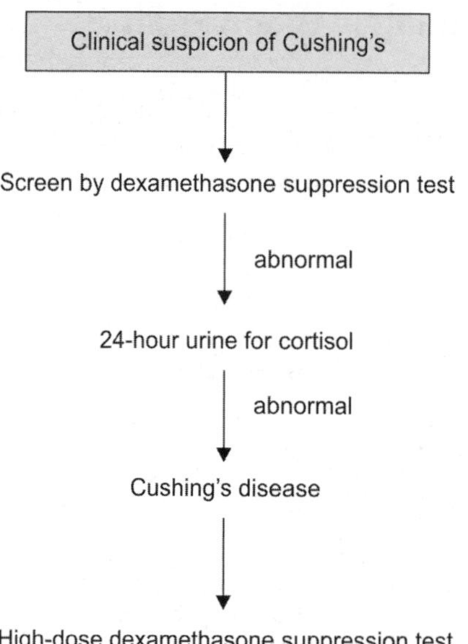

Cushings disease

Cushing's syndrome	Addison's syndrome
Weight gain	Weight loss
Hypertension	Hypotension
↓ K^+, ↓ Cl^-	↓ Na^+, ↑ K^+
Obesity	Weakness, asthenia
No salt craving	Salt craving

Difference

Thyroid Endocrinology

Wolff-Chaikoff Effect

- Excess iodide transiently inhibits thyroid iodide organification, a phenomenon known as the **Wolff-Chaikoff effect**

Sick euthyroid syndrome

- Any acute, severe illness can cause abnormalities of circulating TSH or thyroid hormone levels in the absence of underlying thyroid disease, making these measurements potentially misleading
- The major cause of these hormonal changes is the release of cytokines. Unless a thyroid disorder is strongly suspected, the routine testing of thyroid function should be avoided in acutely ill patients

The most common hormone pattern in sick euthyroid syndrome (SES) is a **decrease in total and free T3 levels**

(Low T3 syndrome) with normal levels of T4 and TSH

HYPERTHYROIDISM:

- **Wide pulse pressure**
- **AF**
- **Tachycardia**
- **Cardiomyopathy**
- **Diarrhea**
- **Heat intolerance**
- **Improper tissue handling in surgeries of thyroid can lead to thyroid storm**

Hormonal changes in Primary Thyrotoxicosis are:

- TSH↓
- T_3 and T_4↑
- RAIU↑

Hormonal changes in Secondary Hyperthyroidism are:

- TSH↑
- T_3 and T_4↑
- RAIU↑

Drugs for Hyperthyroidism

- Propyl thiouracil is unique in the fact that in addition to inhibiting other steps of thyroid hormone synthesis, **it blocks peripheral conversion of T_4 to T_3**
- Propyl thiouracil **can be given in pregnancy**
- Propyl thiouracil is **not associated with fetal aplasia cutis** like methimazole and carbimazole

T4 to T3 conversion is effected by:

- Fasting
- Systemic illness or acute trauma
- Oral contrast agents, and a variety of medications, (e.g. propylthiouracil, propranolol, amiodarone, glucocorticoids)

Subacute Thyroiditis or De Quervain's Thyroiditis or Granulomatous Thyroiditis or Giant Cell Thyroiditis

- Leads to transient hyperthyroidism in early phase and hypothyroidism in late phase
- WCC is normal in viral causes, increased in bacterial causes
- **Myopathy, diffuse goiter, myxedema** are found
- Present with fever, malaise, tender neck swelling
- ESR is increased

- Radio-iodide scan **shows reduced uptake:**
- **It is self-limited inflammation with complete recovery in 6 months**
- Main long-term complication is hypothyroidism which develops after the initial hyperthyroid phase
- **Microscopy reveals:**
  - Initial phase: Acute inflammation
  - Later: Granulomatous reaction
  - More advanced: Fiberoblastic proliferation
- Treat with NSAIDs and steroids if severe.

Hypothyroidism

- **Hung-up reflexes**
- **Carpal tunnel syndrome**
- **Menorrhagia**
- **Constipation**
- **Subnormal body temperature**
- **Tendency for↑ sleep**
- **Cold intolerance**
- **↑TSH**
- **Lithium, PAS, Amidarone implicated in causation**

Commonest cause of congenital hypothyroidism is thyroid agenesis

↓T3↓T4↑TSH are a feature of primary hypothyroidism

Hashimoto's disease is autoimmune throiditis

Thyroxine is used for treatment

Severe cases lead to myxedemic coma characterized by:

- **Slow pulse**
- **Hypotension**

Treated with:

- **IV fluids**
- **Hydrocortisone**
- **T3 injections**

- **Childhood hypothyroidism is treated with levothyroxine**
- **Hyperthyroidism during lactation is treated with propyl thiouracil.**

Primary Hyperparathyroidism

Primary hyperparathyroidism is stereotypically seen in elderly females with an unquenchable thirst and an inappropriately **normal or raised parathyroid hormone level**. It is most commonly due to a **solitary adenoma**

Causes of Primary Hyperparathyroidism:

- 80%: solitary adenoma
- 15%: hyperplasia
- 4%: multiple adenoma
- 1%: carcinoma

Features—'bones, stones, abdominal groans and psychic moans'

- Polydipsia, polyuria
- Peptic ulceration/constipation/pancreatitis
- Bone pain/fracture

- Bone cysts (brown tumors)
- Renal stones
- Depression
- Hypertension
- Impaired glucose tolerance

Associations

- Hypertension
- Multiple endocrine neoplasia: MEN I and II

Investigations

- **Raised calcium, low phosphate**
- PTH may be raised or normal
- Normal alkaline phosphatase
- Technetium-MIBI subtraction scan

Treatment

- Total parathyroidectomy

Hypoparathyroidism

Primary hypoparathyroidism

- Decrease PTH secretion, e.g. secondary to thyroid surgery
- **Low calcium, high phosphate**
- Treat with alfacalcidol

Pseudohypoparathyroidism

- Target cells being insensitive to PTH
- Due to abnormality in a G protein
- Associated with low IQ, short stature, **shortened 4th and 5th metacarpals**
- **Low calcium, high phosphate, high PTH**
- Diagnosis is made by measuring urinary cAMP and phosphate levels following an infusion of PTH. In hypoparathyroidism this will cause an increase in both cAMP and phosphate levels. In pseudohypoparathyroidism type I, neither cAMP nor phosphate levels are increased whilst in pseudohypoparathyroidism type II, only cAMP rises

Pseudo-pseudo-hypoparathyroidism

- **Similar phenotype to pseudohypoparathyroidism but normal biochemistry.**

Conn's Syndrome

- **Hyperaldosteronism**
- **↑Aldosterone↑renin**
- **Hypertension**
- **↑sodium**
- **↓potassium**
- **Polyuria, polydipsia**
- **Weakness**
- **Proximal myopathy**

Addison's Disease

- Addison's disease is **primary** adrenocortical **insufficiency**. Associated electrolyte abnormalities:
  - **Hyperkalemia, hyponatremia**

  - **Hypoglycemia**
  - **Metabolic acidosis**
- **90% gland** must be destroyed to manifest the disease
- Autoimmune causes are responsible for most cases
- Clinical signs include: fatigability, weakness, anorexia, weight loss, **cutaneous and mucosal pigmentation,** hypotension and hypoglycemia
- **Pigmentation** is **usually increased except in adrenal insufficiency secondary** to pituitary failure. Increased pigmentation is characterized by **diffuse tanning of both exposed and nonexposed portions of the body**, especially on pressure points (bony prominences), skin folds, scars, and extensor surfaces
- **Black freckles** over the forehead, face, neck, and shoulders; **areas of vitiligo**; and **bluish-black discolorations of the areolae and of the mucous membranes** of the lips, mouth, rectum, and vagina are common
- In a patient with suspected Addison's disease, the **definite investigation is a short ACTH test**. Plasma cortisol is measured before and 30 minutes after giving Synacthen 250 mg IM. Adrenal autoantibodies such as anti-21-hydroxylase may also be demonstrated
- **Busulfan causes Addisonian-like features.**

Adrenal Insufficiency

A 44-year-old female from Ohio has unexplained fatigue, weight loss, and diffuse muscle pains over the last 4 months. She has been using oral prednisone (10 mg/day) that was started early this year. Three months ago her breathing seemed to be getting a lot better, so she decided to stop the prednisone. Her temperature is 37.0 °C (98.6 °F), blood pressure is 90/40 mm Hg, pulse is 100/min, and respirations are 14/min. On physical examination, she has a tanned appearance with an otherwise normal skin examination. Her heart is tachycardic and regular without murmurs. Her lungs have a few scattered wheezes. Laboratory studies show: hypoglycemia, hyponatremia, and hyperkalemia.

Waterhouse-Friderichsen Syndrome

Fulminant, life-threatening meningitis caused by meningococcus is with a vasculitic purpura and disseminated intravascular coagulation. Complicated by adrenal involvement with coagulopathy, hypotension, adrenal cortical necrosis, and sepsis is Waterhouse-Friderichsen syndrome.

SIADH

CAUSED BY:

- **Carbamezapine**
- **Vincristine**
- **Chlorpropamide**
- **Oxytocin**
- **Head injury**
- **Encephalitis**
- **Oat cell carcinoma of lung**
- **Hypothyroidism**
- **Hyponatremia is a feature**

Concentrated urine, dilute serum: SIADH
Dilute urine-concentrated serum: Diabetes insipidus

Polyglandular Autoimmune Syndrome Type I

PGA type I is usually recognized in the first decade of life and requires two of the three components for diagnosis:

- **Mucocutaneous candidiasis**
- **Hypoparathyroidism and**
- **Adrenal insufficiency**

This disorder is also called **autoimmune polyendocrinopathy-candidiasis-ectodermal dystrophy (APECED)**

Other endocrine defects can include gonadal failure, hypothyroidism, anterior hypophysitis, and, less commonly, destruction of the β cells of the pancreatic islets and development of insulin-dependent (Type 1) diabetes mellitus. Additional features include hypoplasia of the dental enamel, ungual dystrophy, tympanic membrane sclerosis, vitiligo, keratopathy, and gastric parietal cell dysfunction resulting in pernicious anemia

Some patients develop autoimmune hepatitis, malabsorption (variably attributed to intestinal lymphangiectasia, IgA deficiency, bacterial overgrowth, or hypoparathyroidism), asplenism, achalasia, and cholelithiasis.

Polyglandular Autoimmune Syndrome Type II

PGA type II is characterized by:

- **Primary adrenal insufficiency**
- **Graves' disease or autoimmune hypothyroidism**
- **Type 1 diabetes mellitus and**
- **Primary hypogonadism**

Other associated conditions include hypophysitis, celiac disease, atrophic gastritis, and pernicious anemia. Vitiligo, caused by antibodies against the melanocyte, and alopecia are less common than in the type I syndrome. Mucocutaneous candidiasis does not occur.

Insulinomas

- Insulinomas are **endocrine tumors** of the pancreas derived from **β cells** that autonomously secrete insulin, which results in hypoglycemia
- The most common clinical symptoms are due to the effect of the **hypoglycemia** on the central nervous system (neuroglycemic symptoms) and include confusion, headache, disorientation, visual difficulties, irrational behavior, or even coma
- Also, most patients have symptoms due to **excess catecholamine release** secondary to the hypoglycemia, including sweating, tremor, and palpitations. Characteristically these attacks are associated with fasting.
- Insulinomas are **generally small (> 90% are < 2 cm in diameter)**
- Usually solitary (90%), and only 5 to 15% are malignant
- They almost invariably occur only in the pancreas, **distributed equally in the pancreatic head, body and tail**
- Insulinomas should be suspected in all patients with hypoglycemia, especially with a history suggesting attacks provoked by fasting or with a family history of MEN-1
- In insulinomas, in addition to **elevated plasma insulin levels, elevated plasma proinsulin levels are found and C-peptide levels can be elevated**.

Glucagonomas

- Glucagonomas are **endocrine tumors of the pancreas** that secrete **excessive amounts of glucagon that causes a distinct syndrome characterized by dermatitis, glucose intolerance or diabetes, and weight loss**
- Glucagonomas mainly occur in persons between 45 and 70 years old. They are heralded clinically by a characteristic dermatitis **(migratory necrolytic erythema**; accompanied by **glucose intolerance weight loss , anemia, diarrhea and thromboembolism**
- The characteristic rash usually starts as an **annular erythema at intertriginous and periorificial sites,** especially in the groin or buttock. It subsequently becomes raised and bullae form; when the bullae rupture, eroded areas form. The lesions can wax and wane.

- A characteristic laboratory finding is **hypoaminoacidemia**
- Glucagonomas are generally **large tumors at diagnosis**, with an average size of 5 to 10 cm. Between 50 and 80% occur in the **pancreatic tail** and 50 to 82% have evidence of metastatic spread at presentation, usually to the liver
- Glucagonomas are **rarely extrapancreatic and usually occur singly**.

Somatostatinoma Syndrome

- Somatostatinomas are **endocrine tumors that secrete excessive amounts of somatostatin**, which causes a syndrome characterized by **diabetes mellitus, gallbladder disease, diarrhea, and steatorrhea**
- Somatostatinomas occur primarily in the pancreas and small intestine, and the frequency of the symptoms differs in each
- Somatostatinomas occur in the pancreas in 56 to 74% of cases, with the primary location being in the **pancreatic head.**

VIPomas

- These are endocrine tumors that secrete excessive amounts of **VIP**, which causes a distinct syndrome characterized by **large-volume diarrhea, hypokalemia,** and **dehydration**
- This syndrome is also called **Verner-Morrison syndrome, pancreatic cholera, or WDHA syndrome (watery diarrhea, hypokalemia,** and **achlorhydria).**

Important Enzymes and Clinical Correlations

17-Alpha-hydroxylase deficiency: Hypertension is the hallmark of this congenital adrenal hyperplasia disorder, but these patients are **unable to produce sex hormones and glucocorticoids**. Excess mineralocorticoids cause hypertension via sodium and water retention.

3-Beta-hydroxysteroid dehydrogenase: This enzyme metabolizes pregnenolone to progesterone. **No sex hormones, glucocorticoids, or mineralocorticoids may be produced. Excretion of salts is prominent. Prognosis is poor.**

11-Beta-hydroxylase: Virilization, hypertension, and cortisol deficit are the presenting factors in 11-beta-hydroxylase deficiency. Deoxycorticosterone is a mineralocorticoid that causes fluid retention despite aldosterone absence. Sex hormones are produced excessively, as the cortisol feedback needed to decrease ACTH production is lacking.

21-Alpha-hydroxylase: This type of deficiency is the most common congenital adrenal hyperplasia. Laboratory results should reveal decreased cortisone and aldosterone, but deoxycorticosterone should be diminished as well. Promotion of the pituitary-adrenal axis by ACTH promotes virilization by excess sex hormones. Hypotension is common in 21-alpha-hydroxylase deficiency.

Aromatase: The hallmark of aromatase deficiency is **ambiguous genitalia in 46, XX patients**, with progressive virilization. **In 46, XY patients, normal male genitalia are observed, but these individuals are very tall**, possibly eunuchoid, and have an increased risk of osteoporosis. Hypertension has not been associated with aromatase deficiency.

NEUROLOGY

Alzheimer's Disease

- **Mc cause of dementia in elderly**
- **Cortical** Dementia **not Subcortical Dementia**
- Causes **brain atrophy** in advanced cases
- Atrophy usually involves **frontal, temporal and parietal** lobes
- **Neurofibrillary tangles, Neuritic plaques, Granulovacuolar degeneration, Hirano bodies** are pathological features
- **Nucleus Basalis of Meynert** is effected
  - **Aphasia**
  - **Amnesia**
  - **Agnosia**
  - **Acalculia**
  - **Alexia are features**

- There is reduction in **acetylcholine** concentration
- Presenile dementia occurs before 60 years of age
- Associations with:
  - **Down's syndrome, APP** (Amyloid Precursor Protein gene on Chromosome 21)
    - **Presinilin 1** on chromosome 14
    - **Presinilin 2** on chromosome 1
- Treatment is by **Tacrine, Donepezil, Memantine**
  - **Neurofibrillary tangles** are intracytoplasmic filamentous inclusions found in Alzheimer disease and, to a lesser extent, in normal aging brains
  - **Granulovacuolar degeneration**
  - **Hirano Bodies:** They are specific protein deposits associated with **AGE (**Advance Glycosylation End-products localized within soma of neurons
  - **Amyloid Plaques:** They represent fragmented accumulations of proteins which are normally broken down but accumulate in Alzheimer's disease
  - **Alzheimer's Cells (special cells)**
  - **Neurofibrillary tangles:** are insoluble twisted fibrils composed of **Tau proteins**
- **Mini-Mental status examination** is useful screening test for Dementia
- **Maximum score in Mini-Mental examination is 30**

Frontotemporal Dementia and Pick's Disease

Imaging studies reveal **atrophy confined to the frontal or frontal and temporal lobes.** The condition is heterogenous, and the broad designation FTD usually includes Pick's disease

Microscopic findings include gliosis, neuronal loss, and swollen or ballooned neurons, which frequently contain **silver-staining cytoplasmic inclusions referred to as Pick bodies.**

Diffuse Lewy Body Disease

- Lewy bodies are **intraneuronal cytoplasmic inclusions that stain with periodic acid-Schiff and ubiquitin**. They contain epitopes recognized by antibodies against phosphorylated and nonphosphorylated neurofilament proteins, ubiquitin, and a presynaptic protein called α-synuclein.
- Lewy bodies are traditionally found in the substantia nigra of patients with idiopathic Parkinson's disease. Large numbers of such inclusions have also been discovered in cortical neurons in patients with dementia. In patients without other pathologic features, the condition is referred to as **diffuse Lewy body disease**
- In patients whose brains also contain amyloid plaques and NFTs, the condition is called the **diffuse Lewy body variant of Alzheimer's disease.**

Normal Pressure Hydrocephalus

The clinical triad includes an:

- **Abnormal gait (ataxic or apractic)**
- **Dementia (usually mild to moderate)**
- **Urinary incontinence**
- Neuroimaging studies of the brain **reveal enlarged lateral ventricles (hydrocephalus)**

Huntington's Disease

- Huntington's disease (HD) is a **autosomal dominant, degenerative brain disorder**
- The two clinical hallmarks of the disease are **chorea and behavioral disturbance**, the movement disorder is usually slowly progressive and eventually may become disabling.

- There are frequent, irregular, sudden jerks and movements of any of the limbs or trunk. Grimacing, grunting, and poor articulation of speech may be prominent
- The gait is disjointed and poorly coordinated and has a so-called **dancing (choreic) quality**.

MS (Multiple Sclerosis)

- **Multiple scarred are as visible on macroscopic examination of the brain**
  - These lesions, **termed plaques**, are sharply demarcated gray or pink areas easily distinguished from surrounding white matter
  - Plaques vary in size from 1 or 2 mm to several centimeters
  - CSF abnormalities consist of:
    - **Abnormally increased levels of intrathecally synthesized IgG, oligoclinal banding, and mononuclear cell pleocytosis**
    - The ratio of IgG to albumin in the CSF is divided by the ratio in the serum **'the CSF IgG index'**. Oligoclonal banding of CSF IgG is detected by agarose gel electrophoresis techniques
- Optic neuritis is the mc manifestation
- **Also seen are:**
  - **Nystagmus on adducting eye**
  - **One and half syndrome**
  - Pendular nystagmus
- **Two or more oligoclonal bands are found in 75 to 90% of patients with MS.** Three treatment options for patients with RRMS are approved for use:
  - IFN-1b
  - IFN-1a (Avonex) and
  - Glatiramer acetate

Neuromyelitis optica (Devic's syndrome) is characterized by **separate attacks of acute optic neuritis and myelitis.** Optic neuritis may be unilateral or bilateral and precede or follow an attack of myelitis by days, months or years

Acute MS

(Marburg's variant) is a **rare acute fulminant process** that generally **ends in death from brainstem involvement within one year**. There are no remissions. Diagnosis can be established only at postmortem examination; widespread demyelination, axonal loss, edema, and macrophage infiltration are characteristic.

Learn to Differentiate

- **Normal pressure hydrocephalus** is a **potentially reversible cause of dementia** that causes **gait disturbances (unsteady or shuffling gait), urinary incontinence, and dementia. Enlargement of the ventricles** with **increased cerebrospinal fluid (CSF) pressure** is found, and therapeutic lumbar punctures may significantly improve symptoms.
- **Creutzfeldt-Jakob disease** is a **rare diffuse degenerative disease** that usually affects people in their 50s, and the usual course is about one year. The **terminal stage is characterized by severe dementia, generalized hypertonicity, and profound speech disturbances**. It is one of the several diseases **caused by prions.**
- **Huntington's disease** is a **hereditary disease** associated with **progressive degeneration of the basal ganglia and the cerebral cortex.** It is transmitted in **an autosomal dominant** pattern. The onset of Huntington's disease occurs between 35 and 50 years of age, or later in rare cases. This disease is characterized by **progressive dementia, muscular hypertonicity, and bizarre choreiform movements.**
- **Parkinson's disease** is characterized primarily by **motor dysfunction**, but dementia may be a part of the disorder. The characteristic motor symptoms **(bradykinesia, flat facies, resting tremor, shuffling gait, etc. are caused by degeneration of the nigrostriatal dopaminergic tract.**

- **Pick's disease** causes a **slowly progressive dementia**. It is associated with **focal cortical lesions, primarily of the frontal lobe.** Pathological examination of the brain reveals **intraneuronal inclusions called Pick bodies.**

- **Tumor of the Falx** or the parasagittal meninges typically produces **sensory or motor dysfunction of the leg.**
- **Tumor of hippocampus** might produce **memory problems or seizures.**
- **Tumor of the posterior fossa** produces **unilateral deafness, tinnitus, vertigo, and sometimes sensory loss in the distribution of cranial nerves V or VII.**
- **Tumor of the sphenoidal ridge** can cause cranial nerve palsies involving **III, IV, V, or VI.**

Bulbar palsy
- B/L **LMNL of 9,10,11,12 Cranial Nerves**

Features:
- **Dysarthria**
- **Dysphagia**
- **Dysphonia**

Pseudobulbar palsy:
- B/L **UMNL of 9, 10, 11, 12 Cranial Nerves**

Syringomyelia:
- **Dissociated sensory loss**
- **Wasting of small muscles of hand**
- **Charcot's joints**

Syringobulbia:
- **Facial pain/Sensory loss**
- **Facial Palsy**
- **Vertigo, Nystagmus, Horner's Syndrome**

Remember Epilepsy Syndromes Given Below

Juvenile Myoclonic Epilepsy
- Juvenile myoclonic epilepsy (JME) is a **generalized seizure disorder** of unknown cause
- Appears in **early adolescence** and is usually characterized by **bilateral myoclonic jerks** that may be single or repetitive
- The **myoclonic seizures** are most frequent in the morning after awakening and can be provoked by sleep deprivation
- **Consciousness is preserved** unless the myoclonus is especially severe
- Many patients also experience **generalized tonic-clonic seizures, and up to one-third have absence seizures**
- The condition is otherwise benign, and although complete remission is uncommon, the seizures respond well to appropriate anticonvulsant medication (**VALPROIC ACID**)
- There is often a family history of epilepsy, and genetic linkage studies suggest a polygenic cause.

Lennox-Gastaut Syndrome
- Lennox-Gastaut syndrome occurs in children and is defined by the following **triad:**
  - **Multiple seizure types** (usually including generalized tonic-clonic, atonic, and atypical absence seizures);
  - An EEG showing **slow (<3 Hz) spike-and-wave discharges** and a variety of other abnormalities;
  - **Impaired cognitive function in most** but not all cases
- Lennox-Gastaut syndrome is associated with **CNS disease or dysfunction from a variety of causes, including developmental abnormalities, perinatal hypoxia/ischemia, trauma, infection, and other acquired lesions.**

Mesial Temporal Lobe Epilepsy Syndrome
- Mesial temporal lobe epilepsy (MTLE) is the most common syndrome associated with **complex partial seizures** and is an example of symptomatic, partial epilepsy.

- High-resolution magnetic resonance imaging (MRI) can detect the **characteristic hippocampal sclerosis** that appears to be an essential element in the pathophysiology of MTLE for many patients.
- Recognition of this syndrome is especially important because it tends to be **refractory to treatment with anticonvulsants** but **responds extremely well to surgical intervention.**

Progressive Multifocal Leukoencephalopathy

- Characterized pathologically by **multifocal areas of demyelination** of varying size distributed throughout the CNS
- Caused by **JC virus**
- Disease of white matter
- Follows **indolent course** and is fatal. Within a year or so, patients often present with **visual deficits (45%), typically a homonymous hemianopia, and mental impairment (38%) (Dementia, confusion, personality change)**
- Motor weakness may not be present early but eventually occurs in 75% of cases
- Almost all patients (> 95%) have an **underlying immunosuppressive disorder**
- The diagnosis of PML is frequently suggested by MRI or less commonly CT
- MRI is more sensitive than CT and reveals multifocal asymmetric, coalescing white matter lesions located **periventricularly, in the centrum semiovale, in the parietal-occipital region, and in the cerebellum**
- The **CSF is typically normal**, although mild elevation in protein and/or IgG may be found. Pleocytosis occurs in < 25% of cases, is predominantly mononuclear, and rarely exceeds 25 cells/ml
- The presence of a **positive CSF PCR for JC virus DNA in association with typical MRI** lesions in the appropriate clinical setting is diagnostic of PML
- Patients with negative CSF PCR studies may require brain biopsy for definitive diagnosis.

SSPE

- SSPE is a **chronic, progressive, demyelinating, late** CNS complication of Measles.
- It appears after a latent periods of 6–8 years.
- It was first described by Dawson in 1933.
- The incidence of SSPE has decreased over years since the introduction of live attenuated measles vaccine.

Early in the course of disease, the electroencephalogram (EEG) may be normal or show only moderate nonspecific slowing.

- In the myoclonic stage, most patients with SSPE have **'burst-suppression' episodes**. However, this pattern is not unique to SSPE.
- Later in the illness, EEG becomes increasingly disorganized.
- Diagnosis is confirmed by elevated levels of measles antibodies in the serum and CSF. CSF also shows elevated oligoclonal bands (IgG). CSF pleocytosis is absent or minimal.'
- MRI or CT scans of patients with SSPE show variable cortical atrophy and ventricular enlargement
- Myoclonic seizures are a feature.
- No definitive therapy is available.
- **Inosoplex alone** or win combination with interferon has been shown to be beneficial.

- Burst suppression pattern in EEG is seen in SSPE
- **Burst suppression pattern is seen in 'SSPE' and 'Creutzfeldt-Jakob Disease'**
- It is characterized by **high-voltage slow and sharp wave complexes** superimposed on a relatively flat background

Remember:

- Absence seizures show 'three per second spike and wave pattern' on EEG
- **HSV encephalitis** displays **'high-voltage sharp waves'** over temporal lobes at regular three second's interval. (TEMPORAL ENHANCEMENT ON MRI)
- **Hepatic encephalopathy** shows **'synchronous triphasic'** waves
- Burst suppression pattern is seen in 'SSPE' and 'Creutzfeldt-Jakob Disease.'

Prion Diseases

- Prions are a unique class of infectious proteins associated with a group of neurodegenerative diseases, the transmissible spongiform encephalopathies
- **In humans**, these diseases include:
  - **Kuru**
  - **Creutzfeldt-Jakob disease**
  - **Gerstmann-Straussler-Scheinker syndrome and**
  - **Fatal familial insomnia**
- **In animals:**
  - **Scrapie and**
  - **Bovine spongiform encephalopathy (madcow disease)**
- PrP^{Sc} is a pathogenic, transmissible spongiform encephalopathy-specific form of the host-encoded prion protein (PrP);
- PrP^{Sc} differs from PrP in that it contains **a high amount of b-pleated sheet structure and is insoluble and resistant to proteolytic enzymes**
- PrP^{Sc} deposits either consist of or can be readily converted to amyloid fibrils.

Creutzfeldt-Jakob Disease

- Caused by Prion Protein (Infectious proteins)
- **Most common infectious prion disease in humans**
- **Neurodegenerative disease**
- On light microscopy, the pathologic hallmarks of **CJD** are **spongiform degeneration and astrogliosis**
- The **lack of an inflammatory response** in **CJD** and other prion diseases is an important pathologic feature of these degenerative disorders
- Spongiform degeneration is characterized by many 1- to 5-mm **vacuoles in the neuropil between nerve cell bodies**
- **In (new variant) nvCJD**, a characteristic feature is the presence of **'florid plaques'.** These are composed of a central core of PrP amyloid surrounded by vacuoles in a pattern suggesting petals on a flower

Features:
  - **Rapidly progressive dementia**
  - **Myoclonus**
  - **Rapid progression are common features**
  - **Can be transmitted by corneal implants and is inheritable**
- **Brain biopsy is diagnostic**

Guillain-Barré Syndrome

Guillain-Barré syndrome is characterized by the three As: acute, areflexic, ascending. It is an autoimmune-mediated, demyelinating ascending paralysis that is often idiopathic but is also associated with HIV and Campylobacter infections. A lumbar puncture can often help clinch the diagnosis, although nerve conduction studies, if available, are often more consistent, as CSF findings can be ambiguous early in the disease. The classic finding is CSF with few cells and a high total protein

Remember the disease by features:
- **Motor paralysis**
- **Ascending type**
- **Areflexia seen**

- **No sensory loss**
- **Flaccidity seen**
- **Legs affected more than arms**
- **Deep tendon reflexes absent usually**
- **Albumin cytological dissociation seen**

Plasmapheresis and immunoglobulins used for treatment

A 28-year-old man of weakness. He reports a 4-day history of weakness and tingling in his legs, which has since progressively involved his upper body. Physical examination is remarkable for profound weakness in his lower extremities and torso, with normal cranial nerves and moderately reduced strength in his upper extremities. Deep tendon reflexes are absent in his lower extremities and reduced in his upper extremities. All findings are symmetrical. Cerebrospinal fluid (CSF) analysis shows increased total protein.

Guillain-Barre-syndrome is characterized by the three **As: Acute, areflexic, ascending**. It is an autoimmune-mediated, demyelinating ascending paralysis that is often idiopathic but is also associated with HIV and campylobacter infection. A lumbar puncture can often help clinch the diagnosis, although nerve conduction studies, if available, are often more consistent, as CSF findings can be ambiguous early in the disease. The classic finding is CSF with few cells and a high total protein.

Miller-Fisher Syndrome

- **Variant of Guillain-Barre syndrome**
- Associated with **areflexia, ataxia, ophthalmoplegia**
- **Anti-GQ1b** antibodies are present in 90% of the cases

Friedreich's Ataxia

- **Most common** form of inherited ataxia
- **AR Inheritance**
- The classic form of Friedreich's ataxia has been mapped to **(Ch 13)**
- And the mutant gene, **frataxin** contains **expanded GAA triplet repeats** in the first intron
- Earliest feature is **ataxia**
- **Dorsal root ganglia are affected earliest**
- Presents before 25 years of age with progressive staggering gait, frequent falling, and titubation. The lower extremities are more severely involved than the upper ones
- **The neurologic examination** reveals nystagmus, loss of fast saccadic eye movements, truncal titubation, dysarthria, dysmetria, and ataxia of extremity and truncal movements
- Extensor plantar responses (with normal tone in trunk and extremities), absence of deep tendon reflexes, and weakness (greater distally than proximally) are usually found. Loss of vibratory and proprioceptive sensation occurs
- **Absent knee jerk and extensor plantar response are features**
- **Pyramidal tract is involved**
- **Cardiac involvement** occurs in 90% of patients. Cardiomegaly, symmetric hypertrophy, murmurs, and conduction defects are reported. **(CARDIOMYOPATHY)**
- **Musculoskeletal deformities** are common and include **pes cavus, pes equinovarus,** and **scoliosis**.

A 13-year-old boy having difficulty in running and a staggering gait, poor articulation in speech. The physical examination revealed an unsteady, broad-based stance and sudden lurching when walking. Loss of vibratory and position sense was observed bilaterally in all extremities. There was a tremor of the upper extremity as the patient reached for objects. Speech was slurred, slow and with an uneven pattern. Hyporeflexia was present but there was only a slight indication of muscle atrophy, though there were bilateral Babinski's signs.

Ataxia-telangiectasia

- Patients usually present in the first decade of life with **progressive telangiectatic** lesions **associated with deficits in cerebellar function** and **nystagmus**
- Truncal **ataxia**, extremity **ataxia**, dysarthria, extensor plantar responses, myoclonic jerks, areflexia, and distal sensory deficits may develop
- There is a high incidence of:
  - **Recurrent pulmonary infections**
  - **Neoplasms of the lymphatic and reticuloendothelial system and**
  - **Increased incidence of cancer**
- **Especially** an **increased incidence of lymphomas, Hodgkin's disease, and acute leukemias** of the T cell type
- **Thymic hypoplasia with cellular and humoral (IgA and IgG2) immunodeficiencies, premature aging**, and endocrine disorders such as insulin-dependent diabetes mellitus are described
- The immunologic defects and **increased susceptibility to cancer** have been causally linked to cellular disorders in AT. **Exposure of cultured cells to ionizing radiation slows the rate of DNA replication and increases the frequency of chromosomal aberrations**
- The most striking neuropathologic changes include:
  - Loss of Purkinje, granule, and basket cells in the cerebellar cortex as well as of neurons in the deep cerebellar nuclei
  - Loss of anterior horn neurons in the spinal cord and of dorsal root ganglion cells associated with posterior column spinal cord demyelination
- A poorly developed or absent thymus gland is the most consistent defect of the lymphoid system
- The gene for AT (the ATM gene) has been positionally mapped to chromosome 11
- **Defective DNA repair in AT fibroblasts exposed to ultraviolet light has been demonstrated.**

Choreoathetoid movements, slurred speech, ophthalmoplegia, and progressive mental retardation characterize the disease at it advances. Telangiectasias are a helpful diagnostic clue. These children also have vulnerable recurrent sinopulmonary infections. Immunologic evaluation may demonstrate a lack of IgA and IgE, cutaneous anergy, and a progressive cellular immune defect. Other features of the syndrome include endocrine disorders and a predisposition for certain cancers (leukemias, brain cancer, and gastric cancer).

Newer Concepts

Mitochondrial Ataxias

- **Spinocerebellar syndromes** have been identified with mutations in mitochondrial DNA (mtDNA)

Xeroderma Pigmentosum

- Xeroderma pigmentosum is a rare **autosomal recessive neurocutaneous disorder**
- Caused by the inability to repair damage to DNA, such as that produced by ultraviolet radiation
- In addition to skin lesions, patients may show **progressive mental deterioration, microcephaly, ataxia, spasticity, choreoathetosis, and hypogonadism**
- Nerve deafness, peripheral neuropathy (predominantly axonal), electroencephalographic abnormalities and seizures are reported

Cockayne Syndrome

- This is a rare **autosomal recessive** disorder first described by Cockayne in 1936
- Clinical features are **mental retardation, optic atrophy, dwarfism, and neural deafness, hypersensitivity of skin to sunlight, cataracts, and retinal pigmentary degeneration**
- Cerebellar, pyramidal, and extrapyramidal deficits and peripheral neuropathy may occur, with a **'bird-headed' facial appearance** and normal-pressure hydrocephalus
- Skin fibroblasts exposed to ultraviolet light demonstrate **defective DNA repair.**

Marinesco Sjogren Syndrome
- This rare syndrome, in which **progressive cerebellar deficits** begin early in childhood, is another example in which a **Friedreich's syndrome is associated with additional specific features**
- **In this case, cataracts, mental retardation, multiple skeletal abnormalities, hypogonadotropic hypogonadism, and severe cerebellar atrophy are associated**
- The syndrome is likely a **lysosomal storage disorder**

Central Pontine Myelinolysis
- **Demyelination of the central basal pons** can appear in chronically ill patients subjected to sudden fluxes in electrolyte and water metabolism, especially **when hyponatremia is corrected too rapidly**
- Quadriparesis, weakness of lower face and tongue, can evolve over a few days or weeks
- The lesion may extend dorsally to involve sensory tracts and leave the patient with a **'locked-in' syndrome** (an awake and sentient state in which the patient, because of motor paralysis in all parts of the body, cannot communicate except possibly by coded eye movements)

Marchiafava-bignami Disease
- A rare **demyelination of the corpus callosum** that occurs in **chronic alcoholics**, predominantly males
- Patients become agitated and confused and show progressive dementia with frontal release signs.

Diseases of the Cerebellum

- Diseases of the cerebellum result in inability to do movements smoothly and accurately. This condition is called **cerebellar ataxia or cerebellar asynergia.**
- **Disturbance of Gait:** Gait is similar to that of a drunken person; Lesion in one cerebellar hemisphere results in a tendency to fall towards that side. Right side of body is under the control of right cerebellar hemisphere. Lesions of cerebellar ataxia are not corrected by vision
- **Decomposition of movements:** A movement is broken into components, i.e. the shoulder, elbow and the wrists move separately and not in a synchronized way
- **Dysmetria**: Inability to stop a movement at a desired point, i.e. overshooting, past pointing, etc.
- **Dysdiadochokinesia:** Inability to stop one movement and immediately to follow it up with other movement of opposite nature, i.e. rapid pronation and supination.
- **Scanning speech:** Due to lack of synergy of muscles used in speaking, the spacing of sounds is irregular with pauses at wrong places.
- Hypotonia
- Decreased tendon reflexes
- Intention tremor (NOT RESTING TREMOR)
- Sometimes Nystagmus

Bacterial Meningitis

- ***S. pneumoniae*** is the most common cause of meningitis in adults > 20 years
- ***N. meningitidis*** accounts for nearly 60% of bacterial meningitis cases **in children and young adults**
- ***Staphylococcus aureus*** **and coagulase-negative staphylococci** are predominant organisms causing meningitis that follows invasive **neurosurgical procedures**, particularly shunting procedures for hydrocephalus
- **Group *B-streptococcus* or *S. agalactiae*** is responsible for meningitis predominantly in neonates
- ***L. monocytogenes*** has emerged as an important cause of bacterial meningitis in the elderly and in individuals with impaired cell-mediated immunity.
  - Purulent exudates seen
  - Cloudy CSF
  - Ventricular spread seen
  - Ventricular enlargement seen

The **classic clinical triad of meningitis** is fever, headache, and nuchal rigidity **(stiff neck)**. Each of these signs and symptoms occurs in > 90% of the cases.

Alteration in mental status occurs in >75% of patients and can vary from lethargy to coma. Nausea, vomiting, and photophobia are also common complaints.

Nuchal rigidity is the pathognomonic sign of meningeal irritation and is present when the neck resists passive flexion.

Kernig's sign is elicited with the patient in the supine position. The thigh is flexed on the abdomen, with the knee flexed; attempts to passively extend the leg elicit pain when meningeal irritation is present.

Brudzinski's sign is elicited with the patient in the supine position and is positive when passive flexion of the neck results in spontaneous flexion of the hips and knees.

The Classic CSF Abnormalities in Bacterial Meningitis are

- Polymorphonuclear leukocytosis (>100 cells per microliter in 90%)
- ↓glucose concentration [< 2.2 mmol/l (< 40 mg/dl) and/or CSF/serum glucose ratio of < 0.4 in ~ 60%]
- ↑protein concentration [> 0.45 g/l (> 45 mg/dl) in 90%], and
- ↑opening pressure (> 180 mm H_2O in 90%).
- CSF bacterial cultures are positive in > 80% of patients, and CSF Gram's stain demonstrates organisms in > 60%.

Commonest Causes of Meningitis

Commonest causes of meningitis:

- **Neonates: Gram-negative bacilli**
- **Adults: *S. pneumoniae***
- **Epidemics: *N. meningitidis***
- **Head trauma: *S. pneumoniae***
- **Infective endocarditis *Staph aureus***
- **CSF shunts: *Staph epidermis***

Unlike meningitis occurring in normal children, ventriculoperitoneal shunt infections are most commonly caused by coagulase-negative *Staphylococcus*, such as *Staphylococcus epidermidis*. *S. epidermidis* causes 40 to 60% of all CSF infections in persons with ventriculoperitoneal shunts. Coagulase-negative *Staphylococcus* presents a significant threat to people who have indwelling devices or catheters. Most *S. epidermidis* isolates are resistant to multiple antibiotics, including nafcillin and oxacillin. Vancomycin is the drug of choice to *S. epidermidis* infection. Removal of the indwelling medical device and parenteral antibiotic treatment are often necessary.

Viral Meningitis

Enteroviruses account for 75 to 90% of aseptic meningitis cases in most series. Viruses belonging to the *Enterovirus* genus are members of the family Picornaviridae and include the **coxsackieviruses, echoviruses, polioviruses, and human enteroviruses 68 to 71**

The most important laboratory test in the diagnosis of meningitis is examination of the CSF. The typical profile in cases of viral meningitis is:

- Lymphocytic pleocytosis (25 to 500 cells per microliter)
- A normal or slightly elevated protein level [0.2 to 0.8 g/l (20 to 80 mg/dl)]
- A normal glucose level
- **A normal or mildly elevated opening pressure (100 to 350 mm H_2O)**
- **Organisms are not seen** on Gram's or acid-fast stained smears or India ink wet mounts of CSF

CSF polymerase chain reaction (PCR) tests, culture, and serology, a specific viral cause can be found in 75 to 90% of cases of viral meningitis

CSF cultures are positive in 30 to 70% of patients, the frequency of isolation depending on the specific viral agent.

HIV meningitis
- Should be suspected in any patient with known or identified risk factors for HIV infection
- **Aseptic meningitis** is a common manifestation of primary exposure to HIV and occurs in 5 to 10% of cases
- In some patients, seroconversion may be delayed for several months; however, detection of the presence of HIV genome **by PCR or p24 protein** establishes the diagnosis
- HIV can be cultured from CSF in some patients
- Cranial nerve palsies, most commonly involving cranial nerves V, VII, or VIII, are more common in HIV meningitis than in other viral infections.

Fungi causing meningitis: *Cryptococcus,* candida, sporothrix
Viruses causing meningitis: HSV, (Enterovirus) polio, mumps coxsackie

Cryptococcus Neoformans Meningitis

A 44-year-old AIDS patient presents to OPD complaining of fever for the past week and an increasing headache. His past medical history is significant for pneumocystis pneumonia and a total CD4 count of 66. Cerebrospinal fluid (CSF) reveals 4 WBC, and budding encapsulated yeast forms grow on Sabouraud's agar.

Neuroimaging

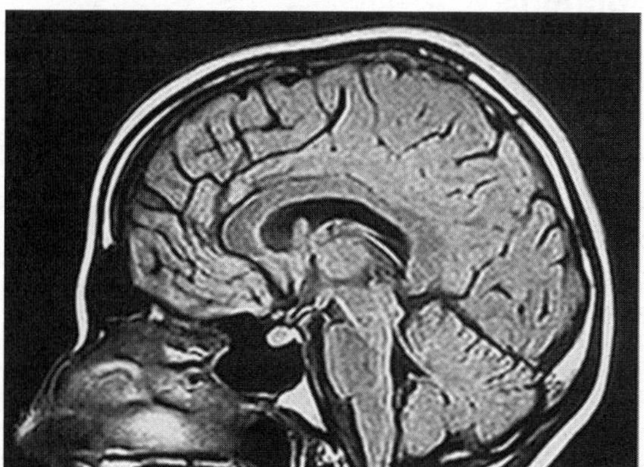

This is a normal sagittal MRI scan demonstrating the midline with the **frontal lobe** and **parietal lobe** and **occipital lobe** and **cerebellum** and **genu of corpus callosum** and **splenium of corpus callosum** and **mammillary body** and **thalmus** and **midbrain** and **pons** and **medulla** and **cervical spinal cord** and **tongue** and **nasal cavity**

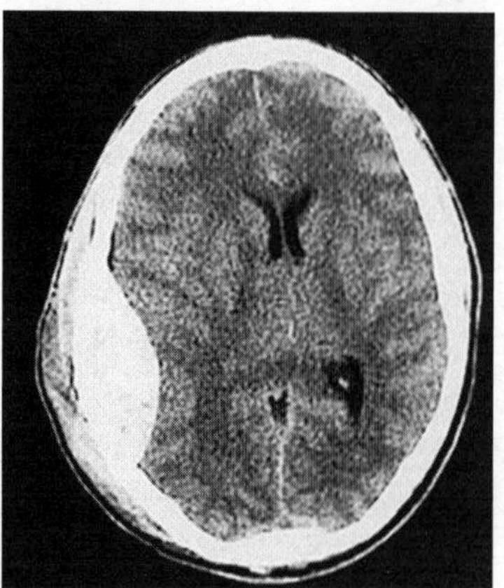

TCT scan without contrast demonstrating a large epidural hematoma with right to left shift and ventricular narrowing

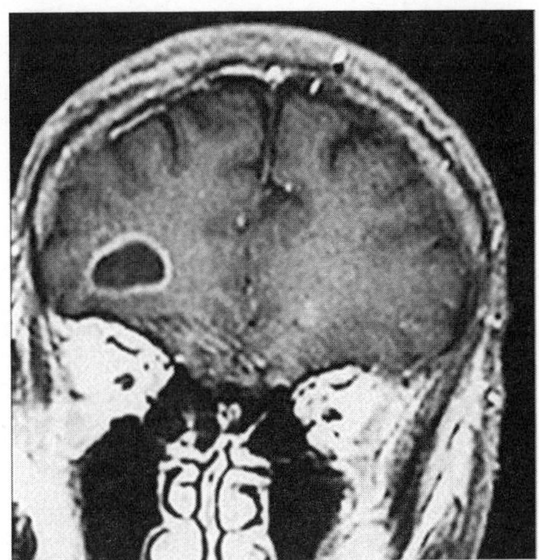

MRI scan of the head in coronal view demonstrates a cysticercus cyst of the brain

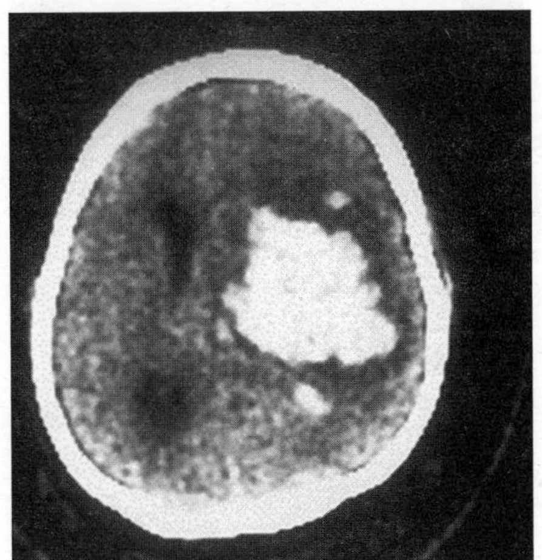

This computed tomographic (CT) scan of the head in transverse view demonstrates an area of hemorrhage arising in the basal ganglia on the left

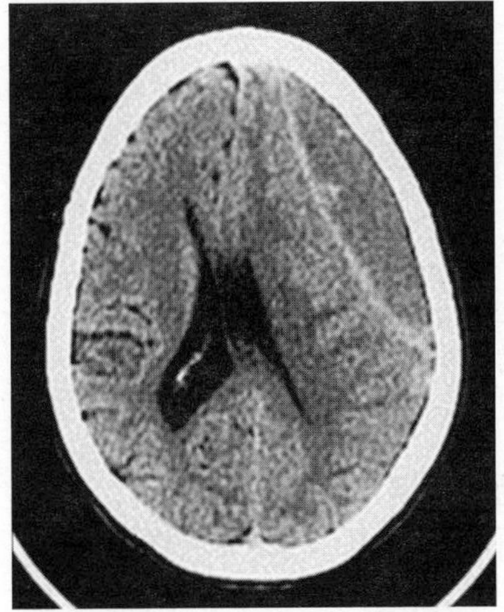

CT scan without contrast demonstrating a large subdural hematoma with left to right shift and ventricular narrowing

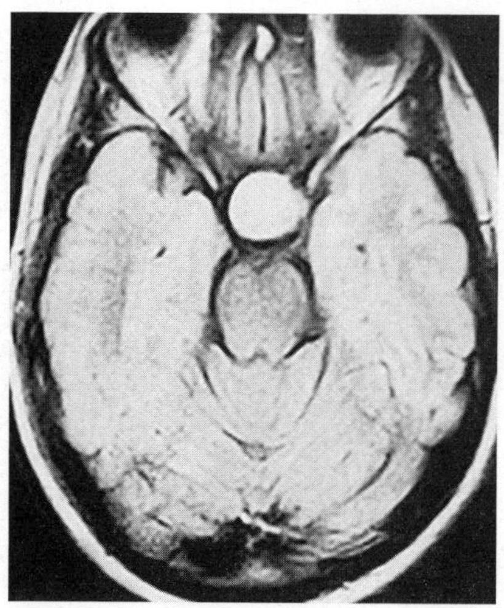

MRI scan in axial view here demonstrates a **macroadenoma** of the pituitary

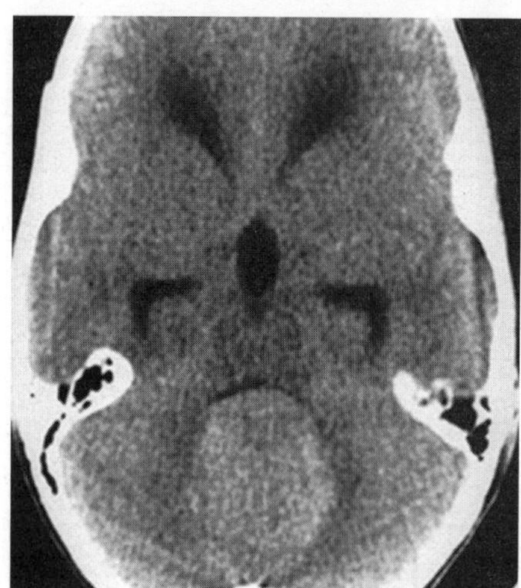

CT scan, there is a **midline cerebellar mass** in a child

Encephalitis

In distinction to meningitis, where the infectious process and associated inflammatory response are limited largely to the meninges, in encephalitis, the **brain parenchyma is also involved**. Many patients with encephalitis also have evidence of associated meningitis (meningoencephalitis) and, in some cases, involvement of the spinal cord or nerve roots (**encephalomyelitis, encephalomyeloradiculitis**)

- HSV is the mc cause of sporadic viral encephalitis
- Hemorrhagic lesions seen
- Temporal lobe involvement is common
- PCR of HSV virus is diagnostic

Progressive Rubella Panencephalitis

Clinical Features and Epidemiology: This is an extremely rare disorder that primarily affects children with congenital rubella syndrome, isolated cases have been reported following childhood rubella

After a latent period of 8 to 19 years, patients develop progressive neurologic deterioration.

The initial manifestations are **similar to those seen in SSPE** and include decline in school performance, behavioral alterations, and seizures, followed by severe progressive dementia, prominent ataxia, pyramidal signs (spasticity, hyperreflexia, extensor plantar responses), and visual deterioration

In the terminal stages of the illness, patients are globally demented, mute, and quadriparetic, often with associated ophthalmoplegia

Diagnostic Studies: CSF **shows a mild lymphocytic pleocytosis, slightly elevated protein level, and rubella virus-specific oligoclonal bands**. CT scan may show enlarged ventricles, cortical and cerebellar atrophy, and hypodensity in the white matter.

Herpes simplex virus (HSV): It is the most common etiologic agent of sporadic viral encephalitis. The clinical presentation is variable but usually abrupt, and the rapid onset of confusion and seizures are frequent manifestations. The most characteristic pathologic lesions, which are demonstrated by CT studies, consist of hemorrhagic necrosis of the temporal lobes. Herpes encephalitis is almost always due to HSV type 1 and affects previously healthy individuals. Up to 50% of newborns delivered vaginally from mothers with active HSV infection develop a severe generalized form of herpetic encephalitis.

Arbovirus encephalitis: It is the most important cause of epidemic viral encephalitis. Many different species may be involved, each with a specific regional geographic distribution. The clinical course is milder and prognosis is better than herpetic encephalitis.

Echovirus encephalitis: It is one of the most common etiologic agents of the so-called **lymphocytic meningoencephalitis**, Symptoms are mild, often limited to headache and malaise. CSF is usually normal or shows mild lymphocytosis.

- **Septic cavernous sinus thrombosis: The oculomotor nerve, the trochlear nerve, the abducens nerve, the ophthalmic and maxillary branches of the trigeminal nerve, and the internal carotid artery** all pass through the cavernous sinus
- The symptoms of septic cavernous sinus thrombosis are fever, headache, frontal and retroorbital pain, and diplopia. The classic signs are ptosis, proptosis, chemosis, and extraocular dysmotility due to deficits of cranial nerves III, IV, and VI
- Hypo- or hyperesthesia of the ophthalmic and maxillary divisions of the fifth cranial nerve and
- A decreased corneal reflex may be detected
- There may be evidence of dilated, tortuous retinal veins and papilledema.
  - **Gradiengo's Syndrome:** It is irritation of ophthalmic division of Trigeminal **(V) nerve** and Abducens **(VI) nerve** in which **Petrositis of petrous temporal** bone occurs.
  - **Tolsa-hunt Syndrome:** Inflammatory condition involving Cavernous Sinus presenting with pain, loss of ocular movements and loss of sensations in territory of ophthalmic division of Trigeminal (V) nerve.
- **Raeder's Syndrome:**
  - It is **Paratrigeminal Syndrome**
  - Pain in **Ophthalmic and Maxillary Divisions** of Trigeminal Nerve
  - Ptosis and Miosis±IV and VI Cranial Nerve involvement
  - It occurs in lesions of Middle Cranial Fossa
- **Costen's Syndrome:** Aching pain around ear aggravated by chewing due to malalignment of Temporomandibular joint with **'Altered BITE'**
- **Symptomatic Neurosyphilis:** Although mixed features are common, the major clinical categories of symptomatic neurosyphilis include **meningeal, meningovascular, and parenchymatous syphilis**. The last category includes **general paresis and tabes dorsalis**

Features:

- **Dorsal column involvement**
- **Ptosis**
- **Miosis**
- **Ataxia**
- **Sensory loss**
- **Argyll-Robertson pupil**
- **Bladder dysfunction**

Benign Intracranial Hypertension

- **↑Intracranial pressure**
- **Normal CSF Pressure**

- **Normal CSF protein**
- **Normal ventricles**
- **Normal ventricular position**

Pseudotumor Cerebri

- Increased intracranial pressure
- Papilledema
- 6th cranial nerve palsy
- Visual field defects

Causes:

- Tetracycline
- OCP
- Hypervitaminosis A

Neuropathic Joint Disease

- Neuropathic joint disease **(Charcot's joint)** is a progressive destructive arthritis associated with loss of pain sensation, proprioception, or both
- **Diabetes mellitus** is the most frequent cause of neuropathic joint disease
- **Diabetes affects tarsal joints mainly**

A variety of other disorders are associated with neuropathic arthritis including:

- **Leprosy**
- **Yaws**
- **Syringomyelia**
- **Tabes dorsalis**
- **Meningomyelocele**
- **Congenital indifference to pain**
- **Peroneal muscular atrophy (Charcot-Marie-Tooth disease)**
- **Amyloidosis**
- There is fragmentation and eventual loss of articular cartilage with eburnation of the underlying bone. Osteophytes are found at the joint margins. With more advanced disease, erosions are present on the joint surface. Fractures, devitalized bone, and intra-articular loose bodies may be present. Microscopic fragments of cartilage and bone are seen in the synovial tissue
- CPPD disease resembles charcot joint.

5 Ds of Charcot's joints:

- **D**isorganization
- **D**ensity increased
- **D**ebris within joint capsule
- **D**estruction of bone
- **D**eformity

Clinical Manifestations

- Neuropathic joint disease usually **begins in a single joint** and then progresses to involve other joints, depending on the underlying neurologic disorder
- The involved joint progressively becomes enlarged from **bony overgrowth and synovial effusion**
- **Loose bodies** may be palpated in the joint cavity
- **Joint instability, subluxation, and crepitus** occur as the disease progresses. Neuropathic joints may develop rapidly, and a totally disorganized joint with multiple bony fragments may evolve in a patient within weeks or months
- The amount of pain experienced by the patient is less than would be anticipated based on the degree of joint involvement. Patients may experience sudden joint pain from intra-articular fractures of osteophytes or condyles.

Remember Here: Joint Erosions are seen in

- **Rheumatoid arthritis**
- **Psoriasis**
- **Reticulohistocytosis**
- **Osteoarthritis**
- **Psoriasis**

Intracerebral Leukocytostasis

Ball's disease is a potentially **fatal complication of acute leukemia** (particularly myelogenous leukemia) that can occur when the **peripheral blast cell count is greater than 100,000/ml**

- **High blast cell counts**
- **Blood viscosity is increased**
- **Blood flow is slowed**
- Primitive leukemic cells are capable of invading through endothelium and causing hemorrhage into the brain

Patients may experience **stupor, dizziness, visual disturbances, ataxia, coma, or sudden death.**

• **Putamen hemorrhage**	Hemiparesis, hemisensory loss, homonymous hemianopia
• **Pontine hemorrhage**	Pin-point pupils, reactive to light, no horizontal eye movements
• **Brainstem lesion**	Sensory loss of half of face, contralateral half of body with cranial nerve lesions
• **Thalamic lesion**	Sensory loss of half of face and ipsilateral half of body
• **Cerebellar involvement**	**Hypotonia, tremor, ataxia**

Arterial Territories and Important Points in Blood Supply of Brain

- **Left middle cerebral artery:** Blockage of this vessel would cause, among other effects, **right-sided hemiplegia** and sensory deficits mainly of the face and arms, a right visual field defect with inability to gaze to the right, and aphasia.
- **Right middle cerebral artery:** Blockage of this vessel would cause, among other things, **left-sided hemiplegia** and sensory deficits mainly of the face and arms and left visual field neglect with inability to gaze to the left. In addition, there may be neglect of the left side.
- **Left anterior cerebral artery:** This vessel supplies the medial aspects of the left hemisphere. Blockage may cause a weak, numb **right leg**. The face is typically spared.
- **Right anterior cerebral artery:** This vessel supplies the medial aspects of the right hemisphere. Blockage may cause a weak, numb **left leg**. The face is typically spared.
- **Left posterior cerebral artery:** This lesion presents as a **right-sided visual field deficit**, **alexia without agraphia** (if the corpus callosum is spared), and possible defects in naming colors.
- **Right posterior cerebral artery:** This lesion typically presents as a **left-sided visual field deficit** along with left-sided sensory loss if the thalamus is affected. There may also be left-sided neglect.

Occlusion of the vertebral artery may cause Medial Medullary Syndrome which is characterized by:

Paralysis or atrophy of tongue on the side of lesion (XII nerve involvement)

Paralysis of arm and leg on opposite side

Impaired tactile and proprioceptive sense on opposite side. (involvement of pyramidal tract and medial lemniscus.

The posterior inferior cerebellar artery (PICA)

- It is the **largest** and main branch of the vertebral artery
- It has a **tortuous S-shaped course** immediately after it arises from the vertebral artery
- Damage causes **Lateral Medullary Syndrome/Wallenberg's Syndrome.**

- **Impaired pain and temperature sense on opposite side.**
- Nystagmus (involvement of vestibular nucleus).
- Dysphagia (involvement of nucleus ambigus).
- Nystagmus (involvement of cerebellum).
- Horner's Syndrome (involvement of sympathetic pathway).

Occlusion of the Anterior Spinal Artery May Cause

- **Loss of motor function** below the level of the lesion (due to damage to the corticospinal tracts)
- **Loss of pain and temperature sensation** below the level of the lesion (due to damage to the spinothalamic tracts)
- **Weakness of limbs** (due to damage of the anterior grey horns in the cervical or lumbar regions of the cord)
- **Loss of bowel and bladder control** (due to damage of the descending autonomic tracts).

Occlusion of the Posterior Spinal Artery May Cause

- Loss of position sense, vibration sense and light touch due to damage of the **posterior white columns**

Pyramidal tract lesions cause

- **Clasp knife** spasticity
- Hyperreflexia
- Absent abdominal reflexes
- Positive Babinsiki (Extensor plantar)

Extra pyramidal tract lesions cause (Movement disorders):

- Rigidity
- Tremor
- Hypokinesia
- Chorea/Athetosis/Hemiballismus

Remember Lesions and their Locations

- **Caudate nucleus lesion: Chorea**
- **Subthalamic nucleus: Hemiballismus**
- **Substantia nigra: Parkinson's**
- **Nucleus basalis: Alzheimer's disease**
- **Amygdala: Klüver-bucy syndrome**

Parkinsonism

Parkinson's disease has a classic tetrad of (1) slowness or poverty of movement, (2) muscular ('lead pipe' and 'cog-wheel') rigidity, (3) 'pill-rolling' tremor at rest (which disappears with movement and sleep), and (4) postural instability (manifested by the classic shuffling gait and festination)

Parkinsonism is a syndrome consisting of a combination of:

- **Tremor**
- **Rigidity**
- **Bradykinesia and**
- **Characteristic disturbance of gait and posture**

Associated:

- **On-off phenomenon**
- **Decreased blinking**

- Symptoms of Parkinson's disease are caused by **loss of nerve cells in the pigmented substantia nigra, pars compacta and the locus coeruleus in the midbrain**
- **Parkinsonism** can be induced in primates by exposure to 1-methyl-4-phenyl-1,2,3,6-tetrahydropyridine **(MPTP)**
- The **4- to 6-Hz tremor** is typically **most conspicuous at rest and worsens with emotional stress**
- **Festinating gait is a feature**
- It often begins with rhythmic flexion-extension of the fingers, hand, or foot, or with rhythmic pronation-supination of the forearm
  - There is fixity **of facial expression**, with widened palpebral fissures and **infrequent blinking**
  - There may be:
- **Blepharoclonus (fluttering of the closed eyelids)**
- **Blepharospasm (involuntary closure of the eyelids) and**
- **Drooling of saliva from the mouth**
- **The voice is hypophonic** and poorly modulated. Power is preserved, but fine or rapidly alternating movements are impaired
- They walk with **small, shuffling steps**, have no arm swing, are unsteady (especially on turning), and may have difficulty in stopping. Some patients walk with a **festinating gait,** i.e. at an increasing speed to prevent themselves from falling because of their abnormal center of gravity
- The tendon reflexes are unaltered, and the plantar responses are flexor
- Repetitive tapping (at about 2 Hz) over the glabella produces a sustained blink response **(Myerson's sign)**

Parkinsonism:

The cause is thought to be a loss of dopaminergic neurons, especially in the substantia nigra, which project to the basal ganglia. The result is decreased dopamine in the basal ganglia. Drug therapy, which aims to increase dopamine, includes:

- **Levodopa with carbidopa**
- **Bromocriptine**
- **Pergolide**
- **Monoamine oxidase-B inhibitors (selegiline), and**
- **Amantidine**

USMLE Case Scenario

An 88-year-old patient complains of shaking in his right hand and trouble starting movements. On physical examination, the patient has a resting tremor of 6 Hz of the right hand. Man's face is expressionless (mask-like). Cogwheel rigidity is noted in both arms. He also has a slightly stooped posture, and a slow, shuffling gait. Saliva seems to be drooping from his mouth.

Drugs Causing Parkinsonism

- Methyldopa
- Reserpine
- Haloperidol
- Manganese
- Thiazides
- Metocloperamide
- Chlorpromazine

Remember

- **A resting tremor may be due to: hyperthyroidism, anxiety, drug withdrawal or intoxication, or benign (essential) hereditary tremor**
- **Benign hereditary tremor is usually autosomal dominant; look for a positive family history, and use beta blockers to reduce the tremor**
- **Also watch for Wilson's disease (hepatolenticular degeneration), which can cause chorea-like movements; asterixis (slow, involuntary flapping of outstretched hands) may be seen in patients with liver and kidney failure.**

Clinical Scenarios of Headache

Clinical scenario	Diagnosis	Features
• A patient comes with **severe, unilateral headaches** several times a day with **lacrimation, photophobia**	• **Cluster headache**	• Periorbital • Male predominant
• A person reports with **severe, unilateral, throbbing** headache with aura of **scintilating scotomas**	• **Migraine**	• Lateralized usually • Female predominant • Often preceded by aura, photopsia • Photophobia, nausea, vomiting
• An elderly person reports **scalp tenderness**, intermittent throbbing and **jaw claudication. ESR is↑**.	• **Temporal arteritis**	
• A person reports with prostrating headache associated with **nausea and vomiting.** The history will usually reveal that the headache started with **severe eye pain**. On physical examination, the eye is often red with a **fixed, moderately dilated pupil**	• **Glaucoma**	
• A person reports with chronic head pain syndrome characterized by **bilateral tight, band-like discomfort**	• Tension and headache	• Tight band-like discomfort • Usually generalized with exacerbation by stress, fatigue
• A patient reports with pain located at the **jaw or neck, deep, dull, and aching**, and it becomes pounding or throbbing. There are often superimposed **sharp, ice pick-like jabs**. Tenderness and **prominent pulsations of the cervical carotid artery** and soft tissue swelling	• Caritodynia	
• A patient reports with **vertigo, dysarthria, or diplopia, tinnitus, distal and perioral paresthesia**, and occipital headache	• Basila-migraine	
• A 56-year-old female presents with **severe headache and neck stiffness of abrupt onset**. She tells she never had such a headache before. She is **nauseated and has photophobia**	• SAH	

Subarachnoid Hemorrhage (SAH)

- **Most aneurysms** present as a **sudden SAH**
- **Berry's aneurysms in anterior circulation are frequent cause**
- **Sudden loss of consciousness may be preceded by a brief moment of excruciating headache, but most patients first complain of headache upon regaining consciousness**
- **The patient often calls the headache 'the worst headache of life'. The headache is usually generalized, and vomiting is common**
- Although sudden headache in the absence of **focal neurologic symptoms is the hallmark of aneurysmal rupture,** focal neurologic deficits may occur. The common deficits that result include hemiparesis, aphasia, and abulia
- **A third cranial nerve palsy, particularly when associated with pupillary dilatation, loss of light reflex, and focal pain above or behind the eye,** may occur with an expanding aneurysm at the junction of the posterior communicating artery and the internal carotid artery
- **A sixth nerve palsy** may indicate an aneurysm in the cavernous sinus, and visual field defects can occur with an expanding supraclinoid carotid or anterior cerebral artery aneurysm
- Occipital and posterior cervical pain may signal **a posterior inferior cerebellar artery or anterior inferior cerebellar artery aneurysm (rarer)**
- **Rebleed and vasospasm are responsible for clinical deterioration in a week following**
- Pain in or behind the eye and in the low temple can occur with an expanding MCA aneurysm. Growing aneurysms rarely cause head pain in the absence of neurologic symptoms and signs.

- Aneurysms can undergo small ruptures and leaks of blood into the subarachnoid space, so-called **sentinel bleeds**
- **Noncontrast CT** is used as best initial investigation. **Nimodepine** is used to prevent vasospasm
- **Surgical clipping of aneurysm** is the modality of treatment used.

Headache of sudden onset ('thunderclap' headache), rapid deterioration of mental status and blood in the CSF are virtually diagnostic of ruptured berry aneurysms. Note the characteristic hyperdensity on CT of the suprasellar cistern, indicating blood in the subarachnoid space. Rupture of a berry aneurysm is the most common cause of subarachnoid bleeding. Berry aneurysms develop as a result of congenital weakness at branching points of the arteries in the circle of Willis. These outpouchings tend to expand progressively, but in most cases they remain asymptomatic. Hypertension facilitates development and rupture of berry aneurysm. One-third of patients recover, one-third die, and one-third develop re-bleeding. Rapid onset of coma is an ominous sign.

- **Basilar migrane seen in adolescent females beginning with total blindness: Bickersaffs migrane**
- **Cluster headache: Reader's syndrome, sphenopalatine neuralgia.**

CRANIAL NERVE DISORDERS

Trigeminal Neuralgia

- **Tic Douloureux**
  - A disorder of the trigeminal nerve producing bouts of severe, lancinating pain lasting seconds to minutes in the distribution of one or more of its sensory divisions, most often the mandibular and/or maxillary. Adults usually are affected, especially later in life
  - The pain is often set off by touching a **trigger point** or by activity (e.g. chewing or brushing the teeth). Although each bout of intense pain is brief, successive bouts may incapacitate the patient
- **Treatment:**
  - **Carbamazepine**
  - **Phenytoin, baclofen, amitriptyline** or **trazodone** is occasionally helpful.

Glossopharyngeal Neuralgia

- A rare syndrome characterized by **recurrent attacks of severe pain in the posterior pharynx, tonsils, back of the tongue, and middle ear**
- As in trigeminal neuralgia, intermittent attacks of:
  - **Brief**
  - **Severe**
  - **Excruciating pain occurs paroxysmally**, either spontaneously or
  - **Precipitated by movement** (e.g. chewing, swallowing, talking, sneezing)
  - **The pain, lasting seconds to a few minutes, usually begins in the tonsillar region or at the base of the tongue and may radiate to the ipsilateral ear. The pain is strictly unilateral. Occasionally, increased vagus nerve activity causes cardiac sinus arrest with syncope. Attacks may be separated by long intervals**
- **Treatment:**
- As in trigeminal neuralgia, **carbamazepine is the drug of choice**
- **Phenytoin, baclofen, amitriptyline, or trazodone** may be added if necessary.

Facial Nerve Disorders: Bell's Palsy

- **Usually unilateral facial paralysis of sudden onset** and unknown cause
- The mechanism is presumed to involve **swelling of the nerve** due to immune or viral disease, with **ischemia and compression of the facial nerve** in the narrow confines of its course through the temporal bone
- Pain behind the ear may precede the facial weakness that develops within hours, sometimes to complete paralysis
- **It is a type of LMNL**

- The involved side is flat and expressionless, but patients may complain instead about the seemingly twisted intact side
- In severe cases, the palpebral fissure is wide, and the eye cannot be closed
- **Corneal protection** is necessary
- The patient may complain of a numb or heavy feeling in the face, but no sensory loss is demonstrable
- A proximal lesion may affect salivation, taste, and lacrimation, and may cause hyperacusis.

PERIPHERAL NEUROPATHY

Peripheral neuropathy may be divided into conditions which predominately cause a motor or sensory loss.

Diseases with Predominately Motor Loss

- **Guillain-Barré syndrome**
- **Porphyria**
- **Lead poisoning**
- **Hereditary sensorimotor neuropathies (HSMN)—Charcot-Marie-Tooth**
- **Inflammatory demyelinating polyneuropathy (IDP)**
- **Diphtheria**

Diseases with Predominately Sensory Loss

- **Diabetes**
- **Uremia**
- **Leprosy**
- **HIV**
- **Alcoholism**
- **Vitamin B12 deficiency**
- **Amyloidosis**
- **Alcoholic neuropathy**
- **Secondary to both direct toxic effects and reduced absorption of B vitamins**
- **Cisplatinum and suramin**
- **Sensory symptoms typically present prior to motor symptoms**

Vitamin B12 Deficiency

- **Subacute combined degeneration of spinal cord** (SACD)
- **Dorsal column** usually affected first (joint position, vibration) prior to distal paresthesia

Amyotrophic Lateral Sclerosis

- Amyotrophic lateral sclerosis is an idiopathic, degenerative, neurological disorder affecting **both upper and lower motor neurons**
- Usually anterior horn cells are affected
- **Corticospinal tracts are involved**
- **Sensory nerves are usually spared**
- **Hyporeflexia is seen**
- **Ocular muscles are spared.** Muscle wasting or atrophy is due to LMNL and brainstem motor nuclei degeneration
- **Combination of upper motor neuron lesions in lower extremity and lower motor neurons in upper extremity is seen.** Typically involvement is asymmetric
- **Riluzole** presynaptically inhibits glutamate release in the central nervous system (CNS) and postsynaptically interferes with the effects of excitatory amino acids.

Remember

- **Balaclava type of sensory loss: Syringomyelia**
- **Dissociated sensory loss: Syringomyelia**
- **Mask-like facies: Parkinsonism**
- **Tic douloureux: Trigeminal neuralgia**
- **Punch drunk: Alcoholism**
- **Picket fence fever: Lateral sinus thrombosis**
- **Astasia-Abasia: Hysterical conversion**
- **Opsoclonus/myoclonus: Neuroblastoma**

Pearls about Brain Tumors

- **Astrocytomas: MC brain tumors**
- **Gliomas: MC intracranial neoplasms**
- **Astrocytomas: MC glial tumors**
- **Medulloblastomas: MC malignant brain tumor in children**
- **Craniopharyngioma: MC supratentorial tumor in children**
- **Medulloblastomas: MC midline cerebellar tumors**
- **Medulloblastomas: Most radiosensitive tumor**
- **Astrocytomas: MC posterior fossa tumors (CEREBELLAR)**

Brain Tumors are associated with

- **von Hippel-Lindau syndrome**
- **Tuberous sclerosis**
- **Neurofibromatosis**

- **Optic nerve glioma is the mc tumor associated with NF1**
- **Bilateral acoustic neuromas are a feature of NF 2**
- **Craniopharyngiomas are derived from Rathke's pouch**

Fevers

Fever	Causative Organism
• **Sandfly fever**	• Arbovirus
• **Lassa fever**	• Arena virus
• **Glandular fever**	• Ebstein-barr virus
• **Boutonneuse fever**	• Rickettsiae conorii
• **Oroya fever**	• Bartonella
• **Pretibial fever**	• Leptospirosis
• **Canicola fever**	• Leptospirosis
• **Swamp fever**	• Leptospirosis
• **Seven-day fever**	• Leptospirosis
• **Haverhill fever**	• *Streptobacillus moniliformis*
• **Scarlet fever**	• Streptococci
• **Pontiac fever**	• *Legionella*

Parasitic Diseases

Parasitic Diseases	
'Most Likely' clinical scenarios associated with parasitic diseases	
Type of Schistosomiasis presenting predominantly with **pulmonary hypertension**	• **Schistosoma mansoni**
Type of Schistosomiasis presenting predominantly with **portal hypertension**	• **Schistosoma japonicum**
Type of Schistosomiasis presenting predominantly with **hematuria**	• **Schistosoma hematobonium**
Parasitic disease in which **pruritis ani** is a feature	• **Pinworm infection**
Parasitic disease in which **rectal prolapse** is a feature	• **Whipworm**
Parasitic disease in which **intestinal obstruction** is a feature commonly	• **Roundworm**
Parasitic disease in which **megaloblastic anemia** is a feature	• **Diphyllobathrium latum**
Parasitic disease in which **cholangitis or cholangiocarcinoma** is a complication	• **Clonorchis sinesis**
Parasitic disease in which **megaesophagus** is a feature	• **Chagas disease**
Parasitic disease in which **anchovy sauce expectoration** is seen	• **Amebic abscess**
Parasitic disease in which **tennis racket-shaped organisms produce malabsorption**	• **Giardiasis**
Parasitic disease in which **hemoptysis** is a feature	• **Paragonimiasis**
Parasitic disease in which **elephantiasis** occurs is a feature	• **Filariasis**

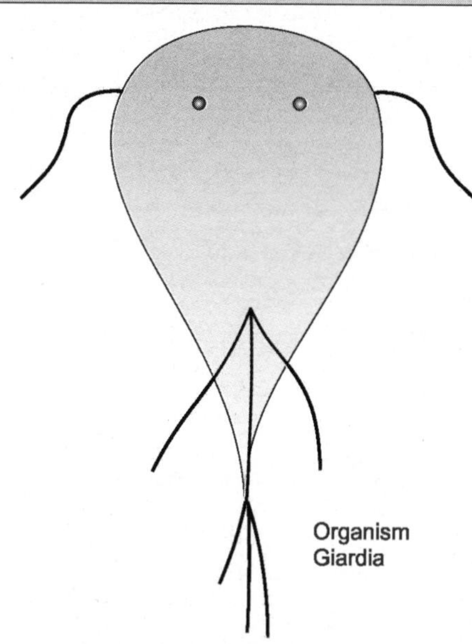

Antibody Target	**Disease**
• **Nicotinic acetyl choline receptor**	• Myasthenia gravis
• **Intrinsic factor**	• Pernicious anemia
• **Proteinase 3 (ANCA)**	• Wegner's granulomatosis
• **Alpha 3 chain of Collagen Type IV**	• Goodpasteur's syndrome
• **Thyroid peroxidase**	• Hashimoto's thyroiditi's

- ANA: SLE
- Anti-smith, anti-dsDNA: Specific for SLE
- Anti-histone: Drug induced SLE
- Anti-centromere: CREST Syndrome (c-c)
- Anti-Scl 70: Scleroderma (scl-scl)
- Anti-SSA, Anti-SSB: Sjogren's syndrome (s-s)
- Anti-Jo 1: **Polymyositis**
- Anti-mitochondrial: Primary biliary cirrhosis
- Anti-glidian, Anti-transglutaminase: Celiac disease
- Anti-GIL: Hemolytic transfusion reactions
- Anti-sacchromyces cerevisiae: Crohn's disease
- Anti-epithelial cell: Pemphigus vulgaris
- Anti-IgG: Rheumatoid arthritis
- Antibodies to filaggrin
- Antibodies to citrulline
- Antibodies to calpastatin
- **Antibodies to components of the spliceosome (RA-33), and an unknown antigen, Sa**

Enzyme Deficiencies in Porphyrias

• **Erythropoietic porphyria**	• **Ferrochelatase**
• **Hereditary porphyria**	• **Coproporphynogen oxidase**
• **Variegate porphyria**	• **Protoporphyrinogen oxidase**
• **Acute Intermittent porphyria**	• **Porphobilinogen deaminase**
• **Porphyria cutanea tarda**	• **URO decarboxylase**
• **Congenital erythropoietic porphyria**	• **URO III CoA synthase**

Eponym Spots in Medicine

• **Koplik spot**	Measeles
• **Roth Spots**	SABE
• **Bitot's Spots**	Vitamin A deficiency
• **Herald Spot**	Pitryriasis rosea
• **Café au lait spots**	Peutz-jegher's syndrome

Important Eponyms

• **Hebra nose**	Rhinoscleroma
• **Rubber man**	Ehler-Danlos syndrome
• **Sailors skin**	Solar elastosis
• **Petrified man**	Myositis ossificans

Gamma heavy chain disease:	**Franklin's disease**
Alpha heavy chain disease:	**Seligmann's disease**

- **Swimming pool granuloma:** Mycobacterium marinum
- **Swimmer's itch:** Schistosomiasis
- **Swimming pool conjunctivitis:** Adenovirus

Rare Syndromes

LEOPARD syndrome:
- **Lentiges**
- **ECG abnormalities**
- **Ocular hypertelorism**
- **Pulmonary stenosis**
- **Abnormal genitalia**
- **Retarded growth**
- **Deafness**

LAMB syndrome:
- **Lentiges**
- **Atrial myxoma**
- **Blue nevus**

NAME syndrome:
- **Nevus**
- **Atrial myxoma**
- **Myxoid neurofibroma**
- **Ephelids**

Carney syndrome: LAMB and NAME syndrome

POEMS syndrome:
- **Polyneuropathy**
- **Organomegaly**
- **Endocrinopathy**
- **M protein**
- **Skin change**

Important Triads and Pentads to be remembered

Triad of Alport's Syndrome: Sensorineural deafness, Progressive renal failure, Ocular anomalies

Triad of Behçet's Syndrome: Recurrent oral ulcers, Genital ulcers, Iridocyclitis

Beck's Triad: Muffled heart sound, Distended neck veins, Hypotension (cardiac tamponade)

Gradenigo's Triad: Sixth Cranial N palsy, Persistent ear discharge, Deep-seated retro-orbital pain

Hutchinson's Triad: Hutchison's teeth, Interstitial keratitis, Nerve deafness

Saint's Triad: Gallstones, Diverticulosis, Hiatus hernia

Trotter's Triad: Conductive deafness, immobility of homolateral soft palate, trigeminal neuralgia

Virchow's Triad: Stasis, Hypercoagulability, Vessel injury

Whipple's Triad: Hypoglycemia during attacks, S. glucose 10%, Hypergammaglobulinemia

Hemolytic Uremic Syndrome Triad: Anemia,Thrombocytopenia, Renal failure

Fanconi Syndrome Triad: Aminoaciduria, Proteinuria, Phosphaturia

Alkaptonuria Triad: Ochronotic arthritis, Ochronotic pigmentation, Urine darkens on standing.

- **Anderson Triad:** Bronchiectasis, Cystic fibrosis, Vitamin A deficiency
- **Pentad of TTP:** Microangiopathic hemolytic anemia, Fever, Disturbed neurological function, Renal failure, Thrombocytopenia
- **O'Donoghue Triad:** Twisting force in a weight-bearing knee joint causes injury to Medial collateral ligament, Anterior cruciate ligament, Medial meniscus
- **Cushing's Triad of Increased Intracranial Pressure:** Bradycardia, Bradypnea, Hypertension
- **Hemobilia:** Malena, Obstructive jaundice, Biliary colic
- **Kartagener's Syndrome Triad:** Triad of bronchiectasis, Recurrent sinusitis, and Situs inversus.

Concept Clarifications

• Hutchinson's freckle	Lentigo maligna (melanoma variant)
• Hutchinson's pupil	Blown pupil in uncal herniation
• Hutchinson's sign	Herpes zoster ophthalmicus, vesicles at tip of nose
• Hutchinson's teeth	Small, widely spaced teeth in congenital syphilis
• Hutchinson's triad	Interstitial keratitis, notched incisors, VIII nerve deafness
• Hutchinson's #	# radial styloid process
• Hutchinson's book	Book on medicine (not asked in exams)

• Charcot's crystals	In bronchial asthma
• Charcot's disease	ALS
• Charcot's joint	Neuropathic joints in leprosy, syphilis
• Charcot's triad	Seen in multiple sclerosis, cholangitis
• Charcot's aneurysm	Brain aneurysm

CD Markers

• Hairy cell leukemia	CD 103+
• Mantle cell lymphoma	CD 5+, CD 103–
• CLL	CD 23+
• Apoptosis	CD 95+

- **Brainstem lesion:**

Cranial nerve involvement+sensory loss of ½ of face+contralateral ½ of body

- **Thalamic lesion:**

Sensory loss of ½ of face+same ½ of body

- **Internal capsule lesion:**

Loss of face, arm, leg without higher cortical dysfunction

- **Renkies edema:** It is edema of vocal cords
- **Angioneurotic edema:** Due to C1 esterase inhibitor deficiency
- **Berlins edema:** Blunt trauma to eye
- **Quincke's edema:** Generalized anasarca

Remember

• Nonenhancing lesion in AIDS	PML
• Solitary weakly ring-enhancing lesion	CNS lymphoma
• Multiple ring-enhancing lesions	Toxoplasmosis

USMLE Case Scenario

Toxoplasmosis

A 44-year-old patient diagnosed with AIDS develops right-sided weakness involving the lower limb. MRI scans reveal two ring-enhancing lesions within the white matter of the left frontal lobe. A biopsy shows coagulative necrosis of brain parenchyma with macrophage-rich chronic inflammatory infiltration admixed with microscopic cysts that contain characteristic bradyzoites.

- This patient has cerebral toxoplasmosis, which represents one of the most common opportunistic infections in AIDS
- Toxoplasma gondii is a protozoon that infects humans who ingest the oocysts from cat feces or incompletely cooked lamb or pork
- Only immunodepressed patients and fetuses are vulnerable to this infection. In the fetus, toxoplasmosis causes extensive damage to brain parenchyma and retina
- Toxoplasmosis associated with AIDS manifests with necrotizing lesions surrounded by chronic inflammation
- A ring-enhancing lesion is a mass that contains a rim of contrast enhancement (bright signal on MRI) surrounding a dark core corresponding to central necrosis
- In AIDS, the most frequent causes of a ring-enhancing lesion are primarily brain lymphoma and toxoplasmosis.

USMLE Case Scenario

A 55-year-old man at home develops hemiparesis, ataxia, homonymous hemianopia, and cognitive deterioration. He was taken to a neurologist In New York. An MRI of the brain demonstrates widespread areas of abnormal T2 signal in the white matter. Brain biopsy reveals demyelination with abnormal giant oligodendrocytes, some of which contain eosinophilic inclusions. Most likely cause is:

1. Chickenpox
2. Progressive multifocal leukoencephalopathy
3. Multiple sclerosis
4. Syphilis
5. Tuberculosis

Ans. 2. Progressive multifocal leukoencephalopathy

Progressive Multifocal Leukoencephalopathy

- It is a rapidly progressive demyelinating disorder
- JC virus (a papovavirus) infects oligodendroglial cells in the brain
- The eosinophilic inclusions represent accumulations of JC virus
- PML occurs in about 1% of AIDS patients, and is the AIDS-defining illness in half of the patients who develop the condition.

- **Pott's puffy tumor** — **Osteomyelitis of skull**
- **Cock's peculiar tumor** — **Complicated, infected sebaceous cyst**

- **Hemoptysis normally is due to bronchial artery**
- **Hempotysis in Mitral stenosis is due to pulmonary artery**

Familial breast cancer: BRCA1
Sporadic breast cancer: p53

- **HTLV1: Adult T cell leukemia/lymphoma, Tropical spastic paraplegia**
- **HTLV2: Hairy T cell leukemia**
- **HTLV3: HIV/AIDS**

- **Rebound hypertension: Clonidine**
- **Postural hypotension: Prazosin**

Cardiac Tamponade

- **X-descent**
- **Pulsus paradoxus**

Constrictive Pericarditis

- **Kussmaul sign**
- **Steep y-descent**
- **Square root sign**
- **M contour sign**
- **Pericardial knock**

- **Myelodysplastic syndrome: 5q**
- **Cri-du-chat syndrome: 5p**

- **S100, TA 90: Melanoma**
- **CA 27.29: Breast Ca**
- **CA 72.4: Ovarian Ca, pancreatic Ca**
- **LASA P: Ovarian Ca**

- **<u>Mycotic aneurysm</u> is due to bacteria**
- **<u>Mycotic abscess</u> is due to fungal infection**

'Quick wrap-up': Important Points Highlighted

USMLE Case Scenarios

• An organism is found to be a **pleomorphic, gram-negative rod that causes a localized skin infection** and seems to be a cause of **an occupational disease of fishermen, fish handlers, and butchers. Most likely disease is caused by:**	**Erysipelothrix**
• **A nematode infection** is caused by taking **undercooked Pork** with symptoms of **diarrhea, periorbital edema, myositis, fever, and eosinophilia. Most likely organism is:**	**Trichinella**
• An organism occurs in the **immunocompromised population** and may cause **severe diarrhea**. The organism presents as **minute (2–5 mm) intracellular spheres or arc-shaped merozoites** under normal mucosa. **Most likely disease is:**	**Cryptosporidiosis**
• A 44-year-old patient from Central America presents with **facial edema and nodules, fever, lymphadenopathy, and hepatosplenomegaly**. The disease also affects **cardiac muscle most severely.** It is most prevalent in **Central and South America;** with rare cases in the southern **US. The disease is:**	**Chagas disease**
• A 35-year-old female says she had a **protozoan infection** and used to **eat undercooked meat** and **had exposure to cat feces**. The organism can also cause a **heterophile-negative, mononucleosis-like syndrome**. In patients with AIDS, it causes **ring-enhanced focal brain lesions and pneumonia**. Most likely the disease is:	**Toxoplasmosis**
• **An African child** develops massive unilateral **enlargement of his lower face in the vicinity of the mandible.** Biopsy demonstrates **sheets of medium-sized blast cells with admixed larger macrophages. This type of tumor has been associated with viral infection. Most likely disease is:**	**Burkitt's lymphoma**
• A **disease is found to be due to reactivation of epidemic typhus infection caused by *Rickettsia prowazekii*.** It can occur many years after an **infection that was not been treated with antibiotics. The most likely disease is:**	**Brill-zinsser disease**
• **A gram-positive coco-bacillus** is causing Infection **during pregnancy** that may result in **sepsis, abortion or premature delivery**. Infection in the neonate may **produce meningitis.** In immunocompromised adults, **either meningitis or sepsis may occur. The organism is:**	**Listerosis**

• **A 3-year-old boy** from rural America is brought to the ENT emergency room in extreme **respiratory distress, with a temperature of 104 degrees Fahrenheit.** He is **drooling and has great difficulty swallowing** and on physical examination, **an inspiratory stridor is noted.** An immediate lateral X-ray done shows **swelling of the epiglottis. He has had no previous vaccinations. Most likely disease is:**	**Epiglottitis**
• **A highly encapsulated organism is found to cause bronchopneumonia** with patchy infiltrates involving one or more lobes with **red sputum** in a **debilitated alcoholic. Most likely disease is:**	**Klebsiella pneumoniae**
• **An 8-year-old girl is bitten in the leg by a dog. She presents the next day with fever and bone pain localized to her right calf. X-ray reveals a lytic lesion of the left femur**. Results of the bone culture are pending. Infecting organism is most likely to be:	**Pasteurella**
• **An organism is causing urinary tract infections.** It has **ability to break down urea and** is thought to contribute to the development of **struvite kidney stones** due to the elevation of urine pH by production of ammonia. The said organism is also **having swarming motility. The organism is identified as:**	**Proteus species**
• A 44-year-old man from rural Indian village is brought to a rural hospital with **severe bronchopneumonia**. He suffered **sudden onset of chills, fever, and headache** several days ago. Two days later, he complained of chest pain and **difficulty breathing, and coughed up blood-tinged sputum. Chest X-ray reveals patchy infiltrates and segmental consolidation. The most likely cause of this man's pneumonia and the disease itself is due to yersinia. Disease itself is:**	**Plague**
• **A disease is caused in a gardener by virtue of organism entering through skin breaks in the fingers or hands, causing a chancre, papule, or subcutaneous nodule with erythema and fluctuance.** Ulcerating lesions appear along **lymphatic channels**, but the lymph nodes are not commonly infected. **Potassium iodide** is used for the treatment of the subcutaneous manifestations. The disease is common in gardeners. Most likely disease is:	**Sporotrichosis**
• A 66-year-old alcoholic man from New with brain and pulmonary abscess and is treated with antibiotics for last two weeks. He develops nausea, vomiting, abdominal pain, and voluminous green diarrhea. The condition is diarrhea due to:	**Clostridium difficile**
• An organism identified on dark ground microscopy caused **testicular involvement with gumma formation**, **endarteritis, and/or a prominent plasma cell infiltrate**. Most likely disease is:	**Syphilis**
• **A disease which may be spread by handling rabbits or rabbit skins**, or by bites from ticks that feed on the blood of wild rabbits, **a gram-negative coccobacillus**. The disease **begins as a rupturing pustule followed by an ulcer, with involvement of regional lymph nodes.** More serious cases can be complicated by **bacteremia, splenomegaly, rash, pneumonia, or endotoxemic shock. Most likely disease is:**	**Tularemia**
• **A gram-positive spore-forming anaerobic rod causing (a spastic paralysis** caused by toxin which blocks the release of the inhibitory neurotransmitters **glycine and gamma-aminobutyric acid [GABA]) is most likely:**	**Tetanus caused by clostridia tetani**
• **A gram-negative rod that is a zoonotic agent causing an undulating febrile disease with malaise, lymphadenopathy and hepatosplenomegaly.** The normal route of exposure is via ingestion of the organism. Most likely disease is:	**Brucellosis**

• A 65-years-old male from Chicago presents with **low back pain, anemia and fatigability**. **ESR** is 90 and **serum creatinine**: 3.2 mg%. Likely diagnosis is:	• **Multiple myeloma**
• A child brought by his mother from Mexico presents with **ascending flaccid paralysis**. There is subsequent respiratory muscle involvement. CSF examination shows **albuminocytological dissociation**. Likely diagnosis is:	• **Guillain-Barré syndrome**
• A 56-year-old engineer from Michigan presents with **pain, numbness and impaired sensation** over half of the face along with **ataxia, nystagmus, dysphagia and hoarseness of voice.** His pain and thermal sensations over opposite half are impaired. **Horner's syndrome** is present. Likely cause is:	• **Wallenberg's syndrome**

• A 25-year-old male scholar from New Zealand had **pigmented macules over the palm, sole and oral mucosa.** He also had **anemia and pain in abdomen**. The most probable diagnosis is:	• **Peutz-Jeghers syndrome**
• A 64-year-old lady admitted in neurology unit of Philadelphia complains of **severe unilateral headache on the right side and blindness for 2 days**. On examination, there is **a 'thick cord' like structure** on the lateral side of the head. The **ESR** is 80 mm/hr in the first hour. The most likely diaganosis is:	• **Temporal arteritis**
• A 45-years-old female in Texas presented with **hypertension, palpitation.** CT scan finds 7 cm **suprarenal mass**. Most likely diagnosis is:	• **Pheochromocytoma**
• A young female presents with history of dyspnea on exertion. On examination, she has **wide, fixed split S2 with ejection systolic murmur** (III/VI) in left second intercostal space. Her EKG shows **left axis deviation.** The most probable diagnosis is:	• **Ostium primum atrial septal defect**
• A 29-year-old woman from Ohio was found to have **hemoglobin of 7.8 g/dl** with a **reticulocyte count of 0.8%.** The peripherial blood smear **showed microcytic hypochromic anemia**, hemoglobin A_2 and hemoglobin F levels were 2.4% and 1.3% respectively. **The serum irom and the total iron-binding capacity were 15 micro g/dl, and 420 micro g/dl, respectively**. The most likely cause of anemia is:	• **Iron-deficiency anemia**
• A 33-year-old lady working as a manager in Ohio presents with **polydipsia and polyuria**. Her symptoms started soon after a road traffic accident 6 months ago. The blood pressure is 120/80 mm Hg with no postural drop. The daily urinary output is 6–8 liters. Investigation showed, Na 130 mEq/l, K.3.5 mEq/l, urea 15 mg/dl, sugar 65 mg/dl. The plasma osmolality is 268 mosmol/l and urine osmolality 45 mosmol/l. The most likely diagnosis is:	• **Psychogenic polydipsia**
• A 4½-year-old girl brought by her dear mother from Washington always had to wear warm socks even is summer season. On physical examination, it was noticed that she had **high blood pressure and her femoral pulse was weak as compared to radial and carotid pulse.** A chest radiograph showed remarkable **notching of ribs** along with their lower borders. The most likely diagnosis is:	• **Coarctation of aorta**
• A 56-year-old immunocompromised man who was given steroids by his physician in Ohio has **painful vesicular rash** over his right upper eyelid and forehead for the last 48 hours. He underwent chemotherapy for nonhodgkin's lymphoma one year ago. His tepmperature is 98 °F, blood pressure 138/76 mm Hg and pulse is 80/minute. Examination shows no other abnormalities. Which of the following is the most likely diagnosis:	• **Herpes zoster**
• A 40-years-male from Calafornia presents with **polyuria, pain abdomen, nausea, vomiting, altered sensorium** was found to have **Bronchogenic carcinoma**. The electrolyte abnormality seen in him would be:	• **Hypercalcemia**
• A 65-year-old female is seen in surgical casualty of New Orleans. The patient has a **progressive skin pigmentation, amenorrhea, and visual field disturbances from a functioning pituitary tumor**. A CT scan shows a pituitary tumor. History is significant for **bilateral adrenalectomy for Cushing's disease.** High plasma concentrations of ACTH and MSH were demonstrated by bioassay. Most likely diagnosis is:	• **Nelson's syndrome**
• A 75-year-old working in some factory in China presents with symptoms of **nonpleuritic chest pain, dyspnea secondary to pleural effusion, weight loss, fever, and cough** also occur with high frequency. Physical examination is notable for dullness to percussion and diminished breath sounds. They **stain positive for keratin**. The chest X-ray shows pleural plaques, pleural effusion. Computed tomography demonstrates extrapleural soft tissue invasion and diaphragmatic involvement. The most likely diagnosis is:	• **Mesothelioma**
• A 55-year-old man has **abdominal fullness, nonspecific symptoms of fatigue, weakness, and weight loss, easy bruising**. It is found that he has a type of leukemia. This leukemia is characterized by **presence of malignant cells that have irregular, filamentous cytoplasmic projections** on light microscopy that give the cells a hairy appearance. The most likely diagnosis is:	• **Hairy cell leukemia**
• In a 55-year-old of Chicago, a **painless firm fibrotic thickening** of the **fascia of the corpora cavernosa** is observed involving the dorsolateral aspects of the penile shaft or the intracavernous septum between the corpora cavernosa. Most likely diagnosis is:	• **Peyronie's disease**

• A 54-year-old alcholic after a **trauma on the highway** in California has **hypoxia, confusion. Petechiae are found over the chest, conjunctivae, and uvula.** Neurological examination shows confusion, agitation, stupor. **Respiratory abnormalities include tachypnea, profound hypoxia.** Blood examination shows thrombocytopenia, hypofibrinogenemia, and prolongation of the partial thromboplastin time. **Electrocardiogram shows prominent S waves in lead 1, prominent Q waves in lead 3, ST segment depression, and right axis strain.** Arterial PO_2 is 50 mm Hg on room air. Most likely diagnosis is:	• **Fat embolism**
• A pathologist from Leicester (UK) reports that a disease is **confined to the mucosal and submucosal layers** of the colonic wall, with superficial ulcers, increased cellular infiltration of the lamina propria, and **crypt abscesses** beginning in the rectum and advancing proximally to involve the entire colon. On gross inspection, the colonic mucosa demonstrates healed **granular superficial ulcers superimposed on a friable and thickened mucosa with increased vascularity.** The most likely cause is:	• **Ulcerative colitis**
• A syndrome is associated with the rare occurrence of **malignant infiltration of the colonic sympathetic nerve** supply in the region of the celiac plexus in which **sometimes massive cecal and colonic dilation** is seen in **the absence of mechanical obstruction**. Such an entity is described as:	• **Ogilvie syndrome**
• **A 6-year-old boy** seen by a neurologist in Washington DC has been complaining of **headache, ignoring to see the objects on the sides for four months.** On examination, he is not mentally retarded, his grades at school are good, and visual acuity **is diminished in both the eyes.** Visual charting showed significant field defect. CT scan of the head showed suprasellar mass with calcification. Most probable diagnosis is:	• **Craniopharyngioma**
• A patient from National Athletic Association of New York has **nuchal lymphedema** at birth, **short stature, webbed neck, widely spaced nipples, and primary ovarian failure.** A buccal smear done would classically reveal **absent Barr bodies.** Most likely diagnosis is:	• **Turner's syndrome**
• A tall Patient from Third year Class of a medical school with **arachnodactyly, hyperextensible joints, mitral valve prolapse, dislocation of the lens of the eye,** and a high risk for **thoracic aortic dissection** is most likely having:	• **Homocystinuria**
• **CD 19 positive, CD 22 positive, CD 103** positive monoclonal B-cells with **bright kappa positivity** were found to comprise 60% of the peripheral blood lymphoid cells on flow cytometric analysis in a **55-year-old man with massive splenomegaly** and a total leucocyte count of 3.3×10^9/l. Most likely diagnosis is:	• **Hairy cell leukemia**
• A 36-year-old female with symptoms of hyperparathyroidism, tumor in pancreas, adrenal cortical hyperplasia, pituitary adenomas, islet cell tumor with cutaneous angiofibromas. Most likely diagnosis is:	• **MEN I**
• A 30-year-old male patient presents with complaints of **weakness in right upper and both lower limbs** for the last 4 months. He developed **digital infarcts** involving **2nd and 3rd fingers on right side and 5th finger** on left side. On examination, BP was 160/140 mm Hg, all peripheral pulses were palpable and there was asymmetrical neuropathy. Investigations showed Hb 12 gm%, TLC 12,000 per cu mm platelets 4,30,000 and ESR 49 mm. Urine examination showed **Proteinuria** and RBC-10–15/hpf with no casts. The most likely diagnosis:	• **Polyarteritis nodosa**
• A 34-year-old female, nonhypertensive working in White House presents with severe headache and neck stiffness of abrupt onset. She tells she never had 'such a severe headache' before. On further asking, she tells she is nauseated and has photophobia. Diagnosis is:	• **Subarachnoid hemorrhage**
• A 16-year-old girl from Texas with **primary amenorrhea** attends OPD. She has **normal sexual development and normal breast** but with **absent pubic and axillary hair**. Examination shows B/L inguinal hernias • USG shows absent uterus and blind vagina. Diagnosis will be:	• **Androgen insensitivity syndrome**

• A 20-year-old male comes to the physician for a routine physical examination. **His height is 198 cm. He has long fingers and toes. Blood pressure is 150/65 mm Hg, and pulse is 66/min.** On auscultation, there is a **grade 2/6, long, high-frequency diastolic murmur** at the second right intercostal space. Echo would reveal most likely a diagnosis of valvular lesion of:	• **Aortic regurgitation**
• A 66-year-old woman reports to a physician because of **aches and stiffness in her neck, shoulders, and hips for two-and-a-half months.** Her symptoms are more in the morning hours. She has had **chronic fatigue and low-grade fever** during this period. **Range of motion of the neck, shoulders, and hips is normal.** The muscles are minimally **tender to palpation.** Muscle strength, sensation, and deep tendon reflexes are normal. Erythrocyte sedimentation rate is 88 mm/h. **Serum rheumatoid factor and antinuclear antibody assays are negative**. The most likely diagnosis is:	• **Polymyalgia**
• A 20-year-**young man** presents with **exertional dyspnea, headache, and giddiness**. On examination, there is hypertension and **LVH.** X-ray picture shows **notching of the anterior ends of the ribs**. The most likely diagnosis is:	• **Coarctation of the aorta**
• A 30-year-old HIV-positive patient from New York robbery gang presents with fever, dyspnea and nonproductive cough. Patient is cyanosed. His chest X-ray reveals **bilateral, symmetrical interstitial infiltrates**. The most likely diagnosis is:	• **Pneunocystis carinii pneumonia**
• A 40-year-old male working as a bartender in a local pub, with history of daily alcohol consumption for the last 7 years, is brought to the hospital with acute onset of not recognizing family members, violent behavior and tremulousness for few hours. There is history of his having missed the alcohol drink since 2 days. Examination reveals increased blood pressure, tremors, increased psychomotor activity, fearful affect, hallucinatory behavior, disorientation, impaired judgment and insight • He is most likely to be suffering from:	• **Delerium tremens**
• **A 50-year-old man, an alcoholic and a smoker** presents with a 3-hour history of **increasing shortness of breath.** He started having this pain while eating, which was constant and **radiated to the back and interscapular region.** He was a known hypertensive. On examination, he was cold and clammy with a **heart rate of 130/min, and a BP of 80/40 mm Hg. JVP was normal. All peripheral pulses were present and equal. Breath sounds were decreased at the left lung base and chest X-ray showed left pleural effusion.** The most likely diagnosis is:	• **Acute aortic dissection**
• A patient **with 'leukemia on chemotherapy' in a Chemotherapy unit of Washington** develops **acute right lower abdominal pain associated with anemia, thrombocytopenia and leukopenia**. The most likely diagnosis is:	• **Neutropenic colitis**
• A patient presents with chronic **small bowel diarrhea,** duodenal biopsy shows **villous atrophy. Antiendomysial antibodies are positive**. Most likely diagnosis is:	• **Gluten enteropathy**
• A **24-year-old** male presents with **abdominal pain, rashes, palpable purpura and arthritis.** The most probable diagnosis is:	• **Henoch-Schonlein Purpura (HSP)**
• A 7-year-old girl presents with **repeated episodes of bleeding into joints. APTT is prolonged and PT is normal.** The most likely diagnosis is:	• **von Willebrand disease**
• In a lady with **bilateral superior temporal quadrantopia** and **galactorrhea**, the most probable cause is:	• **Pituitary macroadenoma**
• **A 40-year-old** engineer presented with **hepatosplenomegaly, hilar lymphadenopathy and hypercalcemia. Most probable diagnosis is:**	• **Sarcoidosis**
• A man with fever, dull-aching retrosternal chest pain reported to the emergency. On examination, he was found to show pulsus paradoxus, Kussmaul's sign and increased jugular venous pressure. His apex beat was impalpable and heart sounds were muffled. Probable diagnosis is:	• **Pericardial effusion**

• A 33-year-old lady presents with **polydipsia and polyuria**. Her symptoms started soon after a **road traffic accident** 6 months ago. The blood pressure is 120/80 mm Hg with no postural drop. The **daily urinary output is 6–8 liters**. Investigation showed **Na 130 mEq/l, K.3.5 mEq/l, urea 15mg/dl, sugar-65 mg/dl. The plasma osmolality is 268 mosmol/l and urine osmolality 45 mosmol/l**. The most likely diagnosis is:	• **Psychogenic polydipsia**
• A 33-year-old HIV-positive male from New York complains of pain on swallowing. Physical examination is remarkable for white plaque-like material on his tongue and buccal mucosa, which is scraped and sent to the laboratory. The man is diagnosed with acquired immunodeficiency syndrome (AIDS) • The most likely diagnosis is:	• **Candidiasis**
• **A 4-year-old boy presents with a 1-day history of loose stools, fever, abdominal cramping, headache, and myalgia. He has no blood in the stool.** The incubation period is **36 hours after ingestion of contaminated food or water. Most likely the causative agent of his diarrhea is:**	• **Salmonella**
• **A 4-year-old girl with a history of hydrocephalus** is brought to the neurologist by her parents with a severe headache and fever. The girl underwent a surgery for a **ventricular-peritoneal shunt 2 months ago,** and the neurologist suspects that an infection has occurred. **Infection is most likely due to:**	• **Staph epidermis infection**

USMLE Case Scenario

Thrombotic thrombocytopenic purpura (TTP, Moschcowitz's syndrome) is a syndrome characterized by:

1. Thrombocytosis, microangiopathic hemolytic anemia, fluctuating neurologic abnormalities, progressive hepatic failure, and fever
2. Thrombocytosis, microangiopathic hemolytic anemia, nonfluctuating neurologic abnormalities, progressive renal failure, and fever
3. Thrombocytopenia, macroangiopathic hemolytic anemia, fluctuating neurologic abnormalities, progressive renal failure, and fever
4. Thrombocytopenia, microangiopathic hemolytic anemia, fluctuating neurologic abnormalities, progressive renal failure, and fever

Ans. 4. Thrombocytopenia, microangiopathic hemolytic anemia, fluctuating neurologic abnormalities, progressive renal failure, and fever

USMLE Case Scenario

Features of tumor lysis syndrome are:

1. Hyperuricemia, hyperphosphatemia, hypercalcemia
2. Hyperuricemia, hypophosphatemia, hypocalcemia
3. Hyperuricemia, hyperphosphatemia, hypercalcemia
4. Hyperuricemia, hyperphosphatemia, hypocalcemia

Ans. 4. Hyperuricemia, hyperphosphatemia, hypocalcemia

USMLE Case Scenario

A 66-year-old man from New Jersy with known hepatitis C and cirrhosis complains of confusion over the past week. He has had a declining urinary output. On physical examination, he is jaundiced, has tense ascites. Laboratory results reveal a WBC count of 4500/mm^3, An Hb of 8.4 g/dl, and a hematocrit of 31%. His KFT reveals a BUN of 37mg/dl and a creatinine of 3.3 mg/dl. Urinary sodium is less than 11 mEq/l. Which of the following is the most appropriate treatment for his elevated BUN and creatinine?

1. Large volume paracentesis
2. Hemodialysis
3. Portocaval shunt
4. Kidney transplantation
5. Liver transplantation
6. Peritoneal dialysis
7. Sodium restriction

Ans. 5. Liver Transplantation

This patient with well-advanced cirrhosis and portal hypertension has developed the onset of renal insufficiency consistent with hepatorenal syndrome. This occurs during the end-stages of cirrhosis and is characterized by diminished urine output and low urinary sodium. Liver transplantation is a viable option which will reverse this clinical scenario and kidney function will return to normal.

USMLE Case Scenario

An elderly patient presents with pallor, fever, recurrent infections, oral ulcerations, ecchymoses, and petechiae. Preliminarily hypersplenism is suspected. Criteria for diagnosis include:

1. Anemia, leukopenia, thrombocytopenia, or combinations, bone marrow hypoplasia, splenomegaly, improvement after splenectomy
2. Erythrocytosis, leukocytosis, thrombocytosis, or combinations, compensatory bone marrow hyperplasia, splenomegaly, improvement after splenectomy
3. Erythrocytosis, leukocytosis, thrombocytosis or combinations, bone marrow hypoplasia, splenomegaly, improvement after splenectomy
4. Anemia, leukopenia, thrombocytopenia, or combinations, compensatory bone marrow hyperplasia, splenomegaly, improvement after splenectomy

Ans. 4. Anemia, leukopenia, thrombocytopenia, or combinations, compensatory bone marrow hyperplasia, splenomegaly, improvement after splenectomy

USMLE Case Scenario

In Hodgkin's Lymphoma, constitutional symptoms (B symptoms) may appear simultaneously with lymph node enlargement or may precede development of lymphadenopathy. Truth about these B symptoms is that they include:

1. Fever, night sweats, weight loss, and pruritus and indicative widespread involvement and are favorable prognostic signs
2. Fever, night sweats, weight gain, and pruritus and indicative widespread involvement and are favorable prognostic signs
3. Fever, night sweats, weight gain, and pruritus and indicative local involvement and are unfavorable prognostic signs
4. Fever, night sweats, weight loss, and pruritus and indicative widespread involvement and are unfavorable prognostic signs

Ans. 4. Fever, night sweats, weight loss, and pruritus and indicative widespread involvement and are unfavorable prognostic signs.

USMLE Case Scenario

Hodgkin's disease involving lymph node regions on both sides of the diaphragm is classified as:

1. Stage I
2. Stage II
3. Stage III
4. Stage IV

Ans. 3. Stage III

- Stage I disease indicates nodal involvement in only one lymph node region
- Stage II disease is limited to two or more lymph node regions on the same side of the diaphragm
- Stage III refers to disease involving lymph node regions on both sides of the diaphragm (the spleen is considered a lymph node)
- Stage IV disease encompasses diffuse or disseminated involvement of one or more distant extranodal organs with or without associated lymph node involvement
- Stage IV is further classified as A (absence) or B (presence) with regard to fever, night sweats, weight loss, and pruritus

USMLE Case Scenario

A 55-year-old man has abdominal fullness nonspecific symptoms of fatigue, weakness, and weight loss, easy bruising. It is found that he has a type of leukemia. This leukemia is characterized by presence of malignant cells that have irregular, filamentous cytoplasmic projections on light microscopy that give the cells a hairy appearance. Truth about it is that it is:

1. Common form of leukemia characterized by pancytopenia, splenomegaly without significant lymphadenopathy
2. Common form of leukemia characterized by pancytopenia, splenomegaly with significant lymphadenopathy
3. Uncommon form of leukemia characterized by pancytopenia, splenomegaly with significant lymphadenopathy
4. Uncommon form of leukemia characterized by pancytopenia, splenomegaly without significant lymphadenopathy

Ans. 4. Uncommon form of leukemia characterized by pancytopenia, splenomegaly without significant lymphadenopathy

Hairy cell leukemia (leukemic reticuloendotheliosis) is an uncommon form of leukemia characterized by pancytopenia, splenomegaly without significant lymphadenopathy, and characteristic mononuclear cells in the blood and bone marrow.

USMLE Case Scenario

Truth about pigment gallstones in patients with sickle-cell anemia is:

1. Incidence of pigment gallstones in patients with sickle-cell anemia decreases with age. Calculi appear first in childhood and are present in approximately 70% of adult patients
2. Incidence of pigment gallstones in patients with sickle-cell anemia increases with age. Calculi appear first in adulthood and are present in approximately 70% of adult patients
3. Incidence of nonpigment gallstones in patients with sickle-cell anemia increases with age. Calculi appear first in childhood and are present in approximately 70% of adult patients
4. Incidence of pigment gallstones in patients with sickle-cell anemia increases with age. Calculi appear first in childhood and are present in approximately 70% of adult patients

Ans. 4. Incidence of pigment gallstones in patients with sickle-cell anemia increases with age. Calculi appear first in childhood and are present in approximately 70% of adult patients

USMLE Case Scenario

The physiologic mechanisms affected by medical strategies for the management of osteoporosis include:

1. Decreased apoptosis of osteoclasts by bisphosphonates
2. Increased activation of osteoclast activity by calcitonin
3. Increased osteoblast differentiation by selective estrogen receptor modulators
4. Decreased intestinal Ca2+ secretion by vitamin D

Ans. 3 Increased osteoblast differentiation by selective estrogen receptor modulators

USMLE Case Scenario

An 88-year-old female smoked cigarettes for 20 years but stopped smoking 5 years ago. She has increasing dyspnea for months with a nonproductive cough. A chest radiograph shows prominent hilar lymphadenopathy. A transbronchial biopsy is performed, and the microscopic findings include interstitial fibrosis and small noncaseating granulomas. This disease is believed to be caused by:

1. Delayed hypersensitivity response to an unknown antigen
2. Immediate hypersensitivity response to an unknown antigen
3. Immune complexes formed in response to inhaled antigens
4. Diffuse alveolar damage (DAD)
5. Smoke inhalation for many years
6. Infection with atypical mycobacteria

Ans. 1. Delayed hypersensitivity response to an unknown antigen

USMLE Case Scenario

Which of the following is LEAST likely to be associated with cystic fibrosis?

1. Intestinal obstruction
2. Sinusitis
3. Steatorrhea
4. Dextrocardia
5. Clubbing

Ans. 4. Dextrocardia

USMLE Case Scenario

Methylphenyltetrahydropyridine is taken by a 25-year-old male from California complaining of uncontrollable shaking in his hands. Most likely pathology he might have as a result of the above-mentioned features is:

1. Lewy bodies
2. Pick bodies
3. Negri bodies
4. Neurofibrillary tangles

Ans. 1. Lewy bodies

USMLE Case Scenario

A 55-year-old alcoholic. Comes to your office complaining of cough, chills and fever. He has a 'cold' for 4 days and has been coughing up yellow-thick tenacious sputum with jelly-like consistency and reddish color. He denies shortness of breath and chest pain. Temperature is 39.6 °C and expiratory rales are heard over both lung fields. Among the following, the most likely causative organism is:

1. Klebsiella pneumonia
2. *E. coli*
3. Pseudomonas pneumonia
4. Mycoplasma pneumonia
5. Pneumocystis carinii pneumonia
6. Pulmonary tuberculosis

Ans. 1. Klebsiella pneumonia

USMLE Case Scenario

Dominantly inherited disease associated with progressive chorea and dementia; related to neurotransmitter imbalance:

1. Wilson's disease
2. Tardive dyskinesia
3. Tourette's syndrome
4. Huntington's disease
5. Shy-Drager syndrome

Ans. 4. Huntington's disease

USMLE Case Scenario

It is found that the mean corpuscular hemoglobin concentration is elevated and cells are resistant to osmotic lysis:

1. Hereditary xerocytosis
2. Hereditary spherocytosis
3. Hereditary elliptocytosis
4. Aplastic anemia

Ans. 1. Hereditary xerocytosis

Hereditary hydrocytosis and xerocytosis are rare forms of hemolytic anemia that result from a primary alteration in red cell membrane monovalent cation permeability. Xerocytosis is differentiated from hereditary spherocytosis, elliptocytosis, or other conditions where the mean corpuscular hemoglobin concentration is elevated by red cell morphology and resistance of the cells to osmotic lysis.

USMLE Case Scenario

Howell-Jolly bodies are:

1. Nuclear remnant
2. Denatured hemoglobin
3. Iron granules
4. Organelles

Ans. 1. Nuclear remnant

- Howell-Jolly bodies are (nuclear remnant)
- Heinz bodies are (denatured hemoglobin)
- Pappenheimer bodies are (iron granules)

USMLE Case Scenario

After splenectomy, suspicion of splenosis is made. This is demonstrated by:

1. Absence of Howell-Jolly bodies, siderocytes
2. Presence of Howell-Jolly bodies, siderocytes
3. Absence of target cells, reticulocytes
4. Presence of target cells, reticulocytes

Ans. 1. Absence of Howell-Jolly bodies, siderocytes

The absence of Howell-Jolly bodies, siderocytes, and other postsplenectomy blood changes as well as the recurrence of the hematologic disease for which splenectomy was performed should raise suspicion of splenosis or the presence of accessory splenic tissue.

USMLE Case Scenario

A 66-year-old has malaise, dyspnea, and weight with abdominal fullness and discomfort, early satiety. Older records suggest that he has had episodes of bone pain, pruritus and hyperuricemia. Pathologist reports he has myeloid metaplasia. Characteristic features of myeloid metaplasia are:

1. Fibrosis of the bone marrow, no extramedullary hematopoiesis, presence in the peripheral blood of mature erythroid and granulocytes and no splenomegaly

2. Fibrosis of the bone marrow, extramedullary hematopoiesis, presence in the peripheral blood of immature erythroid and granulocyte precursors and massive splenomegaly
3. No fibrosis of the bone marrow, no extramedullary hematopoiesis, presence in the peripheral blood of immature erythroid and granulocyte precursors and massive splenomegaly
4. No fibrosis of the bone marrow, extramedullary hematopoiesis, presence in the peripheral blood of immature erythroid and granulocyte precursors and no splenomegaly

Ans. 2 Fibrosis of the bone marrow, extramedullary hematopoiesis, presence in the peripheral blood of immature erythroid and granulocyte precursors and massive splenomegaly

USMLE Case Scenario

A 44-year-old has a long history of arthritis. The patient fails to show a substantial granulocytosis in response to infection, and severe, persistent, and recurrent infections are characteristic. Antibody directed against granulocytes is demonstrable in the patient. Mild anemia and thrombocytopenia are present in some cases. Moderate splenomegaly is seen. Most likely arthritis is:

1. Osteoarthritis
2. Gouty arthritis
3. Gonococcal arthritis
4. Syphilitic arthritis
5. Rheumatoid arthritis
6. Septic arthritis

Ans. 5. Rheumatoid arthritis

Felty's syndrome consists of the triad of severe rheumatoid arthritis, granulocytopenia and splenomegaly

USMLE Case Scenario

A 24-year-old college student is brought to the Emergency Room by her parents who state that the patient vomited all night. Examination reveals an ill-appearing woman. Her temperature is 37.8 °C, blood pressure is 110/70 mm Hg, pulse is 154/min, and respirations are 28/min. The patient is dehydrated. Chest and CVS Examination are normal. Laboratory analysis shows:

Sodium .... 131 mEq/l
Potassium .... 6.4 mEq/l
Chloride .... 101 mEq/l
Bicarbonate .... 8.5 mEq/l
Urea nitrogen .... 10 mg/dl
Creatinine .... 1.1 mg/dl
Glucose .... 777 mg/dl
pH.......................... 7.13
pCO_2 .... 30 mm Hg
pO_2 .... 85 mm Hg
Urinalysis is positive for ketones
Which of the following is the most appropriate initial step in management?

1. Ion exchange resins
2. IV diazepam
3. Intravenous insulin
4. Streptokinase
5. Put her on ventilator
6. IV potassium
7. Mannitol

Ans. 3. Intravenous insulin

Diabetic ketoacidosis (DKA) is a life-threatening complication of diabetes mellitus. DKA exists if there is hyperglycemia (glucose >300), ketonemia, acidosis (pH < 7.30, HCO_3 < 15) with clinical symptoms of diabetes. The mainstay of treatment for DKA is intravenous insulin.

USMLE Case Scenario

A 12-year-old Ashkenazi Jew presents with massive splenomegaly. He is having a disease which is genetically transmitted as an autosomal recessive trait caused by a deficiency of an enzyme responsible for breaking down certain lipid complexes. On biopsy of macrophages, cells are seen to contain dense fibrillar deposits of glucocerebroside in the cytoplasm. Diagnosis is made by finding the typical cells in biopsied tissues. These cells are:

1. Ito cells
2. Gaucher cells
3. Kuffer cells
4. Adipocytes

Ans. 2. Gaucher cells

USMLE Case Scenario

A 66-year-old person from Wales imitates movements of his friend. This implies he has:

1. Echopraxia
2. Echolalia
3. Cataplexy
4. Stereotypy
5. Stereotaxy

Ans. 1. Echopraxia

USMLE Case Scenario

A disease of defect in platelet adhesion with abnormally large platelets and lack of platelet-surface glycoprotein is:

1. Glanzmann's disease
2. ITP
3. TTP
4. Hemophilia
5. Myelofibrosis
6. von Willebrand's disease
7. Bernard-Soulier disease

Ans. 7. Bernard-Soulier disease

USMLE Case Scenario

A 71-year-old man with a 70-pack-year smoking history comes to the physician after he notes that his right eye has a lagging lid. The physician has been seeing this patient for more than 10 years for management of his symptoms of chronic obstructive pulmonary disease (COPD). On physical examination, he has ptosis of the right eye with a constricted right pupil. The remainder of the ophthalmologic examination is normal. Cranial nerve function is otherwise normal. Which of the following would most likely be expected on a chest X-ray film?

1. A normal chest X-ray film
2. An irregularly shaped mass at the apex of the right lung
3. A calcified granuloma in the left mid-lung field
4. A left-sided pleural effusion
5. A right upper lobe pneumonia

Ans. 2. An irregularly shaped mass at the apex of the right lung. This patient has physical findings consistent with right-sided **Horner's syndrome, which consists of a triad of ptosis, miosis, and anhidrosis. This results from a lung cancer in this long-time smoker at the apex of the right lung, which causes compression of the cervical sympathetic plexus. These patients may also complain of scapular pain and a radiculopathy in the ulnar nerve distribution.**

USMLE Case Scenario

Alport's syndrome is:

1. Hereditary nephritis with goiter
2. Hereditary nephritis with nerve deafness

3. Hereditary nephritis with nerve blindness
4. Hereditary nephritis with gynecomastia

Ans. 2. Hereditary nephritis with nerve deafness

USMLE Case Scenario

A 34-year-old Philipino nurse has loss of carotid, radial pulse with night sweats. Most likely diagnosis is:

1. Temporal arteritis
2. Wegener's disease
3. Kawasaki disease
4. Takayasu's arteritis

Ans. 4. Takayasu's arteritis

USMLE Case Scenario

Munchausen syndrome is:

1. Nonfactitious disorder, unconsciously creates symptoms, but doesn't know why
2. Nonfactitious disorder, consciously creates symptoms, but knows why
3. Factitious disorder, consciously creates symptoms, but knows why
4. Factitious disorder, consciously creates symptoms, but doesn't know why

Ans. 4. Factitious disorder, consciously creates symptoms, but doesn't know why

USMLE Case Scenario

A 35-year-old patient has severe muscle discomfort and restlessness that causes him agitation, pacing, and anxiety. He has used antipsychotics for a pretty long period now. Most likely diagnosis is:

1. Dystonia
2. Chorea
3. Hemiballismus
4. Akathisia
5. Akinesia

Ans. 4. Akathisia

It is a subjective feeling of muscle discomfort and restlessness that can cause agitation, pacing, anxiety, and dysphoria. It is related to the use of antipsychotics

USMLE Case Scenario

A 44-year-old presents to medicine clinic with seizures. There is no aura. No EEG abnormalities are seen on further evaluation. The movements are asynchronous and nonstereotyped and they occur when the person is awake. Most likely diagnosis is:

1. Dystonia
2. Chorea
3. Hemiballismus
4. Pseudoseizures
5. Akathisia
6. Akinesia

Ans. 4. Pseudoseizures

USMLE Case Scenario

A middle-aged, itchy woman having CREST has jaundice, pruritus, and hepatomegalies are common. The liver function tests show a mild transaminitis with # alkaline phosphatase and # bilirubin. Diagnosis would be suggested by ordering for:

1. Antimicrosomal antibody
2. Antikidney antibody

3. AntiLKM antibody
4. Antiphospholipid antibody
5. Antimitochondrial antibody

Ans. 5. Antimitochondrial antibody

USMLE Case Scenario

A severely ill HIV-affected patient has evidence of destruction of myelin at multiple sites in the CNS pointing to a diagnosis of progressive multifocal leukoencephalopathy (PML). PML is caused by:

1. JC virus which is a papovavirus
2. JC virus which is a parvovirus
3. HTLV1 virus which is a rhabdovirus
4. HTLV2 virus which is a papovavirus

Ans. 1. JC virus which is a papovavirus

USMLE Case Scenario

Bracht-Wachter lesions are seen in:

1. Subacute bacterial endocarditis
2. Syphilis
3. Dermoid cyst
4. Leprosy
5. Tuberculosis

Ans. 1. Subacute bacterial endocarditis

USMLE Case Scenario

A young girl presents with polyostotic fibrous dysplasia, precocious puberty, café au lait spots, short stature. Most likely the diagnosis is:

1. von Recklinghausen's disease
2. Tuberous sclerosis
3. Stein-Leventhal syndrome
4. Wermer's syndrome
5. Sipple syndrome
6. Albright's syndrome

Ans. 6. Albright's syndrome

USMLE Case Scenario

A 55-year-old male, who was hypertensive and diabetic, developed unconsciousness. It was found that he had paramedian infarct of midbrain with ipsilateral mydriasis, contralateral UMN paralysis of lower face and body. Most likely he is having:

1. Weber's syndrome
2. Wallenberg's syndrome
3. Medial medullary syndrome
4. Argyll Robertson syndrome

Ans. 1. Weber's syndrome

USMLE Case Scenario

The risk of acquiring hepatitis B is significantly higher than the risk for HIV, and somewhat higher than the risk for hepatitis C. Thus, it is essential that health care workers be immunized against the hepatitis B virus. The immunization schedule is for administration of the vaccine at:

1. 1, 2, and 6 months
2. 1, 3, and 6 months

3. 1, 4, and 6 months
4. 0, 3, and 6 months

Ans. 1. 1, 2, and 6 months

USMLE Case Scenario

A patient of 44 years, who recently had a head trauma, is clinically euvolemic and has a high urine osmolality and specific gravity. He responded to demeclocycline. Most likely he is having:

1. SIADH
2. Diabetes mellitus
3. Diabetes insipidus
4. Latent diabetes

Ans. 1. SIADH

USMLE Case Scenario

Pain reproduced by ulnar deviation to stretch the affected tendons is positive Finkelstein sign. It is seen in:

1. de Quervain's tenosynovitis
2. Dupuytren's contracture
3. Carpal tunnel syndrome
4. Bursitis

Ans. 1. de Quervain's tenosynovitis

USMLE Case Scenario

In the 3rd week of life, a baby presents with projectile non-bilious vomiting and on palpation, an olive-sized mass is palpable in the epigastrium. Plain radiographs demonstrate the absence of air distal to the obstructed pylorus. Regarding this condition:

1. Male infants are less commonly affected than female infants and the incidence is far greater in full-term infants than in preterm infants
2. Male infants are more commonly affected than female infants and the incidence is far less in full-term infants than in preterm infants
3. Male infants are less commonly affected than female infants and the incidence is far less in full-term infants than in preterm infants
4. Male infants are more commonly affected than female infants and the incidence is far greater in full-term infants than in preterm infants

Ans. 4. Male infants are more commonly affected than female infants and the incidence is far greater in full-term infants than in preterm infants.

USMLE Case Scenario

An infant presents with a superficial cellulitis of the skin with marked lymphatic involvement, caused by beta-hemolytic group. A streptococci begins with an area of redness and enlarges to form the typical tense, painful, bright red, shiny, brawny, infiltrated plaque with a well-demarcated, distinct, and slightly raised border. Most likely the diagnosis is:

1. Botromycosis
2. Gangrene
3. Rodent ulcer
4. Varicose ulcer
5. SSSS
6. Erysipelas

Ans. 6. Erysipelas

USMLE Case Scenario

A physician diagnoses a boy with Duchenne muscular dystrophy. Which of the following signs is most consistent with Duchenne muscular dystrophy:

1. Wrist drop
2. Foot drop
3. Gower's sign
4. Festinant gait
5. Waddling gait
6. Positive Babinski sign

Ans. 3. Gower's sign

The Gower's sign is very characteristic of Duchenne muscular dystrophy. It is considered positive if the patient uses his hands to 'walk' up the legs when going from a prone to an upright sitting position because he does not have enough proximal muscle power to get-up in a normal fashion.

USMLE Case Scenario

Lucio phenomenon is a widespread diffuse infiltration of the skin with secondary alopecia of the hair, eyebrows and eyelashes, and generalized sensory loss. The patients are systemically ill with fever, chills, malaise, arthralgias, myalgias, and tender cutaneous lesions that are responsive to steroids but not to thalidomide. Lucio phenomenon is usually associated with:

1. Mycoplasma
2. Chlamydia
3. Mycobacterium avium
4. Mycobacterium africanum
5. Mycobacterium tuberculosis
6. Mycobacterium leprae

Ans. 6. Mycobacterium leprae

USMLE Case Scenario

Irregular, unpredictable, involuntary muscle contractions:

1. Athetosis
2. Dystonia
3. Tics
4. Chorea
5. Akinesia

Ans. 4. Chorea

USMLE Case Scenario

A disease characterized by chronic, multiple tics:

1. Parkinson's disease
2. Wilson's disease
3. Shy-Drager syndrome
4. Tourette's syndrome

Ans. 4. Tourette's syndrome

USMLE Case Scenario

Donovanosis is caused by encapsulated, gram-negative bacterium Calymmatobacterium granulomatis. Infection results in a painless papule that eventually ulcerates over the course of days or weeks. Donovan bodies are seen. They are:

1. Leukocytes that contain the organism, Calymmatobacterium granulomatis

2. Eosinophils that contain the organism, Calymmatobacterium granulomatis
3. Monocytes that contain the organism, Hemophilus influenza
4. Monocytes that contain the organism, Calymmatobacterium granulomatis

Ans. 4. Monocytes that contain the organism, Calymmatobacterium granulomatis

USMLE Case Scenario

A 44-year-old male has intense pruritus over bilaterally symmetrical lesions. Patient uses the terms 'coin-shaped' and 'discoid' which are used to describe skin lesions. Microscopically, the dominant feature is a localized spongiosis of the epidermis, containing minute fluid-filled holes that correspond to the tiny vesicles seen clinically in early lesions. Patient gets relief with high-potency steroids. Most likely diagnosis is:

1. Psoriasis
2. Pompholyx
3. Pemphigus vegetans
4. Nummular eczema
5. Seborrhea

Ans. 4. Nummular eczema

USMLE Case Scenario

A 33-year-old woman, who is otherwise well, consults an ophthalmologist because of seeing double and droopy eyelids. She also has complaints of generalized muscle weakness. IV injection of edrophonium dramatically, but only briefly, reverses her symptoms. Most likely cause is:

1. Erb's palsy
2. Erb-Duchenne Paralysis
3. Myotonia
4. Inclusion body myositis
5. Lambert-Eaton syndrome
6. Myasthenia gravis

Ans. 6. Myasthenia gravis. It is an autoimmune disease in which antibodies directed against the acetylcholine receptor of the muscle side of the neuromuscular junction block the ability of the receptor to bind to acetylcholine.

USMLE Case Scenario

Ménétrier's disease is:

1. Atrophic gastritis, small rugae, plasma protein loss
2. Atrophic gastritis, enlarged rugae, plasma protein loss
3. Giant hypertrophic gastritis, small rugae, plasma protein loss
4. Giant hypertrophic gastritis, enlarged rugae, plasma protein loss

Ans. 4. Giant hypertrophic gastritis, enlarged rugae, plasma protein loss

USMLE Case Scenario

ECG manifestation of WPWS is:

1. Long PR interval, delta wave, slight shortening of the QRS complex
2. Long PR interval, delta wave, slight widening of the QRS complex
3. Short PR interval, delta wave, slight shortening of the QRS complex
4. Short PR interval, delta wave, slight widening of the QRS complex

Ans. 4. Short PR interval, delta wave, slight widening of the QRS complex

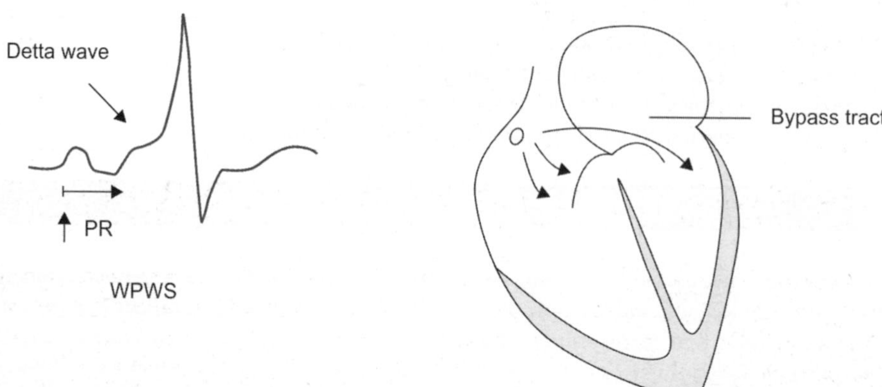

USMLE Case Scenario

A 54-year-old was admitted to hospital and found to have severe symmetrical distal limb weakness and 'glove and stocking' sensory loss to the elbows and knees. Nerve conduction studies showed evidence of a mixed motor and sensory neuropathy. A diagnosis was made of the Guillain-Barré syndrome. Investigation of the patient would demonstrate:

1. Low titers of IgE and IgG antibodies to *Campylobacter jejuni* were found in his peripheral blood
2. Low titers of IgE and IgD antibodies to *Campylobacter jejuni* were found in his peripheral blood
3. High titers of IgE and IgD antibodies to *Campylobacter jejuni* were found in his peripheral blood
4. High titers of IgM and IgG antibodies to *Campylobacter jejuni* were found in his peripheral blood

Ans. 4. High titers of IgM and IgG antibodies to *Campylobacter jejuni* were found in his peripheral blood

USMLE Case Scenario

A 23-year-old woman goes to the emergency department because she feels weak, having muscle cramping and fasciculations. Blood chemistry studies demonstrate plasma potassium of 1.5 mEq/l. She admits to chronic use of laxatives and diuretics to control her weight. Which of the following ECG changes would be most characteristic of changes related to her K+ level?

1. ST segment elevation
2. Decreased U wave amplitude
3. Increased U wave amplitude
4. Prolongation of the P wave
5. Shortening of the QT interval
6. Tall, symmetric, peaked T waves
7. Widening of the QRS complex

Ans. 3. Increased U wave amplitude

Severe hypokalemia, with plasma potassium < 3 mEq/l, can markedly affect skeletal, smooth, and cardiac muscles. Skeletal muscle effects can include:

- Weakness
- Cramping
- Fasciculations
- Paralysis (with risk of respiratory failure), tetany, and rhabdomyolysis
- Smooth muscle effects include hypotension and paralytic ileus
- Cardiac muscle effects include premature ventricular and atrial contractions, tachyarrhythmias, and AV block. Additional ECG changes can include ST segment depression, increased U wave amplitude, and T wave amplitude less than U wave.

USMLE Case Scenario

A 53-year-old woman presents complaining of fatigue, pruritus and weight loss for the last 6 months. There are excoriations noted on all four extremities and trunk and back. The liver edge is smooth and nontender and measures 9.2 cm at the midclavicular line. There is no ascites, splenomegaly, or peripheral edema. Laboratory results reveal a normal complete blood count, normal electrolytes, and liver function tests with an alkaline phosphatase of 288 U/L (Normal, < 110 U/L), total bilirubin of 3.5 mg/dl and normal transaminase levels. Which of the following would be associations of the disease:

1. Iron-deficiency anemia
2. Wegner's granulomatosis
3. Sjögren's syndrome
4. Osteoarthritis
5. Thrombophlebitis

Ans. 3. Sjögren's syndrome

This woman has a classic presentation of primary biliary cirrhosis. Primary biliary cirrhosis is often seen in individuals with other autoimmune diseases, such as Sjögren's syndrome, pernicious anemia and Hashimoto thyroiditis.

USMLE Case Scenario

A 65-year-old female is seen in surgical casualty. The patient has a progressive skin pigmentation, amenorrhea, and visual field disturbances from a functioning pituitary tumor. A CT scan shows a pituitary tumor. History is significant for bilateral adrenalectomy for Cushing's disease. High plasma concentrations of ACTH and MSH were demonstrated by bioassay. Most likely diagnosis is:

1. Liddle's syndrome
2. Barter's syndrome
3. Craniopharyngoma
4. Nelson's syndrome
5. Conn's syndrome
6. Prolactinoma syndrome

Ans. 4. Nelson's syndrome

USMLE Case Scenario

A 40-year-old man with adult polycystic kidney disease is brought to the emergency room in a coma. CT scan of the head demonstrates a subarachnoid hemorrhage without parenchymal hemorrhage. Which of the following is the most likely source of bleeding?

1. AV malformation
2. Bridging veins
3. Charcot-Bouchard aneurysm
4. Circle of Willis
5. Middle meningeal artery

Ans. 4. Circle of Willis

USMLE Case Scenario

A bone marrow examination showed a pleomorphic cellular infiltrate composed of a mixture of small lymphocytes, plasma cells and cells of an intermediate appearance, called lymphoplasmacytoid cells. These are features of :

1. Gaucher's disease
2. Krabe's disease
3. Fabry's disease
4. Hairy cell leukemia
5. Waldenström's macroglobulinemia
6. Sézary syndrome

Ans. 5. Waldenström's macroglobulinemia

USMLE Case Scenario

A 55-year-old gentleman has pickwickian syndrome. He has poor exercise tolerance and often feels lethargic at work. Which of the following is the best investigation?

1. Echocardiography to assess cor pulmonale
2. CT scan of the chest

3. Blood gas
4. Sleep study
5. Exercise tolerance test

Ans. 4. Sleep study

The diagnosis of obstructive sleep apnea can be made with a sleep study. In sleep apnea, there is gross obesity and airways obstruction, occasionally leading to type II respiratory failure.

USMLE Case Scenario

A 67-year-old man after a long-standing illness, has been on hemodialysis for 22 years due to diabetic nephropathy. He now has joint pains in the shoulders and knees. His blood test reveals:
Hb 10 g/dl, ESR 54 mm/hr, urea 19 μmol/l, creatinine 257 μmol/l, sodium 143 mmol/l, potassium 4.2 mmol/l, urate 0.7 (< 0.45)
What is the likely diagnosis?

1. Gout
2. Myeloma
3. Polymyalgia rheumatica
4. Conn's disease
5. Addison's disease
6. Rheumatoid arthritis
7. Calcium pyrophosphate deposition
8. B2 microglobulin amyloidosis
9. Cystinuria

Ans. 8. B2 microglobulin amyloidosis

The history of joint pains in a dialysis patient suggests amyloidosis. Amyloid deposits composed of b2-microglobulin are laid down in periarticular surfaces of joints.

USMLE Case Scenario

An HIV patient complains of visual disturbances. Fundal examination shows bilateral retinal exudates and perivascular hemorrhages. Which of the following viruses are most likely to be responsible for this retinitis:

1. Herpes simplex virus
2. Human herpes virus 8
3. Cytomegalovirus
4. Epstein-Barr (EB) virus

Ans. 3. Cytomegalovirus

USMLE Case Scenario

A chronic inflammatory condition having features of a mass of granulation tissue around the carotid artery in the cavernous sinus with symptoms simillar to cavernous sinus thrombosis associated with painful acute ophthalmoplegia and MRI findings suggesting cavernous sinus enlargement are a feature of:

1. Weber's syndrome
2. Tolsa-Hunt syndrome
3. Benedict's syndrome
4. Nothangel's syndrome
5. Millard-Gubler syndrome

Ans. 2. Tolsa-Hunt syndrome

USMLE Case Scenario

A 59-year-old man driving on highway has been involved in a car accident and is admitted for assessment. His attendants are told by the attending physician that he may have frontal lobe damage. Which of the following might be associated with frontal lobe damage?

1. Left-right disorientation
2. Tremor of tongue

3. Homonymous hemianopia
4. Dressing apraxia
5. Finger agnosia
6. Chorea
7. Perseverance
8. Total blindness

Ans. 7. Perseverance

Deficits following frontal lobe damage are attention disorder (distractibility and poor attention), aphasia, reduced activity, particularly a diminution of spontaneous activity, lack of drive, inability to plan ahead, and lack of concern.

USMLE Case Scenario

A 20-year-old male has presented with repeated episodes of hematemesis. There is no history of jaudice or liver decompensation. On examination, their significant findings include splenomegaly (8 cms below costal margin), and presence of esophageal varices. There is no ascites or peptic ulceration. The liver function tests are normal. The most likely diagnosis is:

1. Extrahepatic portal venous obstruction
2. Noncirrhotic portal fibrosis
3. Cirrhosis
4. Hepatic venous outflow tract obstruction

Ans. 2. Noncirrhotic portal fibrosis

USMLE Case Scenario

After a cardiac catheterization in a 56-year-old patient from New Jersy, a female presents with of a pulsatile mass, femoral bruit, and compromised distal pulses. Most likely diagnosis is:

1. Cholesterol embolization syndrome
2. Femoral pseudoaneurysms
3. Retroperitoneal bleed
4. Femoral hernia
5. Saphena varix

Ans. 2. Femoral pseudoaneurysms

USMLE Case Scenario

A 16-year-old girl was brought by her mother and both have similar skin appearance for soft, pink tumors distributed all over the body. Multiple light brown macules are also seen. Slit lamp examination of eye reveals iris hamartomas. Most likely disease is:

1. Tuberous sclerosis
2. Wilson's disease
3. Sturge-Weber syndrome
4. Neurofibromatosis
5. SABE

Ans. 4. Neurofibromatosis

USMLE Case Scenario

A 20-year-old female with frequent urination, increased thirst with serum osmolality of 350 mOsm/l and 24-hour urine osmolality of 50 mOsm/l improving upon giving desmopressin has most likely:

1. Diabetes insipidus
2. Diabetes mellitus
3. SIADH
4. DIDMOAD syndrome

Ans. 1. Diabetes insipidus

USMLE Case Scenario

A 44-year-old man from New York reports with lethargy and confusion followed by hypotension, bradycardia, AV block and cardiac arrest. After giving IV fluids, next line of treatment would be:

1. Hemodialysis
2. Calcium chloride
3. Digoxin
4. Hemoperfusion

Ans. 2. Calcium chloride

USMLE Case Scenario

A 33-year-old female comes to you with bruising, epistaxis, mennorrhagia. Further examination reveals fever, thrombocytopenia, anemia, hematuria and intravascular hemolysis and confusion. Most likely she is having:

1. ITP
2. TTP
3. Hemophilia
4. von Willebrand disease

Ans. 2. TTP

USMLE Case Scenario

A 44-year-old American male presents with sudden onset lightning-like pain pattern on his face with about 30 episodes in a day. There are no other associated medical problems. The male is nonhypertensive, nondiabetic and afebrile. The complaint described is most likely associated with which of the following disorders:

1. Pick's disease
2. Parkinson's disease
3. Huntington's chorea
4. Multiple sclerosis

Ans. 4. Multiple sclerosis

The condition is bilateral trigeminal neuralgia and multiple sclerosis is associated with it

USMLE Case Scenario

A 75-year-old patient presents with mask-like facies, expression less face, bradykinesia, festinant gait. The disease involves substantia nigra. He is diagnosed with parkinsonism. The aid disease is due to:

1. Overactivity of cholinergic neurons and overactivity of dopaminergic neurons
2. Underactivity of cholinergic neurons and underactivity of dopaminergic neurons
3. Underactivity of cholinergic neurons and overactivity of dopaminergic neurons
4. Overactivity of cholinergic neurons and underactivity of dopaminergic neurons

Ans. 4. Overactivity of cholinergic neurons and underactivity of dopaminergic neurons

USMLE Case Scenario

A 66-year-old male presents with history of frequent falls and nausea. There is no history of alcohol intake. He has difficulty in remaining erect and tends to fall to his right side. He is hypertensive; diabetic. He is currently taking lisinopril and aspirin. On ophthalmological examination, nystagmus is present. Most likely diagnosis is:

1. Parkinsonism
2. Huntington's chorea
3. Tabes dorsalis
4. Hydrocephalus
5. Cerebral disease
6. Pontine lesion

7. Pseudotumor cerebri
8. Normal pressure hydrocephalus
9. Cerebellar disease
10. Midbrain infarct

Ans. 9. Cerebellar disease

USMLE Case Scenario

A 74-year-old man comes to a hematology clinic for a routine check-up. On the peripheral smear, anisocytosis, poikilocytosis nucleated red blood cells, giant platelets, and tear drop-shaped red blood cells are seen. Most likely diagnosis is:

1. Pernicious anemia
2. Iron-deficiency anemia
3. Alpha thalassemia
4. Beta thalassemia
5. ALL
6. AML
7. Myelophthisic anemia
8. Lymphoma
9. Sezary syndrome

Ans. 7. Myelophthisic anemia

USMLE Case Scenario

A 45-year-old female from Toledo has developed a small nodule at a site of previous injury with granulation tissue formation. The lesion is neither nonbacterial nor a true granuloma. Microscopically, proliferating blood vessels in an immature fibrous stroma are seen. Most likely the lesion is a:

1. Wart
2. Keloid
3. Keratocanthoma
4. Basal cell cancer
5. Squamous cell cancer of skin
6. Pyogenic granuloma

Ans. 6. Pyogenic granuloma

USMLE Case Scenario

After a snake bite, a 55-year-old victim was immediately transported to the nearest medical facility. Earlier he had developed diplopia, dysphagia and ptosis after snake bite. Most likely cause is:

1. Myotoxic envenomation by a coral snake
2. Cytolitic envenomation by a pit viper snake
3. Cytolitic envenomation by a rattle snake
4. Neurotoxic envenomation by a coral snake

Ans. 4. Neurotoxic envenomation by a coral snake

USMLE Case Scenario

A 45-year-old patient reports to dermatology clinic after an HSV infection manifests with lesions on the palms and soles with mucosal blisters and a widespread vesicular/bullous skin eruption. Lesions consist of a dusky red center with a central vesicle surrounded by an erythematous halo. Most likely he is having:

1. Erythema multiforme
2. Erythema nodosum
3. Erythema migrans
4. Erythema ab igne

Ans. 1. Erythema multiforme

USMLE Case Scenario

A 66-year-old presents with bilateral knee pain for 6 months. Knee joints are tender with narrow joint space, subchondral bone cysts. Best management is by:

1. Oral NSAIDs
2. Oral acetaminophen
3. Steroids
4. Weight loss

Ans. 4. Weight loss

Obesity being the major risk factor, weight loss is the best management

USMLE Case Scenario

Occlusive arterial occlusion, superficial thrombophlebitis and Raynaud's phenomenon are a feature of:

1. Buerger's disease
2. Beurger's disease
3. Kawasaki disease
4. Takayasu's disease

Ans. 2. Buerger's disease

Buerger's disease is IgA Nephropathy

USMLE Case Scenario

A 40-year-old presents with pain, redness and swelling of external ear. He has joint pains and episcleritis. Most likely diagnosis is:

1. Polychondritis
2. Polyarteritis
3. Rheumatoid arthritis
4. Otitis externa

Ans. 1. Polychondritis

USMLE Case Scenario

A 35-year-old presents with a painful ulcer in mouth. She presented to ophthomologist and gynecologist two days back for uveitis and ulcer on genital respectively. The most likely diagnosis is:

1. Herpes simplex infection
2. Reiter's disease
3. Behçet's disease
4. Sjögren's disease

Ans. 3. Behçet's disease

USMLE Case Scenario

Clear vesicles with red base developing into macules on palms and soles in a patient with Reiter's syndrome are:

1. Pompholyx
2. Keratoderma
3. Circinate balanitis
4. Herpes Zoster

Ans. 2. Keratoderma

USMLE Case Scenario

A 45-year-old female presents with swelling of her right wrist. Her MCP and PIP joints are tender and swollen. She has an oral ulcer with low platelets. Her APTT is prolonged with positive rheumatoid factor and negative anti-Sm antibodies. Lupus anticoagulant is positive. She is most likely having:

1. Rheumatoid arthritis

2. SLE
3. Polymyositis
4. Mixed connective tissue disease

Ans. 2. SLE

Rheumatoid factor is not specific for Rheumatoid arthritis. Combination of oral ulcer, thrombocytopenia, prolonged APTT suggests SLE. Anti-Sm antibodies are not sensitive for SLE.

USMLE Case Scenario

A 60-year-old woman develops multiple organ failure 3 weeks following a pneumonia complicated by septicemia. Antibiotic therapy has resulted in sputum and blood cultures that are now without growth of organisms. Nevertheless, she requires intubation with mechanical ventilation, but it becomes progressively more difficult to maintain her oxygen saturations. Ventilatory pressures must be increased. A portable chest radiograph shows increasing opacification of all lung fields. Which of the following pathologic processes is most likely now to be present in her lungs?

1. Diffuse alveolar damage
2. Extensive neutrophilic alveolar exudates
3. Extensive intra-alveolar hemorrhage
4. Widespread bronchiectasis

Ans. 1. Diffuse alveolar damage (DAD) is the pathologic term for adult respiratory distress syndrome (ARDS) that is the final common pathway for many acute lung injuries. DAD produces increasing interstitial thickening with mixed inflammation and features of an acute restrictive lung disease.

USMLE Case Scenario

A 22-year-old female with low backache for last 7 months presents to orthopedic clinic in Washington DC which improves with physical activity. There is reduced forward flexion of lumbar spine. There is no history of pain in joints, rash, fever, weight loss, decreased appetite. Most likely diagnosis is:

1. Osteoarthritis
2. Ankylosing spondylitis
3. Rheumatoid arthritis
4. Reiter's disease

Ans. 2. Ankylosing spondylitis

USMLE Case Scenario

A rheumatoid arthritis patient presents to OPD clinic with improvement of her symptoms. Blood investigations reveal.

Hb=9.8

Serum Na=141

Serum K=3.7

Calcium=9.9

BUN=15

MCV=14

Most likely medication the patient is taking is:

1. Corticosteroid
2. Chloroquine
3. Cyclosporine
4. Methotrexate

Ans. 4. Methotrexate

Megaloblastic anemia

USMLE Case Scenario

A patient presents to Doctor in a New York's leading orthopedic clinic with pain in her both ankles and lesions on the skin suggesting erythema nodosum and chest radiography revealing bilateral hilar prominence most probably due to hilar lymphadenopathy. Most likely correct diagnosis a specialist makes is:

1. Sarcoidosis
2. Lofgren's syndrome
3. Heerd Ford Waldenstroms syndrome
4. Tuberculosis

Ans. 2. Lofgren's syndrome

USMLE Case Scenario

A 33-year-old woman from New Jersey presents to her physician with complaints of severe heartburn with or without meals. She has a history of hypertension, multiple facial telangiectasias, and very taut skin on the dorsum of both hands. She has failed to obtain relief for her heartburn with large doses of antacids, ranitidine, or omeprazole. Esophageal manometry is ordered. Which of the following would be the most likely results of this test?

1. Decreased esophageal peristalsis and decreased LES pressure
2. Decreased esophageal peristalsis and increased LES pressure
3. Increased esophageal peristalsis and decreased LES pressure
4. Increased esophageal peristalsis and increased LES pressure
5. Normal esophageal peristalsis and normal LES pressure

Ans. 1. Decreased esophageal peristalsis and decreased LES pressure. Patient has GERD secondary to scleroderma

USMLE Case Scenario

A 55-year-old patient presents orthopedic clinic with pain and stiffness in shoulder girdle. However, on examination, no tender spots can be found. However, occasional headaches and fever are noted by the patient who has all investigations within normal except for raised ESR. Most likely diagnosis is:

1. Fibromyalgia
2. Chronic fatigue syndrome
3. Polymyalgia rheumatica
4. Rheumatoid arthritis

Ans. 3. Polymyalgia rheumatica

USMLE Case Scenario

A 72-year-old male presents with headaches and myalgias. On examination, there is tenderness in scalp on right side with visual field defect in the right eye. He is a smoker for the last 35 years. His investigations reveal:

Hb = 12
Serum Na = 141
Serum K = 3.7
Calcium = 9.9
BUN = 15
ESR = 65
He is most probably having:

1. Reiter's arthritis
2. Giant cell arteritis
3. Reactive arthritis
4. Takayasu's arteritis

Ans. 2. Giant cell arteritis

USMLE Case Scenario

Abdominal pain, diarrhea, weight loss and joint pains suggesting bacterial infection represents:

1. Celiac disease
2. Whipple's disease
3. Inflammatory disease
4. Reactive arthritis

Ans. 2. Whipple's disease

USMLE Case Scenario

A 66-year-old female from Kansas complains of pain. She describes the pain as sudden onset, severe, electric shock-like pain occurring in paroxysms multiple times a day at infrequent intervals not responding to conventional NSAIDs without any rash. The doctor traces the path of pain along the branches of Cranial Nerve V. Most likely the pain represents:

1. Carotidodynia
2. Giant cell arteritis
3. Migraine
4. Herpes zoster
5. Neuralgia

Ans. 5. Neuralgia

USMLE Case Scenario

A 45-year-old patient presents orthopedic clinic with widespread pain. He complains of poor sleep, fatigue and depression. Multiple trigger points of tenderness are found. The patient most likely represents:

1. Fibromyalgia
2. Chronic fatigue syndrome
3. Polymyalgia rheumatica
4. Rheumatoid arthritis

Ans. 1. Fibromyalgia

USMLE Case Scenario

Subchondral sclerosis, narrow joint space, osteophytes are a radiological feature of:

1. Hemochromatosis
2. Reactive arthritis
3. Gouty arthritis
4. Osteoarthritis
5. Spondylitis

Ans. 4. Osteoarthritis

USMLE Case Scenario

A 25-year-old man from Chicago comes to the emergency department with a 4-day history of fever, chills, cough, pleuritic chest pain. His friends were caught by police for drug-trafficking. His temperature is 103.2 °F, blood pressure is 120/70 mm Hg, pulse is 71/min, and respirations are 15/min. Physical examination shows oval, retinal hemorrhages with a clear, pale center and marks over his arm. Blood cultures are drawn. A chest X-ray film shows multiple patchy infiltrates. Laboratory studies show high ESR. Most likely the causative organism is:

1. *E. coli*
2. Candida albicans
3. Pseudomonas aeruginosa
4. HACEK
5. Serratia marcescens
6. *Staphylococcus*
7. *Streptococcus*

Ans. 6. *Staphylococcus*

This patient has acute bacterial endocarditis, most likely due to *Staphylococcus aureus*, the most common organism causing endocarditis in intravenous drug abusers. The marks on his arm are signs of injection drug abuse. Acute endocarditis in drug abusers typically presents with a high fever, pleuritic chest pain, and cough.

USMLE Case Scenario

A dusky malar rash and periorbital edema and scaly patches over MCP joints in a 40-year-old female with symmetrical weakness of her proximal muscles is most likely:

1. Malar rash of SLE
2. Rash of psoriasis
3. Rash of scabies
4. Heliotrope rash of dermatomyositis

Ans. 4. Helitrope rash of dermatomyositis

USMLE Case Scenario

Fibromyalgia is usually treated by:

1. Colchicine and NSAIDs
2. Oxycodone
3. Counseling
4. Amitryptiline and cyclobenzapyrine

Ans. 4. Amitryptiline and cyclobenzapyrine

USMLE Case Scenario

A 45-year-old female from Ohio is suspected to have porphyria. Porphyria is evaluated by measuring:

1. Copper protoporphyrin levels in blood
2. Selenium protoporphyrin levels in blood
3. Cadmium protoporphyrin levels in blood
4. Zinc protoporphyrin levels in blood
5. Iron protoporphyrin levels in blood

Ans. 4. Zinc protoporphyrin levels in blood

USMLE Case Scenario

A 45-year-old nonhypertensive has had severe headache. Headache of sudden onset ('thunderclap' headache), rapid deterioration of mental status and blood in the CSF are diagnostic of:

1. Migraine
2. Tension headache
3. Cluster headache
4. Trigeminal neuralgia
5. Ruptured berry aneurysms

Ans. 5. Ruptured berry aneurysms

USMLE Case Scenario

An 86-year-old lady who usually stays indoors with restricted mobility presents with frequent episodes of back pains. Lateral spine X-rays and pelvic X-rays show osteopenia. A serum-corrected calcium is 1.9 mmol/l and phosphate is 0.7 mmol/l. Alkaline phosphatase is 369 U/l. Which of the following diagnosis is most likely?

1. Infantile rickets
2. Myeloma
3. Metastasis
4. Osteoporosis
5. Osteomalacia
6. Paget's disease
7. Ankylosing spondylitis

Ans. 5. Osteomalacia

Osteomalacia is likely due to the low calcium, low phosphate and raised ALP.

USMLE Case Scenario

An 18-year-old man from Texas has had type 1 diabetes for 5 years. He now presents with leg edema. After reporting to a physician, on investigation, he was found to have an urinary protein of 5.5 g/24 hours and serum cholesterol was 8.2 mmol/l. The histology will show fusion and deformity of the foot processes under the electron microscope. The most likely diagnosis is:

1. RPGN
2. MPGN
3. Diabetic nephropathy
4. IgA nephropathy
5. Minimal change disease
6. Alport's syndrome
7. SLE
8. Poststreptococcal glomerulonephritis

Ans. 5. Minimal change disease

USMLE Case Scenario

A 79-year-old lady complains of a headache for 2 days in the left side of the head. The pain is worse when she is chewing or talking. Her ESR is 95 mm/hr. The vision in the right eye is 6/18 and her left eye is 6/6. What is the best course of action?

1. Start aspirin immediately
2. Start IV methylprednisolone
3. Do nothing till temporal artery biopsy
4. CT of the head to exclude space-occupying lesion
5. MRI of the brain
6. PET scan immediately
7. Refer to an ophthalmologist

Ans. 2. Start IV methylprednisolone

There are early signs of visual loss. So high-dose steroids should be commenced with the suspicion of temporal arteritis.

USMLE Case Scenario

A 68-year-old man with severe aortic stenosis presented with melena. Upper GI endoscopy was normal. What may be the cause of bleeding?

1. Hemorrhoids
2. Cecal carcinoma
3. Angiodysplasia
4. Duodenal ulcer
5. Ulcerative colitis

Ans. 3. Angiodysplasia

Angiodysplasia is the most common vascular abnormality of the GI tract. After diverticulosis, it is the second leading cause of lower GI bleeding in patients older than 60 years. Angiodysplasia has been reported to be associated with aortic stenosis.

USMLE Case Scenario

A 65-year-old has colonic cancer. Pathologist states that no single genetic defect has been identified that is common to all cancers. The process of carcinogenesis is believed to be due to a sequence of genetic alterations, which ultimately result in both the activation of oncogenes and the inactivation of tumor suppressor genes. The loss of tumor suppressor gene function serves to promote carcinogenesis. The K-ras oncogene, the DCC (deleted in colon cancer) and the p53 tumor suppressor gene are implicated. The true for these genes is:

1. The K-ras oncogene is located on chromosome 12, the DCC (deleted in colon cancer) located on chromosome 18 and the p53 tumor suppressor gene located on chromosome 17p
2. The K-ras oncogene is located on chromosome 13, the DCC (deleted in colon cancer) located on chromosome 19 and the p53 tumor suppressor gene located on chromosome 17p
3. The K-ras oncogene is located on chromosome 14, the DCC (deleted in colon cancer) located on chromosome 19 and the p53 tumor suppressor gene located on chromosome 17p

4. The K-ras oncogene is located on chromosome 15, the DCC (deleted in colon cancer) located on chromosome 20 and the p53 tumor suppressor gene located on chromosome 17p

Ans. 1. The K-ras oncogene is located on chromosome 12, the DCC (deleted in colon cancer) located on chromosome 18 and the p53 tumor suppressor gene located on chromosome 17p

USMLE Case Scenario

A patient has nuchal lymphedema at birth, short stature, webbed neck, widely spaced nipples, and primary ovarian failure. A buccal smear done would classically reveal:

1. Absent Barr bodies
2. One Barr body
3. Two Barr bodies
4. Three Barr bodies

Ans. 1. Absent Barr bodies

USMLE Case Scenario

Classic electrolyte and vitamin/mineral abnormalities in alcoholics are:

1. High magnesium, high potassium, low sodium, deficiencies of folate and thiamine
2. High magnesium, low potassium, high sodium, deficiencies of folate and thiamine
3. High magnesium, high potassium, low sodium, deficiencies of folate and thiamine
4. Low magnesium, low potassium, low sodium, deficiencies of folate and thiamine

Ans. 4. Low magnesium, low potassium, low sodium, deficiencies of folate and thiamine

USMLE Case Scenario

A 33-year-old patient presents with a sore throat fever, malaise, pharyngitis, rash, lymphadenopathy. As a doctor, you should be concerned about a sexually transmitted disease. The disease which you should be concerned most about is:

1. Syphilis
2. LGV
3. Chancroid
4. HIV

Ans. 4. HIV

Human immunodeficiency virus infection, because initial seroconversion may present as a mononucleosis-like syndrome (e.g. fever, malaise, pharyngitis, rash, lymphadenopathy).

USMLE Case Scenario

Samter's triad is a triad consisting of:

1. Rectal polyp, angioedema, aspirin intolerance
2. Colonic polyp, urticaria, aspirin intolerance
3. Nasal polyp, asthma, aspirin intolerance
4. Hamatomatous polyp, urticaria, aspirin intolerance

Ans. 3. Nasal polyp, asthma, aspirin intolerance

USMLE Case Scenario

A 25-year-old man presents with episodes of light headedness. He has no significant past medical history. Cardiac examination reveals no heart murmurs, chest X-ray and ECG are normal. A 24-hour tape is requested. Which arrhythmia might cause these symptoms?

1. Atrial extrasystole
2. Supraventricular tachycardia
3. Wenkebach

4. Ventricular extrasystole
5. First-degree heart block

Ans. 2. Supraventricular tachycardia

Out of the following options, the most likely rhythm which may cause symptoms are supraventricular tachycardia. The other rhythms may cause palpitations but would be unusual to cause light-headedness/presyncope.

USMLE Case Scenario

A 45-year-old tennis player presents with shoulder pains especially whilst serving the ball. He has limited passive and active shoulder abduction to less than 55°. His temperature is 36.5 °C and he has a normal white cell count. There is tenderness around the anterior portion of the shoulder joint. Which of the following diagnoses is likely?

1. Glenohumeral joint osteoarthritis
2. Bursitis
3. Tennis elbow
4. Supraspinatus tendonitis
5. Septic arthritis

Ans. 4. Supraspinatus Tendonitis

Supraspinatus tendonitis. Pain during abduction with limitation of movement is suggestive of supraspinatus tendonitis. Palpation or compression around the greater tubercle of the humerus is particularly tender.

USMLE Case Scenario

A 40-year-old man presented with painless hematuria. Bimanual examination revealed a ballotable mass over the right flank. Subsequently, right nephrectomy was done and mass was seen to be composed of cells with clear cytoplasm. Areas of hemorrhage and necrosis were frequent. Cytogenic analysis of this mass is likely to reveal an abnormality of:

1. Chromosome 1
2. Chromosome 3
3. Chromosome 11
4. Chromosome 17

Ans. 2. Chromosome 3

USMLE Case Scenario

A 75-year-old lady has sudden movements of her arm where she throws her arm outwards, and uncontrollably injures herself. Which one of the following areas could have sustained an infarct?

1. Globus pallidus
2. Pontine nucleus
3. Corpus callosum
4. Subthalamic nucleus
5. Thalamus

Ans. 4. Subthalamic nucleus

Hemiballismus is caused by a subthalamic nucleus lesion, which is commonly due to an infarct.

USMLE Case Scenario

A 55-year-old man is referred to the dermatologist for further assessment having noticed a growth of papules from the nailfolds. A doctor confirms that they are subungual fibromas. There is also a history of seizures and renal impairment. The likely diagnosis is:

1. NF 1
2. NF 2
3. Tuberous sclerosis
4. Sturge-Weber disease
5. Weber-Christian disease
6. Wilson's disease

7. Normal pressure hydrocephalus
8. Motor neuron disease
9. Multiple sclerosis

Ans. 3. Tuberous sclerosis

The diagnosis is tuberous sclerosis. This is an inherited (autosomal dominant) hamartomatous condition in which there are facial angiomas (adenoma sebaceum), subungual fibromas, angiomyolipomas, cardiac rhabdomyomas, pulmonary lymphatic involvement, skin changes such as shagreen patches and ash leaf macules.

USMLE Case Scenario

A 32-year-old lady has difficulty with her vision. On examination, she has impaired adduction of the left eye looking right. The right eye has jerky nystagmus. Which investigation is most likely to yield a diagnosis?

1. Nerve conduction studies
2. X-ray of the head
3. CSF and serum for oligoclonal bands
4. Serum copper
5. Serum ceruloplasmin
6. Visual evoked potentials

Ans. 3. CSF and serum for oligoclonal bands

The clinical scenario is internuclear ophthalmoplegia. This is most commonly seen in multiple sclerosis.

USMLE Case Scenario

A 22-year-old veterinary surgeon presents with a 2-week history of high fevers, night sweats. He also had dry cough, and myalgia. On examination, the patient had a palpable splenic tip. Blood films for malaria parasites were negative. Liver function tests showed a raised serum alkaline phosphatase, raised serum aspartate aminotransferase concentration, ↑serum bilirubin concentration Likely cause is:

1. Salmonella
2. Chlamydia
3. Bartonella
4. Francisella
5. Mycoplasma
6. Brucella
7. Legionella

Ans. 6. Brucella

The occupation suggests Brucella. It is transmitted through milk and meat, especially in abattoirs. The commonest cause is Brucella melitensis. Detection of brucella may require extended culture of 6 weeks and blood agar plates. Detection of Brucella agglutinins (with the Coombs' test) also helps confirm the diagnosis

Fever and rigors, followed by possible osteomyelitis, polyarthritis, endocarditis, pneumonia, hepatitis/jaundice, splenic abscess, meningitis/encephalitis, skin changes, orchitis/cervicitis and retinitis.

USMLE Case Scenario

A 38-year-old lady from Mexico presents with myalgia and lethargy. Her blood tests show a positive ANA and rheumatoid factor is negative. The CK is raised at 360 U/l. Extranuclear antigen tests show a negative Ro and negative La, negative Scl 70 and positive ribonuclear protein antibody. Most likely diagnosis is:

1. Sjögren's syndrome
2. Polymyalgia rheumatica
3. Polymyositis
4. Scleroderma
5. Systemic lupus erythematosus
6. Mixed connective tissue disease

Ans. 6. Mixed connective tissue disease

Positive ANA (speckled pattern), raised CK and positive anti-RNP antibody suggests mixed connective tissue disease

USMLE Case Scenario

A 69-year-old man from Ohio presents with muscle weakness and difficulty swallowing. On neurological examination, he has proximal and distal upper and lower limb weakness. Antibody profile is normal. There is wasting of the intrinsic muscles of the fingers and thigh muscles. CK is elevated and EMG findings are consistent with a myopathic process. Most likely diagnosis is:

1. Localized sclerosis
2. Myasthenia gravis
3. Lambert-Eaton crisis
4. Polymyositis
5. Dermatomyositis
6. Inclusion body myositis
7. Motor neuron disease
8. Duchenne muscular dystrophy

Ans. 6. Inclusion body myositis

Muscle biopsy shows intracellular inclusions (amyloid precursor protein, ubiquitins) and inflammatory infiltrates, connective tissue disease.

USMLE Case Scenario

A 3-week-old girl is brought by her parents to the emergency room. She looks severly ill. She is pale and dyspneic with a respiratory rate of 80 breaths per min. Heart rate is 210 bpm, heart sounds are distant, a gallop is heard, and she has cardiomegaly on X-ray. An echo demonstrates poor ventricular function, dilated ventricles, and dilation of the left atrium. An electrocardiogram shows ventricular depolarization complexes that have low voltage. Most likely she is suffering from:

1. Pericarditis
2. Myocarditis
3. Libman-Sacks endocarditis
4. Cardiac tamponade
5. Tuberculous pericardial effusion

Ans. 2. Myocarditis

The findings of pallor, dyspnea, tachypnea, tachycardia, and cardiomegaly are common in congestive heart failure regardless of the cause. The most common causes of myocarditis include adenovirus and coxsackievirus B, although many other viruses can cause this condition.

USMLE Case Scenario

A 55-year-old immunosuppressed HIV-positive man presents with episodes of breathlessness. He has a temperature of 38 °C. The blood gases show a pH of 7.30, pO_2 of 8kPa and pCO_2 of 3 kPa. CXR shows bilateral interstitial and alveolar consolidation. Which of the following medications should be used?

1. Quadruple anti-TB therapy
2. Pencillin
3. Cephalosporine
4. Amphotericin
5. Pyridium
6. Cotrimoxazole
7. Foscarnet
8. Teicoplanin

Ans. 6. Cotrimoxazole

The patient has pneumocystis carinii pneumonia and is hypoxic on the blood gases. IV cotrimoxazole, clindamycin or pentamidine can be used to treat this.

USMLE Case Scenario

A 25-year-old man presented with fever, cough, expectoration and breathlessness of 2 month's duration. Contrast-enchanced computed tomography of the chest showed bilateral upper lobe fibrotic lesions and mediastinum had enlarged necrotic nodes with peripheral rim enhancement. Which one of the following is the most probable diagnosis?

1. Sarcoidosis
2. Tuberculosis
3. Lymphoma
4. Silicosis

Ans. 2. Tuberculosis

USMLE Case Scenario

In acute pancreatitis, a diverse spectrum of illness is seen, varying from a mild, short-lived, self-limited disease to a severe toxic condition associated with shock, hypovolemia, multiple metabolic derangements, and ultimate death. Typical findings on physical examination in patients with acute pancreatitis include fever, tachycardia, epigastric tenderness, and abdominal distention. It is characterized by:

1. Turner's sign (bluish discoloration in the flanks) and Cullen's sign (bluish discoloration of the periumbilical region)
2. Turner's sign (bluish discoloration in the periumbilical region) and Cullen's sign (bluish discoloration of the flanks)
3. Turner's sign (reddish discoloration in the flanks) and Cullen's sign (bluish discoloration of the periumbilical region)
4. Turner's sign (bluish discoloration in the periumbilical region) and Cullen's sign (reddish discoloration of the flank region)

Ans. 1. Turner's sign (bluish discoloration in the flanks) and Cullen's sign (bluish discoloration of the periumbilical region)

USMLE Case Scenario

A 35-year-old man presents with malaise and is found to be anemic clinically. His blood tests reveal: Blood film shows spherocytosis. Hereditary spherocytosis is diagnosed. Which of the following tests is most appropriate for diagnosis?

1. FISH
2. ELISA
3. Direct antiglobulin test
4. G6PD activity
5. Hb electrophoresis
6. Urinary hemosiderin
7. Methemoglobin levels

Ans. 3. Direct antiglobulin test

The blood tests with high bilirubin, reticulocyte count and high LDH suggests hemolysis. Spherocytes on blood film suggest hereditary spherocytosis. In HS, the red cells are smaller, rounder, and more fragile than normal. The condition is commoner among Northern Europeans. The direct antiglobulin test will help to confirm this.

USMLE Case Scenario

A pregnant 18-year-old woman came to the clinic with a low-grade fever, malaise, and headache. Few days later, she presented with a macular rash on her trunk, arms, hands, and feet. Further examination revealed that one month previously, she had a painless ulcer on her vagina that healed spontaneously. Most likely diagnosis is:

1. Lyme disease
2. Lymphogranuloma venereum
3. Behçet's disease
4. Endocarditis
5. Syphilis

Ans. 5. Syphilis

The initial lesion of primary syphilis develops at the site of transmission after an incubation period of 10–90 days, with a mean of about 21–28 days, and then heals spontaneously in 3–7 weeks. ***T. pallidum*** **is sensitive to the penicillins and is easily treatable in the early stages.**

USMLE Case Scenario

The commonest cause of traveler's diarrhea is:

1. Giardia
2. Shigella

3. Pseudomonas
4. Salmonella
5. Campylobacter
6. EHEC
7. EIEC
8. ETEC

Ans. 8. ETEC

USMLE Case Scenario

A 35-year-old woman presented with a 5-month history of weight loss (half a stone), anorexia and generalized pruritus. On examination, she was jaundiced with numerous spider nevi, scratch marks, palmar erythema and hepatosplenomegaly. Investigations showed:
Hemoglobin 9.5 g/dl
White-cell count 7 x 10^9/l
Erythrocyte sedimentation rate 140 mm/h
Serum albumin 42 g/l
Serum bilirubin of 37 µmol/l
Alanine transaminase of 122 IU/l
Aspartate transaminase of 154 IU/l
Alkaline phosphatase level 83 IU/l
Which one of the following findings is suggestive of autoimmune hepatitis?

1. High IgG
2. HLA DR2
3. HLA DR6
4. Antimitochondrial antibodies
5. Antineutrophil cytoplasmic antibodies

Ans. 1. High IgG

Antinuclear antibodies of IgG class are frequently strongly positive (e.g. to a titer of 1/10000) in autoimmune hepatitis. Antibodies to dsDNA and to smooth muscle are also good markers. HLA-DR3 and DR4 antigen are associated with autoimmune hepatitis.

USMLE Case Scenario

A 44-year-old woman presented with unusual feelings like tingling, numbness and clumsiness of both hands for 2 weeks. Earlier she had experienced paresthesia in the feet. On neurological examination, she had absent abdominal reflexes with brisk tendon jerks and bilateral extensor plantar responses. Blood investigations were normal, including hemoglobin, white-cell count and differential, erythrocyte sedimentation rate, vitamin B12 and folate levels and syphilis serology. Oligoclonal IgG bands were found in CSF. The most likely diagnosis is:

1. SAH
2. Guillain-Barré syndrome
3. Multiple sclerosis
4. Subacute degeneration of cord
5. Hysteria
6. Empty sella syndrome

Ans. 3. Multiple sclerosis

USMLE Case Scenario

An 88-year-old man presents to the physician with a 3-day history of headache, fever and profound malaise. Tenderness over the right temple is appreciated on palpation. The right temporal artery is tender and slightly nodular. Neurologic examination is normal, including funduscopic examination. However, visual acuity is reduced. Laboratory studies show: Erythrocyte sedimentation rate 88 mm/hr. Which of the following is the most appropriate next step in management?

1. Measurement of intraocular pressure
2. Give lithium
3. Give sumatriptan

4. Give ergometrine
5. Give latanoprost
6. Low-dose prednisone treatment
7. High-dose prednisone treatment
8. Temporal artery biopsy

Ans. 7. High-dose prednisone treatment

The patient needs urgent treatment with high-dose prednisone for giant cell arteritis (i.e. temporal arteritis)

USMLE Case Scenario

A 25-year-old woman in New Jersey presented with a 1-day history of fever and chills. On examination, she was febrile with a blood pressure of 70/40 mm Hg. Over several hours, a widespread erythrodermic rash developed. The female collapses. Further questioning revealed that the patient had removed a tampon shortly before presentation, as she had just ceased menstruating

1. Streptococcus bovis infection
2. Hemolytic uremic syndrome
3. *E. coli* sepsis
4. Fungal infection
5. Toxic shock syndrome
6. Meningococcal septicemia
7. Staph epidermis infection
8. Pseudomonas-induced shock

Ans. 5. Toxic shock syndrome

Toxic shock syndrome is due to toxin-1 (TSST-1), a protein secreted by *S. aureus* **or streptococci, was the first of many toxins associated with the syndrome to be identified.**

USMLE Case Scenario

A 45-year-old man was brought by ambulance into hospital. He was found by his friends on a rooftop with unusual position of his legs and was reported to have stood there without moving in a stuporose state for three hours. This implies:

1. Cerebral palsy
2. Lissencephaly
3. Porencephaly
4. Paralysis
5. Narcolepsy
6. Cataplexy
7. Catalepsy
8. Mannerisms

Ans. 7. Catalepsy

Catalepsy is a type of catatonia. It a disorder of muscle tone in which uncomfortable positions can be maintained for a long time. It is a feature of schizophrenia

Cataplexy is the sudden loss of motor tone associated with the sleep disorder narcolepsy.

USMLE Case Scenario

A 55-year-old man presents with severe hemoptysis. An organism is isolated and it is found that it has a tendency to invade pre-existing pulmonary cavities and form a rounded necrotic mass of matted hyphae, fibrin and inflammatory cells. This mass usually lies free in the cavity and can change its location as the patient moves from an upright to a recumbent position. On the chest X-ray, a crescentric radiolucency adjacent to a rounded mass within a cavitary lesion is seen. A filamentous organism with coarse, septate, fragmented hyphae is isolated. Most likely organism is:

1. Cryptococcus neoformans
2. Candida albicans
3. Blastomyces dermatitidis
4. Paracoccidioides brasiliensis

5. Coccidioidomycosis
6. Aspergillus fumigatus

Ans. 6. Aspergillus fumigatus

USMLE Case Scenario

A 44-year-old man working as a manual laborer injures his foot. He develops swelling, erythema and pain in all the digits of his foot. The pain is severe and burning in nature. He cannot sleep due to severity of pain. He has an ESR of 22 mm/hour and a temperature of 36 °C. Most likely cause could be:

1. Hysteria
2. Sepsis
3. Cellulitis
4. Gout
5. Raynaud's phenomenon
6. Reflex sympathetic dystrophy
7. Phantom limb

Ans. 6. Reflex sympathetic dystrophy occurs following trauma, can progress to other parts. It is due to autonomic nervous system dysfunction. Symptoms of extreme pain and burning can occur.

USMLE Case Scenario

A 75-year-old man presents to New York City Hospital unwell with diarrhea. He has a BP of 110/70, heart rate 120 and temperature 38 °C. A diastolic murmur is heard in aortic area. Which organism is likely to grow in the blood cultures?

1. MRSA
2. Listeria
3. *Streptococcus mitis*
4. *Staphylococcus aureus*
5. *Streptococcus bovis*
6. *Escherichia coli*
7. *Brucella melitensis*

Ans. 5. *Streptococcus bovis* usually enters the bloodstream via the gastrointestinal tract. There is also an association with malignancy of the GI tract.

USMLE Case Scenario

A 28-year-old man has come from suburban Mexico 6 years ago. Since a year ago, he has had three tonic clonic seizures a week. On examination, he appears well, with no focal neurological deficit. A CT scan shows multiple calcified cystic lesions in the brain. Which diagnosis is there likely?

1. PML
2. Cerebral malaria
3. SAH
4. Encephalitis
5. MID (Multi-infarct dementia)
6. Neurocysticercosis
7. Multiple sclerosis
8. Cerebral toxoplasmosis
9. Tuberculosis

Ans. 6. Neurocysticercosis is caused by *Tenia solium* (pork tapeworm)

USMLE Case Scenario

A 45-year-old woman has Z deformity of her hands. She was asked to see a pulmonologist because of breathlessness. She has a known history of rheumatoid arthritis and is on leuflunomide. She has a CXR and lung function tests. Which one of the following can be associated with rheumatoid arthritis?

1. Small cell carcinoma
2. Adenocarcinoma

3. Asthma
4. Fibrotic lung
5. Pulmonary eosinophilia
6. Pulmonary embolus

Ans. 4. Fibrotic lung

- In rheumatoid arthritis:
- Exudative pleural effusions
- Fibrotic lung disease
- Caplan's syndrome (pneumoconiosis, pulmonary nodules)
- Obstructive lung disease in the form of bronchiolitis obliterans (obstruction of bronchiolar lumen with inflammatory exudate) may occur

USMLE Case Scenario

A 53-year-old man working in India for the last two years presents with a 4-month history of cough and breathlessness. Mantoux test done is negative. He was apyrexial on admission to the hospital. His blood tests shows: ESR 68 mm/hr. Chest X-ray shows bilateral hilar lymphadenopathy and egg shell calcification. What is the likely diagnosis?

1. Churg-Strauss syndrome
2. Extrinsic allergic alveolitis
3. Tuberculosis
4. Sarcoidosis
5. Allergic bronchopulmonary aspergillosis
6. Farmer's lung
7. Cat-scratch disease

Ans. 4. Sarcoidosis

Bilateral hilar lymphadenopathy in sarcoidosis

USMLE Case Scenario

A 58-year-old woman seen by a rheumatologist in Washington is suspected of having polymyalgia rheumatica. Which of the following features supports the diagnosis?

1. Low ESR
2. Stiffness around the shoulders
3. Muscle weakness
4. Iritis
5. Mania
6. Weight gain
7. Glaucoma

Ans. 2. Stiffness around the shoulders

Polymyalgia Rheumatica (PMR) typically produces pain and stiffness, especially around the shoulders. There is associated polyarthritis.

USMLE Case Scenario

A 26-year-old man from New Orleans developed flu-like symptoms, severe diarrhea and abdominal pain 4 days after attending a dinner party at which he had eaten a chicken. Stool cultures taken from all four individuals grew *Campylobacter jejuni*. Over the next week, the sensory changes worsened and spread to involve his arms and legs. He was admitted to hospital and found to have severe symmetrical distal limb weakness and 'glove and stocking' sensory loss to the elbows and knees. Nerve conduction studies showed evidence of a mixed motor and sensory neuropathy. High titers of IgM and IgG antibodies to *Campylobacter jejuni* were found in his peripheral blood. A diagnosis was made of the Guillain-Barré syndrome. His CSF would show:

1. A very low total protein level but without any increase in the number of cells in the CSF
2. A normal protein level with an increase in the number of cells in the CSF

3. A very high total protein level but without any increase in the number of cells in the CSF
4. A very high total protein level along with an increase in the number of cells in the CSF

Ans. 3. A very high total protein level but without any increase in the number of cells in the CSF

USMLE Case Scenario

A 66-year-old lady from Texas is investigated for recurrent episodes of gouty arthritis. On examination, she looked plethoric and has a 6 cm splenomegaly. She has the following results:
Hb 19.9 gm/dl
Hct 0.632
Platelet count 468 x 109/l
ESR 2 mm/1st hour
Coagulation screen normal
AST normal
ALT normal
BUN: Normal
Creatinine: Normal
What is the diagnosis?

1. B-cell lymphoma
2. Aplastic anemia
3. Multiple myeloma
4. Polycythemia
5. Acute myeloid leukemia
6. Sickle-cell disease

Ans. 4. Polycythemia

USMLE Case Scenario

A 6-year-old boy has been complaining of headache, ignoring to see the objects on the sides for four months. On examination, he is not mentally retarded, his grades at school are good, and visual acuity is diminished in both the eyes. Visual charting showed significant field defect. CT scan of the head showed suprasellar mass with calcification. Which of the following is the most probable diagnosis?

1. Astrocytoma
2. Craniopharyngioma
3. Pituitary adenoma
4. Meningioma

Ans. 2. Craniopharyngioma

USMLE Case Scenario

A 27-year-old woman presented with a 6-month history of extreme fatigue, lethargy and difficulty in concentration following a flu-like illness. She was unable to work as a manager. Clinical examination was unremarkable with the exception of reduced muscle strength; the rest of the neurological examination was normal. She was assessed by several physicians with no explanation being found for her extreme lethargy. Likely diagnosis is:

1. Polymyalgia
2. Reiter's disease
3. Myopathy
4. Neuropathy
5. Chronic fatigue syndrome (CFS)

Ans. 5. Chronic fatigue syndrome (CFS)

USMLE Case Scenario

A 35-year-old man from New Zealand working as a nurse has been having dysuria previously. Now he has renal colic. Ultrasound of the abdomen confirms renal calculi. Urinalysis showed typical hexagonal or benzene crystals. The most likely diagnosis is:

1. Calcium stones
2. Oxaluria
3. Calcium carbonate stones
4. Adult polycystic kidney disease
5. Cystinuria
6. Uric acid stones
7. Pigment stones
8. Cholesterol stones

Ans. 5. Cystinuria is a disorder of proximal tubular cells
Urinalysis may show typical hexagonal which are pathognomonic of cystinuria

USMLE Case Scenario

A 66-year-old man working as an automobile engineer in Texas presents with pain in his left foot. Examination reveals a swollen ankle. Neurological examination reveals absent ankle jerk and weak foot flexion/extension on the left. His ESR is 32 mm/hr, CRP is < 5 mg/l. Joint X-ray reveals subchondral fractures, soft tissue swelling and a narrowed joint space. The likely diagnosis is:

1. Rheumatoid arthritis
2. Caplan's syndrome
3. Reiter's arthritis
4. Neuropathic joint
5. Osteoarthritis
6. Gouty arthritis
7. Juvenile chronic arthritis

Ans. 4. Charcot joint or neuropathic joint disease can be caused by:

- Diabetic neuropathy
- Syphilis
- Syringomyelia or
- Leprosy

USMLE Case Scenario

A 63-year-old man complains of trouble swallowing and hoarseness. On physical exam, he is noted to have ptosis and a constricted pupil on the left, and a diminished gag reflex. Neurological examination shows decreased pain and temperature sensation on the left side of his face and on the right side of his body. Which of the following vessels is most likely occluded?

1. Internal carotid
2. External carotid
3. Anterior inferior cerebellar artery
4. Anterior spinal artery
5. Middle cerebral artery
6. Posterior cerebral artery
7. Posterior inferior cerebellar artery
8. Subclavian
9. Axillary

Ans. 7. Posterior inferior cerebellar artery (PICA)

USMLE Case Scenario

A 40-year-old man has genital ulceration and uveitis. His GP suspects Behçet's syndrome and is referred to the rheumatologist. Which one of the following is a feature of Behçet's syndrome?

1. Facial asymmetry
2. Receding hair line

3. Hirsutism
4. Malignant melanoma
5. Arterial thrombosis

Ans. 5. Arterial thrombosis

Behçet's syndrome is inflammatory disorder (associated with certain HLA B and DR types) causing:

- Mouth ulceration
- Arthritis
- Eyes (anterior uveitis, retinal vein occlusion)
- Vasculitis (thrombophlebitis) and thrombosis
- CNS vasculitis involvement may lead to TIA, meningoencephalitis, Parkinson's and dementia

USMLE Case Scenario

A 20-year-old female presents with history of dyspnea on exertion. On examination, she has wide, fixed split of S2 with ejection-systolic murmur (III/VI) in left second intercostal space. Her EKG shows left axis deviation. The most probable diagnosis is:

1. Total anomalous pulmonary venous connection
2. Tricuspid atresia
3. Ostium primum atrial septal defect
4. Tetralogy of Fallot

Ans. 3. Ostium primum atrial septal defect

USMLE Case Scenario

A 20-year-old man is referred for investigation of abnormal liver function tests. His ophthalmological check-up reveals some abnormality which he does not remember. He has a previous history of diabetes diagnosed 5 years ago. His albumin is 35 g/l, bilirubin elevated at 15 μmol/l, ALP is 390 U/l and ALT is 350 U/l. He has a serum copper of 30 μmol/l (12–26) and cerulloplasmin of 90 μmol/l (200–350). What is the diagnosis?

1. Cholangiocarcinoma
2. Autoimmune hepatitis
3. Primary biliary cirrhosis
4. Hemochromatosis
5. Wilson's disease
6. Menke's disease

Ans. 5. Wilson's disease

Wilson's disease is described. The abnormal gene is the ATP7B gene on chromosome 13. It is autosomal recessive. Kayser-Fleischer rings are often seen on slit lamp, but not always. Ceruloplasmin levels are low in 95% of patients, but can be normal in acute liver failure when there is a hypoproteinemic state. The best test is hepatic copper concentration (> 250 μg/g of dry weight).

USMLE Case Scenario

A 35-year-old secretary has jaundice and lethargy. Her blood tests show Bilirubin 110 μmol/l (1–22), AST of 240 U/l (1–30) and ALP of 650 U/l (5–35 U/l). AMA is positive. If she has primary biliary cirrhosis, what is the liver biopsy likely to show?

1. Granulomatous changes of hepatocytes
2. Fatty changes of the liver parenchyma
3. Piecemeal necrosis and fibrosis around portal veins
4. Collagen layering around bile ducts
5. White cell infiltrates causing biliary duct destruction

Ans. 5. White cell infiltrates causing biliary duct destruction

Inflammatory changes with biliary destruction are suggestive of primary biliary cirrhosis. Granulomatous changes would suggest sarcoidosis or Wegener's granulomatosis. Piecemeal necrosis and fibrosis suggest chronic hepatitis.

USMLE Case Scenario

A 20-year-old man is referred for investigation of abnormal liver function tests. His ophthalmological check-up reveals some abnormality which he does not remember. He has a previous history of diabetes diagnosed 5 years ago. His albumin is 35 g/l, bilirubin elevated at 15 µmol/l, ALP is 390 U/l and ALT is 350 U/l. He has a serum copper of 30 µmol/l (12–26) and cerulloplasmin of 90 µmol/l (200–350). Abnormality is in:

1. Iron metabolism
2. Calcium metabolism
3. Sodium metabolism
4. Potassium metabolism
5. Zinc metabolism
6. Copper metabolism
7. Phosphorus metabolism

Ans. 6. Copper metabolism

Wilson's disease is described. The abnormal gene is the ATP7B gene on chromosome 13. It is autosomal recessive. Kayser-Fleischer rings are often seen on slit lamp, but not always. Ceruloplasmin levels are low in 95% of patients, but can be normal in acute liver failure when there is a hypoproteinemic state.

USMLE Case Scenario

A 40-year-old man presented 14 days after return from a 6-week field trip to New Guinea. He had a six-day history of high fevers and rigors which upset him terribly On the day of presentation, he had become lethargic, vague and slightly confused. He had taken antimalarials as prophylaxis. He does not remember any incidence of bite by mosquito or flea

His temperature was 40 °C

Pulse rate 140 bpm

Respiratory rate 28 per minute and

Blood pressure 100/60 mm Hg

He had dry mucous membranes, mild jaundice, pallor and splenomegaly and generalized crackles in both lungs

Full blood examination revealed:

6.5 g/dl

WCC 2.5 x 10^9/l

Platelet 10 x 10^9/l

Bilirubin 60 µmol/l (3–20 µmol/l)

Lactate dehydrogenase 489 U/l (100–225 U/l) creatinine 250 umol/l

What is the likely diagnosis?

1. Leishmaniasis
2. Tick bite fever
3. Endocarditis
4. Falciparum malaria
5. Viral hemorrhagic fever

Ans. 4. Falciparum malaria

This patient has severe malaria suggested by altered consciousness, focal neurological signs, jaundice, oliguria, severe anemia, hypoglycemia, hypotension and acidosis. Severe malaria requires treatment with intravenous quinine. Not remembering mosquito bite is a distractor and is not essential.

USMLE Case Scenario

A 40-year-old man has been to Malaysia for 6 months. He has an erythematous, serpiginous, pruritic, cutaneous eruption on the medial side of the ankle. What is the diagnosis?

1. Lyme disease
2. Cutaneous larval migrans
3. Leishmaniasis
4. Sarcoidosis
5. Tuberculosis

Ans. 2. Cutaneous larva migrans

Cutaneous larva migrans is caused by the penetration through intact skin of larval animal hookworms, (e.g. *Ancylostoma braziliense*)**. Diagnosis is predominantly clinical**

Treatment is often necessary because of intense pruritus, long duration (over a year) and complications, such as impetigo and allergic reactions. Therapy comprises ivermectin, albendazole or thiabendazole.

USMLE Case Scenario

A 35-year-old man presents with lethargy and pruritus. He has had no abdominal pains and he is not jaundiced on examination. Blood tests show an increased bilirubin of 16.68 μmol/l, albumin 35 g/l, ALT 350 U/l, ALP 1200 U/l Antibody profile of ANA and AMA is negative

Ultrasound of the liver shows normal intrahepatic bile ducts and increased echotexture of liver parenchyma. Which is the likely diagnosis?

1. Primary biliary cirrhosis
2. Chronic active hepatitis
3. Autoimmune hepatitis
4. Primary sclerosing cholangitis
5. Cholangiocarcinoma

Ans. 4. Primary sclerosing cholangitis

Primary sclerosing cholangitis is usually seen in males. It is typically associated with ulcerative colitis. A positive pANCA can occur. The best investigation to confirm this is ERCP, which will reveal multiple strictures in the biliary system. 10% of patients with PSC will progress towards developing cholangiocarcinoma.

USMLE Case Scenario

A 44-year-old man was found to have heaviness in his left hypochondrium. Clinical exam reveals an enlarged spleen. USG scan followed by CT scan of abdomen shows gross splenomegaly. Further Investigation showed normal hemoglobin. The hematologist reports: On the blood film, cells are mainly small mononuclear cells resembling lymphocytes, but having a spiky or 'hairy' appearance, have B-cell markers on their surface and are positive for kappa but not lambda light chains. The cells stain positively for tartrate-resistant acid phosphatase (TRAP positivity) Most likely diagnosis is:

1. Mantle cell lymphoma
2. Glandular fever
3. Littoral cell angioma
4. Portal hypertension
5. Acute leukemia
6. Follicular cell lymphoma
7. Hairy cell leukemia
8. CML
9. Kala-Azar

Ans. 7. Hairy cell leukemia

USMLE Case Scenario

A 12-year-old child of a family from Malta has had recurrent episodes of bone pain and mild fever. He has X-rays which show necrosis of the hip. Examination also reveals proliferative retinopathy. Which of the following diagnoses is likely to be there?

1. Multiple myeloma
2. Paget's disease
3. Pernicious anemia
4. Osteopetrosis
5. Sickle-cell disease
6. Thalassemia

Ans. 5. Sickle-cell disease

Aseptic necrosis of the hip, cholecystitis, renal papillary necrosis and proliferative retinopathy are clinical features of sickle-cell disease.

USMLE Case Scenario

An 18-year-old male presented with acute onset descending paralysis of 3 day's duration. There is also a history of blurring of vision for the same duration. On examination, the patient has quadriparesis with areflexia. Both the pupils are non-reactive. The most porbable diagnosis is:

1. Poliomyelitis
2. Botulism
3. Diphtheria
4. Porphyria

Ans. 2. Botulism

USMLE Case Scenario

A 73-year-old woman is referred for investigation of a creatinine of 255 mmol/l. She also has had episodes of hematuria. She has a long history of low back pain treated with a combination of painkillers. An ultrasound shows two irregular-shaped kidneys sized 8.3 and 9.1 cm. Which of the following is the most likely diagnosis?

1. Minimal change nephropathy
2. ATN
3. Diabetic nephropathy
4. Membranous glomerulonephritis
5. IgA nephropathy
6. RPGN
7. Analgesic nephropathy

Ans. 7. Analgesic nephropathy

There is interstitial nephritis and renal papillary necrosis, eventually leading to acute renal failure or chronic renal failure. There may be hematuria but minimal or no proteinuria.

USMLE Case Scenario

A 26-year-old lady from Michigan has been repeatedly attending a physician. Eventually the physician orders investigations which reveal:

Hb: 13 g/l
PH 7.20
Sodium 141 mmol/l
Potassium 2.7 mmol/l
Urea 6.6 mmol/l
Creatinine 92 μmol/l
Chloride 119 mmol/l (95–107)
Bicarbonate 13 mmol/l

Which of the following is likely to be there?

1. Diabetic ketoacidosis
2. Type I renal tubular acidosis
3. Type II renal tubular acidosis
4. Overdose of ibuprofen
5. Lactic acidosis

Ans. 2. Type I renal tubular acidosis

There is a hypokalemic, hyperchloremic acidosis. The anion gap is normal (Na+ K– Cl– Bicarb) – normal range is 10–16. This is most likely to represent distal (type I) renal tubular acidosis.

USMLE Case Scenario

A 21-year-old man presented with acute pain in the iliac region. A year later, he developed an iritis in his left eye, low back pain and stiffness. His peripheral joints were normal but pain could be elicited in both sacroiliac joints. On investigation, he had a raised erythrocyte sedimentation rate of 102 mm/h, a mild anemia (Hb 106 g/l) but no detectable serum rheumatoid factor. Tissue typing would reveal:

1. HLA-DR4 positivity
2. HLA-B27 positivity
3. HLA-DR2 positivity
4. HLA-DR5 positivity

Ans. 2. HLA-B27 positivity

USMLE Case Scenario

A 66-year-old man from Illinois while reading the morning newspaper suddenly becomes completely blind in one eye. The report of angiography demonstrates occlusion of the central retinal artery. Which of the following is the most likely cause of the occlusion?

1. Atheroma or embolism
2. Cranial (temporal) arteritis
3. Hypertension
4. Polycythemia vera
5. Tumor

Ans. 1. Atheroma or embolism is the most common cause of central retinal artery occlusion

USMLE Case Scenario

A 52-year-old man while driving rashly on a highway has an automobile accident. He sustains a closed head injury. On arriving at a hospital, his CT scan of head was done. CT scan does not show any intracranial hemorrhage or contusion, but reveals a small tumor at the cerebellopontine angle of the brain. Which of the following nerves is most likely to be affected by this tumor?

1. Facial nerve and vestibular nerve
2. Glossopharyngeal nerve and vestibular nerve
3. Optic nerve and facial nerve
4. Trigeminal nerve and abducens nerve
5. Vagus nerve and vestibular nerve

Ans. 1. Facial nerve and vestibular nerve

USMLE Case Scenario

A 35-year-old man presented with decreasing vision and painful swollen knees. He had a six-year history of relapsing and remitting mouth ulcers and frequent episodes of genital ulceration. On examination, he had retinal vasculitis, few mouth ulcers and synovitis in both knees. Investigations show a raised erythrocyte sedimentation rate at 99 mm/h but a normal blood count and negative tests for rheumatoid factor, antinuclear antibodies, cytomegalovirus and HIV infection. A clinical diagnosis suggests:

1. Reiter's syndrome
2. Ankylosing spondylitis
3. Psoriatic arthritis
4. Pseudogout
5. CPPD deposition disease
6. Polymyalgia
7. Behçet's syndrome

Ans. 7. Behçet's syndrome
Remember in nutshell
ORO-OCCULO-GENITAL SYNDROME

USMLE Case Scenario

A 30-year-old veterinarian on a cattle farm presents with a 1 to 2-month history of malaise, chills, drenching malodorous sweats, fatigue, and weakness. He has anorexia and has lost 15 pounds. He has intermittent fevers that range up to 103 °F (39.4 °C) There is no accompanying skin lesion. He has no pets. He complains of visual blurring. A physical examination reveals mild lymphadenopathy, petechiae and a cardiac murmur consistent with aortic insufficiency. The most likely diagnosis is:

1. Anthrax
2. Trichinosis
3. Brucellosis
4. Leptosporiosis
5. Toxoplasmosis
6. Histoplasmosis

Ans. 3. Brucellosis

Brucellosis abortus is the most common species to cause endocarditis. The aortic valve is most commonly involved, followed by the mitral valve, and then both valves. Most cases of brucellosis are associated with occupational exposure in persons such as veterinarians.

USMLE Case Scenario

A 45-year-old woman who works in a grocery shop presents to her physician with 'double vision'and is unable to adduct her right eye on attempted left lateral gaze

Convergence is intact. Both direct and consensual light reflexes are normal. Which of the following structures is most likely to be affected?

1. Left oculomotor nerve
2. Medial longitudinal fasciculus
3. Occipital cortex
4. Pretectal area
5. Right abducens nerve
6. Right oculomotor nerve
7. Right trochlear nerve

Ans. 2. Medial longitudinal fasciculus

The medial longitudinal fasciculus (MLF) connects the oculomotor (III), trochlear (IV), and abducens (VI) nuclei and is essential for conjugate gaze. A lesion in the MLF will result in the inability to medially rotate the ipsilateral eye on attempted lateral gaze.

USMLE Case Scenario

A 58-year-old woman, who is a bit nervous, presents with a 3-year history of headaches, generalized tonic-clonic seizures and bilateral leg weakness. Skull X-ray films reveal hyperostosis of the calvarium. Biopsy of the responsible lesion shows a whorling pattern of the cells. Which of the following is the most likely diagnosis?

1. Medulloblastomas
2. Arachnoid cyst
3. Glioblastoma multiforme
4. Meningioma
5. Neurosarcoid
6. Metastatic breast cancer
7. Oligodendroglioma

Ans. 4. The most likely diagnosis is an intracranial meningioma

Microscopically, the meningioma cells have a tendency to encircle one another, forming whorls and psammoma bodies

USMLE Case Scenario

A 25-year-old man comes to the Medical Emergency department because of dyspnea, palpitations, and a headache. These symptoms came on soon after he took Trimethoprim-sulfamethoxazole for a urinary tract infection. Laboratory studies show a normochromic, normocytic anemia with the peripheral blood smear revealing Heinz bodies. Which of the following is the most likely cause of this patient's anemia?

1. Lead poisoning
2. Folate deficiency
3. Pyruvate kinase deficiency
4. Thalassemia
5. Glucose-6-phosphate dehydrogenase (G6PD) deficiency
6. Hereditary spherocytosis
7. Blood loss

Ans. 5. Glucose-6-phosphate dehydrogenase deficiency

This patient has glucose-6-phosphate dehydrogenase (G6PD) deficiency, which is an X-linked disorder that leads to hemolytic crises within hours of exposure to oxidant stress. The most common stressors are:

- Viral and bacterial infections
- Sulfa drugs
- Quinines and
- Fava beans

During an acute hemolytic crisis, hemoglobin becomes denatured and leads to the formation of Heinz bodies. The diagnosis is made by the demonstration of Heinz bodies during an acute crisis and low levels of G6PD during normal times. The treatment includes maintaining adequate urine output and the prevention of future episodes.

USMLE Case Scenario

High blood levels of homocysteine are known to increase severity of atherosclerosis and frequency of both arterial and venous thrombosis. The reason is:

1. Homocysteine promotes the formation of microaggregates of clotting protiens
2. Homocysteine is linked to the formation of anticardiolipin antibodies
3. Homocysteine causes decreased levels of proteins C and S
4. This is in fact completely wrong, homocysteine is protective

Ans. 3. Homocysteine causes decreased levels of proteins C and S

USMLE Case Scenario

A 22-year-old male from Kansas comes to the medicine OPD for a follow-up examination. He has taken paracetamol for chronic headaches and phenytoin for a seizure disorder for 3 years. Examination shows 4 cm nontender axillary lymph nodes. A lymph node biopsy shows hyperplasia. Most likely the cause is:

1. Toxoplasmosis
2. Cat-scratch disease
3. Tuberculosis
4. CLL
5. ALL
6. Hodgkin's disease
7. Drug reaction

Ans. 7. Drug reaction

USMLE Case Scenario

A 75-year-old woman from Illinois reports to a physician saying that she has had increasing difficulty swallowing solids and liquids over the past one year. She has noticed that her fingers change color when exposed to cold. Examination shows tightness of the skin over the face with tightening of oral cavity. Barium swallow shows a dilated esophagus with loss of peristalsis. Most likely diagnosis is:

1. Pharyngoesophageal (Zenker's) diverticulum
2. Plummer-Vinson syndrome
3. Polymyositis
4. Systemic sclerosis
5. Diffuse esophageal spasm
6. Esophageal cancer
7. Esophageal candidiasis
8. Globus hystericus
9. Lower esophageal web
10. Paraesophageal hernia
11. Peptic stricture of the esophagus

Ans. 4. Systemic sclerosis

USMLE Case Scenario

A 77-year-old man from Missouri is brought to the medicine OPD by his wife because she is concerned about his memory loss over the past two years. Few days back, he could not remember his daughter's name. Although he himself denies that there is any problem, she says he has been forgetful and becomes easily confused. There is no history of alcohol abuse
His temperature is 37 °C
Blood pressure is 120/80 mm Hg
Pulse is 72/min
On mental status examination, his mood is normal
He is oriented to person and place but initially gives the wrong year, which he is able to correct
He has difficulty recalling the names of common objects he uses in day-to-day life and does not remember the name of his son, who lives with him. The most likely cause is:

1. Generalized anxiety disorder
2. Depression
3. Normal age-associated memory decline
4. Normal pressure hydrocephalus
5. Parkinson's disease
6. Pick's disease
7. Multi-infarct (vascular) dementia
8. Alcohol withdrawal
9. Apathetic hyperthyroidism
10. Bipolar disorder, depressed
11. Dementia, alcohol-related
12. Dementia, Alzheimer's type

Ans. 12. Dementia, Alzheimer's type

USMLE Case Scenario

A 34-year-old G1P0 at 34 weeks' gestation presents to a maternity clinic with chief complaints of four days' history of generalized malaise, anorexia and vomiting. She has also complains of abdominal discomfort, a poor appetite. On physical exam, she has mild jaundice. Her vital signs indicate a temperature of 101 °F, pulse of 74, and BP of 100/70. She has no significant edema, and in fact appears very dehydrated.
Blood results are obtained:

- **WBC: 22,000**
- **HCT: 41.0**
- **Platelets: 45,000**
- **SGOT/PT: 292/334**
- **Glucose: 45**
- **Creatinine: 2.0**
- **Fibrinogen: 125**
- **PT/PTT: 12/50 s**
- **Serum ammonia level: 80 mol/l (n 11–35)**
- **Urinalysis is positive for protein and ketones**

The patient's most likely diagnosis is:

1. Hepatitis A
2. Hepatitis B
3. Acute fatty liver of pregnancy
4. Intrahepatic cholestasis of pregnancy
5. Severe preeclampsia
6. Hyperemesis gravidarum

Ans. 3. Acute fatty liver of pregnancy

USMLE Case Scenario

CAH (congenital adrenal hyperplasia) is a medical emergency. Which one is the fact about CAH?

1. CAH is an autosomally inherited disease of adrenal hyperfunction that causes hyponatremia and hyperkalemia because of lack of mineralocorticoids
2. CAH is an autosomally inherited disease of adrenal failure that causes hypernatremia and hyperkalemia because of lack of mineralocorticoids
3. CAH is an autosomally inherited disease of adrenal failure that causes hyponatremia and hyperkalemia because of lack of mineralocorticoids
4. CAH is an autosomally inherited disease of adrenal failure that causes hyponatremia and hypokalemia because of lack of mineralocorticoids

Ans. 3. CAH is an autosomally inherited disease of adrenal failure that causes hyponatremia and hyperkalemia because of lack of mineralocorticoids.

USMLE Case Scenario

The second most common site in the gastrointestinal tract for non-Hodgkin's lymphoma is:

1. Stomach
2. Small intestine
3. Colon
4. Rectum

Ans. 2. Small intestine

The stomach is the most common site in the gastrointestinal tract for non-Hodgkin's lymphoma, followed by the small intestine and the colon.

USMLE Case Scenario

MHC class II molecules with a bound antigen are recognized by:

1. T-cell receptor on CD41 cells
2. B-cell receptor on CD81 cells
3. B-cell receptor on CD81 cells
4. T-cell receptor on CD41 cells

Ans. 1. T-cell receptor on CD41 cells

- Major histocompatibility complex (MHC) proteins are polymorphic cell surface molecules that are important in lymphocyte-lymphocyte and lymphocyte-target interactions
- All nucleated cells express MHC class I proteins. B lymphocytes, macrophages, antigen-presenting cells, vascular endothelium, and activated T lymphocytes express both MHC class I and class II. MHC class I proteins are encoded by the HLA-A, B, and C loci, and MHC class II proteins are encoded by the HLA-D locus. Classically, MHC class I molecules with a bound antigen are recognized by the T-cell receptor on CD81 cells, and MHC class II molecules with a bound antigen are recognized by the T-cell receptor on CD41 cells.

USMLE Case Scenario

Graft-versus-host disease (GVHD) is:

1. Donor-type lymphoid cells transplanted may recognize the host's tissue as nonforeign and mount an immune response against the host
2. Donor-type lymphoid cells transplanted may recognize the host's tissue as foreign and mount an immune response against the host
3. Host-type lymphoid cells transplanted may recognize the tissue as nonforeign and mount an immune response against the donor
4. Host-type lymphoid cells transplanted may recognize the donor's tissue as foreign and mount an immune response against the donor

Ans. 2. Donor-type lymphoid cells transplanted may recognize the host's tissue as foreign and mount an immune response against the host.

USMLE Case Scenario

A 19-year-old young boy presents with low back pain for the past 7months accompanied by stiffness of the lumbar spine. He denies any gastrointestinal or genital infections. Examination reveals moderate limitation of back motion and tenderness of the lower spine. X-ray films of the vertebral column and pelvic region show flattening of the lumbar curve and subchondral bone erosion involving the sacroiliac joints. Which of the following is the most likely diagnosis?

1. Psoriatic arthritis
2. Gout
3. Caplan's syndrome
4. Ankylosing spondylitis
5. Degenerative joint disease
6. Reiter's syndrome
7. Seronegative rheumatoid arthritis
8. Still disease

Ans. 4. Ankylosing spondylitis. It should be suspected in any young person complaining of chronic lower back pain and confirmed by radiographs or CT scans of sacroiliac joints.

USMLE Case Scenario

A 44-year-old man with alcoholic cirrhosis is ordered some investigations. A screening battery of tests is ordered, revealing a decreased total thyroxine (T4). Physical examination of the thyroid gland is unremarkable. Follow-up studies showed a decreased total triiodothyronine (T3) and normal TSH. Which of the following is the most likely diagnosis in this patient?

1. Digeorge syndrome
2. Pappilary thyroid cancer
3. Euthyroid sick syndrome
4. Graves' disease
5. Hashimoto disease
6. Medullary carcinoma of the thyroid
7. Lymphocytic thyroiditis

Ans. 3. Euthyroid sick syndrome

This patient is seriously ill, with low T4 and low T3, but normal TSH. This is typical for euthyroid sick syndrome, which occurs in many seriously ill patients who do not have clinical hypothyroidism.

USMLE Case Scenario

Overall, 30–40% of all infections contracted in the postrenal transplant period are viral. The most common viral infections are by:

1. DNA viruses
2. RNA viruses
3. Retroviruses
4. Arboviruses

Ans. 1. DNA viruses

The most common viral infections are DNA viruses of the herpes virus family and include cytomegalovirus (CMV), Epstein-Barr virus, herpes simplex virus, and varicella zoster virus.

USMLE Case Scenario

The treatment modalities used for acute rejection are high-dose steroids, antilymphocyte globulin and OKT3. OKT3 is:

1. Murine monoclonal antibody to the human CD3 complex
2. Murine monoclonal antibody to the human CD8 complex
3. Equine monoclonal antibody to the human CD9 complex
4. Equine monoclonal antibody to the human CD10 complex

Ans. 1. Murine monoclonal antibody to the human CD3 complex

USMLE Case Scenario

Tumor necrosis factor (TNF) is a peptide hormone produced by endotoxin-activated monocytes/macrophages and has been postulated to be the principal cytokine mediator in gram-negative shock and sepsis-related organ damage. Biologic actions of TNF do not include:

1. Polymorphonuclear neutrophil (PMN) deactivation
2. Increased nonspecific host resistance
3. Increased vascular permeability
4. Lymphopenia
5. Promotion of interleukins 1, 2, and 6
6. Capillary leak syndrome
7. Microvascular thrombosis; anorexia and cachexia

Ans. 1. Polymorphonuclear neutrophil (PMN) deactivation

USMLE Case Scenario

The classic triad hemoptysis, pleuritic chest pain, and dyspnea can be seen in:

1. Esophagitis
2. Pulmonary embolism
3. Pneumothorax
4. Asthma
5. Mediastinitis

Ans. 2. Pulmonary embolism

USMLE Case Scenario

A 52-year-old, tall male presents to the Accident and Emergency department complaining of shortness of breath. He denies chest pain. He has no significant past medical history and takes no medications. A chest X-ray shows clear lung fields, mild cardiomegaly and a widened thoracic aorta with linear calcifications. An MRI of the chest shows aortic dilatation in the thorax, extending proximally,with atrophy of the muscularis and wrinkling of the intimal surface. The most likely etiology of this condition is:

1. Syphilis
2. Tuberculosis
3. Atherosclerosis
4. Hypertension
5. Noonan's syndrome
6. Marfan's syndrome
7. Syphilis infection
8. Takayasu's arteritis

Ans. 6. Marfan's syndrome. An autosomal dominant connective tissue disorder

USMLE Case Scenario

A 66-year-old professor from Michigan, concerned about his recent complaints, presents to a physician because of difficulty in coming downstairs, which he attributes to an inability to 'look down'. A complete Physical examination reveals that the patient looks around by moving his head rather than his eyes and also shows a distinctive axial rigidity of neck, trunk, and proximal limb muscles. He shows poverty of movement and dysarthric speech. Mentally, the patient responds very slowly but has better memory and intellect than are initially apparent. Most likely diagnosis is:

1. Pick's disease
2. Alzhiemer's disease
3. Multiple sclerosis
4. Progressive supranuclear palsy
5. PML
6. CJD
7. Kuru disease
8. Parkinson's disease

Ans. 4. Progressive supranuclear palsy

USMLE Case Scenario

CD19 positive, CD22 positive, CD103 positive monoclonal B-cells with bright kappa positivity were found to comprise 60% of the peripheral blood lymphoid cells on flow cytometric analysis in a 55-year-old man with massive splenomegaly and a total leucocyte count of 3.3 x 109/L. Which one of the following is the most likely diagnosis?

1. Splenic lymphoma with villous lymphocytes
2. Mantle cell lymphoma
3. B-cell prolymphocytic leukemia
4. Hairy cell leukemia

Ans. 4. Hairy cell leukemia

USMLE Case Scenario

A 24-year-old man presented to an ophthalmologist with a severe painful left eye for 38 hours. There is marked redness around the cornea which developed into iritis. Three days later, the right eye also became involved. One week after the onset of the eye symptoms, the patient complained of pain after and during micturation. No chlamydia, viruses or bacteria were isolated from his urinary discharge. He was treated with tetracycline and his eye signs gradually cleared. Subsequently, several joints were similarly involved. He was found to be HLA-B27-positive. Most likely diagnosis would be:

1. Behçet's disease
2. Ankylosing spondylitis
3. Reiter's disease
4. Gonococcal arhrtitis
5. Rheumatoid arthritis
6. Gouty arthritis

Ans. 3. Reiter's disease

USMLE Case Scenario

A 25-year-old male had pigmented macules over the palm, sole and oral mucosa. He also had anemia and pain in abdomen. The most probable diagnosis is:

1. Albright's syndrome
2. Cushing's syndrome
3. Peutz-Jegher's syndrome
4. Turcot's syndrome
5. Incontinentia pigmenti
6. FAP
7. HNPCC
8. Gardener's syndrome

Ans. 3. Peutz-Jegher's syndrome

USMLE Case Scenario

A 22-year-old student has been diagnosed with Type 1 diabetes mellitus for the last 3 years. Which of the following is the best early indicator for diabetic nephropathy?

1. Hematuria
2. WBC casts
3. Bence Jones proteins
4. Albuminuria
5. Hypertension
6. Rising blood urea nitrogen
7. Rising creatinine
8. Urinary tract infection

Ans. 4. Albuminuria

The spilling of albumin into the urine and, more specifically, the spilling of very small levels of albumin (microalbuminuria) are the best markers for significant diabetic nephropathy.

USMLE Case Scenario

Familial polyposis coli is a rare condition inherited as autosomal dominant, with equal sex incidence. Hundreds of adenomas develop throughout the colon and rectum. The gene responsible for FAP is:

1. On the short arm of chromosome 5
2. On the long arm of chromosome 5
3. On the short arm of chromosome 15
4. On the long arm of chromosome 15

Ans. 1. On the short arm of chromosome 5

USMLE Case Scenario

Exudate within the pleural cavity can be a result of:

1. Bacterial pleuritis
2. Cirrhosis of the liver
3. Congestive heart failure
4. Nephrotic syndrome
5. Protein-losing enteropathy

Ans. 1. Bacterial pleuritis

An exudate results from leakage of protein-rich fluid from the plasma into the interstitium. It is usually the result of increased vascular permeability caused by inflammation. Exudates also contain numerous acute or chronic inflammatory cells.

USMLE Case Scenario

A 77-year-old man residing in a suburban area presented with lumbago. He was mildly anemic but had no lymphadenopathy and no fever. There were no signs of bruising, no finger-clubbing, no hepatosplenomegaly and no abdominal or pelvic masses. On investigation, his hemoglobin was low 102 g/l. He had a normal differential white-cell count and a normal platelet count but his ESR was 94 mm/h

- **Total serum proteins were raised with rouleaux seen on the blood film**
- **His serum albumin, creatinine and urea were normal**
- **He had a raised serum calcium level (3.2 mmol/l) but a normal alkaline phosphatase**
- **Serum protein electrophoresis revealed a monoclonal band in the gamma region**
- **Diagnosis of myeloma is established. Findings would be:**

1. Raised serum calcium level, a raised alkaline phosphatase, raised platelets usually
2. Normal serum calcium level, a normal alkaline phosphatase, normal platelets usually
3. Raised serum calcium level, a normal alkaline phosphatase, elevated platelets usually
4. Raised serum calcium level, a normal alkaline phosphatase, normal platelets usually

Ans. 4. Raised serum calcium level, a normal alkaline phosphatase, normal platelets usually

USMLE Case Scenario

A 45-year-old woman has had a long history of frequent fractures to the long bones, deafness and recurrent osteomyelitis. She is told she has osteopetrosis. Which one of the following is a description of the pathology?

1. Mixed osteolytic and osteoblastic defect
2. Increased bone density due to defective osteoclastic activity
3. Increased bone density due to defective osteoblastic activity
4. Decrease in bone density
5. Decrease in bone mineralization
6. Decreased collagen turnover

Ans. 2. Increased bone density due to defective osteoclastic activity

Osteopetrosis is caused by increased bone density due to defective osteoclastic activity. Paget's disease is due to high turnover due to osteoblastic and osteoclastic activities. Osteoporosis causes decreased bone density. Osteomalacia causes decrease in bone mineralization.

USMLE Case Scenario

An 88-year-old patient was admitted in ICU with Herpes simplex encephalitis. Part of brain effected most specfically would be:

1. Hippocampus
2. Cerebellum
3. Basal ganglia
4. Brainstem
5. Spinal cord
6. Temporal lobes

Ans. 6. Temporal lobes

USMLE Case Scenario

Physical examination of a 55-year patient from Philadelphia demonstrates a pulsatile abdominal mass. Radiographic studies demonstrate a 9 cm diameter aneurysm of the abdominal aorta with foci of calcification in the walls. Which of the following is the most common etiology for this aneurysm?

1. Mucocutaneous disease
2. Atherosclerosis
3. Congenital weakness
4. Cystic medial necrosis
5. Syphilis
6. Vasculitis

Ans. 2. Atherosclerosis

USMLE Case Scenario

Myxopapillary ependymoma is a variant of ependymoma, a tumor arising from ependymal cells. Histologically, myxopapillary ependymoma contains a myxoid intercellular matrix, in which spindly neoplastic ependymal cells are arranged in a fascicular and papillary pattern. They are mostly found in:

1. Cerebrum
2. Cerebellum
3. Arachnoid cap cells
4. Sella turcica
5. Conus medullaris
6. 4th ventricle
7. Lateral ventricles
8. Midbrain

Ans. 5. Conus medullaris

It is a benign tumor that almost always occurs in the distal segment of the spinal cord, i.e. the conus medullaris

USMLE Case Scenario

A 46-year-old who was nonhypertensive with adult polycystic kidney disease is brought tot he emergency room in a coma. CT scan of the head demonstrates a subarachnoid hemorrhage without parenchymal hemorrhage. Which of the following is the most likely source of the bleeding?

1. Thrombosis
2. AV malformation
3. Bridging veins
4. Charcot-Bouchard aneurysm
5. Middle meningeal artery
6. Berry aneurysm

Ans. 6. Berry aneurysm

USMLE Case Scenario

A 58-year-old man has been reported by a physician to have bitemporal hemianopia. He also has elevated IGF-1 levels in the serum and an enlarged pituitary seen on MRI. Which one of the following is an associated feature?

1. Hypolipidemia
2. Hypoglycemia
3. Rheumatoid arthritis
4. Myocarditis
5. Carpal tunnel syndrome
6. Hypotension

Ans. 5. Carpal tunnel syndrome

The diagnosis is acromegaly. Impaired glucose tolerance, carpal tunnel syndrome and high cardiac output, cardiac failure are associated.

USMLE Case Scenario

A 26-year-old student of biochemistry after his return from India reports that he was bitten by flies while he was there in the Indian city of Delhi. He has been lethargic for two-and-a-half months and has a fever. Clinical examination reveals hepatomegaly with splenomegaly. Ultrasound of the abdomen reveals lymphadenopathy as well. One of the lymph nodes is biopsied which shows amastigotes within a macrophage. Most likely diagnosis is:

1. Brucellosis
2. Schistosomiasis
3. Malaria
4. Amebiasis
5. Leptosporiosis
6. Chlamydia infection
7. Kala azar
8. Babesiosis

Ans. 7. Leishmaniasis or Kala azar

The smears can show Donovan bodies (amastigotes of Leishmania donovani)

USMLE Case Scenario

A 24-year-old female who is working as a secretary in Honduras has had a diagnosis of pulmonary embolus. She has the following investigations: Hemoglobin 10.3 g/dl, white cell count 4.0 x 109/L, platelet count 45 x 109/L. Which of the following diagnoses is likely to be there?

1. Homocystinuria
2. Protein C deficiency
3. Factor V Leiden deficiency
4. DIC
5. Antiphospholipid syndrome
6. Protein S deficiency

Ans. 5. Antiphospholipid syndrome

USMLE Case Scenario

A 66-year-old man who was hypertensive, smoker for the last 20 years and also had raised serum cholesterol, was admitted to the coronary care unit in New Texas with a diagnosis of a large myocardial infarct (MI) of the left ventricle. On his 6th postinfarct day, he goes into shock and dies, manifesting signs and symptoms of cardiac tamponade. The most likely cause of this patient's death is:

1. HOCM
2. Aortic dissection
3. AV block
4. Extension of previous MI
5. Fatal arrhythmia
6. Rupture of the left ventricular wall
7. Rupture of papillary muscle

Ans. 6. Rupture of the left ventricular wall

USMLE Case Scenario

A 67-year-old patient had lymphoma and, after few months, developed herpes simplex encephalitis. Which of the following would you expect a CT scan of the patient's brain to show?

1. Generalized volume loss in cerebral hemispheres
2. Volume loss selectively in the basal ganglia and thalamus
3. Volume loss selectively in the medulla
4. Volume loss selectively in the cerebellar vermis
5. Volume loss selectively in the temporal and frontal lobes

Ans. 5. Volume loss selectively in the temporal and frontal lobes

Herpes simplex can cause anecrotizing, hemorrhagic, acute encephalitis that may rapidly produce death. The encephalitis characteristically involves the lower portions of the cerebral cortex, notably the temporal lobes and the base of the frontal lobes, possibly because the infection spreads from the oropharynx.

USMLE Case Scenario

A young male had a polymorphic ventricular tachycardia with syncopal episodes. He died of a sudden death. The features of the disease he died of are that it has an autosomal dominant inheritance and the abnormality is in the cardiac sodium channel. The most likely disease is:

1. Chaga's disease
2. Floppy valve disease
3. Holt oram disease
4. Wenkeback's disease
5. Brugada syndrome
6. Leigh's disease
7. NARP syndrome

Ans. 5. Brugada syndrome

USMLE Case Scenario

A 45-year-old man came to see an immunologist who has noted several 1 to 2 cm reddish purple, nodular lesions present on the skin of his right arm which have increased in size and number over the past 3 months. The lesions do not itch and are not painful. He has had a watery diarrhea for the past month. On physical examination, he has generalized lymphadenopathy and oral thrush. Which of the following infections is most likely to be related to the appearance of these skin lesions?

1. Candida albicans
2. Human herpesvirus 8
3. Mycobacterium tuberculosis
4. Pseudomonas aeruginosa
5. Pneumocystis jiroveci

Ans. 2. Human herpesvirus 8

Lesions of Kaposi sarcoma in an immunodeficient HIV patient.

USMLE Case Scenario

A 35-year-old female presented with one year history of menstrual irregularity and galactorrhea. She also had off-and-on headache. Her examination revealed bitemporal superior quadrantopia. Her fundus examination showed primary optic atropy. Which of the following is the most likely diagnosis in this case:

1. Craniopharyngioma
2. Pituitary macroadenoma
3. Pineal tumor
4. Frontal lobe tumor
5. Occipital infarct
6. Ophthalmic ICA aneurysm
7. Chiasmal glioma

Ans. 2. Pituitary macroadenoma

USMLE Case Scenario

Needle-shaped, strongly negatively birefringent crystals are seen from synovial fluid of a patient with pain in his joints. These crystals most likely are composed of:

1. Cysteine
2. Calcium phosphate
3. Oxalate
4. Calcium pyrophosphate dihydrate
5. Cholesterol
6. Monosodium urate

Ans. 6. Monosodium urate

USMLE Case Scenario

A patient presents with a platelet count of 700 × 109/L with abnormalities in size, shape and granularity of platelets, WBC count of 12 x 109/L, hemoglobin of 11 g/dl and the absence of the Philadelphia chromosome. The most likely diagnosis would be:

1. Polycythemia vera
2. Essential thrombocythemia
3. Chromic myeloid leukemia
4. Leukemoid reaction

Ans. 2. Essential thrombocythemia

USMLE Case Scenario

Lyme disease caused by Borrelia burgdorferi presents with a red macule or papule at the site of the tick bite. The initial lesion slowly expands to form a large annular lesion with a red border and central clearing. The lesion is warm, but usually not painful. This initial lesion is called:

1. Erythema nodosum
2. Erythema gyrum repens
3. Erythema chronicum migrans
4. Erythema multiforme
5. Erythema ab igne

Ans. 3. Erythema chronicum migrans

USMLE Case Scenario

A 28-year-old student from New York presented with a 1-week history of a sore throat, stiffness and tenderness of his neck and extreme malaise. On examination, he was mildly pyrexial with posterior cervical lymphadenopathy, palatal petechiae and pharyngeal inflammation without an exudate. Abdominal examination showed mild splenomegaly. There was no evidence of a skin rash or jaundice. Feature seen in him would be:

1. Atypical lymphocytosis and his serum contains IgE antibodies to CMV viral capsid antigen
2. Atypical lymphocytosis and his serum contains IgM antibodies to CMV viral capsid antigen
3. Atypical lymphocytosis and his serum contains IgM antibodies to Epstein-Barr viral capsid antigen
4. Atypical lymphocytosis and his serum contains IgE antibodies to Epstein-Barr viral capsid antigen

Ans. 3. Atypical lymphocytosis and his serum contains IgM antibodies to Epstein-Barr viral capsid antigen

USMLE Case Scenario

A 23-year-old engineer from New York presented with a 1-week history of a sore throat, stiffness and tenderness of his neck, and extreme malaise. On examination, he was mildly pyrexial with posterior cervical lymphadenopathy, palatal petechiae and pharyngeal inflammation without an exudate. Abdominal examination showed mild splenomegaly. There was no evidence of a skin rash or jaundice. The clinical diagnosis is:

1. Hay fever
2. Glandular fever

3. Lymphoma
4. Tonsillitis
5. Retropharyngeal abscess
6. Ludwig's angina
7. Quinsy

Ans. 2. Glandular fever

USMLE Case Scenario

A 30-year-old lady presents with features of malabsorption and iron-deficiency anemia. Duodenal biopsy shows complete villous atrophy. Which of the following antibodies is likely to be present?
1. Antiendomysial antibodies
2. Antigoblet cell antibodies
3. Anti-Saccharomyces cerevisae antibodies
4. Antineutrophil cytoplasmic antibodies

Ans. 1. Antiendomysial antibodies

USMLE Case Scenario

An 89-year-old elderly patient suffering from Pick's disease also has multiple small strokes. During her stay in the nursing home, on multiple occasions she aspirated food, and neurological examination reveals that her gag reflex is absent. These findings suggest involvement of the nucleus of which of the following cranial nerves?
1. Facial (VII)
2. Glossopharyngeal (IX)
3. Hypoglossal (XII)
4. Spinal accessory (XI)
5. Vestibulocochlear (VIII)

Ans. 2 Cranial nerve IX is the glossopharyngeal nerve, which has a nucleus in the medulla and is necessary for the gag reflex

USMLE Case Scenario

A 16-year-old boy on a routine health check-up by a physician in New York is said to have systolic murmur preceded by a distinct click on auscultation. The patient has unusually long legs and long, tapering fingers. An ocular examination reveals dislocation of the lens. An abnormality of which of the following gene products is thought to underlie this condition?
1. Collagen
2. Dystrophin
3. Elastin
4. Fibrillin
5. Myosin b-chain

Ans. 4. Fibrillin

The genetic condition is Marfan syndrome, which is characterized by skeletal, ocular, and cardiovascular abnormalities. The gene mutated in Marfan syndrome encodes fibrillin protein that serves as scaffolding for the deposition of elastin and formation of elastic fibers.

USMLE Case Scenario

A 37-year-old man with Wegener's granulomatosis (WG) was admitted to hospital with a 2-week history of fever and shortness of breath. The diagnosis of WG had been made 19 months earlier when he presented with hemoptysis and glomerulonephritis. Disease remission will be achieved with aggressive immunosuppressive therapy using:
1. A combination of pulse hydrocortisone and nitrogen mustard
2. A combination of pulse hydrocortisone and cyclosporine
3. A combination of pulse methylprednisolone and cyclophosphamide
4. A combination of pulse cyclosporine and cyclophosphamide

Ans. 3. A combination of pulse methylprednisolone and cyclophosphamide

USMLE Case Scenario

A clinical condition as seen in a 24-year-old male from New Orleans is characterized by a facial palsy and is often associated with facial pain and the appearance of vesicles on the ear drum, ear canal and pinna. Vertigo and sensorineural hearing loss (VIII nerve) accompanying it are suggestive of:

1. Down's syndrome
2. Turner's syndrome
3. Bell's palsy
4. Pendred syndrome
5. Ramsay-Hunt syndrome
6. Goldenhar syndrome
7. Alport's syndrome
8. Pierre Robin syndrome
9. Treacher collins syndrome

Ans. 5. Ramsay-Hunt syndrome

USMLE Case Scenario

CREST syndrome (calcinosis, Raynaud's phenomenon, esophageal motility syndrome, sclerodactyly, and telangiectasia) which is also called limited scleroderma This would be associated with:

1. Anti-Ro
2. Anti-SS-B
3. Decreased ESR
4. Anticentromere antibody

Ans. 4. Anticentromere antibody

USMLE Case Scenario

An infection is transmitted by inhaling dust or drinking milk from infected mammals, especially sheep and cows. The disease in humans, Q fever, is marked by mild nonspecific symptoms or pneumonia, and may progress to myocarditis or hepatitis. The causative organism is:

1. Moraxella
2. Bordetella
3. Coxiella
4. Francisella
5. Salmonella
6. Kingella

Ans. 3. Coxiella

USMLE Case Scenario

A 50-year-old male presents with bilateral weakness of upper limbs for the last one-and-a-half weeks. He has blood pressure of 130/80 mm Hg. He got a flu three weeks back followed by paresthesias. There is no history of alcohol intake. Neurological examination of face reveals facial palsy on both sides. CSF shows a normal cell count. A doctor starts him on plasmapheresis and his condition improves. He is most likely suffering from:

1. Brain metastasis
2. Putamen hemorrhage of left side
3. Botulism
4. Guillain-Barré syndrome
5. Herpes encephalitis
6. Tuberculous meningitis
7. Polio
8. Wegener's granulomatosis
9. Sarcoidosis
10. Multiple sclerosis

Ans. 4. Ramsay-Hunt syndrome

USMLE Case Scenario

A solitary weakly ring-enhancing lesion without demyelination is seen in MRI of a 45-year-old man from Kansas. The patient is on HAART for HIV for the last 3 months. After a check-up in a medical clinic. He was given Trimethoprim but failed to respond to the medication. What can be expected in this patient:

1. SSPE after measles infection
2. A positive toxoplasma serology
3. Cytoalbuniological dissociation
4. Response to plasmapheresis
5. Progressive multifocal leukoencephalopathy
6. EBV DNA in CSF
7. CSF suggestive of bacterial meningitis

Ans. 6. EBV DNA in CSF

Explanation: Case is suggestive of CNS lymphoma in a HIV infected patient. Exclude other options.

USMLE Case Scenario

A 34-year-old female is not able to work in her office, says she can't sleep either. She has not taken her meals the nicely for the last 20 hours because of severe nature of her pain. The pain is described as electric with about 20–30 episodes for the last two days. She was given oral Paracatemol and later Piroxicam for the pain which failed to respond. There is no obivious precipitant for the said pain. Her psychiatric check-up reveals nothing abnormal. She does not take alcohol or any other drug. Which drug would be most effective for her complaint?

1. Low-flow oxygen
2. High-flow oxygen
3. Levodopa
4. Ergot
5. Sumatriptan
6. Steroids
7. Acyclovir
8. Lithium
9. Carbamazepine
10. Histocalamine lotion

Ans. 9. Carbamazepine

USMLE Case Scenario

After suffering from a stroke, a 36-year-old man from New Jersey is reported by his wife to be shaving only right side of his face. He is asked to lift his left hand and he lifts his right hand. Hemineglect is due to involvement of:

1. Left parietal lobe (dominant)
2. Right parietal lobe (dominant)
3. Right parietal lobe (nondominant)
4. Left parietal lobe (nondominant)

Ans. 3. Right parietal lobe (nondominant)

USMLE Case Scenario

A 52-year-old male presents with bilateral weakness of upper limbs for the last one-and-a-half weeks. He has blood pressure of 120/80 mm Hg. He got a flu three weeks back followed by Parasthesias. There is no history of alcohol intake. Neurological examination of face reveals facial palsy on both sides. CSF shows a normal cell count. He is said to have Guillain-Barré syndrome. Guillain Barré syndrome is:

1. Acute idiopathic noninflammatory demyelinating polyneuropathy
2. Chronic idiopathic inflammatory demyelinating mononeuropathy
3. Chronic idiopathic noninflammatory demyelinating polyneuropathy
4. Acute idiopathic inflammatory demyelinating polyneuropathy

Ans. 4. Acute idiopathic inflammatory demyelinating polyneuropathy

USMLE Case Scenario

A 66-year-old man from Downtown, Chicago develops severe, acute, excruciating chest pain that radiates to his back. On the way to the emergency room, he collapses after a spell of becoming unresponsive, and is pulseless on arrival Several resuscitation attempts are unsuccessful. Autopsy reveals massive hemoperitoneum due to a ruptured aortic dissection. There is an intimal tear in the ascending aorta, with a dissecting hematoma in the media, extending from the aortic valve to the renal arteries. Which feature of this scenario most strongly suggests hypertension as the cause of the aortic dissection?

1. Adventitial tear above renal arteries
2. Dissection through media
3. Involvement of major aortic branches
4. Origin at the ascending aorta
5. Rapid exsanguination

Ans 4. Origin at the ascending aorta

The two most common causes of aortic dissection are hypertension and atherosclerosis. An important distinction between the two is that hypertensive dissections generally originate in the ascending aorta, at an intimal surface free of atherosclerosis Dissection secondary to atherosclerosis is typically the consequence of a ruptured aortic aneurysm, which originates in the abdominal aorta at the iliac bifurcation.

USMLE Case Scenario

Which of the following is an example of disorders of sex chromosomes?

1. Marfan's syndrome
2. Testicular feminization syndrome
3. Klinefelter's syndome
4. Down's syndrome

Ans. 3. Klinefelter's syndrome

USMLE Case Scenario

A history of a new kitten in the house and the papule in a child at the site of a scratch with regional painful adenopathy defines:

1. Rat bite fever
2. Bacillary angiomatosis
3. Cat-scratch disease
4. Pausterulla infection
5. Cat-cry syndrome
6. Tularemia

Ans. 3. Cat-scratch disease

This patient has the classic symptoms of cat-scratch disease caused by the bacillus Bartonella henselae.

USMLE Case Scenario

An organism is a part of the normal flora of the oral cavity of pets. A splenectomized patient develops cellulitis and fulminant septicemia after a bite of a cat. An organism is identified as the causative agent. The likely organism is:

1. Capnocytophaga canimorsus
2. Bartonella
3. Pasteurella
4. Spirillum

Ans. 1. Capnocytophaga canimorsus

This organism is associated with cat bites, but the patient develops cellulitis and fulminant septicemia, especially in asplenic patients.

USMLE Case Scenario

Listeriosis is caused by the gram-positive rod listeria monocytogenes. Meningitis and bacteremia are common clinical manifestations. Most at risk are:

1. Young, nonpregnant, immunocompetent
2. Elderly, neonates, pregnant women
3. Nonpregnant females, middle-aged
4. Immunocompetent, pregnant and young

Ans. 2. Elderly, neonates, pregnant women

USMLE Case Scenario

Feature of X-linked recessive diseases is that:

1. Carrier mothers cannot pass the disease to their sons; nonaffected fathers can have carrier daughters but not affected sons
2. Carrier mothers pass the disease to half their daughters; affected fathers cannot have carrier daughters but affected sons
3. Carrier mothers pass the disease to half their sons; affected fathers can have carrier daughters but not affected sons
4. Carrier mothers pass the disease to half their sons; affected fathers can have carrier sons

Ans. 3. Carrier mothers pass the disease to half their sons; affected fathers can have carrier daughters but not affected sons.

USMLE Case Scenario

A 55-year-old man while reading newspaper in the morning suddenly becomes completely blind in one eye, and angiography demonstrates occlusion of the central retinal artery. Which of the following is the most likely cause of the occlusion?

1. Atheroma or embolism
2. Cranial (temporal) arteritis
3. Hypertension
4. Polycythemia vera
5. Tumor

Ans. 1. Atheroma or embolism

Simple explanation. Occlusion of the central retinal artery rapidly causes irreversible blindness with loss of the inner retinal layers. (The photoreceptor rod and cone cells are maintained by the pigment epithelium.) The site of occlusion is typically just posterior to the cribriform plate. A garden-variety atheroma or embolism is overwhelmingly the most common cause of central retinal artery occlusion.

USMLE Case Scenario

A 35-year-old woman with known HIV comes to her physician with a 3-month history of watery diarrhea, severe weakness, and a 22-pound weight loss. Multiple stool tests for bacteria, ova, and parasites are repeatedly negative. A colonoscopy is normal, as are biopsies of the colon. Which of the following is the most likely explanation for her diarrhea?

1. Cryptosporidiosis
2. Cytomegalovirus infection
3. Entameba histolytica
4. Enterotoxigenic *Escherichia coli*
5. Shigella dysenteriae

Ans. 1 Cryptosporidiosis

This patient has a typical small bowel-type diarrhea seen in HIV with watery diarrhea, weakness, and weight loss. The most common etiology for this syndrome is cryptosporidiosis infection of the small intestine, where the spores can be seen on the tips of the villi on biopsy. This organism can be demonstrated with special culture media. Other organisms in the same family, such as microsporidia and isospora belli, produce identical syndromes.

USMLE Case Scenario

A 49-year-old woman meets with an automobile accident and sustains a closed head injury. A CT scan does not show any intracranial hemorrhage, but reveals a small tumor at the cerebellopontine angle of the brain. Which of the following nerves is most likely to be affected by this tumor?

1. Facial nerve
2. Glossopharyngeal nerve
3. Optic nerve
4. Trigeminal nerve
5. Vagus nerve
6. Abducens nerve

Ans. 1. Facial nerve

The facial nerve and the vestibulocochlear nerve emerge from the brainstem at the cerebellopontine angle. These are the two nerves which will be initially affected by a tumor in this region.

USMLE Case Scenario

A 58-year-old woman from Chicago seen previously by a physician presents with an eight-year history of headaches, generalized tonic-clonic seizures, and bilateral leg weakness. X-ray skull films reveal hyperostosis of the calvarium. Biopsy of the responsible lesion shows a whorling pattern of the cells. Which of the following is the most likely diagnosis?

1. Arachnoid cyst
2. Glioblastoma multiforme
3. Meningioma
4. Metastatic breast cancer
5. Oligodendroglioma
6. Ependymoma

Ans. 3. Meningioma

The most likely diagnosis is an intracranial meningioma. Meningiomas are slow-growing, benign tumors comprising 15% of intracranial tumors; seen mostly in elderly. They originate from meninges, either the dura mater or the arachnoid matter

- **Meningiomas often incite an osteoblastic reaction in the overlying cranial bones. Microscopically, the meningioma cells have a tendency to encircle one another, forming whorls and psammoma bodies**
- **Clinically, they present as mass lesions; seizures may occur**
- **The superior parasagittal surface of the frontal lobes is a favorite site of origin**
- **This can often produce leg weakness, since the leg motor fibers that pass down through the internal capsule originate in parasagittal cortical regions**
- **Treatment of meningiomas is usually surgical.**

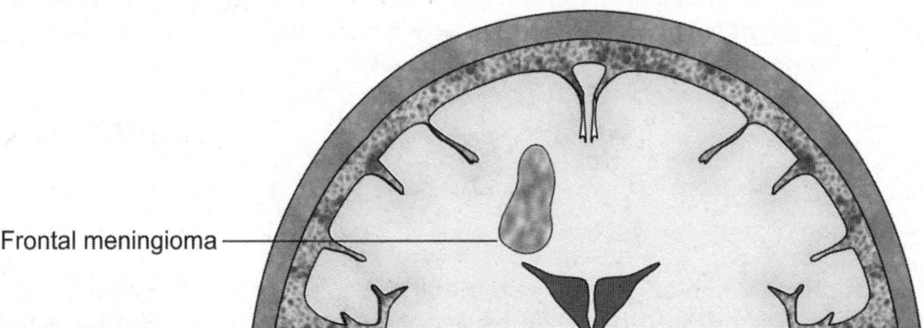

USMLE Case Scenario

A 72-year-old woman was commenced on oral corticosteroids for giant cell arteritis. Over the next 6 months, she had three episodes of a painful, vesicular rash over the ophthalmic division of the right trigeminal nerve. Virus implicated is:

1. CMV
2. Polio

3. EBV
4. HPV
5. HIV
6. Herpes

Ans. 6. Herpes

USMLE Case Scenario

A 2-year-old boy presents with fever for 3 days which responded to administration of paracetamol. Three days later, he developed acute renal failure, marked acidosis and encephalopathy. His urine showed plenty of oxalate crystals. The blood anion gap and osmolal gap were increased. Which of the following is the most likely diagnosis?

1. Paracetamol poisoning
2. Diethyl glycol poisoning
3. Severe malaria
4. Hanta virus infection
5. Sulfuric acid poisoning
6. Dengue fever

Ans. 2. Diethyl glycol poisoning

USMLE Case Scenario

A 68-year-old, well-developed, well-nourished black male presents to the emergency department complaining of shortness of breath. He denies chest pain. He has no significant past medical history and takes no medications. A chest X-ray shows clear lung fields, mild cardiomegaly and a widened thoracic aorta with linear calcifications. An MRI of the chest shows aortic dilatation in the thorax, extending proximally, with atrophy of the muscularis and wrinkling of the intimal surface. What is the most likely etiology of this condition?

1. Atherosclerosis
2. Hypertension
3. Marfan's syndrome
4. Syphilis infection
5. Takayasu's arteritis

Ans. 4. Syphilis infection

USMLE Case Scenario

A 41-year-old man with no previous medical history presents to the emergency department with chest pain and shortness of breath. An ECG done in the emergency department shows normal sinus rhythm with no ST-T segment changes. Cardiac enzymes are negative. He is admitted to the telemetry unit for monitoring. Six hours after admission, he begins to feel dizzy. The telemetry monitor shows the patient is in atrial fibrillation with a pulse of 160/min. His blood pressure is 70/40 mm Hg. Which of the following is the most appropriate next step in management?

1. DC cardioversion
2. Intravenous digoxin
3. Start coumadin
4. Start intravenous diltiazem drip
5. Start intravenous heparin drip

Ans. 1. DC cardioversion

In patients with atrial fibrillation and hemodynamic instability, the treatment of choice is immediate cardioversion. Hemodynamic compromise may be manifested clinically by hypotension and shock and by worsening angina pectoris, shortness of breath, or heart failure.

USMLE Case Scenario

A 35-year-old woman has a dry mouth and pain during sexual intercourse, most probably attributed to genital dryness with a raised ESR (53 mm/h). Schirmer's test was performed. The test was markedly abnormal. Her rheumatoid factor titer is increased and ANA and antibodies to the extractable nuclear antigens Ro and La are detectable. Now she also has development of the dry mouth and dry eyes and bilateral nonerosive polyarthritis of her hands, wrists and knees. Likely diagnosis is:

1. SLE
2. Dermatomyositis
3. Polymyositis
4. Sjögren's syndrome
5. MCTD
6. Amyloidosis

Ans. 4. Sjögren's syndrome

USMLE Case Scenario

A 13-year-old boy from Chicago has a small tumor in the wall of the left lateral ventricle of brain. A biopsy of this tumor is consistent with pathologic diagnosis of subependymal giant cell astrocytoma. Which of the following lesions may also be present in this patient?

1. Café au-lait spots
2. Renal angiomyolipomas
3. Sesamoid bones
4. Hemangioblastoma
5. Wickham's striae
6. Lisch nodules
7. Cancers of genital tract
8. Schwannoma of the VIII cranial nerve

Ans. 2. Renal angiomyolipomas

Tuberous sclerosis: It manifests with multiple hamartomatous lesions in the skin, CNS, and visceral organs. Cortical tubers are malformed (hamartomatous) nodules of the cortex, probably resulting from faulty cortical development

Other lesions include:

- **Shagreen patches**
- **Ash leaf spots on the skin**
- **Cardiac myomas**
- **Renal angiomyolipomas**

USMLE Case Scenario

In a 34-year-old female with Raynaud's phenomenon, tethering and thickening of skin, dysphagia soft-tissue, calcified nodules, increasingly shortness of breath would indicate:

1. Sjögren's syndrome
2. Rheumatoid arthritis
3. Localized sclerosis
4. Systemic sclerosis
5. SLE
6. Polymyositis

Ans. 4. Systemic sclerosis

USMLE Case Scenario

In a 34-year-old female Raynaud's phenomenon, tethering and thickening of skin, dysphagia soft-tissue, calcified nodules, increasingly shortness of breath showed the patient to systemic sclerosis. Lung function tests would show:

1. An obstructive defect with only a slight reduction in transfer factor
2. An obstructive defect with elevation in transfer factor
3. A restrictive defect with only a slight reduction in transfer factor
4. A restrictive defect with elevation in transfer factor

Ans. 3. A restrictive defect with only a slight reduction in transfer factor

USMLE Case Scenario

A 25-year-old Asian presented with a 4-week history of coughing, breathlessness and malaise. He had lost 4 kg in weight, but had no history of night sweats or hemoptysis. He had returned from holiday in India 2 months earlier. Crepitations were audible over both the lung apices; there were no other physical signs. His hemoglobin and white cell count were normal but the CRP was 239 mg/l. The chest X-ray showed bilateral upper- and middle-lobe shadowing but no hilar enlargement. Correct statement would be:

1. Noncaseating granuloma
2. BAL showing pneumocystis carinii
3. Red currant sputum
4. Sputum was found to contain acid-fast bacilli
5. Frothy sputum would be a feature

Ans. 4. Sputum was found to contain acid-fast bacilli

USMLE Case Scenario

A 38-year-old man from Washington complained of breathlessness. On examination, he had no clubbing and no abnormal chest signs. A chest X-ray showed fine, diffuse radiological shadows, predominantly in the mid zones, and bilateral hilar lymphadenopathy. Lung function tests were normal and a Mantoux test was negative. ACE levels and calcium levels are increased. A clinical diagnosis suggests:

1. Pneumonia
2. Tuberculosis
3. Sarcoidosis
4. Cat-scratch disease
5. Coal worker's lung
6. Caplan's syndrome

Ans. 3. Sarcoidosis

USMLE Case Scenario

A 22-year-old primigravida from New Texas had been well once she had recovered from morning sickness during the first 4 weeks of gestation. She had been drinking unpasteurized milk for 5 weeks when she developed fever, vomiting and diarrhea followed by headache, myalgia and low back pain which persisted for 5 days. Four weeks later, at 28 weeks gestation, she went into premature labor and a stillborn, jaundiced child was delivered after 36 hrous. At the post-mortem of the child, there was evidence of hepatitis, purulent pneumonia, conjunctivitis and meningitis. Most likely organism would be:

1. *E. coli*
2. Pseudomonas
3. Legionella
4. Streptococci
5. Anthrax bacillus
6. Listeria
7. Measles
8. Toxoplasma

Ans. 6. Listeria

USMLE Case Scenario

A 33-year-old business-class woman was admitted with a 3-week history of increasing bloody diarrhea and abdominal pain; she had lost 5 kg in weight. She smoked 25 cigarettes a day. On examination, she was having tenderness over the right iliac fossa. Sigmoidoscopy showed a red, granular mucosa with mucous and contact bleeding. Ulceration of the surface epithelium, noncaseating granulomas and skip lesions. Most likely cause is:

1. Ischemic colitis
2. Gluten enteropathy
3. Crohn's disease

4. Ulcerative colitis
5. Pseudomembranous colitis

Ans. 3. Crohn's disease

USMLE Case Scenario

CSF analysis of a 55-year-old man presenting with numbness and parasthesis off and on reveal:

- **Protein concentration 0.4 g/l (NR 0-0.4 g/l)**
- **Red blood cells: None**
- **Lymphocytes 4 × 106/l (NR < 5 × 106/l)**
- **IgG concentration 120 mg/l (NR < 60 mg/l)**
- **Albumin concentration 488 mg/l (NR < 400 mg/l)**
- **IgG/albumin ratio 28% (NR 4–22%)**
- **IgG index 1.17 (NR < 0.7)**
- **Isoelectric focusing oligoclonal bands present**

The most likely diagnosis is:

1. SAH
2. Guillain-Barré syndrome
3. Multiple sclerosis
4. Subacute degeneration of cord
5. Hysteria
6. Empty sella syndrome

Ans. 3. Multiple sclerosis

- MS is a disorder of unknown cause, defined clinically by characteristic symptoms, signs, and progression and pathologically by scattered areas of inflammation and demyelination affecting the brain, optic nerves, and spinal cord
- After separating CSF gamma globulin fractions by agarose or polyacrylamide gel electrophoresis, separate discrete 'oligoclonal' bands (OCB) can be detected in 70 to 80% of patients. The sensitivity for detecting OCB can be increased by separating CSF by isoelectric focusing or by staining the gels or nitrocellulose blots with anti-immunoglobulin antibodies

USMLE Case Scenario

A 57-year-old mechanical engineer from rural Mexico complains of seeing double, was found to have bilateral ptosis, covering most of the pupil on the right side and partially obscuring that on the left. He admitted to tiredness in the arms and legs on exercise, which recovered with resting. A clinical diagnosis of ocular myasthenia gravis was made. His Tensilon test was positive but electromyography was inconclusive. His serum would contain:

1. Antibodies to adrenergic receptors of smooth muscle
2. Antibodies to acetylcholine receptors of smooth muscle
3. Antibodies to acetylcholine receptors of skeletal muscle
4. Antibodies to acetylcholine receptors of both skeletal and smooth muscle

Ans. 3. Antibodies to acetylcholine receptors of skeletal muscle

USMLE Case Scenario

A 58-year-old man made repeated visits to a dermatologist after being referred to a physician. He presented with mild itching and redness of his skin for 2 months, with severe keratosis on the soles of his feet and the palms of his hands. On examination, he had characteristic exfoliative dermatitis with bilateral axillary lymphadenopathy but no hepatosplenomegaly. Investigation showed that his hemoglobin was normal (139 g/l) but he had a raised white-cell count (12.8 × 109/l). A blood film showed an increase of small cleaved lymphocytes, 90% of which were T-lymphocytes. Electron microscopy of buffy coat cells confirmed that the nuclei of these cells had multiple clefts. The patient was treated with PUVA therapy to the skin. Most likely diagnosis is:

1. Mantle cell lymphoma
2. Glandular fever

3. Littoral cell angioma
4. Portal hypertension
5. Acute leukemia
6. Sezary syndrome
7. Follicular cell lymphoma
8. Hairy cell leukemia
9. CML

Ans. 6. Sezary syndrome

USMLE Case Scenario

A 33-year-old nervous and anxious woman presented with a 3-month history of increased sweating and palpitations with weight loss of 7 kg despite a relatively good appetite. On examination, she had a diffuse, nontender, smooth enlargement of her thyroid, over which a bruit could be heard. She had a fine tremor of her fingers and a resting pulse rate of 159/minute. On investigation, she had:

- **Serum T3 of 5.2 nmol/l (NR 0.8-2.4)**
- **T4 of 59 nmol/l (NR 9-23)**
- **Measurement of her thyroid-stimulating hormone showed that this was low normal, 0.4 mU/l (NR 0.4 – 5 mU/l)**
- **Circulating antibodies to thyroid peroxidase were detected by agglutination**

Most likely cause is:

1. Hashimoto's disease
2. Wolff-Chaikkoff effect
3. Pendred syndrome
4. Autoimmune thyrotoxicosis
5. De Quervian's disease

Ans. 4. Autoimmune thyrotoxicosis

USMLE Case Scenario

A 44-year-old woman from a hilly area presented with a large, painless swelling in her neck. Thyroid function tests showed that she was euthyroid; however, her serum contained high titer antibodies to thyroid peroxidase. Most likely cause is:

1. Hashimoto's thyroiditis
2. Wolf-chaikkoff effect
3. Pendred syndrome
4. Autoimmune thyrotoxicosis
5. De Quervian's disease
6. Pendred syndrome
7. Basedow phenomenon
8. Dawn phenomenon

Ans. 1. Hashimoto's thyroiditis

USMLE Case Scenario

A 15-year-old girl presented with vague abdominal discomfort for 3 months. She had noticed occasional diarrhea but had not passed any blood. She admitted to weight loss and anorexia. On examination, she was pigmented with her buccal mucosa and gums were also brown. She had a low cortisol level and her response to the adrenocorticotrophic hormone in a Synacthen test was poor. Most likely cause is:

1. Parathyroid hyperactivity
2. Parathyroid underactivity
3. Thyroid overactivity
4. Thyroid underactivity
5. Adrenal medulla failure
6. Adrenal cortical failure

Ans. 6. Adrenal cortical failure

USMLE Case Scenario

A 70-year-old female presented in hospital with increasing tiredness, exertional dyspnea and ankle swelling for a few years. Two years earlier, she had been found to be anemic and had been treated with oral iron without symptomatic improvement. Laboratory investigations showed:

- Hemoglobin of 62 g/l with a reduced white-cell count of 3.8 x 109/l (and a platelet count of only 32 × 109/l)
- A blood film showed marked macrocytosis with a mean cell volume of 112 fl
- Bone marrow examination revealed marked megaloblastic erythropoiesis with abundant iron stores
- Serum vitamin B12 was decreased but serum folate, serum iron and total iron-binding capacity were normal
- Her serum contains positive gastric parietal cell antibodies of IgG class and blocking antibodies to intrinsic factor. The patient would respond to:

1. Thiamine
2. Hydroxocobalamin
3. Ascorbate
4. Tocopherol
5. Pantothenic acid

Ans. 2. Hydroxocobalamin

USMLE Case Scenario

A 58-year-old female presented in hospital with increasing tiredness, exertional dyspnea and ankle swelling for few years. Two years earlier, she had been found to be anemic and had been treated with oral iron without symptomatic improvement. She responded to hydroxycobalamine. Most likely cause was:

1. Hemolytic anemia
2. Iron-deficiency anemia
3. Pernicious anemia
4. Aplastic anemia

Ans. 3. Pernicious anemia

USMLE Case Scenario

A 44-year-old female developed loose stools and generalized but vague abdominal pain. On questioning, she had felt tired for 3 years and had lost about five kg in weight during the preceding 7 months despite a good appetite. Laboratory investigations showed:

- A macrocytic anemia but normal white-cell, platelet and reticulocyte counts
- The blood film showed many Howell-Jolly bodies

Bone marrow examination revealed active erythropoiesis with early megaloblastic features. Her serum was positive for IgA antibodies to endomysium and she had high levels of IgA and IgG antibodies to gliadin, strongly supporting the clinical diagnosis. A jejunal biopsy was performed: this showed a convoluted pattern of stunted villi under the dissecting microscope and subtotal villous atrophy with marked increase in intraepithelial lymphocytes and chronic inflammation in the lamina propria. The patient should be started on:

1. A high-carbohydrate diet
2. A low-iron diet with high gluten content
3. A high-calorie diet
4. A gluten-free diet with folic acid and iron supplements
5. Total parenteral nutrition
6. Intravenous iron only

Ans. 4. A gluten-free diet with folic acid and iron supplements

USMLE Case Scenario

A 44-year-old lady had nephrotic syndrome. On further investigations, warm sample of ladies blood serum contained a mixed cryoglobulin. A skin biopsy showed scattered deposits of IgM, IgG and C3 in dermal blood vessels. The final diagnosis was mixed cryoglobulinemia. It is seen in association with:

1. Perihepatitis by chlamydia
2. Hepatitis A infection

3. Chronic hepatitis C infection
4. Hepatitis B
5. Lichen planus
6. Psoriasis

Ans. 3. Chronic hepatitis C infection

USMLE Case Scenario

The most common malignancy found in Marjolin's ulcer is:

1. Basal cell carcinoma
2. Squamous cell carcinoma
3. Malignant fibrous histiocytoma
4. Neurotrophic malignant melanoma

Ans. 2. Squamous cell carcinoma

USMLE Case Scenario

A 25-year-old woman was admitted in the neurology department with a stroke due to a cerebrovascular thrombosis. She had three spontaneous abortions in the past. She was a nonsmoker. Antibodies to nuclei, extractable nuclear antigens and double-stranded DNA were negative, but she did have high-titer antiphospholipid antibodies. A diagnosis of primary antiphospholipid antibody syndrome was made. Lab tests would suggest:

1. ↑Hemoglobin, ↑platelet and ↑white-cell counts↑C3 and C4 levels. A normal kaolin-cephalin clotting time
2. ↓Hemoglobin, ↓ platelet and ↓white-cell counts↓C3 and C4 levels. A ↓ kaolin-cephalin clotting time
3. Normal hemoglobin, platelet and white-cell count, normal C3 and C4 levels. A normal kaolin-cephalin clotting time
4. Hemoglobin, platelet and white-cell counts were normal, normal C3 and C4 levels. A prolonged kaolin-cephalin clotting time

Ans. 4. Hemoglobin, platelet and white-cell counts were normal, normal C3 and C4 levels. A prolonged kaolin-cephalin clotting time

USMLE Case Scenario

A bone marrow examination showed only 12% plasma cells. X-ray done showed absence of osteolytic lesions, the absence of monoclonal free light chains in the urine and normal serum IgA and IgM levels. These findings support a diagnosis of:

1. Myeloma
2. Amyloidosis
3. MGUS
4. Histiocytosis X

Ans. 3. MGUS

USMLE Case Scenario

A 64-year-old man presents to a physician because of difficulty in reading newspapers and coming downstairs, which he attributes to an inability to 'look down'. Physical examination reveals that the patient looks around by moving his head rather than his eyes and also shows a distinctive axial rigidity of neck, trunk, and proximal limb muscles. He shows decrease of movement and altered dysarthric speech. Mentally, the patient responds very slowly but has good short-term as well as long memory and his intellectectual capabilities are apparently normal. Which of the following pathologic findings of the brain would most likely be present?

1. Depigmentation of the substantia nigra
2. Widespread cortical atrophy
3. Temporal lobe atrophy
4. Degeneration of the caudate nucleus and putamen
5. Widespread neuronal loss and gliosis in subcortical sites

Ans. 5. Widespread neuronal loss and gliosis in subcortical sites

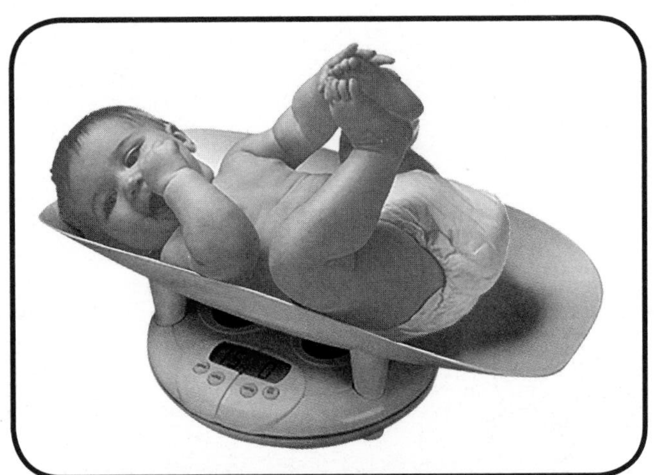

PEDIATRICS

Pediatrics 2

Intrauterine Growth Retardation: IUGR

Causes:
- Alcohol
- Smoking
- CRF
- Propranolol
- **Fetal growth is maximally affected by insulin**
- **Fetal well-being in IUGR is assessed by:**
  - Amniocentesis
  - NST (Nonstress Test)
  - AF (Amniotic Fluid) Volume

Small for Date Babies

- **'Any infant whose weight is below the 10th percentile for gestational age, whether premature, full-term, or postmature.'**
- Despite his small size, a full-term SGA infant **does not have the problems related to organ system immaturity** that the premature infant has
- Causes: An infant may be small at birth because of **Genetic factors** (short parents or a genetic disorder associated with short stature) or from other factors that can retard intrauterine growth. These intrauterine (nongenetic) factors usually are not operative before 32 to 34 weeks' gestation, and include **placental insufficiency** that often results from maternal disease involving the small blood vessels (as in **preeclampsia, primary hypertension, renal disease, or long-standing diabetes**); placental involution accompanying postmaturity; or infectious agents such as **cytomegalovirus, rubella virus, or Toxoplasma gondii**
- An infant may be SGA if the mother is a **narcotic or cocaine addict or a heavy user of alcohol and, to a lesser degree, if she smokes** cigarettes during pregnancy.

Full-Term Small for Date Babies are at a Risk For

- IUFD (Intrauterine fetal death)
- Perinatal asphyxia

Hypoglycemia:
The SGA infant is very prone to hypoglycemia in the first hours and days of life because of lack of adequate glycogen stores

- Polycythemia-Hyperviscosity
- Hypothermia
- Dysmorphology
- Pulmonary hemorrhage

COMPLICATIONS OF LBW (LOW BIRTH WEIGHT)

Immediate

- Hypoxia/ischemia
- IVH

• Sensorineural injury
• Respiratory failure
• Necrotizing enterocolitis
• Cholestatic liver disease

Late

Neurological: • Mental retardation • Seizures • Microcephaly • Poor school performance • Hearing impairment, visual impairment, myopia
Respiratory: • Bronchopulmonary dysplasia • Cor pulmonale, recurrent pneumonia
GIT: • Short bowel syndrome • Malabsorption • Infectious diarrhea
Liver: Cirrhosis, liver failure, carcinoma
Nutrient deficiency: Osteopenia, anemia, growth failure
Others: • SIDS • Inguinal hernia • GERD • Hypertension • Craniosynostosis • Nephrocalcinosis

Differentiate Between

Cephalohematoma	Caput succedaneum
• **Not present** at time of birth • **Subperiosteal** swelling • **Does not cross** suture lines • **Disappears late** (2 weeks–3 months)	• Present over presenting part • Soft, boggy swelling • Can cross suture line • Disappears early

Causes of Macrocephaly are:

• Caput succedaneum • Cephalohematoma • Subgaleal hematoma • Hydranencephaly • Subdural collections • Sotos syndrome • Canavan's disease • Alexander disease

Causes of Microcephaly are:

There are about more than 200 causes of 'microcephaly'. However, the most important ones are:

- Down's syndrome
- Congenital Rubella syndrome
- Edward's syndrome
- Patau's syndrome
- Beckwith-Wiedemann syndrome
- Cornelia de Lange syndrome
- Velocardiofacial syndrome
- Cockayne syndrome
- Charge syndrome

Teratogens

• Carbamazepine	• Cleft lip, cleft palate
• Valproic acid	• Neural tube defects
• Warfarin	• Chondrodysplasia punctata
• Carbimazole	• Fetal cutis aplasia
• Lithium	• Ebstein's anomaly
• Thalidomide	• Phocomelia
• Chloramphenicol	• Gray baby syndrome
• DES	• Clear-cell cancer

Fetal Alcohol Syndrome

Remember the features:

- Microcephaly
- Retarded growth
- Maxillary hyperplasia (imp)
- Small eyes

- Mental retardation
- Cardiac malformation
- Hyperkinetic movements

Milestones in Children (Try to Memorize as Much as Possible)

Social smile	2 months
Recognizes mother	3 months
Holds object and takes it to mouth	4 months
Sitting on slight support	5 months
Enjoys mirror	6 months
Sits alone momentarily	5–6 months
Transfers object from head to hand	6 months
Rolls over	7 months
Sits steadily	7–8 months
Crawls in bed	8 months

Monosyllabic words (Mama, Dada)	9 months
Creeps	10 months
Cruises around furniture	10 months
Builds a tower of 2 cubes and pincer grasp	12 months
Can turn two or three pages of a book	13 months
Walks alone	13–14 months
Walks sideways and backwards	15 months
Builds a tower of three cubes	18 months
Feeds self	18 months
Can drop and draw a horizontal or vertical line	2 years
Can turn one page at a time	2 years
Able to wear socks or shoes	2 years
Can remove his pants	2½ years
Can draw a circle	3 years
Can dress or undress completely and buckle his shoes	3 years
Knows age and sex	3 years
Can copy and draw a cross (Plus Sign)	4 years
Can draw a rectangle	4 years
Can draw a tilted cross (Multiplication sign)	5 years
Can draw a triangle	5 years
Bladder control—Diurnal	12–16 months
Nocturnal	2½ to 3 years

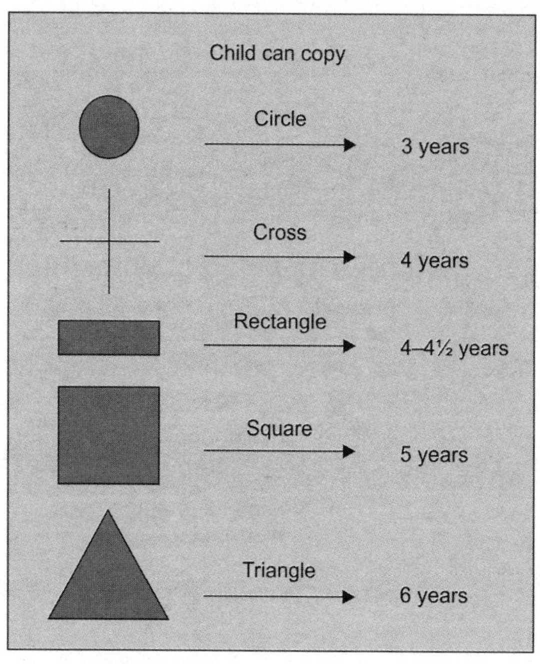

Drawing pattern at different ages

• Draws a **horizontal or vertical line**	• 2 years
• Draws a **circle**	• 3 years
• Draws a **cross**	• 4 years
• Draws a **rectangle**	• 4 years
• Draws a **triangle**	• 5 years

Most Importantly Remember

- **A 2-month-old infant** can lift its head to 45 degrees, eyes follow to the midline, vocalize, smiles and has a state of half-waking consciousness
- **A 6-month-old infant** can roll over, grasp a rattle, turn to voice, feed self and separate the world into a 'parent' and 'not parent' world
- **A 12-month-old child** can sit without support, pull to stand, use a pincer grasp, babble, indicate wants, and have stranger anxiety
- **An 18-month-child** can walk well, make a tower of 2 blocks, say 3 words, use a spoon and a cup, have temper tantrums, and bridge gaps by bringing objects to the caregiver.

Remember the Following Nonpathological Entities

- Erythema toxicum
- Epstein pearls
- Stork bites
- Vaginal bleeding (Maternal hormones)
- Mongolian spots
- Phimosis
- Breast engorgement

Important Clinical Conditions

- **Single umbilical artery:** Very common in infants of **diabetic mothers and trisomies 18 and twins**
- **Hernia:** Has peritoneal layer and skin
- **Omphalocele:** Peritoneal layer but no skin
- **Gastroschisis: Neither peritoneal layer nor skin**

Premature Neonate

Features are:

- Sutures widely separated
- Skin appears shiny
- Abundant lanugo
- Subcutaneous fat is reduced
- Sluggish neonatal reflexes
- Small face

Hemorrhagic Disease of the Newborn

- As a result of vitamin K deficiency. The normal newborn has a moderate deficiency of the vitamin K-dependent coagulation factors
- Prematurity has been associated with hemorrhagic disease of the newborn. Delayed feeding, breastfeeding, vomiting, severe diarrhea, and antibiotics also delay the colonization of the gut by bacteria
- Bleeding is usually severe and occurs most commonly on the 2nd or 3rd day of life. The most common manifestations are melena, large cephalohematomas and bleeding from the umbilical stump and after circumcision
- Generalized ecchymoses, often without petechiae, intracranial bleeding, and large intramuscular hemorrhages, also may develop in severe cases
- In infants with hemorrhagic disease of the newborn, the prothrombin time (PT) is always prolonged. The partial thromboplastin time (PTT) and the thrombin time are also prolonged. Specific factor assays reveal deficiencies of prothrombin; factors VII, IX, and X; and proteins C and S. The bleeding time and the platelet count usually are within normal limits.

Breast Milk

Has got many protective factors against bacteria, viruses, parasites

- **Lactoferrin** is particularly important against *Plasmodium falciparum, E. coli, Giardia*
- **Bile salt-stimulated lipase** is important against ***E. histolytica***
- **Lactadherin** against **Rotavirus**
- **PABA** is also anti-infective for **malaria**
- **Can transmit tuberculosis**

Breastfed infant can be deficient in:

- Vitamin B1
- Vitamin B12
- Vitamin D
- Vitamin K
- Folic acid

- Cow's milk has **more proteins** than breast milk
- Cow's milk has **more calcium** than breast milk
- Cow's milk has **more Vitamin K** than breast milk

- **Oxytocin** is necessary for **ejection/let down**
- **Prolactin** is necessary for **milk synthesis**

Contraindications to Breastfeeding

- **Galactosemia** is an absolute contraindication to breastfeeding
- Chronic medical illness such as **decompensated heart failure**
- **Open tuberculosis** of mother is also a contraindication to breastfeeding in developing countries
- Severe **anemia**
- Chronic nephritis
- Puerperal psychosis
- Patient on **antiepileptic, antithyroid drugs**

Growth and Development

- Thelarche → Pubarche → Menarche
- **Thelarche** is the **first change** occurring at puberty
- It is noticed as appearance of **firm, tender lump under center of nipple**
- It is referred to as **breast budding**
- It is due to rising **estrogen** levels

- **Pubarche** refers to appearance of **pubic hair**
- It results from rising **androgen** levels

- **Menarche** refers to appearance of first menstrual cycle
- **Adrenarche** refers to stage of maturation of adrenal cortex

MALNUTRITION

Marasmus

- It is a state in which virtually all available body fat stores have been exhausted due to starvation. The diagnosis is based on:
  - Severe fat and muscle wastage resulting from prolonged calorie deficiency. Diminished skin-fold thickness reflects the loss of fat reserves
  - Reduced arm muscle circumference with temporal and interosseous muscle wasting reflects the catabolism of protein throughout the body, including vital organs such as the heart, liver, and kidneys
  - The laboratory findings in marasmus are relatively unremarkable
  - The creatinine-height index (the 24-hour urinary creatinine excretion compared with normal values based on height) is low, reflecting the loss of muscle mass, immunocompetence, wound healing, and the ability to handle short-term stress are reasonably well-preserved in most patients with marasmus.

Kwashiorkor

- In contrast to marasmus, kwashiorkor in developed countries occurs mainly in connection with acute, life-threatening illnesses such as trauma and sepsis, and chronic illnesses that involve acute-phase inflammatory responses. In its early stages, the physical findings of kwashiorkor are few and subtle
- Fat reserves and muscle mass are initially unaffected, giving the deceptive appearance of adequate nutrition
- Signs that support the diagnosis of kwashiorkor include easy hair pluck ability, edema, skin breakdown, and poor wound healing
- The major sine qua non is severe reduction of levels of serum proteins such as albumin (< 2.8 g/dl) and transferrin (< 150 mg/dl) or iron-binding capacity (< 200 g/dl).

- Cellular immune function is depressed, reflected by lymphopenia (< 1500 lymphocytes/l in adults and older children) and lack of response to skin test antigens (anergy)
- Unlike treatment in marasmus, aggressive nutritional support is indicated to restore better metabolic balance rapidly.

Marasmic Kwashiorkor

- Marasmic kwashiorkor, the combined form of PEM, develops when the cachectic or marasmic patient experiences acute stress such as surgery, trauma, or sepsis, superimposing kwashiorkor onto chronic starvation
- An extremely serious, life-threatening situation can occur because of the high risk of infection and other complications. It is important to determine the major component of PEM so that the appropriate nutritional plan can be developed
- If kwashiorkor predominates, the need for vigorous nutritional therapy is urgent; if marasmus predominates, feeding should be more cautious.

Features	Marasmus	Kwashiorkor
• Edema	Absent	**Present**
• Wasting	Marked	Less
• Growth retardation	Severe	Less
• Mental changes	Usually absent	Usually **present**
• Hepatomegaly	Absent	**Present**

Remember

- **Gomez syndrome:** It is a **nutritional recovery syndrome** due to sudden rise of estrogen leading to hepatomegaly, jaundice and spider naevi.
- **Keshans disease:** It is cardiomyopathy due to selenium deficiency
- **Kashin-Beck disease:** It is osteoarthritis due to selenium deficiency

PEM

- Hypothermia
- Hypoglycemia
- Hypomagnesemia
- ↑Total body water
- ↑Cortisol and↑GH

Acute malnutrition is judged by: Weight for height

Chronic malnutrition is judged by: Height for age. Features are:

- Hypokalemia
- Hypoglycemia
- Hypothermia are acute complications of PEM
- **Tick sign:** It is seen in Kwashiorkor: Edema disappears on starting treatment
- **Flag sign:** It is seen in Kwashiorkor: Hair is thin, dry, brittle, lusterless, sparse, easily pluckable and hypopigmented

Causes of Delayed Puberty

Delayed puberty with short stature

- Turner's syndrome
- Prader-Willi syndrome
- Noonan's syndrome

Delayed puberty with normal stature

- Polycystic ovarian syndrome
- Androgen insensitivity
- Kallmann's syndrome
- Klinefelter's syndrome

Other causes:

- Chronic diseases
- Hypothyroidism
- Hypopituitarism
- Anorexia nervosa

Rickets

The clinical manifestations of rickets are the result of skeletal deformities:

- **Susceptibility to fractures**, weakness and hypotonia, and disturbances in growth
- **Features:**
  - Parietal flattening
  - **Frontal bossing** develops in the skull
  - **Craniotabes:** The calvariae are softened
  - **Sutures** may be widened
  - **Rachitic rosary:** Prominence of the costochondral junctions is called the **rachitic rosary**
  - **Harrison's groove:** Indentation of the lower ribs at the site of attachment of the diaphragm
  - Knock Nee + Coxa Vara
  - Bow legs
  - Pot belly
  - Forward projection of sternum **(pectus carinatum)**
  - Caput quadratum
  - Lumbar lordosis
  - Short stature, genu valgum, coxa vara, kyphoscoliosis
  - Triradiate pelvis
- Rickets is characterized by **defective mineralization** of bones
- Rickets is seen **before** closure of growth plates

Causes

- Nutritional rickets: Vitamin D deficiency, malabsorption
- Accelerated loss of Vitamin D: Phenytoin, rifampicin, barbiturates
- Impaired hydroxylation in liver and kidney
- Liver disease, hypoparathyroidism, renal failure, renal tubular acidosis
- Vitamin D-resistant rickets Fanconi's syndrome, Wilson's disease

Biochemical

Serum calcium: Normal or low
Serum phosphate: Low
Alkaline phosphatase: High
PTH : High

Scurvy

- Vitamin C deficiency causes **scurvy**
- Symptoms of **scurvy** primarily reflect impaired formation of mature connective tissue and include bleeding into skin **(petechiae, ecchymoses, perifollicular hemorrhages); inflamed and bleeding gums; and manifestations of bleeding into joints,** the peritoneal cavity, pericardium and the adrenal glands
- Wimberger's sign seen
- Rosary seen
- **Pseudoparalysis seen**

Vitamin C, or ascorbic acid, is a necessary cofactor for platelet function. A deficiency, most commonly due to a dietary cause, results in petechiae, microhemorrhages, gingival bleeding, and perifollicular hemorrhages. Classically, this disease was called 'scurvy,' and British sailors who did not have access to fresh fruits and vegetables suffered from this condition. Today, scurvy is rare and is seen mostly in elderly patients with poor dietary habits (such as those who may live alone). Treatment requires the daily administration of vitamin C for 3 to 4 weeks and is quite successful.

Rashes in Infancy and Childhood

Vesicular Rashes

- **Varicella**

Lesions normally appear without a prodromal illness and progress rapidly (within a few hours) from **papules to vesicles surrounded by an erythematous base. Crops of vesicles** appear over 3 days, predominantly on the trunk and proximal limbs. Vesicles may also develop on **mucous membranes.**

- **Herpes zoster**

Lesions similar to those seen in varicella infection may develop over **specific dermatomes or cranial nerves**. Although the immunosuppressed are at increased risk from zoster, this condition is also seen in normal children.

- **Herpes simplex virus**

Although infection is most commonly associated with **gingivostomatitis** during childhood, vesicles are seen on the skin in **eczema herpeticum (Kaposi's varicelliform eruption)**. Pyrexia is followed by the appearance of crops of vesicles on the eczematous skin. Crops of lesions may occur over several days. Correct and rapid diagnosis is essential because untreated severe infection may be fatal.

- **Hand, foot and mouth disease**

This is caused by **enteroviruses**, the commonest being **Coxsackievirus type 16**, and occurs in epidemics. It is associated with a papular-vesicular eruption of the mouth, hands, feet and, sometimes, buttocks.

- **Impetigo**

This condition usually presents as a red macule and then becomes vesicular. The small vesicles burst to leave a honey-colored crust. **Both streptococcal and staphylococcal impetigo** occur commonly around the mouth but can occur elsewhere.

- **Molluscum contagiosum**

This is caused by a **poxvirus**. Flesh-colored papules with a **central dimple** are seen. Although firm initially, they become softer and more waxy with time. Lesions are 2–5 mm in size and may occur anywhere. It is more severe in **HIV** infection.

- **Dermatitis herpetiformis**

This occurs in children from 8 years upwards who develop recurrent crops of pruritic papulovesicles over **extensor surfaces** including the elbows, buttocks and knees. Many of these children also have a **gluten-sensitive enteropathy**.

Maculopapular Rashes

Measles

Measles rash is **blotchy, red or pink in color**, raised in places, and starts **behind the ears and on the face, spreading downwards**. The lesions tend to become confluent on the upper part of the body and remain more discrete lower down. The rash fades, usually after 2–3 days. The skin becomes brown and although desquamation occurs, this is not usually seen on the hands and feet as it is in the case of scarlet fever.

Rubella

Rubella results in a **pink rash which progresses caudally**. The lesions are normally discrete and the rash **develops more quickly** and disappears earlier than in measles. Desquamation is not a characteristic.

Scarlet fever

The eruption is **dark red and punctiform**

The rash tends to be most prominent on the neck and in the major skinfolds

A distinctive feature is **circumoral pallor** as a result of the rash sparing the area around the mouth. As with measles, desquamation is seen but the hands and feet are involved

True scarlet fever is associated with inflammation of the tongue (white and red strawberry tongue)

Scarlatina refers to the rash which may occur alone in milder streptococcal infection, and is often shortlived.

Kawasaki disease
Although several features are required for the diagnosis of this condition, which is of unknown etiology, the rash may be confused with that of scarlet fever. **Discrete red maculopapules are seen on the feet, around the knees and in the axillary and inguinal skin creases. Desquamation** of the hands and feet is a common feature.
Erythema infectiosum or fifth disease
Infection caused by **parvovirus B19** is associated with a rash which develops in two stages
The cheeks appear red and flushed, giving rise to a **'slapped cheek' appearance**. A maculopapular rash develops 1–2 weeks later, predominantly over the arms and legs which, as it fades, **appears lace-like**
Causes nonimmune hydrops is caused by parvo virus.
Roseola infantum
The main cause is **human herpesvirus 6 (HHV-6)**
Roseola infantum is characterized by a widespread **morbilliform (measles-like) rash**, seen in its most florid form on the trunk. The lesions tend to be discrete. As the rash appears, the fever, which is normally present over the previous 4 days, resolves and the child looks well (in contrast to measles, in which the child is febrile and unwell when the rash appears).
Viral infections
Many viral infections, particularly those associated with the enteroviruses, may cause maculopapular rashes.

Kawasaki Disease

A 2-year-old boy was admitted to a pediatric hospital with a 7-day history of high fever, lymphadenopathy, conjunctivitis and an erythematous exfoliative rash affecting his trunk and extremities.

Petechial and Purpuric Rashes

- **Meningococcal Infection**

The first sign of meningococcal septicemia may be a **petechial or purpuric rash** anywhere on the body and often localized. On occasions, these lesions may be preceded by or accompany a maculopapular rash which may blanch

The petechiae will not blanch, and although it is conventional to make a microbiological diagnosis on blood culture, PCR bacteria can also be isolated from these lesions.

- Meningococcal petechiae can be confused with those seen on the face around the eyes following events that result in a transient rise in venous pressure such as vomiting. Rarely petechial rashes are associated with septicemia caused by other bacteria particularly *Hemophilus influenzae*.

- **Henoch-Schönlein purpura**

This condition often follows an **upper respiratory tract** infection but no single infective agent has been implicated. Hemorrhagic macules and papules develop on the **buttocks and extensor surfaces of the limbs,** particularly the knees and ankles. The lesions come in crops and fade over a few days, leaving a brown pigmentation.

- **Idiopathic thrombocytopenic purpura (ITP)**

A purpuric rash sometimes associated with frank bleeding is seen in this condition.

- **Leukemia**

Children with leukemia may present with a hemorrhagic rash as a result of thrombocytopenia but, in addition, the pallor of severe anemia will usually be obvious.

Types of Rash

• Anaphylactoid purpura	• **Vasculitis**
• Dermatomyositis	• **Violaceous**
• Salmonella	• **Evanescent**
• Erythema infectiosum	• **Slapped face appearance**
• Infectious mononucleosis	• **Drug (ampicillin) induced rash**

Henoch-Schönlein Purpura

A 7-year-old boy from Kansas is brought to the emergency department. His parents assert that over the past 3 days, he has become progressively ill with generalized fatigue and mid-abdominal pain that have become steadily worse. On examination, he has a maculopapular rash on his thighs and feet with some spread of the rash to his buttocks. The rash does not blanch and some lesions near the ankles look petechial. His temperature is 103.4 °F. He has dark stool, which is positive for occult blood. The boy has not voided since early morning and is unable to provide a urine sample. The physician determines that the boy is dehydrated.

- Also referred to as **anaphylactoid purpura**, is a distinct **systemic vasculitis syndrome** that is characterized by:
  - **Palpable purpura** (most commonly distributed over the buttocks and lower extremities)
  - Arthralgias
  - Abdominal pain
  - Glomerulonephritis
- It is a **small vessel vasculitis**
- Henoch-Schönlein purpura is **usually seen in children**; most patients range in age from 4 to 7 years
- A seasonal variation with a **peak incidence in spring** has been noted
- **Ig A** is the antibody class most often seen in the immune complexes and has been demonstrated in the renal biopsies of these patients
- Gastrointestinal involvement, which is seen in almost 70% of pediatric patients, is characterized by **colicky abdominal pain** usually associated with **nausea, vomiting, diarrhea, or constipation** and is frequently accompanied by the passage of blood and mucus per rectum; **bowel intussusception** may occur rarely
- It usually **resolves spontaneously** without therapy. Rarely, a progressive glomerulonephritis will develop
- **Renal failure is the most common cause of death** in the rare patient who dies of Henoch-Schönlein purpura
- Routine laboratory studies generally show a **mild leukocytosis, a normal platelet count, and occasionally eosinophilia. Serum complement components are normal, and IgA levels are elevated** in about one-half of patients
- **Treatment:** The prognosis of Henoch-Schönlein purpura is **excellent**. **Most patients recover completely, and some do not require therapy.**

Kawasaki Disease

- Kawasaki disease (also known as **'lymph node syndrome', 'mucocutaneous node disease', 'infantile polyarteritis')**
- Kawasaki disease is an inflammation (vasculitis) of the **<u>middle-sized arteries</u>**
- Kawasaki disease affects many organs, including the skin, mucous membranes, lymph nodes, and blood vessel walls, but the 'most serious' effect is on the heart where it can cause **'severe aneurysmal dilations'.**

Classically, five days of fever plus four of five 'diagnostic criteria' must be met in order to establish the diagnosis

- The criteria are:

• Erythema of the lips or oral cavity or cracking of the lips
• Rash
• Swelling or erythema of the hands or feet
• Red eyes (conjunctival injection)
• Swollen lymph node in the neck of at least 15 millimeters

Treatment:

Intravenous immunoglobulin + aspirin. Long-term therapy: aspirin. Only condition in children in which aspirin is given. (Causes Reye's syndrome.)

Rashes

- Mnemonic "V'ery 'S'ick 'P'atient 'M'ust 'T'ake Double Tea.
- Day 1 of fever: 'v'aricella zoster
- Day 2 of fever: 's'carlet fever
- Day 3 of fever: small'p'ox
- Day 4 of fever: 'm'easles
- Day 5 of fever: 't'yphus
- Day 6th- dengue fever
- Day 7th- typhoid

• First disease	• Rubeola or measles, (koplik's spots)
• Second disease	• Scarlet fever (circumoral pallor, pastia's lines, strawberry tongue)
• Third disease	• Rubella (Forchheimer's spots, posterior cervical lymphadenopathy)
• Fourth disease	• SSSS (Nikolsky's sign)
• Fifth disease	• Erythema infectiosum (parvovirus B19, slapped cheek appearance)
• Sixth disease	• Exanthem subitum, roseola infantum, HHV 6

SSSS (Staphylococcal Scalded Skin Syndrome)

A 3-month-old male infant developed otitis media for which he was given a course of Co-trimoxazole. A few days later, he developed extensive peeling of the skin; there were no mucosal lesions and the baby was not toxic

The most likely diagnosis is:

SSSS

Simple Important Eponyms (WITHOUT CLUES)

- 1st day disease: Measles
- 2nd day disease: Scarlet fever
- 3rd day disease: Rubella
- 5th day disease: Erythema infectiosum
- 6th day disease: Roseola infantum
- 8th day disease: Tetanus

Kawasaki Disease

- It is a systemic vasculitis of unknown origin that remains a leading cause of acquired heart disease in infants and children
- It is a multisystemic disease, also known as mucocutaneous lymph node syndrome. An (unidentified) infectious origin and a T-cell immune activation play a prominent role in disease pathogenesis
- Tumor necrosis factor alpha (TNF-alpha) receptor levels correlate with the degree of vascular damage and likelihood of coronary artery aneurysm formation
- The cardiovascular complications account for most of the morbidity and mortality
- **Fever, bilateral nonexudative conjunctivitis, mucous membrane changes (injected pharynx, cracked lips, or strawberry tongue), extremity changes (edema, desquamation, erythema, or rash), and cervical adenopathy are common at presentation.**

- The acute manifestations include **myocarditis, valvular insufficiency, arrhythmias, pericardial effusion, and congestive heart failure** with coronary abnormalities; these develop in 15% to 25% of patients
- **Leukocytosis and an elevated C-reactive protein are associated with the development of coronary artery aneurysms**
- Treatment includes aspirin at 80-100 mg/kg/day in divided doses and IV immune globulin in high doses
- **Corticosteroids should be avoided** because of the potential link with increasing the likelihood of coronary aneurysm development.

CHROMOSOMAL SYNDROMES

Down's Syndrome

- **Common** trisomy
- Head circumference **is small**
- **Brachycephalic skull**
- The neck is **short and thick**
- Hypotonicity is present
- The **palpebral fissures slope upwards** (i.e. the outer canthus is higher than the inner canthus) and there may be marked epicanthic folds (HYPOTELORISM)
- **Brushfield's spots** (whitish spots scattered round the periphery of the iris)
- ↑ **Nuchal fold thickness**
- There is an increased incidence of **lens opacities**. The ears are small with an overfolding helix. The nasal bridge is flat.
- The **tongu**e appears **large and may protrude** because the mouth is relatively small. Eruption of the teeth is frequently delayed with abnormalities in dental positioning. The hair may be fine and sparse
- Hypothyroidism and VSD can be present
- **Transient myeloproliferative disorder of newborn is seen**
- The hands are short and broad. The fifth finger is short and incurved **(clinodactyly)**. Radiologically this feature is accompanied by shortening of the shaft of the middle phalanx
- **Iliac index < 60**
- A single transverse **palmar** crease **(or simian crease)**
- A deep **plantar** crease **(sandal gap)** between the first and second toe may also be a helpful diagnostic sign

- **Atrioventricular canal** and **ventricular septal defects** are the commonest types of cardiac lesion seen. **Intestinal atresia**, in particular, duodenal atresia. Leukemia (**CML**) is also common
- **Transient myeloproliferative disorder is seen**
- Initially a child with Down may be **hypotonic**, but the early developmental milestones are eventually reached. Hypothyroidism is common
- The ultimate IQ ranges from 20 to 75 with a mean around 50. The earlier assessment of development tends to be more favorable than the formal measurement of IQ in later childhood
- It is associated with Alzheimer's dementia
- Intellectual function shows a decline with age and this has been attributed to a **presenile dementia**
- Triple test is done for Down's syndrome
- ↑nuchal fold thickness is a feature of Down's syndrome
- **Maternal nondisjunction is the mc cause**

A 48-year-old woman from Holland delivers a 3126 g newborn male. Her pregnancy was normal except that she noted decreased fetal movement compared to her previous pregnancies. She declined an amniocentesis offered by her obstetrician. Physical examination of the newborn reveals an infant with facial features suggestive of Down's Syndrome. The infant then has bilious vomiting. An X-ray film showing the kidneys, ureters, and bladder (KUB) is performed, which shows a distended and gas-filled stomach and proximal duodenum and the absence of gas in the distal bowel.

Other causes of mental retardation:

- Fragile X syndrome
- Homocystinemia
- Phenylketonuria
- Tuberous sclerosis

Trisomy 18 (Edward's Syndrome)

- There is often **polyhydramnios** and intrauterine growth retardation.
- The cranium is long and narrow with a prominent occiput. **The ears are low set** and frequently underdeveloped.
- The facies characteristically shows **micrognathia** and narrow-sloping palpebral fissures.
- The **hands are clenched** with the **second and fifth fingers overlapping the third and fourth fingers**. There may be other flexion deformities. The nails are hypoplastic.
- The feet show a **'rocker bottom'** appearance like the shape of the runners of a rocking chair.
- A variety of congenital malformations are present. Anomalies of the gastrointestinal tract are particularly common, e.g. **intestinal atresias, malabsorption** and **exomphalos.**
- **Renal abnormalities** are also frequent with **renal hypoplasia or cystic dysplasia** being one of the commoner and more serious abnormalities. Congenital heart defects, ocular abnormalities and neural tube defects can also occur
- **Most specific marker for neural tube defects is acetylcholine esterase.**

Trisomy 13 (Patau's Syndrome)

- The affected children show **intrauterine growth retardation**.
- There may be marked **microcephaly**
- Structural malformations of the brain are common and this may alter facial development. Instead of two cerebral hemispheres with lateral ventricles, a single forebrain with a single ventricle may form. This malformation sequence is known as **holoprosencephaly**
- The process alters the development and separation of optic vesicles from the forebrain and the migration of the median process from the forehead to form the nose. In its most extreme form, the optic vesicles may fuse to give **cyclopia**
- Marked **hypotelorism** with a small nose and cleft lip and palate. Ocular abnormalities such as **microphthalmos** are common, often reflecting the underlying cerebral abnormality.
- In the hands, postaxial **polydactyly** is frequent.
- **Flexion contractures and 'rocker bottom' feet may also be present**. Scalp defects may be helpful diagnostically as they rarely appear in other abnormalities. Internally, in addition to cerebral malformations, renal and cardiac abnormalities are also frequent.

4p–(WOLF-HIRSCHHORN) Syndrome

- The features include
  - **Microcephaly**
  - **Hypertelorism**
  - **Low set simple ears**
  - **Coloboma cleft palate, renal abnormalities, heart defects and intrauterine growth retardation**
- The facial features are described as resembling a **Greek helmet** since the flat nasal bridge appears to run in continuity from the glabella in much the same way that the protective nose piece is incorporated into a Greek helmet.

5p–(CRI DU CHAT) Syndrome

- It derives its name from the striking **cat-like cry** that is heard in infancy
- This cry is related to the **hypoplastic larynx** and tends to lessen with increasing age and growth of the larynx
- In the newborn, the face is round with **microcephaly, micrognathia and down-slanting palpebral fissures**. With further growth, the microcephaly remains but the face becomes long and narrow
- Survival into adult life with severe mental retardation has frequently been described.

18q–syndrome

- The cardinal features are **intrauterine growth retardation, profound mental retardation and a 'carp-shaped mouth'**
- Cleft palate, heart defects and ocular defects are also common. Genital hypoplasia may occur
- **Serum immunoglobulin A (IgA)** is decreased in about half the affected individuals.

Deletions of 13q

- Deletions of 13q14 are **associated with retinoblastoma**
- They also characteristically have **hypoplastic thumbs and anal atresia**

Digeorge Syndrome 22q11 Deletion

- Different names, e.g. **velocardiofacial syndrome** or **CATCH 22 syndrome**
- About 75% of patients with 22q11 deletion will have **significant congenital heart defects.** The range of defects is wide but **tetralogy of Fallot** and abnormalities in the main arteries are most frequently seen. About 50% of patients will have defects of the palate. This is often **velopharyngeal insufficiency** rather than overt cleft palate
- **Hypocalcemia** may also occur and is a cause for fits. Other feature is **severe immunodeficiency** with T cell depletion.

A 5-year-old boy suffers from a condition characterized by recurrent fungal and viral infections, thymic hypoplasia, tetany, and abnormal facies. Serum levels of immunoglobulins are mildly depressed, and lymph node biopsy shows lymphocyte depletion of T-dependent areas.

- The constellation of **thymic hypoplasia, hypocalcemia with (Tetany) abnormal facies and congenital cardiac anomalies** defines the condition known as DiGeorge syndrome
- This results from a **developmental failure of third and fourth pharyngeal pouches,** which gives rise to congenital absence or anomalies of the parathyroid, thymus, lower face, and cardiac structures
- Immune deficiency results from **failure of T-lymphocytes to mature in the thymus**. Thus, fungal and viral organisms, which are normally controlled by T-mediated mechanisms, become frequent causes of **opportunistic infections**
- The underlying gene defect is **related to 22q11 deletion**, which results in two partially overlapping conditions.

USMLE Case Scenario

Condition resulting from incomplete separation of the cerebral hemisphere along the midline, leading, in its extreme form, to a single midline ventricular cavity enclosed within the forebrain. Associated facial anomaly, often associated with trisomy 13, is:

1. Dandy-Walker malformation
2. Holoprosencephaly
3. Arnold-Chiari malformation
4. Myelomeningocele

Ans. 2. Holoprosencephaly

Williams Syndrome

It was initially referred to as **infantile hypercalcemia** as the biochemical change was the usual presentation, **'elfin facies'**

- Short stature
- Supravalvular aortic stenosis
- Hyperacusis
- Developmental delay

Angelman Syndrome and Prader-Willi Syndrome

Although these are very different clinical disorders, it is important to consider these together as they can both be due to **deletions of chromosome 15** and illustrate an important biological principle known as **genetic imprinting.**

Prader-Willi syndrome usually presents with **neonatal hypotonia with feeding difficulties and in males, undescended testes**

Angelman syndrome presents with severe developmental delay, inappropriate laughter and complex seizures

- Prader-Willi syndrome is due to **paternal deletions**
- Angelman syndrome is due to **maternal deletions**

This phenomenon would not be predicted by Mendelian inheritance where the paternal origin of a mutation does not usually matter and is an example of genetic imprinting. It appears that both paternal and maternal chromosome 15s are required in early embryonic development and that paternal and maternal chromosome 15q12 have different functions. Thus, genetic imprinting may be defined as the determination of gene expression depending on the parental origin.

SEX CHROMOSOME ABNORMALITIES

Turner's Syndrome

- At birth, there is **lymphedema** especially in the dorsum of the hand and there may be redundant skin over the back of the neck. (**Sequestration of jugular lymph sacs**)
- **Hydrops and cystic hygroma** are seen in utero and may occasionally be present in the neonate
- There is a **short stature**
- Webbed neck with low posterior hairline
- The chest is shield-shaped with **widely spaced nipples**
- The carrying angle at the elbow is increased **(Cubitus valgus)**
- Finger deformities
- **Coarctation of the aorta** may also be present
- Renal tract abnormalities, which include **horseshoe kidneys and duplex ureters**
- **At puberty,** it may present for the first time with **primary amenorrhea** and failure of secondary sexual development. **Streak gonads** are found with ultrasound and at laparotomy. The patients are almost invariably sterile, but menstruation and secondary sexual development may be induced by estrogen replacement
- **Short fourth metacarpal**
- Have a **normal life span**
- Patients with Turner's syndrome have a **45XO karyotype**

47XXX

- The majority of girls with triple X (47XXX) will not have been brought to medical attention and have had their chromosomes tested. However, prospective studies have identified some potential differences
- Their **height tends to be greater** than average and in statistical terms, there is a **slight lowering of mean IQ** but no specific abnormal behavioral patterns
- **Fertility is normal**

Klinefelter's Syndrome (47xxy)

- Klinefelter's syndrome of:
  - **Gynecomastia**
  - **Small atrophic testes and**
  - **Absent spermatogenesis (azoospermia)** in phenotypic males
  - It is associated with an abnormal karyotype **(47XXY)**
  - **MC cause of hypergonadotrophic hypogonadism**

- At puberty, however, the **secondary sexual characteristics develop poorly** and body fat tends to take on a feminine distribution with gynecomastia in 50% of cases
- Beard growth is minimal and in adult life, patients will rarely need to shave more than twice a week
- The **testes remain small** and infertility may be the presenting feature in adult males. Sexual function is normal, although the libido is reduced
- **The testosterone levels are low and the gonadotrophin levels elevated** and testosterone replacement may be helpful
- Testicular histology shows an increase in Leydig cells and interstitial fibrosis. Height is usually increased with **relatively long limbs**
- **Subnormal intelligence**

It is best diagnosed with a 47, XXY karyotype, although variants with 46, XY exist. This condition is characterized by small testes, disproportionately long arms and legs (secondary to delayed epiphyseal plate closure in puberty), infertility, and gynecomastia. Mental retardation and learning disability are common. Many men are not diagnosed until adulthood when they seek medical attention for infertility. Our patient clearly has these traits. Patients with Klinefelter's syndrome often have an unexplained increase in follicle-stimulating hormone and luteinizing hormone. This increase occurs even in patients with normal testosterone levels. Low follicle-stimulating hormone, luteinizing hormone and testosterone are typical for a secondary form of hypogonadism. Secondary hypogonadism is not associated with gynecomastia because patients don't have an increase in conversion of testosterone to estradiol, which is stimulated by follicle-stimulating hormone and luteinizing hormone.

Fragile X Mental Retardation

- It is now recognized as the **second commonest cause of mental handicap** in males after Down's syndrome
- Fragile X males have a:
  - Large forehead
  - Large head
  - Prominent chin and
  - Long ears
- Fragile X males tend to be larger at birth
- **Macroorchidism is present:** The size of the testes may be considerably enlarged
- There is a slight increase in the frequency of **mitral valve prolapse, aortic root dilatation and hernias**. More striking clinically is the soft skin and joint hypermobility, which may be helpful diagnostically
- The range of intellectual handicap in fragile X males varies but most are **moderately to severely retarded**.

Torch Infections

The acronym **TORCH** has been used to summarize the infections **toxoplasma, rubella, CMV and herpes, to which should be added human immunodeficiency virus and varicella zoster.**

- Rubella

Rubella infection in the first 16 weeks of pregnancy can result in a severely damaged baby with:

- Cataracts
- Sensorineural deafness
- Congenital heart disease (PDA), ASD, VSD, PDA
- Microcephaly
- Hepatosplenomegaly
- Thrombocytopenia

The condition is preventable by achieving high immunization coverage.

• CMV Can present in a dramatic form with jaundice and petechiae, the 'blueberry muffin' baby. Most babies who are symptomatic at birth will be handicapped. Only small percentage of babies born with congenital CMV infection are symptomatic. However, most babies are being clinically unaffected by the infection.
• Varicella zoster Can result in severe damage with cicatricial skin scarring, cataracts and seizures.
• Herpes simplex virus Can result in severe illness in newborns. There is a high incidence of meningitis and encephalitis.
• Human immunodeficiency virus This retrovirus can cause meningitis and encephalopathy. Neurological manifestations include encephalopathy and microcephaly.
• ***Toxoplasma gondii*** – This protozoan can cause neurological sequelae when acquired in uterine life and the diagnosis is important because the condition is treatable – The organism is mainly acquired from cat litter or consumption of undercooked meat – The classic is of hydrocephalus, chorioretinitis and intracranial calcification is seen – MC Manifestation: Chorioretinitis

Syphilis

Early Congenital Syphilis Snuffles or rhinitis is the early feature

- **Vesico bullous** lesions (not found in any other variety of syphilis)
- **Snail track ulcers** on oral mucosa

Late Congenital Syphilis

- **Hutchinson's triad** (Hutchinson's teeth + 8th cranial nerve deafness+ Interstitial keratitis)
- **Moon's molars** and **maldevelopment of the maxilla** resulting in **'bulldog' facies** are typical
- **Saddle nose**
- **Saber tibia**
- **Mulberry molars**
- **Rhagades** The infant may fail to thrive and have a characteristic 'old man' look, with fissured lesions around the mouth (rhagades) and a mucopurulent or blood-stained nasal discharge causing snuffles
- **Frontal bossing of Parrot**
- **Peroistitis** (Higoumenakis sign)
- **IgM FTA ABS best diagnoses congenital syphilis**

• Cataract, deafness, IUGR, patent ductus arteriosus	• Rubella
• Chorioretinitis, intracerebral calcification, jaundice	• Toxoplasmosis
• Chorioretinitis, periventricular manifestations, microcephaly	• CMV
• Limb hypoplasia, cutaneous scar, microcephaly, cataract	• Varicella

Maternal Serum Screening

- Measurements of alpha-fetoprotein (AFP) and human chorionic gonadotrophin (hCG) in the second trimester constitute the **Double test**
- The addition of unconjugated estriol (μE3) makes the **Triple test**
- The addition of μE3 and inhibin A makes the **Quadruple test**

Jaundice in Pediatrics

Causes of **'Unconjugated'** hyperbilirubenimia are:
- Criggler najar Syndrome I, Criggler najar Syndrome II
- Hemolytic anemia
- Physiological jaundice
- Hypothyroidism
- Breast milk jaundice
- Excessive RBC destruction (Rh incompatibility, G6PD deficiency, spherocytosis, vitamin K, sulfamethoxazole)

Causes of **'Conjugated'** hyperbilirubenemia are:
- Parenchymal diseases (Rubella, Toxoplasmosis, CMV, Herpes infection)
- Neonatal hepatitis syndrome
- Biliary atresia (intrahepatic/extrahepatic)
- Watson-Alagille syndrome
- Choledochal cyst
- Dubin-Johnson syndrome, Rotor syndrome
- Commonest cause in newborn: **Idiopathic infantile hepatitis**

Remember

- Jaundice appearing on the first day in any newborn and a bilirubin concentration >10 mg/dl in premature infants or >15 mg/dl in full-term infants warrant investigation
- Physiological jaundice usually appears on 3rd day and disappears by 7th day
- When the blood level of bilirubin is about 4 to 5 mg/dl, jaundice becomes apparent
- In kernicterus, unconjugated bilirubin is increased
- In kernicterus, staining of brain is more in basal ganglia
- With increasing bilirubin levels, visible jaundice advances in a head-to-foot direction
- MC cause of jaundice in a newborn within 24 hours is erythroblastosis fetalis
- Breast milk jaundice is due to pregnanediole

Physiological Jaundice

- Jaundice not present on day 1
- Total bilirubin level rises < 5 mg/dl/day
- Total bilirubin does not exceed 13 mg/dl in term infants and 15 mg/dl in preterm infants
- Jaundice should not last more than one week in term infants or 2 weeks in preterm infants

Causes of Prolonged Neonatal Jaundice

- Hypothyroidism
- Galactosemia

- Alpha 1 antitrypsin deficiency
- Tyrosenemia
- GH deficiency

Gilbert's Syndrome

- Common, **benign, inherited condition**
- **Unconjugated** hyperbilirubinemia
- Common in males
- **↓UDP glucoronyl transferase activity**
- **Normal LFT**
- **Normal liver histology**
- Stress, fatigue, alcohol use, ↓ caloric intake, illness ↑ serum bilirubin

Idiopathic Neonatal Hepatitis

- Also known as **Giant Cell Hepatitis**
- It is **cholestatic jaundice** in nature
- Cause is **unknown**
- Among all cases of **intrahepatic cholestasis,** it accounts for about of the 50% cases (MC)
- Typical feature in **liver histology** is the appearance of **giant cells**
- Conditions with similar features clinically and histologically:
  - Alpha 1 antitrypsin deficiency
  - Alagille syndrome
  - Byler disease
  - Viral infections

Alagille Syndrome

- Alagille syndrome is an **autosomal dominant** (AD) disorder
- There is an **error in development of bile ducts, heart, CNS and face**
- **Neonatal intrahepatic cholestasis** and **hepatosplenomegaly** with **xanthomas** with **teratology of fallot and coarctation of aorta** are a feature
- **Supplementation of vitamins A, D, E, K and ursodeoxycholic acid** is initially used for treatment
- **Liver transplant** is selectively used
- A liver biopsy may indicate **too few bile ducts (bile duct paucity)**

Other signs of Alagille syndrome include:

- Congenital heart problems, particularly tetralogy of fallot
- Unusual **butterfly shape of the bones of the spinal column**
- Many people with Alagille syndrome have similar facial features, including a broad, prominent forehead, deep-set eyes, and a small pointed chin. The kidneys and central nervous system may also be affected.

A full-term infant is brought to the office on her 6th day of life because her mother noted that she looked 'yellow'. The mother states that the infant is strictly breast-fed and has been eating every 2-3 hours. On examination, she is noted to be jaundiced over her trunk and face. There is no scleral icterus. She is otherwise healthy. Both the mother and baby are Rh positive. Which of the following is the most likely cause of this infant's jaundice?

Breastfeeding jaundice

Infantile Hypertrophic Pyloric Stenosis

- Pyloric stenosis develops in approximately **3 per 1000 live births** with a male to female preponderance of 4:1
- Appears around **2 weeks after birth**
- **A thickening of the pyloric muscle** results in gastric outlet obstruction with resulting vomiting

- Symptoms of **projectile vomiting occurring 10–20 min after a feed** develops between the **second and fourth weeks of life**, although they can occasionally occur either sooner or at up to 4 months of age
- With progressive vomiting, the infants **lose weight and may eventually become dehydrated and alkalotic (hypokalemic metabolic alkalosis)**
- **Compensation is by: paradoxical aciduria with hyponatremia and hypochloremia**
- On clinical examination, **gastric peristaltic activity** may be seen, and palpation of the right upper quadrant of the abdomen during a test feed will reveal the pyloric tumor in most cases
- **The initial management** of the patient after the diagnosis has been confirmed is intravenous rehydration and correction of any acid-base disturbance
- The patient should then undergo a **Ramstedt's pyloromyotomy** where the pyloric muscle is split down to the mucosa.

Pyloric Stenosis

A four-week-old boy is brought to the pediatric emergency department by his father who states that he has been vomiting after being fed for the past several days. She describes the vomitus as nonbilious, and he has had normal stools with no blood in them. On examination, the infant appears to be mildly dehydrated, his abdomen is soft, and there is a palpable, olive-sized, firm movable mass in the right upper quadrant.

USMLE Case Scenario

A 2-week-old boy is brought to the emergency department by his parents. He has become dehydrated during his first few weeks of life and is vomiting frequently. The parents state that the infant vomits after each feeding but he is always hungry. The emesis is nonbilious in color. On examination, the infant is afebrile and the anterior fontanelle is sunken. Abdominal examination shows visible gastric peristaltic waves and a 2.2 cm firm, mobile mass above and to the right of the umbilicus in the midepigastrium beneath the liver edge.

Cystic Fibrosis

- Cystic fibrosis is an **autosomal recessive condition**
- The underlying defect results from one of a number of possible mutations, in a **chloride transporter protein** which lines ductular epithelium
- As a result, **abnormal sweat chloride test**
- **Lung is normal at birth**
- This results in **inspissation of mucus** in the ducts of the pancreas and in the bronchial and biliary trees with the resulting **development of pancreatic insufficiency, chronic respiratory disease and biliary cirrhosis**
- **Causes intractable diarrhea in children**
- **Pancreatic insufficiency:** The inspissated concretions result in distension of the ducts and acini of the pancreas which with time progress to the formation of small cysts with destruction and fibrosis of the exocrine tissue. As a consequence of this, the output of pancreatic enzymes and bicarbonate falls, leading to pancreatic insufficiency
- Patients with cystic fibrosis have pancreatic insufficiency with resulting malabsorption and steatorrhea

Meconium Ileus

- Fibrosis may present in the **first day or two of life with vomiting and abdominal distension due to meconium ileus** (mucoviscidosis)
- This **obstruction to the small intestine with thick tenacious meconium** may be complicated by volvulus, atresia or peritonitis
- Plain abdominal X-ray will show **dilated loops of intestine with meconium**, outlined by trapped air, present in the obstructed segment of bowel and
- Gastrografin enema will reveal a **microcolon distal to the obstruction.**

Shwachman's Syndrome

- This autosomal recessive condition is characterized by the presence of **neutropenia with impairment of neutrophil function**
- The diagnosis should be considered in **any child with pancreatic insufficiency, a normal sweat test and neutropenia.**

(Mucoviscidosis; Fibrocystic Disease of the Pancreas; Pancreatic Cystic Fibrosis)

- An inherited disease of the **exocrine glands**, primarily affecting the GI and respiratory systems, and usually characterized by the **triad of chronic obstructive pulmonary disease, exocrine pancreatic insufficiency, and abnormally high sweat electrolytes**
- CF is carried as an **autosomal recessive trait**
- The gene responsible for CF has been localized to 250,000 base pairs of genomic DNA on **chromosome 7q (the long arm)**
- It encodes a membrane-associated protein called the **cystic fibrosis transmembrane conductance regulator (CFTR)**
- Nearly all exocrine glands are affected in varying distribution and degree of severity

Involved Glands Fall into 3 Types

- Those that **become obstructed by viscid or solid eosinophilic material in the lumen (pancreas, intestinal glands, intrahepatic bile ducts, gallbladder, submaxillary glands)**
- Those that produce an excess of histologically normal secretions (tracheobronchial and Brunner's glands)
- Those that are normal histologically but **secrete excessive Na and Cl (sweat, parotid, and small salivary glands)**

- **Aspermia and infertility** are seen in 98% of adult men secondary to maldevelopment of the vas deferens. In women, fertility is decreased secondary to viscid cervical secretions, but many women with CF have carried pregnancies to term. However, maternal complications and fetal wastage show an increased incidence.
  - In infants without meconium ileus, onset is frequently heralded by a delay in regaining birthweight and inadequate weight gain at 4 to 6 weeks of age.
  - **Pancreatic insufficiency** is clinically apparent in 85 to 90% of patients. It is usually present early in life but may be progressive.
  - Manifestations include the passage of **frequent, bulky, foul-smelling, oily stools; abdominal protuberance; and poor growth pattern** with decreased subcutaneous tissue and muscle mass, despite a normal or voracious appetite.
  - **Rectal prolapse** occurs in 20% of untreated infants and toddlers.
  - In arid climates, infants may present with chronic metabolic alkalosis. Findings of salt crystal formation on the skin and a **salty taste on the skin** are highly suggestive of CF.
  - Fifty percent of all patients present with **pulmonary manifestations** usually consisting of chronic cough and wheezing associated with recurrent or chronic pulmonary infections.

Laboratory Findings

- Since meconium in most neonates with CF contains large amounts of serum proteins (especially albumin), **meconium examination** has been used as the basis of a newborn screening test. Pancreatic insufficiency is present in about 85% of patients with CF
- The serum concentration of **immunoreactive trypsin** is elevated in newborns with CF

Causes of Neonatal Obstruction

Congenital Atresias

- Duodenal (mc)
- Jejunal
- Ileal
- Colonic
  - Arrested rotation
  - Meconium ileus
  - Hirschsprung's disease
  - Volvulus neonatorum (Barium meal follow-through is DOC)

Intussusception

- Intussusception is one of the **acute abdominal emergencies** occurring in children. In children, three months to three years of age without prior abdominal surgery, intussusception is the **most common cause of an acquired intestinal obstruction**. It is believed that enlarged intramural lymphoid tissue (Peyer's patches) in the small bowel may act as a **lead point** for the development of an idiopathic intussusception with invagination of the distal small bowel into the cecum and colon. Other structural lesions such as a **Meckel's diverticulum, duplication cyst, polyp or lymphoma may be lead points** for an intussusception. However, these associated lead points are more frequently identified in children younger than three months of age, older than five years of age, or in children with multiple recurrent episodes of intussusception
- **A child with intussusception typically has intermittent episodes of abdominal pain, emesis and bloody or 'currant jelly' stools.** However, the clinical presentation may be varied, occasionally with diarrhea, a palpable abdominal mass or lethargy with delay in treatment. Plain films may be diagnostic if a soft-tissue mass in the cecum or transverse colon is identified or strongly suggestive of intussusception with a distal small bowel obstruction in a young child with no prior abdominal surgery. However, plain films are frequently unrevealing. Therefore, if intussusception is suspected, clinically further imaging evaluation is warranted
- Intussusception has a **characteristic appearance on ultrasound (US)**. On transverse imaging through an intussusception, a **'target'** or **'donut' sign** is seen with a peripheral rim of hypoechoic tissue and a hyperechoic center. On longitudinal imaging through the intussusception, the intussusceptum can be seen extending into the intussuscipiens.

- Outer tube
- Inner tube
- Most common
- Most infantile cases
- Intussuscipiens
- Intussceptum
- Iliocolic type
- Idiopathic

Secondary causes:
- Meckel's diverticulum
- Polyps/carcinomas
- Duplication cysts
- Lipoma
- Purpura
- Lymphoma

- Intermittent colicky pain with screaming, vomiting with red currant jelly stools
- Sausage-shaped periumbilical mass
- Commonest cause of intestinal obstruction in children: intussusception
- Empty right iliac fossa (signe de dance)
- Step ladder peristalsis
- Initially hydrostatic reduction is done
- Laparotomy with reduction is done in complicated cases and those failing initially

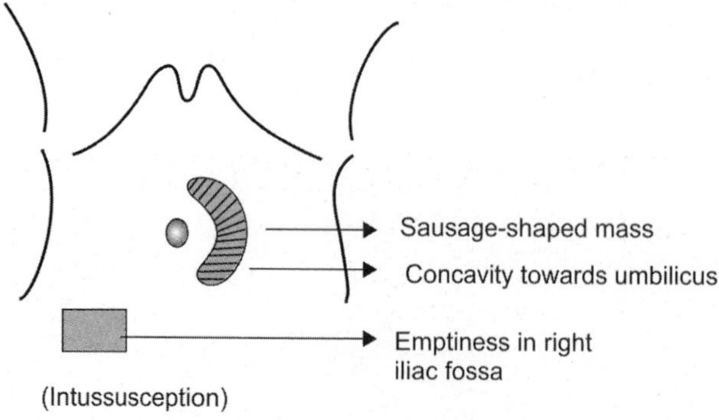

Features of intussusception

- **X-ray features show:**
  - Target sign
  - Meniscus sign
- **Barium enema shows:**
  - Claw sign
  - Coiled spring sign
- **USG signs are:**
  - Target sign
  - Bull's eye sign
  - Pseudokidney sign
  - Hayfork and sandwich appearance

Hirschsprung's Disease

- There is **absence of ganglion cells** in the **myenteric plexuses** (both Auerbach's and Meissner's) of the most distal bowel and extending proximally for a variable distance
- Aganglionosis involving only the rectum or rectosigmoid is often termed **'short segment' Hirschsprung's disease** and **affects males five times more commonly than females**
- **'Long segment' Hirschsprung's disease, extending above the sigmoid**
- Associated congenital anomalies are:
  - **Down's syndrome**
  - **Waardenburg's syndrome**
  - **Cartilage-hair hypoplasia syndrome**
- Usually the symptoms of Hirschsprung's disease are manifest within the first few days of life
- **Failure to pass meconium within the first 24 h,** abdominal distention, bile-stained vomiting and reluctance to feed are the main symptoms
- **Diarrhea may be the presenting feature of Hirschsprung's enterocolitis**, a devastating complication of the condition which has a high mortality
- A plain abdominal X-ray shows distended small and large bowel, sometimes with multiple fluid levels on an erect film. **Distal segment is constricted, proximal segment is dilated**
- A barium enema is best carried out without a previous rectal examination as then the narrow aganglionic bowel with dilation proximally is demonstrated
- Definitive diagnosis is by **rectal biopsy.**

Duodenal Atresia

- Associated with **Down's syndrome**
- Atresia at the level of **ampulla of vater**
- **Double bubble sign** on radiograph
- **Mc cause of acute intestinal obstruction in neonates**
- **Duodenojujenostomy** is the procedure of choice

Reye's Syndrome

Reye's syndrome is the best known example of **secondary mitochondrial hepatopathy**

Mitochondrial changes include:
• Microvesicular steatosis
• Swelling of mitochondrial matrix
• Dissolution of cristae/appearance of granules
• Ameboid shapes

- Reye's syndrome is an **encephalopathy with fatty degeneration of liver**
- In liver **peripheral zonal hepatic necrosis** is seen
- **Liver** is **yellow, enlarged with diffuse microvacuolization of cells**
- **In renal tubules, fatty changes in renal tubular cells** are seen
- **In brain cerebral edema and neuronal degeneration** are seen
- It usually occurs in **children**
- Patients have a history of **recent viral upper respiratory tract infection or varicella**
- **Adeno, herpes, influenza are common precipitants**
- **Use of aspirin** also leads to Reye's syndrome
- **Hypoglycemia, hypoglycorrhea, ↑AST, ALT.**

USMLE Case Scenario

An 8-year-old girl has chickenpox. A week after the onset of the rash, she begins vomiting and becomes lethargic and comatose. Laboratory examination is significant for elevated liver enzymes and ammonia. Which of the following is the most likely diagnosis?

1. Crigler-Najjar syndrome
2. Dubin-Johnson syndrome
3. Gilbert's syndrome
4. Reye's syndrome

Ans. 4. Reye's syndrome

Wilson's Disease

It is an **AR disorder**

- **Chromosome 13** is involved
- The diagnosis is confirmed by the demonstration of either:
  - A serum ceruloplasmin level < 20 mg/dl and Kayser-Fleischer rings or
  - A serum ceruloplasmin level < 20 mg/dl and a concentration of copper in a liver biopsy sample >250 mg/g dry weight
  - Most symptomatic patients excrete > 100 mg copper per day in urine and have histologic abnormalities on liver biopsy

Pathognonic features are:

- **Hepatic dysfunction:** Jaundice, hepatomegaly, cirrhosis, portal hypertension
- **Eye changes:** Brownish or grayish **Kayser-Fleischer ring in Descemet's membrane in cornea**. These golden deposits of copper in Descemet's membrane of the cornea do not interfere with vision but indicate that copper has been released from the liver and has probably caused brain damage
- If a patient with frank neurologic or psychiatric disease does not have Kayser-Fleischer rings when examined by a trained observer using a slit lamp, the diagnosis of Wilson's disease can be excluded
- Rarely, Kayser-Fleischer rings may be accompanied by **sunflower cataracts**
- **The neurologic manifestations** include resting and intention tremors, spasticity, rigidity, chorea, drooling, dysphagia, and dysarthria. Babinski responses may be present, and abdominal reflexes are often absent. **Sensory changes never occur, except for headache**
- **Psychiatric disturbances** are present in most patients with neurologic symptoms. Schizophrenia, manic-depressive psychoses, and classic neuroses may occur, but the commonest disturbances are bizarre behavioral patterns that defy classification

Treatment consists of removing and detoxifying the deposits of copper as rapidly as possible and must be instituted once the diagnosis is secure, whether the patient is ill or asymptomatic

- **Zinc is the DOC**
- **Penicillamine**
- **Trientine**
- **Zinc acetate or gluconate** are effective as maintenance therapy.

Biliary Atresia

- It is a disorder of unknown cause where a destructive **sclerosing inflammatory process causes obstruction of the extrahepatic bile ducts and extends into the major intrahepatic bile ducts**
- By 6–10 weeks of age, the portal blood pressure is increased. Cirrhosis rapidly develops

Clinical features:

- **The first sign is prolongation of jaundice. The urine is always yellow. The stools contain no yellow or green pigment**
- **Conjugated hyperbilirubinemia**
- **Acholic stools**
- Biliary atresia must be considered in any infant remaining jaundiced beyond 14 days of age
- Percutaneous liver biopsy showing the features described above in all portal tracts is suggestive. Diagnosis of it is confirmed at laparotomy
- **Complications:** Cholangitis occurs in a significant minority of cases in the first 2 years after surgery. Portal hypertension is present in almost all cases
- The prognosis is transformed by the Kasai operation and with liver.

A four-month-old presents with cholestasis. Biopsy shows inflammation and fibrosing stricture of the hepatic or common bile ducts; inflammation of major intrahepatic bile ducts, with progressive destruction of the intrahepatic biliary tree, marked bile ductular proliferation, portal tract edema and fibrosis, and parenchymal cholestasis); and periportal fibrosis and cirrhosis.

Choledochal Cyst

- In this disorder, there is enlargement or dilatation of part or all the **extrahepatic biliary system**
- Bile flow may be obstructed with intrahepatic changes similar to those of biliary atresia, **progressing to cirrhosis**
- More common in females
  - Recurrent abdominal pain
  - Episodic jaundice
  - Right upper quadrant mass
  - Or silent up to childhood are features
- Type 1 (dilatation of common bile duct) is commonest
- Cholangitis
- Cyst rupture
- Pancreatitis
- Gallstones
- Carcinoma of the cyst wall
- In infancy, it presents with features of neonatal cholestasis
  - In older children, there may be recurrent upper abdominal pain, recurrent jaundice and/or a palpable cystic mass but the classical triad is rare
  - The treatment is surgical removal wit**h biliary drainage via a Roux-en-Y loop**

USMLE Case Scenario

A 2-week-old infant is jaundiced. Findings include weight and length at the 75th percentile for age; icterus; with hepatosplenomegaly; total bilirubin, 6.8 mg/dl; direct bilirubin, 5.9 mg/dl; alanine aminotransferase activity, 139 U/L; aspartate aminotransferase activity, 149 U/L; and gamma-glutamyl transpeptidase activity, 1050 U/L. Of the following, the BEST study to evaluate the excretion of bile from the liver is:

1. Computed tomography of the liver
2. Hepatic ultrasonography
3. Hepatobiliary scintigraphy
4. Spiral CT
5. Indigo carmine
6. Rose Bengal test

Ans. 3. Hepatobiliary scintigraphy

Caroli's Disease

- **Congenital**, autosomal recessive disorder
- **Communicating cavernous ectasia of intrahepatic biliary ducts. Kindly note this point. It differentiates the disease from choledochal cyst**
- **Cystic structures (multiple)** converging towards porta hepatis
- **Central dot sign on CT scan**
- **Cholangiography most diagnostic**
- **Congenital hepatic fibrosis and cystic (polycystic) kidney disease are associations.**

Clinical Scenarios. Highlighted text underlined. Don't look at the answers initially. Try to make diagnosis reading the left column only.

• Within **6 hours of birth** a baby with **excessive salivation**. NG tube insertion shows **tube coiling back** and air in GIT	• TE fistula
• A **newborn** is found to be **tachypneic, cyanotic** and grunting. **Abdomen is scaphoid with bowel sounds heard in chest**	• Congenital diaphragmatic hernia
• A **newborn** with **green-colored vomitus** in first day of life not passing **meconium. X-ray shows multiple air fluid levels and distended bowel**	• Intestinal atresia
• A **prematurely born** baby has **feeding intolerance and early abdominal distension**	• Necrotizing enterocolitis
• A 2-year-old boy has **fractured humerus, subdural hematoma and retinal hemorrhages**	• Suspect child abuse
• A **3-month**-old has **chronic constipation, abdominal distension.** X-ray shows **dilated bowel loops**	• Hirschsprung's disease
• A **3-week**-old has **non bilious, projectile vomiting** with **visible peristalsis and mass in right upper abdomen**	• Hypertrophic pyloric stenosis
• A **7-year**-old with **bloody bowel movement**	• Meckel's diverticulitis

Common Causes of Chronic Diarrheas

- Lactase deficiency
- Cow's milk intolerance
- Irritable bowel
- Inflammatory bowel
- Giardiasis
- Cystic fibrosis
- Celiac disease

A 12-year-old boy has a productive cough characterized by large volumes of foul-smelling sputum. Three years ago, the patient was diagnosed with pancreatic insufficiency, as evidenced by repetitive gastrointestinal symptoms of steatorrhea. After culture of the sputum, colorless, oxidase-positive colonies with a fruity aroma develop on the agar. Most likely cause is:

Cystic Fibrosis

Pneumatosis Intestinalis

- Pneumatosis intestinalis, defined as gas in the bowel wall, is often first identified on abdominal radiographs or computed tomography (CT) scans
- It is a **radiographic finding** and not a diagnosis, as the etiology varies from benign conditions to fulminant gastrointestinal disease
- In neonates, **pneumatosis is usually secondary to NEC and indicates a later stage of the disease**
- **NEC is seen almost exclusively in premature infants** and is associated with bowel ischemia caused by bacterial invasion and hyperosmolar feeds. Mesenteric vascular occlusion leads to ischemic damage of the mucosa, which allows luminal gas and bacteria to invade the bowel wall
- Pneumatosis intestinalis is considered an **'ominous finding'** in ischemia, especially in association with portomesenteric venous gas.

Pneumatosis Intestinalis occurs in 2 forms

- **Primary pneumatosis intestinalis (15% of cases)** is a benign idiopathic condition in which **multiple thin-walled cysts develop in the submucosa or subserosa of the colon.** Usually, this form has no associated symptoms, and the cysts may be found incidentally through radiography or endoscopy. When the cysts protrude into the lumen, they may mimic polyps or carcinomas, as shown on barium enema studies. This primary form is often termed pneumatosis cystoides intestinalis
- **The secondary form (85% of cases)** is associated with obstructive pulmonary disease, as well as with obstructive and necrotic gastrointestinal disease.

The Disease is seen in Other Conditions, Including

- Chronic obstructive pulmonary disease
- Connective tissue disorders
- Infectious enteritis
- Celiac disease
- Leukemia
- Amyloidosis and
- Acquired immunodeficiency syndrome (AIDS)

It is also found in association with organ transplantation, steroid use and chemotherapy

RESPIRATORY SYSTEM

Choanal Atresia

- This rare anomaly is due to **failure of breakdown of the nasobuccal membrane** which normally occurs at 6 weeks' fetal development
- Of the cases, 50% are associated with the **CHARGE syndrome** – choanal atresia with ear, eye, heart and genital defects
- **Gasping respiration** in a neonate is suggestive of choanal atresia
- Bilateral choanal atresia is a **neonatal emergency**
- The diagnosis is by suspicion, by **inability to pass a catheter along the nose** and confirmation by endoscopic examination
- The treatment consists of **establishment of an airway, either oral or orotracheal.**

A newborn infant is in respiratory distress and requires several attempts at resuscitation in the delivery room because of difficulty breathing and frequent cyanosis. The neonatologist notes that during crying, her breathing improves and breath and heart sounds are normal. Direct laryngoscopy is unremarkable as well. Deep inspirations by the neonate are ineffective. Which of the following is the most effective intervention?

The patient most likely has choanal atresia, which is the presence of a congenital membrane between the nose and the pharynx. Since most newborns are obligate nose breathers, spells of crying force mouth breathing, improving the ventilation. If unilateral, the atresia may not cause symptoms. Intubation via the oropharynx will provide immediate relief and surgery should then be performed to correct the atresia.

• Transient tachypnea of newborn	• Self-limited • Seen after cesarean section • Tachypnea, mild retractions and grunting seen • CXR shows fluid in fissure and prominent vascular markings, air bronchogram and reticular shadows
• Meconium aspiration syndrome	• Meconium aspirated • CXR shows patchy infiltration • Mechanical ventilation, NO, ECMO are used

Foreign-Body Aspiration

A 2-year-old girl is rushed to the emergency department by her parents because of an acute attack of wheezing. At one point, they noticed that something was wrong because she was gasping for breath and became very frightened and quiet. They looked in her mouth, thinking she had swallowed something, as there were lots of snacks and food lying around, but they could not see anything. The patient has an unremarkable medical history with no prior respiratory problems. She is not allergic to any foods or drugs. On physical examination, the patient is in severe respiratory distress, drooling and continuously attempting to swallow. Nasal flaring and intercostal retractions are present. She appears cyanotic. Breath sounds are decreased bilaterally.

Foreign-body aspiration is most commonly seen in children 1 to 3 years of age because of the size of the trachea, the lessening of parental supervision secondary to increased independence of the child, and the tendency of small children to put objects in their mouths. Foreign bodies include hot dogs, peanuts, beans, coins, buttons, nuts, deflated balloons, etc. When aspirated, these items may go to the airway or the esophagus.

USMLE Case Scenario

A 7-month-old child presents with a 4-day history of fever, deepening cough, and dyspnea. A chest X-ray shows multiple interstitial infiltrates and hyperinflation of the lungs. Multinucleated giant cells with cytoplasmic inclusion bodies are seen when a nasal wash is inoculated into culture. Diagnosis is:
Bronchiolitis

USMLE Case Scenario

A 4-week-old infant is brought with a 7-day history of coughing and choking spells. The white blood cell count is elevated with 80% lymphocytes. The child is gasping for breath, experiencing paroxysms of coughing. Encapsulated; gram-negative rods grow out on Bordet-Gengou media. Likely diagnosis is:
Pertusis

Diaphragmatic Hernia

- The commonest herniation is the **Bochdalek type, a posterolateral defect**, possibly a failure of closure of the pleuroperitoneal canal
- A hernia through the **Foramen of Morgagni (Retrosternal) is less common in neonates.** This defect is retrosternal, to the right or left of the midline
- The third site for herniation is the **Esophageal hiatus**—the so-called hiatus hernia
- Majority present with **respiratory distress—cyanosis, dyspnea and tachypnea**—either immediately after birth or **within a few hours**
- **Most common on left side**
- Examination reveals a **scaphoid abdomen, bowel sounds on auscultation of the affected side of the chest** and a **shift of the apex beat to the right** in the case of a left-sided hernia. Once air has been swallowed after birth, a chest X-ray confirms the diagnosis, showing gas-filled loops of bowel on the affected side of the chest with displacement of the mediastinum to the opposite side
- **Treatment:** A nasogastric tube is passed to reduce the gaseous distention of the bowel with air.

Eventration of the Diaphragm

- This is due to a **deficiency in the muscle of the diaphragm**
- The thin layer becomes **attenuated and bulges up into the thorax**
- Extensive eventrations are similar to diaphragmatic hernia presenting in the neonatal period
- Smaller eventrations present later and require localized plication
- Congenital diaphragmatic hernia are present along with polyhydramnios.

HMD (Hyaline Membrane Disease)

- Most neonates with HMD demonstrate clinical findings of respiratory distress in the delivery room or during the **first few hours of life**. (6) HOURS

HM is made of fibrin

- The condition starts with an **increase in breathing rate**, with respiration then becoming labored and more rapid
- It is due to surfactant deficiency resulting in **poor lung compliance and atelectasis**
- Seen in diabetics, premature babies
- In addition to the early onset of respiratory distress, clinical features include:
  - Tachypnea
  - Intercostal and sternal retractions, expiratory grunt
  - Nasal flaring
  - Decreased lung compliance.

Four Radiographic Features Characteristic of HMD are

- **Reduced lung volume**, with expansion only to the fifth, sixth or seventh thoracic vertebrae, rather than to the eighth or ninth, as found in the normally expanded chest. The reduced lung expansion is **a consequence of atelectasis**, which occurs due to a lack of surfactant. Also, the diaphragms will appear unusually high and sometimes domed, and the intercostal spaces will appear narrow
- **Air bronchograms** or the outlines of air-filled secondary and tertiary bronchi are seen over abnormal lung fields. Because normally expanded lungs and the overlying bronchi are of air density, air bronchograms are not generally seen in the lung fields on a normal chest X-ray
- **A reticulogranular/reticulonodular pattern, or ground glass appearance**, uniformly distributed throughout both the lung fields. Because of surfactant deficiency, some alveoli in the lung collapse from high surface tension. The alveoli that remain distended have lower surface tension. Air entering the lung goes only to the area of lowest pressure, creating the image of ground glass
- **Increased lung opacification**. When diffuse lung opacification becomes visible, it usually is the result of nonexpanded alveoli with little or no terminal airway aeration. The heart borders may be visible initially, but the X-ray may progress to a complete loss of visualization of the heart borders, called a **'whiteout'**

- Confirmed by chest X-ray
- L/S > 2 indicates lung maturity

Pulmonary Alveolar Proteinosis (PAP)

- PAP presents in infancy with **progressive respiratory distress**
- In some children, it may be related to a form of immune deficiency, such as **thymic atrophy, lymphopenia and immunoglobulin deficiency**
- **CXR shows a ground glass appearance**
- **HRCT, a typical cobblestone appearance.**

USMLE Case Scenario

A male born at term after an uncomplicated pregnancy, labor and delivery develops severe respiratory distress within a few hours of birth. Results of routine culture were negative. The chest roentgenogram reveals a normal heart shadow and fine reticulonodular infiltrates radiating from the hilum. ECHO findings reveal no abnormality. Family history reveals similar clinical course and death of a male and female sibling at 1 month and 2 months of age respectively.

Bronchiolitis

- Caused by RSV mainly. Commonly in children less than 2 years
- Self-limiting

- Ribavirin DOC
- Leads to asthma
- Humidified oxygen

Distinct Symptoms of RSV Bronchiolitis Include

- Rhinorrhea (runny nose)
- Wheezing and coughing (can persist for several months in severe infections)
- Irritability and restlessness (usually in those with impending respiratory failure)
- Low-grade fever (102 °F); but temperatures can be as high as 104 °F when another illness, such as otitis media is present
- Nasal flaring and retractions (intercostal, subcostal, and sternal) are indicative of airway obstruction. The chest may appear hyperexpanded and be hyper-resonant to percussion. As a result of hyperexpansion of the lungs, the liver and spleen may be palpable several centimeters below the costal margins
- X-ray findings are not pathognomonic, but often show air trapping and hyperinflation or appear normal
- Apnea, usually as an initial presenting symptom in short episodes. It occurs in approximately 20 to 25% of young infants
- Circumoral and nailbed cyanosis (severely affected infant).

USMLE Case Scenario

A 7½-month-old child with cough, mild stridor is started on oral antibiotics. The child showed initial improvement but later developed wheeze, productive cough, and mild fever. X-ray shows hyperlucency and PFT shows an obstructive curve.

Integrated Management of Childhood Illness Includes

- Malaria
- Diarrhea
- Acute respiratory infections

Bronchiolitis (Detailed Overview, Important Topic)

The infecting organism in around 75% cases is respiratory syncytial virus (RSV) and *H. influenzae*

- More common in boys
- Infants at high risk of severe RSV include those born prematurely, and those with cardiovascular disease, chronic respiratory disease including bronchopulmonary dysplasia (BPD) and cystic fibrosis or immunosuppression
- Characteristically there is a **short prodromal upper respiratory tract illness** with coryzal symptoms and low-grade pyrexia, followed by a relatively sudden onset of **tachypnea, hypoxia, a moist cough and difficulty with feeding**. Increased work of breathing is reflected by suprasternal, subcostal and intercostal recession with head bobbing and nasal flaring. The predominant feature on auscultation is crackles with or without the presence of wheeze. As the chest becomes hyperinflated, the liver is displaced and is often easily palpable in the abdomen
- CXR show **hyperinflation with multiple areas of interstitial infiltration**
- Current therapy for RSV bronchiolitis is essentially supportive, involving maintenance of hydration and oxygen status. Nasogastric or intravenous feeding is required if the baby is unable to suck
- May lead to asthma in later life
- **Ribavirin inhibits viral replication and is the antiviral agent available against RSV**
- **Oxygen is helpful**
- **RSV immunoglobulin has no role in acute attacks**
- **Antibiotics are not used initially**

Obliterative Bronchiolitis

- Obliterative bronchiolitis (OB) has been described in association with infections caused by **adenovirus types 3, 7 and 21; measles, pertussis, influenza A, mycoplasma; after lung transplantation; and secondary to chronic aspiration**
- The clinical course is one of **cough, wheeze and tachypnea in an infant or young child, which may be static if the cause is an infection, or progress at a variable rate to respiratory failure and failure to thrive if there is ongoing aspiration**
- Chest radiography initially shows **generalized hyperinflation. HRCT demonstrates patchy air trapping, particularly if the scan is expiratory**
- Focal hyperlucency involving a lobe or a whole lung represents the radiological appearance of MacLeod's syndrome, in which the affected lung appears small and hyperlucent
- **Long-term oxygen dependency is common**
- Improvement after 2–3 years may be seen. The condition is usually stable once the initial effects of the devastating infection have burnt out, but some may go on to require lung transplantation. OB developing after lung transplant is eventually fatal and the results of second transplantation are very poor.

Follicular Bronchiolitis

- Follicular bronchiolitis (FB) is part of the **spectrum of lymphoid disorders of the lung, which includes lymphoid interstitial pneumonia (LIP)**
- There is a **polyclonal expansion of lymphoid tissue**, probably part of the bronchus-associated lymphoid tissue (BALT), which causes small airway obstruction
- Presentation is with **chronic respiratory distress, and HRCT demonstrates air trapping, sometimes with associated infiltrates.**

Inhaled Foreign Bodies

- Acute onset cough, stridor, dyspnea in a child indicates foreign body inhalation
- Commonest sign is cough
- Intrabrochial foreign bodies need bronchoscopy/thoracotomy/ lung resection
- Immediate procedure is bronchoscopy.

Pulmonary lymphangiectasia

- This typically presents with **relentlessly progressive respiratory distress in a term baby**
- CXR may show **dilatation of lymphatics and pleural effusions.**

Pulmonary alveolar microlithiasis

- This condition, which may be **inherited, has a nonspecific presentation** but a **classical sandstorm appearance on CXR**
- **Calcium carbonate stones** are formed within the alveoli; the differential diagnosis is other form of pulmonary calcification
- **Pulmonary fibrosis may develop** many years later when the patient becomes symptomatic.
- **Asphyxiating thoracic dystrophy (Jeune's syndrome):** This is a rare disorder of the costal cartilages in which the ribs are shortened and the rib cage narrowed so that lung development is retarded and the lungs are small.

• Bronchiolitis	0–18 months	**Respiratory syncytial virus**	**Hyperinflation**
• Laryngotracheobronchitis	1–2 years	**Parainfluenza virus**	**Steeple sign**
• Epiglottitis	2–5 years	***H. influenzae***	**Thumb sign**

USMLE Case Scenario

A 3-month-old child has moderate fever and nonproductive cough and mild dyspnea. After course of mild antibiotic, the condition of the child improved transiently but he again develops high fever, productive cough and increased respiratory distress. Chest X-ray shows hyperlucency and PFT shows obstructive pattern.

Bronchiolitis

Kartagener's Syndrome

- **Situs inversus in Kartagener's Syndrome**

It is assumed that during early embryonic life, ciliary beats in the growing embryo determine the type of laterality. When ciliary movements are absent, laterality may develop fortuitously, thus affecting a situs inversus in about half the affected cases

- **Infertility in Kartagener's Syndrome**

Infertility is common due to defective ciliary action in the fallopian tube in affected females or diminished sperm motility in affected males

- **The Chest in Kartagener's Syndrome**

Mucociliary clearance is an important primary innate defense mechanism that protects the lungs from deleterious effects of inhaled pollutants, allergens and pathogens (bronchiectasis)

The main consequence of impaired ciliary function is reduced or absent mucus clearance from the lungs, and susceptibility to chronic recurrent respiratory infections, including sinusitis, bronchitis, pneumonia and otitis media.

1. *Ciliated columnar epithelia* move mucus and other substances via cilia, and are found in the upper respiratory tract, the Fallopian tubes, the uterus and the central part of the spinal cord.
2. Mucociliary clearance is an important primary innate defense mechanism that protects the lungs from deleterious effects of inhaled pollutants, allergens, and pathogens.
3. Ciliated columnar epithelium lines the lumen of the uterine tube, where currents generated by the cilia propel the egg cell, toward the uterus.
4. Cilia are also involved in maintaing left-right axis during embryogenesis.

Pediatric Cardiology

• A 10-year-old girl with **pulmonary flow systolic murmur and fixed split second hear sound**	ASD
• A 3-year-old girl with failure to thrive **has pansystolic murmur on left sternal border with prominent pulmonary vascular markings**	VSD
• A 5-day-old girl with **machinery-like heart murmur** and bounding peripheral pulses	PDA
• A 6-year-old with **clubbing, cyanosis improved by squatting, systolic ejection murmur** in 3rd intercostal space with right ventricular hypertrophy.	Tetralogy of Fallot

• Alcohol	• VSD mainly
• Lithium	• Ebstein's anamoly
• Phenytoin	• Pulmonic stenosis, aortic stenosis, coarctation, PDA

Right to left shunts:

- TOF
- Transposition of great vessels
- Tricuspid atresia

Left to Right shunts (when Eisenmenger's complex) is not developed:

- ASD
- VSD
- PDA

Cardiac tumors in childhood:

- Rhabdomyoma
- Myxoma
- Fibroma

ASD:
- Commonest: **Ostium secondum defects**
- **Systolic ejection murmur in left, mid and upper sternal borders**
- **A wide fixed split of S2**
- **Left parasternal heave is seen**
- CXR: Enlarged RA, RV not LA
- Seen in **Holt-Oram syndrome**

VSD:
- **Holosystolic murmur at left lower sternal border**
- Thrill associated
- **LVF, biventricular hypertrophy with left axis deviation**
- Close spontaneously in 30-50% cases

PDA:
- **Failure of closure of ductus arteriosus**
- Blood flows from **aorta to pulmonary artery** both **during systole and diastole**
- **Wide** pulse pressure
- **Seen in rubella**
- **Hypoxia and prematurity** predispose
- **'Differential cyanosis'** is seen
- **'Machinery murmur'** which is continuous. Heard at 2nd left intercostal space
- **CXR:** Prominent pulmonary artery
- PG inhibitors stimulate closure of PDA

Coarctation of Aorta

- **Mostly below** origin of left subclavian artery
- **Acyanotic**
- Seen in **Turner's syndrome** and associated with bicuspid aortic valve
- **Upper extremity, hypertension, headache, dizziness, intermittent claudication**
- **Lower extremity hypotension**
- **Ribnotching** due to increased flow through collaterals
- **Ribnotching with double buldging is seen**
- **Cause of death is usually complication of hypertension, CHF, endocarditis.**

USMLE Case Scenario

A 4½-year-old girl brought by her deer mother from Washington always had to wear warm socks even is summer season. On physical examination, it was noticed that she had high blood pressure and her femoral pulse was weak as compared to radial and carotid pulse. A chest radiograph showed remarkable notching of ribs along with their lower borders. The most likely diagnosis is:

Coarctation of aorta

Trilogy of Fallot:
- Pulmonary valve stenosis
- Atrial septal defect
- Right ventricular hypertrophy

Tetralogy of Fallot:
- Ventricular septal defect, communication between the two ventricles
- Pulmonary stenosis, narrowing at the pulmonary valve or at the level of right ventricular infundibulum, which lies just below the pulmonary valve
- Overriding of the aorta, the aorta being positioned over the ventricular septal defect instead of in the left ventricle
- Right ventricular hypertrophy

Pentalogy of Fallot:
- The four characteristics of Fallot's tetralogy syndrome, **plus a patent foramen ovale or atrial septal defect.**

TOF: Tetrology of Fallot
- Boot-shaped heart, Corn en Sabot heart
- ↓ Pulmonary blood flow
- Ejection systolic mumur, single S2
- Associated with right-sided aortic arch
- Right axis deviation and RVH
- **Blue spells** seen
- **TOF with ASD = Pentology of Fallot**

TGA (Transposition of Great Vessels)
- **Aorta arises from right ventricle and pulmonary artery from left ventricle**
- Common in **infants of diabetic mothers**
- **Presents with cyanosis** in first 24 hours of life
- **Egg on string appearance**
- PGE_1 is used.

Tricuspid atresia:
- Single S_2
- **Pansystolic murmur**
- **LVH and LAD**

Total anomalous pulmonary venous return (TAPVR)
- Pulmonary veins drain back into systemic venous circulation
- Right atrial blood goes to left atrium through foramen ovale/ASD
- **Pulmonary hypertension occurs**
- **Mc Type issu pracardiac**
- **Infracardiac type is invariably always obstructive**
- **Snowman pattern of figure 8 occurs.**

USMLE Case Scenario

A two-month-old infant born to a mother who was taking lithium for BPD was noted at birth to have an upper left sternal border ejection murmur. The infant at that time was not cyanotic, but slowly developed cyanosis over the next two months. ECG shows right axis deviation and right ventricular hypertrophy. A chest X-ray film showed a small heart with a concave main pulmonary artery segment and diminished pulmonary blood flow. Most likely diagnosis is: TOF
Tetralogy of Fallot

Important Points about ASD

Most common type of ASD is	**Ostium secondum type**
S_2 is fixed and widely split in	**ASD**
There is	**Delayed diastolic murmur (Tricuspid)**
ASD+Mitral stenosis	**Ejection systolic murmur (Pulmonary)**

• ASD+Single atrium	• **Lutembacher's syndrome**
• ASD+Bony abnormalities	• **Ellis-van Creveld Syndrome**
	• **Holt-Oram Syndrome**

- **Carey Coombs Murmur:** Transient Soft **middiastolic murmur** of acute rheumatic fever due to mitral valvulitis, low-pitched
- **Austin Flint Murmur:** Murmur of **mitral stenosis** at apex
- **Graham Steell Murmur:** Early diastolic murmur of **Pulmonary Regurgitation**
- **Means Murmur: Pulmonary Systolic murmur** in Thyrotoxicosis
- **Seagull's Murmur: Aortic regurgitation** murmur.

Carcinoid Syndrome and Heart

- **ENDOCARDIUM** is most commonly involved
- Involvement of tricuspid valve cause **TRICUSPID REGURGITATION**
- Involvement of pulmonary valve cause **PULMONARY STENOSIS**
- **MITRAL VALVE** is most commonly involved valve on left side (not the commonest overall)
- If cardiac lesions are present in carcinoid syndrome, it causes **heart failure in 80% patients**
- Cardiac effects in carcinoid are due to **serotonin.**

Major Cardiovascular Manifestations of Some Important Diseases

- Progeria: Accelerated atherosclerosis
- Cystic fibrosis: Cor pulmonale
- Friedreich's ataxia: Cardiomyopathy
- William's syndrome: Supravalvular aortic stenosis
- Cornelia de Lange syndrome: VSD

Kindly Memorize

• Turner's syndrome	• Coarctation of aorta
• Noonan syndrome	• Pulmonary stenosis, ASD
• Congenital rubella	• PDA
• Marfan's syndrome	• MVP
• William's syndrome	• Supravalvular aortic stenosis
• Digeorges's syndrome	• Aortic arch abnormalities

Marfan's syndrome

- It is an autosomal dominant disorder of the **connective tissues**
- The genetic defect results in abnormal synthesis and secretion of **fibrillin**, which is an essential component in connective tissues
- Patients with Marfan's syndrome often have involvement in the **skeletal, ocular and cardiovascular systems**
- Most of the morbidity and mortality with this disease are related to the cardiovascular manifestations; patients develop aortic root dilatation. This may be associated with **aortic insufficiency and aortic arch dissection.** They may also have mitral valve prolapse with significant hemodynamic consequences. Aortic root, aortic valve and mitral valve replacement may be needed during the lifetime of the patient.

- Patients with Marfan's syndrome may frequently complain of chest pain; these patients must be viewed as having aortic dissection until proven otherwise. In this population, a spontaneous pneumothorax is another potential cause of chest pain
- Patients must avoid contact sports that cause acceleration-deceleration injury and isometric maneuvers that tend to increase central blood pressure. Aerobic activity is encouraged, but those with established aortic root dilatation should have adequate heart rate control with beta-blockers.

Hypoplastic Left Heart (HLH) Syndrome

- It is a group of closely related cardiac anomalies characterized by underdevelopment of the left cardiac chambers, atresia or stenosis of the aortic and/or the mitral orifices, and hypoplasia of the aorta
- These anomalies are an especially common cause of heart failure in the 1st week of life
- The left atrium and ventricle often exhibit endocardial fibroelastosis. Pulmonary venous blood traverses a patent foramen ovale and a dilated and hypertrophied right ventricle acts as the systemic, as well as pulmonary, ventricle; the systemic circulation receives blood by way of a patent ductus arteriosus
- Infants who have HLH syndrome develop poor perfusion and metabolic acidosis when systemic blood flow decreases. When the ductus closes, inadequate blood flow to the body occurs because the ductus is the only path for blood to flow from the right ventricle to the body. Even if the ductus remains open, when the infant is given oxygen, the oxygen will dilate the vasculature of the pulmonary circulation and blood will preferentially flow to the lower pressure pulmonary system, depriving the systemic circulation of adequate perfusion
- **ECG usually shows** right axis deviation, right atrial and ventricular enlargement, and nonspecific ST and T-wave abnormalities in the left precordial leads
- **Chest radiography** may show only slight enlargement shortly after birth, but with clinical deterioration, there is marked cardiomegaly with increased pulmonary vascular markings
- **Echocardiography is diagnostic** and will show a diminutive aortic root and left ventricular cavity and absence or poor visualization of aortic and mitral valves
- An infant with HLH syndrome has a **hyperdynamic precordium** because the enlarged right ventricle is contracting against systemic pressure. The infant also has a loud, or even palpable, second heart sound (S2) because the pulmonary artery acts as the aorta by pumping blood to the systemic circulation through the ductus arteriosus.

Blood

- Hematopoiesis is the process by which formed elements of the blood are produced
- In the BM (Bone Marrow) first morphologically recognizable precursor is the **PRO** normoblast and **'not normoblast'**
- Erythropoietin is produced by the peritubular cells within the kidney
- There is daily replacement of 0.8–1% of all circulating red cells
- **'Hematopoiesis'** is the process by which formed elements of the blood are produced. Stem cells are capable of producing all classes of cells
- In the BM (Bone Marrow), first morphologically recognizable precursor is the'**PRO** normoblast.' This cell can undergo **4–5 cell divisions** that result in production of 16–32 mature red cells
- Hemoglobin first to appear in fetus: **Hb Gowers**
- Switch over of fetal Hb to adult Hb begins at **14 week's gestation**
- Fetal Hb is completely replaced by adult Hb by **6 months**
- Increased Fetal Hb is a feature of **CML.**

Iron-deficiency Anemia

Commonest type of anemia in children

Iron deficiency in children can be due to causes **slightly different** from adults:

- Cow's milk (poor source of iron)
- Hookworm infestation
- Polyposis colon
- Meckel's diverticulum
- Malabsorption syndrome

- Prematurity and low birthweight
- Red cell distribution width (RDW) in iron-deficiency anemia is increased
- Iron supplementation should be started to a term breastfed baby **at 6 weeks**
- **Lab features of iron-deficiency anemia:**

↓Iron strores
↓Serum iron
↑Free erythrocyte porphyrin
↑TIBC (Total iron-binding capacity)
↑RDW

- **Increased reticulocyte is the first indicator of response after iron therapy**
- **Iron requirement: 4x wt (kg) × Hb deficit (gm/dl)**

	Iron deficiency	Thalassemia	Sideroblastic anemia	Chronic anemia
Sr Fe	↓	ν	ν	↓
TIBC	↑	ν	ν	↓
% Saturation	↓	↑	↑	↓
Ferritin	↓	↑	↑	↑

Hypochromic microcytic anemia with ↓srFe, ↑TIBC: Iron-deficiency anemia ↑RDW, ↓MCH↓MCV↓MCHC
Hypochromic microcytic anemia with ↓srFe, ↓TIBC: Anemia of chronic disease.
↓ Sr Ferritin is the early indicator of iron deficiency.

Thalassemias

(Mediterranean Anemia; Hereditary Leptocytosis; Thalassemia Major and Minor)

- A group **of chronic, inherited, microcytic anemias**
- Characterized by **defective Hb synthesis and ineffective erythropoiesis**
- They are **particularly common in persons of Mediterranean, African, and South-east Asian ancestry**
- Clinical features of all thalassemias are similar but vary in severity
- Symptoms of **severe anemia occur in ß-thalassemia major (Cooley's anemia).** Clinical features result from anemia, markedly expanded marrow space, and transfusional and absorptive Fe overload. Patients are jaundiced, and leg ulcers and cholelithiasis occur (as in sickle cell anemia)
- **Splenomegaly is common**, and the spleen may be huge. If splenic sequestration develops, the survival time of transfused, normal RBCs is shortened. Bone marrow hyperactivity causes thickening of the cranial bones and malar eminences, producing '**hemolytic facies**'
- Long-bone involvement makes pathologic fractures common
- Osmotic fragility **decreased**. NOT INCREASED
- Growth rates are impaired, and puberty may be significantly delayed or absent

- Fe deposits in heart muscle may cause dysfunction and ultimately heart failure
- **Hair on end** appearance seen
- Hepatic siderosis occurs typically, leading to functional impairment and cirrhosis
- **Electrophoresis** is the diagnostic test.

Thalassemia Major

- ↑HbF
- Normal Hb A2
- Microcytosis and hypochromia
- Anisocytosis and poikilocytosis
- Target and tear drop RBC
- Howel-Jolly bodies and Heinz bodies
- Erythroblasts seen

- Bone marrow hypercellular
- Hemosiderin deposits↑
- Serum ferritin↑

α Thalassemia

Deletion of one α globin gene	• Silent hematologically
Deletion of two α globin gene	• Called α **Thalassemia triat** • Presents as mild microcytic anemia • ↑HbF • ↑Hb A2
Deletion of three α globin gene	• **Hb H disease** • Cases have chronic hemolysis with jaundice and hepatosplenomegaly • Gallstones and leg ulcers seen
Deletion of four α globin gene	• **Hydrops fetalis** occurs • Profound anemia • Most severe

- **Tear drop cells:** Myelofibrosis, myelophthisic anemia
- **Target cells:** Liver diseases, thalassemia
- **Helmet cells:** DIC, microangiopathic hemolytic anemia
- **Burr cells:** Uremia
- **Bite cells:** G6PD deficiency
- **Smudge cells:** CLL

von Willebrand's Disease

von Willebrand's disease is the most common inherited bleeding disorder. It is inherited in an autosomal dominant fashion and characteristically behaves like a platelet disorder, i.e. epistaxis and menorrhagia are common whilst hemoarthroses and muscle hematomas are rare:

Role of von Willebrand factor:

- Large glycoprotein which forms massive multimers up to 1,000,000 Da in size
- Promotes platelet adhesion to damaged endothelium
- Carrier molecule for factor VIII

Types:

- Type 1: Partial reduction in vW

- Type 2: Abnormal form of vW
- Type 3: Total lack of vWF

Investigation

- Prolonged bleeding time
- APTT may be prolonged
- Factor VIII levels may be moderately reduced
- Defective platelet aggregation with ristocetin

von Willebrand's Disease

- von Willebrand's disease is an **autosomal dominant** disease
- von Willebrand's disease is the **commonest** hereditary bleeding disorder
- von Willebrand's disease is characterized by platelet adhesion defect
- **Postoperative traumaticor mucosal bleeding,** epistaxis, menorrhagia is common
- Hemarthosis or muscle hematomas are rare
- **Increased BT and increased PTT** are findings
- **vWf** (von Willebrand's factor) level which is synthesized in platelets is **low**
- Treatment: **Factor VIII cryoprecipitate, vasopressin**

LABORATORY TESTING: There are five tests commonly used to screen for vWD

- Plasma vWF antigen (vWF:Ag)
- Plasma vWF activity (ristocetin cofactor activity, vWF: RCo)
- Factor VIII activity (FVIII) and activated partial thromboplastin time (APTT)
- Platelet function analyzer (PFA) testing or bleeding time (BT)

If one or more of these tests is abnormal, or if there is still a high index of suspicion for vWD in the face of normal results, further testing is carried out to evaluate the following:

- vWF multimer distribution on gel electrophoresis
- Ristocetin-induced platelet aggregation (RIPA)

Collagen-binding assay: Collagen binding has been introduced as a second type of functional assay for vWF (vWF:CB). The binding of plasma vWF to collagen-coated plates is dependent upon the quantity of vWF in plasma and on the presence of higher molecular weight multimers that bind more readily. This functional assay takes longer to perform, but is gaining wide acceptance in clinical laboratories.

ITP

In many cases, the cause is not actually idiopathic but **autoimmune**, with antibodies against platelets being detected in approximately 60 percent of patients:

Most often these **antibodies are against platelet membrane glycoproteins IIb-IIIa or Ib-IX,** and are of the **IgG type**

- The diagnosis of ITP is a **process of exclusion**
- In approximately one percent of cases, autoimmune hemolytic anemia and immune thrombocytopenic purpura coexist. This condition is called **'Evans syndrome'**
- **Bleeding time is prolonged** in ITP patients

- On examination of the bone marrow, **an increase in the production of megakaryocytes** may be observed and may help in establishing a diagnosis of ITP
- Platelet transfusions are not helpful in immunogenic variety.

TTP (Thrombotic Thrombocytopenic Purpura)

There is widespread formation of platelet thrombi

'Pentad of signs' is:

- Fever
- **Thrombocytopenia**
- **Microangiopathic hemolytic anemia**
- Neurological symptoms
- Renal failure

Lab features:

- Decreased platelet count and **increased bleeding time**
- Normal PT and PTT
- **Normal complement**

Overwhelming Postsplenectomy Infection (OPSI)

- Infection due to **encapsulated bacteria**
- Almost **50% due to strep pneumoniae**
- Other organisms include: *Hemophilus influenzae, Neisseria meningitidis*
- Occurs postsplenectomy in **4% patients** without prophylaxis
- Mortality of OPSI is approximately **50%**
- Greatest risk in **first 2 years postop.**

Renal System

Childhood Hypertension

- Childhood hypertension is defined as **arterial BP above 95th percentile with reference to age and sex**
- Essential hypertension is relatively **uncommon** in children
- Causes of persistent hypertension in children: in decreasing order:
  - Chronic glomerulonephritis
  - Chronic pyelonephritis
  - Essential hypertension
  - Renal artery stenosis
  - Renal arteritis
  - Obstructive uropathy

Liddle's Syndrome

Liddle's **syndrome** is a rare familial disease with a clinical presentation of **'hyperaldosteronism'**, consisting of:

- Hypertension (Compare with Bartter's syndrome)
- Hypokalemia
- Metabolic alkalosis

Bartter's Syndrome

Most cases of classic Bartter's syndrome present during **childhood**

- Symptoms such as **weakness and cramps** are secondary to hypokalemia
- **Polyuria and nocturia** are common due to the hypokalemia-induced nephrogenic diabetes insipidus
- **Growth retardation** may be seen.

Characteristies of Bartter's syndrome:

1. Hypokalemia
2. Metabolic alkalosis
3. Normal to low blood pressure, (compare with Liddle's syndrome)

The Gitelman's variant of Bartter's syndrome presents during **adolescence or adulthood** and generally has a **milder course** than Bartter's syndrome. The dominant features are fatigue and weakness. It is distinguished from Bartter's syndrome by:

- **Hypocalciuria**
- **Hypomagnesemia with hypermagnesuria**
- **Normal prostaglandin production**

Nephrocalcinosis

- Hypercalciuria
- Hyperoxaluria
- Distal renal tubular acidosis
- Bartter's syndrome
- Dent's disease
- Primary hyperparathyroidism

Urachus

The urachus in the embryo connects the bladder to the allantois. It is normally obliterated to form the **median umbilical ligament**. It may, however, persist as a patent urachus in the neonate, requiring repair. Occasionally the two extremities of the urachus close, leaving a cyst in the middle which becomes filled with secretions and may present as a mass or, more commonly, when it becomes infected, as an abscess.

Bladder Exstrophy (Ectopia Vesicae)

- In bladder exstrophy, there is a **lower abdominal wall anomaly** in which there is **wide separation of the pubic bones, the bladder surface being flat and exposed with the two ureteric orifices clearly visible**
- **In the male,** there is **complete epispadias** with a strip of urethral mucosa on the dorsum of a short broadened flattened penis
- **In the female,** there is also an **epispadiac urethra** with a bifid clitoris and separation of the labia anteriorly at the level of the vaginal orifice
- The bladder is best repaired soon after birth
- If necessary, bilateral iliac osteotomies enable the pubic bones to be better approximated, thus facilitating the repair. Careful construction of the bladder neck is vital to achieve subsequent continence and in the male, later repair of the severe epispadiac deformity is required.

VUR

- **Straining and dribbling of urine in a male child with recurrent UTI is suspicious of UTI**
- **Mc cause of renal scarring in CHILDREN**
- Caused by congenital **incompetence of vesicoureteral junction**

Common cause of hypertension and scarring:

- Grade I reflux into an undilated distal ureter
- Grade II reflux into the upper collecting system (ureter plvis calyces) without dilatation of the kidney
- Grade III reflux into the dilated ureter and/or blunting of the calyceal fornices
- Grade IV reflux into a grossly dilated ureter with moderate dilatation of the pelvis, calyces
- Grade V massive rflux, gross dilation, tortuosity of ureter, pelvis, calyces
- Diagnosed by **MCUG**

Acute Nephritic Syndrome

- It is characterized by sudden onset (i.e. over days to weeks) of acute renal failure and **oliguria** (< 400 ml of urine per day)
- Renal blood flow and glomerular filtration rate (GFR) fall
- Extracellular fluid volume expansion, **edema**
- **Hypertension develops** because of impaired GFR and enhanced tubular reabsorption of salt and water
- As a result of injury to the glomerular capillary wall, urinalysis typically reveals **red blood cell casts, dysmorphic red blood cells, leukocytes, and subnephrotic proteinuria of < 3.5 g per 24 h (nephritic urinary sediment)**
- Hematuria is often macroscopic.

Poststreptococcal Glomerulonephritis

- Most cases are **sporadic**, though the disease can occur as an epidemic.
- Glomerulonephritis develops, on an average, **10 days after pharyngitis or 2 weeks after a skin infection** (impetigo) with a **nephritogenic strain of group Ab-hemolytic *streptococcus.***
- The known **nephritic** strains include **M types**
- Epidemic poststreptococcal glomerulonephritis is most commonly encountered in children of 2 to 6 years of age with pharyngitis during the winter months.
- The classic clinical presentation of poststreptococcal glomerulonephritis is full-blown **nephritic syndrome** with oliguric acute renal failure; however, most patients have milder disease
- **Subclinical cases outnumber overt cases** by four- to tenfold during epidemics.

Nephrotic Syndrome

The **nephrotic syndrome** is characterized by **proteinuria** of > 3.5 g per 1.73 m^2 per 24 h (in practice, > 3.0 to 3.5 g per 24 h), **hypoalbuminemia, edema, hyperlipidemia, lipiduria, and hypercoagulability**

- Hyperlipidemia is a consequence of **increased hepatic lipoprotein synthesis**
- Hypercoagulability is caused by **increased urinary loss of antithrombin III, altered levels and/or activity of proteins C and S, hyperfibrinogenemia due to increased hepatic synthesis, impaired fibrinolysis, and increased platelet aggregability. Patients can develop spontaneous peripheral arterial or venous thrombosis, renal vein thrombosis, and pulmonary embolism**
- Clinical features that suggest acute **renal vein thrombosis** include sudden onset of flank or abdominal pain, gross hematuria, a left-sided varicocele (the left testicular vein drains into the renal vein), increased proteinuria, and an acute decline in GFR. Seen most commonly in **membranous glomerulonephritis**
- An increased susceptibility to infection may reflect low levels of IgG that result from urinary loss and increased catabolism
- Low serum calcium is a feature

Six entities account for greater than 90% of cases of **nephrotic syndrome** in adults: **Minimal change disease (MCD) is the commonest cause.** Focal and segmental glomerulosclerosis (FSGS), membranous glomerulopathy, MPGN, diabetic nephropathy, and amyloidosis

Renal biopsy is used for establishing a definitive diagnosis, guiding therapy, and estimating prognosis

Renal biopsy is not required in the majority of children with **nephrotic syndrome** as most cases are due to MCD and **respond to empiric treatment with glucocorticoids**.

Minimal Change Disease

- This glomerulopathy accounts for about 80% of **nephrotic syndrome** in **children**
- MCD (also called **nil disease, lipoid nephrosis, or foot process disease**) is so named because glomerular size and architecture are normal by light microscopy
- **Immunofluorescence studies are typically negative for immunoglobulin and C3**
- Mild mesangial hypercellularity and sparse deposits of C3 and IgM may be detected. Occasionally, mesangial proliferation is associated with scanty IgA deposits, similar to those found in IgA nephropathy.

- Bacterial peritonitis is common (SBP)
- **Electron microscopy reveals characteristic diffuse effacement of the foot processes of visceral epithelial cells**
- MCD is **highly steroid-responsive** and carries **an excellent prognosis.**

HUS (Hemolytic Uremic Syndrome)

- Occurs most commonly in **children**
- Follows gastroenteritis
- **Verocytotoxin producing *E. coli* 0157: H7** is most commonly encountered
- HUS is characterized by:
  - **Microangiopathic hemolytic anemia**
  - **Thrombocytopenia**
  - **Acute renal failure**
- The onset is preceded by acute diarrheal or dysenteric illness by shigella or *E. coli* **(Shigella dysentriae 1, Verocytotoxin producing *E. coli***
- **Serum complement may be low**
- There is no significant direct involvement of CNS. Direct microvascular injury affects kidneys significantly.

Cat-Scratch Disease

- Typical cat-scratch disease presents with **painful regional lymphadenopathy** persisting for weeks to months after a cat scratch
- **Only occasionally** a generalized lymphadenopathy may occur
- Tender regional lymphadenopathy occurs in 1–2 weeks after inoculation
- **Epitrochlear, axillary, pectoral and cervical lymph nodes** may be affected
- Lymph nodes become suppurative occasionally
- Lymphadenopathy persists for weeks

- ***Bartonella henselae*** is the most common organism
- 60% cases occur in children
- Most cases are caused by **scratch**
- CSD is a type of **granulomatous infection**
- **Azithromycin, doxycycline and ciprofloxacin** are used in treatment.

HIV in Pediatric Age Group

- Incubation period is **short**: 6 months to 1 year
- Recurrent infection with **typical organisms**
- **Kaposi sarcoma** is rare
- **NHL is common**
- **Parotid enlargement**

- Polyclonal hyperglobuliemia
- Lymphocytic interstitial pneumonitis is seen
- Ideal mode of delivery is **cesarean section**
- Breastfeeding is **contraindicated**

HIV in Newborn is Diagnosed by

- HIV DNA or RNA PCR
- HIV culture
- HIV p24 antigen
- Immune-dissociated p24 antigen

Commonest viral tumor: Warts
Commonest benign tumor in infancy is hemangiomas
Commonest malignant tumor in childhood: Leukemia

Acute Lymphoblastic Leukemia (ALL)

- Risk factors for ALL: Down's syndrome, Bloom's syndrome, Ataxia, telangiectasia
- ALL is the commonest childhood tumor
- PreB-cell type is the commonest
- CALLA antigen absent
- **TdT positive**
- **Commonest childhood malignancy: leukemia**
- **Mediastinal mass is a feature of T-cell ALL**

Specific cytogenetic abnormalities include:

- **t(15;17)** in **M3**
- **inv(16)** in **M4**
- **t(8;14)** in **mature B cell ALL**

FAB Classification of ALL

- L 1 Lymphoblasts with uniform, round nuclei and scant cytoplasm
- L 2 More variability of lymphoblasts; nuclei may be irregular with more cytoplasm than L 1
- L 3 Lymphoblasts have finer nuclear chromatin and blue-to-deep-blue cytoplasm with cytoplasmic vacuolization

FAB Classification of AML

- M 1 Undifferentiated myeloblastic; no cytoplasmic granulation
- M 2 Differentiated myeloblastic; a few to many cells may have sparse granulation
- M 3 Promyelocytic; granulation typical of promyelocytic morphology
- M 4 Myelomonoblastic; mixed myeloblastic and monocytoid morphology
- M 5 Monoblastic; pure monoblastic morphology
- M 6 Erythroleukemic; predominantly immature erythroblastic morphology, sometimes megaloblastic appearance
- M 7 Megakaryoblastic; cells have shaggy borders that may show some budding.

Favorable Outcome is seen in

Low WBC counts
3–7 years of age
Female gender
No organomegaly

Hyperdiploidy
DNA index >16
PreB-cell type

USMLE Case Scenario

A 4-year-old boy has severe pains in both his legs. On physical examination, his temperature is 37.7°C (99.8°F), blood pressure is 108/68 mm Hg, pulse is 96/min, and respirations are 17/min. He is noted to have marked pallor on his lips and palpebral conjunctiva. Numerous purpura and petechiae are noted on his skin. His spleen is palpable 3 cm below his left costal margin. Laboratory evaluation reveals a white blood cell count of 1600/mm^3; hemoglobin, 6.1 g/dl; and platelets, 36,000/mm^3. Diagnosis is: ALL

Neuroblastoma

- Most frequently presenting as a large abdominal mass and abdominal calcification
- The commonest **primary sites** are the **adrenal glands**
- It arises from **primordial neural crest cells** which form part of the sympathetic and rarely the parasympathetic nervous system
- May present as **lytic lesion in skull with sutural diasthesis**
- **Spontaneous regression** of malignant to benign ganglioneuroma occurs
- It occurs with increased frequency in **Beckwith-Wiedemann's syndrome, neurofibromatosis, nesidioblastosis and in fetal phenytoin syndrome**
- MC mass in **postmediastinum of children**
- The commonest presentation is with a **large firm abdominal mass often crossing the midline** but with the features of marrow infiltration including anemia, bruising, fever, lethargy and irritability. A syndrome **of opsoclonus/myoclonus** in which the patient has acute cerebellar and truncal
- **Metastasize to bones** most often
- **HVA, VMA, Catecholamines in urine are seen**
- **Associated with hypertension**

Wilms' Tumor

- Wilm's tumor is the **most common primary tumor of childhood**
- Wilms' tumor is also called **nephroblastoma**
- An embryonal adenomyosarcoma of the kidneys with **heterogenous** carcinomatous elements; the tumor occurs fetally and may not manifest itself clinically for years
- The diagnosis usually is made in children < 5 years of age, but the tumor occasionally can be detected in older children and rarely in adults
- The **most frequent presenting finding is a palpable abdominal mass**; other findings include abdominal pain, hematuria, fever, anorexia, nausea, and vomiting
- Hematuria (15 to 20% of cases) indicates invasion of the collecting system
- Hypertension may occur secondary to ischemia from renal pedicle or parenchymal compression.

- Wilms' tumor involves **chromosome 11**
- Wilms' tumor on pathology examination shows **tan to gray color** with areas of necrosis, hemorrhage and cyst formation
- Chemotherapy with **actinomycin D and vincristine**, with or without radiation therapy, is used, depending on the stage of the disease
- **It has the highest cure rates.**

- **ISOP (International Staging of Society of Pediatrics) is used for staging**

Wilms' tumor occurs in association with:

- **WAGR syndrome:** Wilms' Tumor, Aniridia, Genitourinary Anomalies, Mental Retardation
- **Denys-Drash syndrome:** Characterized by gonadal dysgenesis and nephropathy
- **Beck-Wiedemann syndrome**: Characterized by hemihypertrophy, renal medullary cysts, enlargement of adrenal cortex. Macroglossia, renomegaly, omphalocele, hypoglycemia (Lancet: 1997, 349 663)

Rhabdomyosarcoma (RMS)

- These are **the commonest soft tissue sarcomas** and arise from tissue which imitates striated muscle
- They make up over **75% of the soft tissue sarcomas**
- **Bladder and vaginal rhabdomyosarcomas predominantly occur in infancy and in the young**
- They are principally embryonal or botryoid in type
- Rhabdomyosarcomas can arise at any site in the body as mass lesions. They are usually nontender and the presentation depends on the site of the tumor
- **Head and neck**—about 10% of tumors arise in the orbit producing proptosis and ophthalmoplegia. These usually present early, before the tumor has metastasized. There is little lymphatic spread from the orbit and the prognosis is good. Parameningeal tumors (about 20%) arise from the nasopharynx, paranasal sinuses, middle ear, mastoid and pterygopalatine fossa, producing nasal airway and ear symptoms often with signs of secondary purulent or even bloody discharge
- **Commonest tumor of face in children**
- **Genitourinary tract**
- These usually arise in the bladder **(commonest)** and prostate (12%) presenting as a **polypoid mass** inside the bladder leading to hematuria, urinary obstruction or even extrusion of the tumor into the urethra in females. They tend to be localized. Prostatic tumors lead to bladder outlet obstruction. Constipation may arise from obstruction of the rectum. Bladder tumors tend to occur in younger patients. Vaginal and uterine rhabdomyosarcomas
- Most **are botryoid (grape-like)** and present with a mucousy and sometimes bloody discharge.

• MC Pediatric malignancy	• Leukemia > Lymphoma
• MC Neoplasm in children < 2 years	• ALL
• MC Solid tumor in children	• Brain tumors
• MC Renal neoplasm in children	• Wilms' tumor
• MC Soft-tissue tumor in children	• Rhabdomyosarcoma

The Eye in Relation to Medical Pediatrics and Clinical Genetics

- Diabetes mellitus
  - Diabetic retinopathy is exceptionally rare before puberty. Retinal screening examinations should be carried out annually from puberty. Cataract may develop as an acute feature of diabetes mellitus.
- Cystinosis
  - Small crystals may develop in the corneal epithelium, which may be painful.

The Eye in Relation to Medical Pediatrics and Clinical Genetics

- Cherry-red spot
  - In Tay-Sachs disease (GM2 type 1) ganglioside accumulation in retinal ganglion cells leads to a 'cherry-red spot' appearance
  - A cherry-red spot is also seen in Niemann–Pick disease type A (sphingomyelinase deficiency) and neuraminidase deficiency (sialidosis types 1 and 2)

- Corneal clouding
  - Mucopolysaccharidoses, all of which show corneal clouding, except MPSII and MPSIII
  - Mucolipidoses
  - Fucosidosis
  - Mannosidosis
- Wilson's disease
  - KF ring. Copper deposition in the peripheral cornea may be detected on slit-lamp examination
- Ophthalmology changes in leukemia
  - Retinal hemorrhages may be found in severe anemia and leukemia

- Marfan's syndrome
  - Screening for lens subluxation, ectopia lentis may be requested
- Neurofibromatosis
  - The ophthalmologist may provide diagnostic information in cases of suspected neurofibromatosis types 1 and 2 (NF1, NF2). **Lisch nodules of the iris** will be present in over 90% of children aged 5 years or more who have NF1. Children with confirmed NF1 also require regular screening examinations for **optic nerve gliomas and optic chiasma gliomas**
- In NF2, **posterior subcapsular cataract** is present in more than 50% of cases and is a useful diagnostic sign. Combined hamartoma of the retina and pigment epithelium is a less common ocular association of NF2.
- Tuberous sclerosis
  - Fundus examination for retinal hamartomas should be performed in children with seizures and delayed cognitive development. Hamartomas will be found in approximately 50% of patients with tuberous sclerosis.
- von Hippel-Lindau disease
  - Retinal angiomas are the earliest and the most common clinical features of von Hippel-Lindau disease. Careful annual fundus examination is required in order to detect early lesions, which are most often found in the mid-periphery.

Endocrinology

Rokitansky–Küster–Hauser Syndrome

- Girls with this condition are phenotypically normal, with a **46XX karyotype** and normal ovaries
- The degree of failure of development varies from total absence of Mullerian duct structures to varying degrees of uterine horn development, very occasionally including endometrium within a small blind uterine horn when the girl will present with severe cyclical abdominal pain
- Vaginal reconstruction either by the use of dilators or surgically using a loop of bowel is required.

Complete Androgen Insensitivity Syndrome (CAIS)

- Girls with CAIS have a **46XY karyotype**
- They are **often slightly taller** than average, have good breast development and sparse pubic and axillary hair
- The condition arises as a result of the cells of the mesonephric duct and genital tubercle **failing to respond to circulating androgens** with the resulting failure of development of male external genitalia
- Production of **Mullerian inhibitory factor (MIF)** causes degeneration of the fallopian tubes, uterus and upper third of the vagina
- Treatment is by **removal of the testes** because of the 5% risk of malignancy and vaginal reconstruction. **Long-term estrogen replacement** is required to protect against osteoporosis.

Glycogen Storage Diseases

1. Von Gierke's disease	• Glucose-6-phosphatase deficiency	• **Protruding abdomen because of marked hepatomegaly, renomegaly, hypotrophic muscles, truncal obesity, a rounded 'doll face'** • **Severe symptomatic hypoglycemia is frequent, often occurring during the night or after even short periods of reduced caloric intake.**

		• **Even minor delays or reduction of carbohydrate intake may provoke hypoglycemic attacks that are accompanied by lactic acidosis and hyperuricemia** • **Muscles not involved**
2. Pompe disease	• Lysosomal alpha-1,4-glucosidase deficiency • (Acid maltase deficiency (AMD)	• **Profound muscle hypotonia, weakness, hyporeflexia, glossomegaly, massive cardiomyopathy without murmurs but no hepatomegaly except with cardiac failure** • The ECG shows a huge QRS complex, **left or biventricular hypertrophy** and shortened PR interval.
3. Cori disease	• Debranching enzyme	• Mild **hypoglycemia, hepatomegaly**
4. Anderson's disease	• Branching enzyme	• **Infantile hypotonia, cirrhosis**
5. McArdle9i's disease	• Muscle phosphorylase	• **Increasing intolerance for strenuous exercise** • Strenuous muscle activity is accompanied by **severe cramps** and may be followed by **myoglobinuria,** which can precipitate **anuria and renal failure**.
6. Hers' disease	• Liver phosphorylase	• **Pronounced hepatomegaly, without splenomegaly** • **Protuberant abdomen due to muscle hypotonia are the most striking features**
7. Tarui's disease	• Phosphofructokinase deficiency	

Glucose-6-Phosphatase Deficiency (GSD Type IA: von Gierke's Disease)

- The most conspicuous clinical findings are a **protruding abdomen because of marked hepatomegaly, hypotrophic muscles, truncal obesity, a rounded 'doll face' and short stature.** Because glucose-6-phosphatase activity is required for both glycogenolysis and gluconeogenesis, severe symptomatic hypoglycemia is frequent, often occurring during the night or after even short periods of reduced caloric intake
- Even minor delays or reduction of carbohydrate intake may provoke **hypoglycemic attacks** that are accompanied by lactic acidosis. The **liver may be enlarged at birth**; its size increases gradually and may achieve a total span of 15–20 cm.

Lysosomal alpha-1, 4-glucosidase deficiency (GSD type II: Pompe Disease)

- Deficiency of this enzyme, also called **acid maltase deficiency (AMD)**, leads to a generalized glycogen storage disease
- Pompe disease is characterized by the rapid onset in the first months of life of **profound muscle hypotonia, weakness, hyporeflexia, glossomegaly, massive cardiomyopathy without murmurs but no hepatomegaly except with cardiac failure**. The ECG shows a huge QRS complex, **left or biventricular hypertrophy** and shortened PR interval. The clinical course is downhill with **cardiopulmonary failure** or pneumonia leading to death in the first 2 years.

McArdle's Disease

- This disorder is characterized by **increasing intolerance for strenuous exercise**
- Strenuous muscle activity is accompanied by **severe cramps** and may be followed by **myoglobinuria**, which can precipitate **anuria and renal failure**. In middle life, the fatigue increases and muscle wasting and weakness predominate.

- The **serum CPK** may be permanently or intermittently **elevated**
- Muscle exercise is normally accompanied by release of lactate and of inosine, hypoxanthine and ammonia through the purine nucleotide cycle. In myophosphorylase deficiency, lactic acid production is blocked and release of the purine nucleotide cycle compounds is exaggerated. The ensuing myogenic hyperuricemia is one of the characteristic features of defects of muscle glycogenosis.

- **Phosphorylase activity must be assayed in muscle;**
- **Liver phosphorylase** is presumably **normal,** as is glucose homeostasis
- DNA mutation analysis is useful in myophosphorylase deficiency as there are common mutations
- Treatment is symptomatic and consists of the avoidance of strenuous exercise. 'Carbo-loading' and a high-protein diet are of some help and glucose should always be taken during exercise. Strenuous exercise is always a risk.

Galactosemia

- Three enzyme deficiencies implicated
  - GPUT deficiency (Galactose 1 Po_4 uridyl transferase) most common
- AR condition:
  - Newborn presents with failure to thrive, vomiting, diarrhea and jaundice
  - Hepatomegaly
  - Cataract (oil-drop cataract)
  - Mental retardation
  - *E. coli* sepsis
- Cataract because of accumulation of galactitol
- Reducing sugar seen in urine
- Rapid diagnosis and rapid removal of galactose from diet are essential.

USMLE Case Scenario

A newborn born to a couple appears normal at birth, but develops mild vomiting and diarrhea accompanied by jaundice and hepatomegaly within the first few weeks of life. Within five months, the baby has obvious difficulty in vision as per mother which was diagnosed as cataracts. By one year of age, he has developed mental retardation.

Lipid Metabolism Disease	Deficiency
• Fabry's	• Alpha galactoside A (Ceramide trihexoside accumulates)
• Niemann-Pick's	• Sphingomyelinase (RBCs appear as foam cells)
• Tay-Sach's	• Hexosaminidase A
• Sandhoff	• Hexosaminidase A and B
• Krabbe leukodystrophy	• Galactocerebrosidase
• Metachromatic leukodystrophy	• Arylsulfatase A
• Gaucher's	• Glucocerebrosidase
• Tangier's	• Lipid metabolism disturbed (Low alpha-lipoprotein)

Fabry Disease

- This is an **X-linked disorder**
- Results from a variety of mutations in the **alphagalactosidase gene**
- Clinically, the disease manifests with:
  - **Angiokeratomas** (telangiectatic skin lesions)
  - Hypohidrosis
  - Corneal and lenticular opacities
  - Acroparesthesia
  - **Small-vessel disease** of the kidney, heart and brain

- **Angiokeratomas** are punctate, dark red to blue-black, flat or slightly raised, usually symmetric, and do not blanch with pressure. They range from barely visible to several millimeters in diameter and have a tendency to increase in size and number with age
- **The acroparesthesia** can be debilitating in childhood and adolescence, with a tendency to decrease after the third decade. **Episodic agonizing, burning pain** of the hands, feet and proximal extremities can last from minutes to days and can be precipitated by exercise, fatigue, or fever. Abdominal pain can resemble that from appendicitis or renal colic
- **Renal:** Casts and microscopic hematuria can occur early, whereas proteinuria, isosthenuria, and progressive renal dysfunction occur in the second to fourth decades. **Progressive renal failure occurs and requires transplantation**
- **CVS:** Hypertension, left ventricular hypertrophy, anginal chest pain with or without myocardial ischemia or infarction, and congestive heart failure can occur in the third to fourth decades
- **Hypohidrosis or anhidrosis, angiokeratomas, and the typical corneal and lenticular lesions provide a presumptive diagnosis in males.**

Amino Acid Metabolism Disease	Deficiency
• Phenylketonuria	• Phenylalanine hydroxylase
• Alkaptonuria	• Homogentisic acid oxidase
• Homocystinuria	• Cystathionine synthetase
• Hartnup	• Decreased trytophan absorption, increased excretion

Phenylketonuria	**Phenylalanine hydroxylase**	• **Mental retardation**, seizures, hyperactivity • Tremor • Microcephaly, hypopigmentation • Failure to grow are features • Convulsions seen • **Musty urine** • **Ferric chloride test+** • **Guthrie's test +**
Alkaptonuria	**Homogentisate oxidase**☞	• **Urine darkens on standing** • Pigmentation of the sclerae and ears • Generalized darkening of the concha, anthelix, and helix of the ear are typical • Pigmentation of heart valves, larynx, tympanic **membranes and skin** • **Arthritis**

Maple syrup urine disease (MSUD)	Branched chain α ketoacid dehydrogenase	• **Valine, leucine, isoleucine defect** • Maple syrup urine • Lethargic baby, loses weight, letosis, coma
Homocystinuria	Cystathionine synthetase	• Mental retardation, MI, osteoporosis • Dislocation of lens • It is inherited as **AR** trait • Patients can be responsive to **Vitamin B6** (pyridoxine)
Albinism	Tyrosinase	• White hair • Photosensitivity • Strabismus • Nystagmus • Photophobia

Alkaptonuria

- Alkaptonuria is inherited as an **autosomal recessive trait**
- Patients have **minimally increased concentrations of homogentisic acid in blood** because it is rapidly cleared by the kidney. However, homogentisic acid accumulates in cells and body fluids.

- Its oxidized polymers bind to collagen, leading to the progressive deposition of a gray to **bluish-black pigment**
- **Clinical Manifestations:** Alkaptonuria may go unrecognized until middle life when degenerative joint disease develops. Prior to this time, the tendency of the **patient's urine to darken on standing** may go unnoticed, as may slight pigmentation of the sclerae and ears. Foci of gray-brown scleral pigment and generalized darkening of the concha, anthelix, and finally, helix of the ear are typical. Ear cartilages may be irregular and thickened
- **Ochronotic arthritis** is heralded by pain, stiffness, and some limitation of motion of the hips, knees, and shoulders. Acute arthritis may resemble rheumatoid arthritis, but small joints are usually spared. Limitation of motion and ankylosis of the lumbosacral spine are common late manifestations. **Pigmentation of heart valves, larynx, tympanic membranes, and skin occurs, and occasional patients develop pigmented renal or prostatic calculi.** Degenerative cardiovascular disease may be increased in older patients

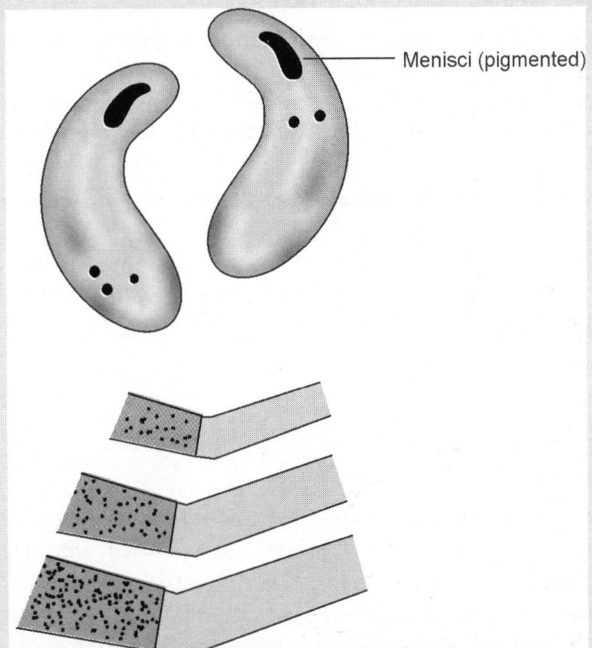

- **Diagnosis:** The diagnosis is usually made from the **triad of degenerative arthritis, ochronotic pigmentation, and urine that turns black upon alkalinization**
- Homogentisic acid in urine may be identified presumptively by other tests: after addition of **ferric chloride**, a purple-black color is observed; treatment with **Benedict's reagent** yields a brown color; addition of a saturated **silver nitrate** solution produces an intermediate black color
- These screening tests can be confirmed by chromatographic, enzymatic, or spectrophotometric determinations of homogentisic acid
- X-rays of the lumbar spine show **degeneration and dense calcification of the intervertebral disks and narrowing of the intervertebral spaces (bamboo-like appearance)**
- There is no specific treatment for ochronotic arthritis. Joint manifestations might be mitigated if homogentisic acid accumulation and **deposition could be curbed by dietary restriction of phenylalanine and tyrosine**. Ascorbic acid impedes oxidation and polymerization of homogentisic acid in vitro, but the efficacy of this form of treatment has not been established.

Homocystinuria

- Homocystinuria (elevated urinary levels of homocysteine) is a hallmark of several disorders in the metabolism of **sulfur-containing amino acids**.

- The classic form of the disease which is caused by **defective activity of the enzyme cystathionine beta-synthase (CBS)**
- This **autosomal recessive enzyme defect** is the most common cause of homocystinuria
- The classic presentation of cystathionine beta-synthase deficiency includes **Marfanoid habitus, developmental delay, lens dislocation and predisposition for blood clotting**.

- Presentation is usually in the first decade with the exception of **embolism which may occur later**
- **The most characteristic feature of this disorder is subluxation of the ocular lens. Mental retardation is common,** although not always present
- Most patients have **osteoporosis and skeletal abnormalities** similar to those seen in Marfan's syndrome. In homocystinuria, however, the joints tend to be limited in mobility rather than hypermobile
- There is also lenticular subluxation in both conditions; however, in Marfan's syndrome, the lens is usually displaced upwards, whereas **in homocystinuria it is displaced downwards and medially**
- **Diagnosis**
- In CBS deficiency, **elevated homocysteine can be detected in both urine and blood**. Levels of methionine are usually also elevated and levels of cystine are reduced. Because homocysteine is unstable, testing should be done on fresh urine
- Screening tests for homocystinuria **using cyanide nitroprusside reagent** are available, but are not completely sensitive. Measurement of total homocysteine in blood is useful
- Because homocystinuria can be caused by several genetic defects, it is important to specifically confirm the diagnosis of **CBS deficiency by measuring the enzyme in liver, cultured skin fibroblasts or lymphoblasts**
- **Treatment**
- **All patients should initially be treated with large doses (100–500 mg/day) of pyridoxine** to determine their degree of vitamin responsiveness
- Those who do not respond may be treated with a diet low in methionine and supplemented with L-cysteine. All patients should probably receive **high doses of folic acid**. In addition, the compound **betaine** may be used to aid in the conversion of homocysteine to methionine.

Cystinuria

- Cystinuria is a complex genetic disorder involving at least three alleles governing **dibasic amino acid COAL (cystine ornithine, arginine and lysine) transport**
- Renal tubular cells demonstrate an inability to take up cystine from their brush border, but can do so from the basolateral surface. Because the excretion of cystine can exceed the amount filtered, there is evidence of net cystine secretion by the tubule
- The clinical manifestations are confined to individuals in whom the cystine concentration in urine exceeds its solubility product and leads to **calculus formation**. Almost all untreated homozygotes will experience calculi at some time in their lives, a quarter of them before 20 years of age. Obstruction and infection cause lasting damage to the urinary tract. Patients present with renal colic or episodes of hematuria
- **The stones are radiopaque** because of their high sulfur content. Ultrasound is a good way of identifying calculi in both the renal collecting system and the bladder but often misses calculi in ureters
- **Microscopy of the urine reveals flat hexagonal birefringent crystals** under polarized light, and the **Nitroprusside test** for urinary disulfides is positive. Confirmation is by quantification of urinary proteins
- The mainstay of treatment is to keep the **urine volume sufficiently high** so that cystine is kept below its solubility maximum
- A second line of treatment, additional to and not a substitute for the first, is to **prescribe bicarbonate or citrate** to ensure that the early morning urine pH is alkaline
- Increase in cystine solubility can be achieved by forming a thiol is cysteine disulfide with agents such as **D-penicillamine.**

Mucopolysaccharidoses (MPS)

The various forms of MPS result from deficiencies of lysosomal enzymes needed for glycosaminoglycan (GAG) catabolism. GAGs are long-chain, complex carbohydrates that are linked to proteins in connective tissue.

MPS IH (Hurler Disease)

- This a severe **autosomal recessive disorder**
- Results from mutations of **L-iduronidase**
- **Progressive mental retardation, hepatosplenomegaly, skeletal malformations, and cardiopulmonary compromise** typically lead to death during the first decade.

- Affected individuals appear normal at birth but exhibit accelerated growth and mild coarsening of facial features in the first year. Subsequently, there is slowing of growth, leading to short stature
- In the first 2 years, clinical diagnosis is suggested by hepatosplenomegaly, **corneal clouding,** coarse features, large tongue, joint stiffness, and characteristic dysostosis multiplex on skeletal X-rays
- Instability of the cervical vertebral bodies can lead to paralysis, particularly with subluxation on hyperextension

MPS II (Hunter Syndrome)

- This is an **X-linked recessive disorder**
- Results from mutations in the gene encoding **iduronate sulfatase**
- Clinically, MPS IH and II are similar, **though corneal clouding is absent in MPS II**
- Clinical manifestations range from severe CNS and visceral involvement with death in late childhood to milder forms with normal CNS function and survival into adulthood

MPS IIIA, IIIB, IIIC, and IIID (the Sanfilippo Syndrome)

- Skeletal defects and hepatosplenomegaly are less pronounced in this group of MPS variants, though progressive behavioral problems, mental retardation, and seizures are present
- Affected patients can survive into the third or fourth decade with progressive CNS disease

MPS IV (Morquio Syndrome)

- These MPS variants are autosomal recessive disorders characterized by **severe skeletal diseases** that resemble the spondyloepiphyseal dysplasias
- There is extreme shortening of the trunk due to multiple vertebral collapses
- The long bones are relatively spared. Joint laxity can lead to osteoarthritis-like destruction of the joints
- Upper cervical spinal cord compression due to atlantoaxial instability predisposes to subluxation and paralysis. Many patients have mitral valve insufficiency that can be functionally significant

MPS VI (Maroteaux-Lamy Disease)

- Mutations in the **arylsulfatase B gene** cause this autosomal recessive disorder. Although clinically variable, the general phenotype resembles Hurler disease. Intelligence is normal, and the life span can extend beyond three decades. Cardiac valvular disease and progressive pulmonary hypertension are frequent causes of death.

Different Skull Appearances

- **Salt and pepper skull**
- **Hair on end appearance of skull**
- **Rain drop pattern of skull**
- **Punched out skull lesions**

Lesch-Nyhan Syndrome

A **complete deficiency of HPRT**, the Lesch-Nyhan syndrome, is characterized by:

- **Hyperuricemia**
- **Self-mutilative behavior**
- **Choreoathetosis**
- **Spasticity**
- **Mental retardation**

Kelley-Seegmiller syndrome

- A **partial deficiency of HPRT**, the **Kelley-Seegmiller syndrome**, is associated with hyperuricemia but no central nervous system manifestations
- In both disorders, the hyperuricemia results from urate overproduction and can cause **uric acid crystalluria, nephrolithiasis, obstructive uropathy, and gouty arthritis**
- **Purine metabolic defect**
- **HPRT catalyzes the reaction that combines PRPP and the purine bases hypoxanthine and guanine to form the respective nucleoside monophosphate IMP or GMP and pyrophosphate.**

Menkes' Disease

- **Menkes' disease is** also known as **kinky hair disease**
- **X-linked neurodegenerative disease**
- **Impaired copper transport.** Occurs Named after noting the similarity of kinky hair to the **brittle wool of Australian sheep raised in areas with copper-deficient soil,** he demonstrated abnormal levels of copper and ceruloplasmin in these patients
- In Menkes' disease, transport of dietary copper from intestinal cells is impaired, leading to the **low serum copper levels.** Abnormal copper transport in other cells leads to **paradoxical copper accumulation in duodenal cells, kidney, pancreas, skeletal muscle, and placenta**
- **Hair changes:** Abnormal kinky hair, eyebrows, and eyelashes. Often lightly or abnormally pigmented; can be white, silver, or gray
- Associated are abnormal **facies, progressive cerebral degeneration, connective-tissue abnormalities. Loose skin** at the nape of the neck and over the trunk
- **Joint hypermobility, polypoid masses, which can be multiple, in the gastrointestinal tract, umbilical and inguinal hernias, which can be bilateral, bladder diverticula, dilated ureters, emphysema, arterial rupture, brachial, lumbar and iliac artery aneurysms, internal jugular vein aneurysms**
- Menkes' kinky hair syndrome is associated with the defecive functioning of several copper-dependent enzymes due to impaired copper absorption, transport, or metabolism. **Lysyl oxidase** is a copper-requiring enzyme
- **Decreased lysyl oxidase (LO) activity** accounts for the **connective-tissue fragility** and **vascular abnormalities** in Menkes' disease.

Congenital Hypothyroidism

- **Open** posterior fontanelle
- **Large** posterior fontanelle, sluggishness are a feature of newborn hypothyroid
- **Absent social smile, absent eyebrows are also features of a hypothyroid**
- **Growth retardation, delayed puberty, umbilical hernia are a feature**

Other important features:

- Constipation
- Pallor
- Hypothermia
- Cold extremeties in children are a common feature
- Large tongue
- Rough, dry skin
- Hypotonia
- Causes prolonged physiological jaundice
- Causes delayed skeletal maturity

- **Epiphyseal dysgenesis** is a feature
- **Seminiferous tubule dysgenesis is also seen**
- **Pendred syndrome is hypothyroidism + deafness**
- **Pendred syndrome has goiter + sensorineural type deafness**

Remember Related Terminology Frequently asked

Arnold-Chiari malformations are congenital herniations of hindbrain structures into the spinal canal

In type I Arnold-Chiari malformation, the **cerebellar tonsils** herniate into the foramen magnum

In type II Arnold-Chiari malformation, **parts of the hindbrain, cerebellar vermis, and fourth ventricle** herniate into the foramen. This second type is commonly associated with meningomyeloceles

Other neonatal presentations associated with Arnold-Chiari malformation include **hydrocephalus** (because of cerebrospinal fluid obstruction) and **brainstem dysfunction** (causing stridor and poor swallowing). Milder cases may present later in life with spinal cord or cerebellar symptoms.

'Holoprosencephaly' is a complex malformation of the brain such that only a single large monoventricular cerebral hemisphere exists. It is characterized by **failed septation of the midline forebrain structures and is frequently accompanied by midfacial abnormalities.** Associated syndromic (including Smith-Lemli-Opitz, Hall-Pallister, pseudotrisomy 13) and structural anomalies are common. **Trisomy 13** is the most commonly identified cause.

'Porencephaly' is a severe cleft in the brain that allows the ventricles to communicate with the subarachnoid space.

It is a vascular malformation

Seen in cerebral infarction, Dandy-Walker syndrome.

Dandy-Walker malformation: Dandy-Walker malformation (DWM) describes **agenesis or hypoplasia of the cerebellar vermis with communication between the fourth ventricle and the cisterna magna, due to obstruction of foramen of Magendie and Lushka.**

Lissencephaly is synonymous with **'smooth brain.'**

- A rare condition in which there is **defective neuronal migration** from 12th week of gestation onwards resulting in **'Agyria'**
- Such children are severely handicapped
- **Viral infections**, mutation of **'Reelin gene'** on **'chromosome 7'** occurs
- It occurs in association with:
  - Miller-Dieker syndrome
  - Walker-Warburg syndrome and
  - Muscle eye brain diseases

Remember the commonest cause of obstructive hydrocephalus in children is aqueductal stenosis.

USMLE Case Scenario

An 8-month-old weak girl is brought to the emergency clinic by her parents because of intractable vomiting. The girl was born at home to a mother who did not receive any prenatal care. MRI studies reveal the following congenital malformations in the CNS: small posterior fossa, downward displacement of the cerebellar vermis and medulla through the foramen magnum, syringomyelia, and myelomeningocele.

Arnold-Chiari malformations

Arnold-Chiari malformations are among the most frequent congenital anomalies of the CNS. The small posterior fossa is a crucial diagnostic feature of Arnold-Chiari type 2. This change is probably responsible for downward displacement of the cerebellar vermis and medulla through the foramen magnum. This leads to obstruction of the CSF flow and hydrocephalus. Important associated abnormalities include lumbar myelomeningocele and syringomyelia.

Hydrocephalus

- **Internal or noncommunicating hydrocephalus:** Excess of CSF **within the ventricular system** up to the level of the outlet foramina of the fourth ventricle. The common sites of obstruction are at the outlet foramina of the fourth ventricle, the aqueduct of Sylvius or at the foramen of Monro
- **External or communicating hydrocephalus:** An **increase in the ventricular volume and the subarachnoid spaces** of the cranium and spine. The sites of obstruction are at the arachnoid villi or in the basal cisterns
- **Panventricular hydrocephalus:** Dilation of the lateral, third and fourth ventricles (in aqueduct stenosis, the fourth ventricle is small or of normal size—**'triventricular hydrocephalus'**). An *isolated fourth ventricle* **('double compartment hydrocephalus' or 'trapped fourth ventricle')** occurs when there is outlet obstruction from that ventricle and stricture of the aqueduct.

- **Unilateral hydrocephalus:** Abnormal dilation of the body, frontal and/or posterior horn of the lateral ventricle on one side. This may be due to compression of the ventricular system on the opposite side, obstruction to one foramen of Monro, slit ventricle syndrome or hemiparenchymal atrophy
- **Slit ventricles:** A **reduction in the size of the ventricular system seen on CT scan, usually in response to excessive CSF drainage**. The slit ventricle *syndrome* is distinguished from radiological slit ventricles by the presence of symptoms and clinical signs attributable to this overdrainage.

Bacterial Meningitis

The classic triad of symptoms of bacterial meningitis includes:
- Fever
- Stiff neck
- Alterations of mental status

Poor feeding is the most common presentation of neonatal meningitis

Physical signs are:

- **Kernig's sign**
- **Brudzinski's sign**
- **Nuchal rigidity**

Rash is present in only **a minority** of cases of bacterial meningitis

Classic cerebrospinal fluid findings among patients with bacterial meningitis include:
- White blood cell count more than 1000 cells per microliter
- More than 80% neutrophils on white blood cell differential
- Elevated protein levels
- Reduced glucose levels
- **Group B *streptococcus*** most common cause in neonates
- ***E. coli* and *listeria* are other common organisms**
- **Aseptic meningitis is caused by: mumps, polio, coxsackie viruses**
- **LOW CSF protein is seen in:**
  - **Infants**
  - **Pseudotumor cerebri**
  - **Recurrent LP**

USMLE Case Scenario

An 18-month-old boy is brought to the emergency room because of fever and rash. Two days ago, he was fine. An ENT physician diagnosed otitis media and prescribed amoxicillin. During the interim period, the child has developed a nonblanching erythematous rash on his face, trunk, and extremities. Currently, the child is very irritable with temperature of 103.5 °F. He turns drowsy.

Meningitis in a young

A febrile, irritable, inconsolable infant with rash and fever with an altered state of alertness even in the absence of meningeal signs should be suspected to have meningitis.

Seizures in Childhood

- **Commonest cause of convulsions in childhood is febrile seizures**
- **Subtle seizures are the commonest type of seizures in newborn**

- **Phenobarbitone is the DOC for neonatal convulsions**
- **Diazepam is the DOC for status epilepticus in childhood**
- **Diazepam is the DOC for prophylaxis of seizures in childhood**

Febrile Seizures

Hypoxic ischemic encephalopathy is mc cause of seizure in newborne

Commonest type of seizure in newborn: Subtle

- **Seen between 9 months and 5 years. Do not usually last more than 10 minutes**
- **Good prognosis**
- **Generalized in nature**
- **EEG normal after 2 weeks**
- **Fifty percent recurrence**

Asterixis:
- Consists of coarse arrhythmic lapses of sustained posture
- It is usually related to metabolic disorders and is most easily seen when the patient's arms are outstretched
- Asterixis occurs bilaterally

Lennox-Gastaut syndrome:
- It is a variant of petit mal epilepsy
- Consists of intellectual impairment, distinctive slow spike and wave pattern, and atonic postural lapses followed by minor tonic-clonic spasms.

Pseudoseizures:
- Are parts of conversion disorder and are not directly related to the use of antipsychotics
- They are very much like real seizures except that there are no aura and no EEG abnormalities
- The movements are asynchronous and nonstereotyped and they occur when the person is awake.

Infantile Spasms

Constitute a unique and very serious epilepsy syndrome confined to infants. The usual characteristic features of this syndrome are:
- **Tonic or myoclonic seizures**
- **Hypsarrhythmic EEGs**
- **Mental retardation**

Infantile spasms may vary considerably in their clinical manifestations. Some seizures are characterized by brief head nods, whereas other seizures consist of violent flexion of the trunk, arms, and legs. Most patients have more than one seizure type. Infantile spasms can be classified into three major groups:
1. **Flexor:** Flexion of the neck, trunk, arms, and legs. Spasms of the muscles of the upper limbs result in either adduction of the arms or a self-hugging motion, or adduction of the arms to either side of the head with the arms flexed at the elbow
2. **Extensor:** A predominance of extensor muscle contractions, which produce abrupt extension of the neck and trunk, along with extensor abduction or adduction of the arms, legs, or both
3. **Mixed flexor-extensor:** Flexion of the neck, trunk, and arms and extension of the legs, or flexion of the legs and extension of the arms with varying degrees of flexion of the neck and trunk.

Electroencephalography

Infantile spasms are usually associated with markedly abnormal EEGs. The most common interictal abnormality is hypsarrhythmia. There are several variations:
- Hypsarrhythmia with interhemispheric synchrony
- Hypsarrhythmia with a consistent focus of abnormal discharge
- Hypsarrhythmia with episodes of attenuation
- Hypsarrhythmia consisting primarily of high-voltage slow activity with few sharp waves or spikes.

Batten's Disease (Neuronal Ceroid Lipofuscinosis, NCL)

- The ceroid lipofuscinoses are characterized by the storage of **lipopigments** that present morphological and tinctorial similarities with **ceroid and lipofuscin**
- The chemical nature of these pigments is unknown
- They normally accumulate in neurones with age and present in external tissues out with the CNS

Twin-Twin Transfusion Syndrome

- The syndrome develops when there is **unbalanced shunting of blood** from one twin (the donor) to the other (the recipient) through arteriovenous anastomoses in the placenta
- **The donor twin** progressively becomes **anemic, growth-restricted, and oliguric.** The resulting oligohydramnios can be so severe that the donor becomes shrouded in the amniotic membrane ('stuck twin')
- **The recipient twin** becomes **plethoric, polyuric, and develops cardiomegaly and cardiac failure** manifest as hydrops. The polyuria leads to hydramnios which predisposes to miscarriage.

The Gray Baby Syndrome

- Immaturity of liver function leads to jaundice and also to the newborn's inability to tolerate drugs which are usually excreted via the biliary tree
- The 'gray baby' syndrome is due to **increased free and conjugated chloramphenicol levels** in the serum, leading to vomiting, poor sucking, respiratory distress, abdominal distention, diarrhea.

Physical Abuse

- A physically abused child is defined as **'any child who receives physical injury (or injuries) as a result of acts (or omissions) usually on the part of his parents or guardians'**
- The definition includes actual or likely physical injury to a child, or failure to prevent physical injury (or suffering) to a child
- Deliberate poisoning, suffocation and Munchausen syndrome by proxy are usually included in this category
- Physical abuse (nonaccidental injury) is usually **perpetrated by the child's carers**. It has been recognized as an assault, i.e. abuse, from when 'battered babies' were first described
- Common pattern of injuries in infancy includes **skull, rib and long bone fractures, bruising anywhere (but note that the head, neck and chest are more common), retinal hemorrhages and subdural hematomas**

Battered child syndrome (BCS) is found at every level of society, although the incidence may be higher in low-income households, where adult caregivers suffer greater stress and social difficulties, without having had the benefit of higher education. The child abuser most often injures a child in the heat of anger that he was also often abused as a child himself. The incessant crying of an infant or child may trigger abuse. Symptoms may include a delayed visit to the emergency room with an injured child; an implausible explanation of the cause of a child's injury; bruises that match the shape of a hand, fist or belt; cigarette burns; scald marks; bite marks; black eyes; unconsciousness; bruises around the neck; and a bulging fontanel in infants.

A four-month-old infant is brought to a physician because of increased lethargy and irritability. The father of the infant says that the child rolled off the bed and fell on the cemented floor. According to the father, the child has been previously healthy and is up-to-date on his vaccinations. He has been meeting his development milestones. While in office, the patient develops a seizure. Initial examination shows tense fontanellae and bruises on limbs.

Shaken Baby Syndromes

- **This term is applied to a clinical picture in which the causative mechanism of injury is thought to be severe repeated shaking, probably with impact in most cases**
- **Important symptoms include drowsiness, unconsciousness, poor feeding, irritability, fits, pallor, floppiness, and vomiting, sudden collapse, breathing difficulties, signs of other injury, large head, apnea and delayed development**
- **Infants may present as 'cot death'**
- **Diagnosis is commonly missed or delayed.**

Sexual Abuse

'The sexual exploitation of children is referred to as the involvement of dependent, developmentally immature children and adolescents in sexual activities that they do not fully comprehend, are unable to give informed consent to and that violates the social taboos of family roles'.

Contact involves touching, fondling or oral contact of breast or genitals. There may be insertion of fingers or objects into vulva or anus. Masturbation may be by adult of him/herself in the presence of the child, including ejaculation onto the child, by adult of child or by child of adult. Intercourse is vaginal, anal or oral, whether actual or attempted in any degree. This is usually with an adult as the active party but, in some cases a child may be encouraged to penetrate the adult. Rape is attempted or achieved penile penetration of the vagina. Other genital contacts include intercrural intercourse where the penis is laid between the legs or genital contact with any part of the child's body, e.g. a penis rubbed on child's thigh

Prostitution involves any of the above abuses which includes the exchange of money, gifts or favors and applies to both boys ('rent boys') and girls

Noncontact abuse involves exhibitionism (flashing), pornography (photographing sexual acts or anatomy), showing pornographic images (photographs, films, videos) and erotic talk (telling children titillating or sexually explicit stories). Other sexual exploitations include sadistic activities, e.g. burning a child's buttocks or genital area.

Refsum Disease

- The cardinal manifestations of Refsum disease include **retinitis pigmentosa, cerebellar ataxia and polyneuropathy**
- The underlying metabolic etiology for Refsum disease is a deficiency of **phytanoyl-coenzyme A (CoA) hydroxylase**, an enzyme that catalyzes an essential step in phytanic acid degradation
- Deficiency of this enzyme results in the **accumulation of phytanic acid**
- **The sensory-motor polyneuropathy** associated with Refsum disease typically begins in the distal lower extremities and, if untreated, progresses to involve the upper extremities and trunk. Usually become evident later than the retinal degeneration and polyneuropathy
- Additional clinical features can include **sensorineural hearing loss, anosmia, cardiac conduction abnormalities and cardiomyopathy and skeletal manifestations (epiphyseal dysplasia, shortening or elongation of the third or fourth metatarsals, hammer toes)**
- **Cardiomyopathy is a frequent cause of sudden death** in untreated patients
- **Therapy: Because phytanic acid is dietary in origin, therapy focuses on diets low in phytanic acid.**

Nail-patella Syndrome

- Nail-patella syndrome is an **autosomal dominant disorder** consisting of **hypoplasia or absence of patellae, dystrophic nails, dysplasia of the elbows and iliac horns, and renal disease**
- The nephropathy is usually benign and includes microhematuria and mild proteinuria, which usually appear in adolescence or young adulthood. Some patients develop nephrotic syndrome and mild hypertension and are at risk of progression to end-stage renal failure
- Remember chronic glomerulonephritis is mc cause of childhood hypertension.

Kasabach–Merritt Syndrome

- In the neonate, **large or multiple hemangiomas are occasionally associated with a generalized bleeding disorder caused by the trapping of platelets within them, which produces a profound thrombocytopenia**
- A course of prednisone, 2–4 mg/kg per 24 h can effect dramatic improvement
- If this fails, embolization of the hemangioma can be considered.

Sacrococcygeal Teratoma

- **The sacrococcygeal teratoma** is the **commonest teratoma** presenting in the **neonatal period**
- They tend to be large and **protrude from the space between the anus and the coccyx**
- The lesion is usually covered in skin but the most protuberant part may be necrotic due to vascular compromise
- The tumor may also extend up into the pelvis and a large retrorectal component is palpable in all the cases. In a presacral teratoma, there is no protrusion behind the anus and the presentation may be later in the first year of life

- The tumor may be both solid and cystic in nature. **A very large tumor may give rise to dystocia** and, if diagnosed antenatally, is best delivered by cesarean section
- **Treatment is excision within the first few days of life**
- **Adulthood recurrence** of benign or malignant elements may occur.

Prune Belly Syndrome (Triad syndrome)

- This consists of **deficiency of the anterior abdominal wall muscles, cryptorchidism and urinary tract deformities.** The abdominal muscular deficiency is mainly in the lower abdomen, the whole abdominal wall taking on the wrinkled appearance of a prune.

Infants of Diabetic Mothers

- **Hypoglycemia**
- **Hypocalcemia**
- **Hypomagnesemia**
- **Respiratory distress syndrome**
- **Hyperbilirubinemia**
- **Polycythemia**
- **HOCM**
- **VSD, ASD, transposition of great vessels, caudal regression**
- **Lazy left colon**

Caudal Regression Syndrome

- It is a rare disorder characterized by abnormal development of the lower spine end of the developing fetus
- A wide range of abnormalities may occur, including partial absence of the tailbone end of the spine causing no apparent symptoms, to extensive abnormalities of the lower vertebrae, pelvis, and spine
- Neurological impairment as well as inability to control urination and bowel movements (incontinence) may occur in severe cases.

Physiological pubertal gynecomastia:
- May involve one or both breasts
- Spontaneous regression may occur
- All hormones are normal

Musculoskeletal System

Systemic Juvenile Rheumatoid Arthritis

- More **common in boys**
- **Maculopapular rash** with clearing in center
- Hepatosplenomegaly and lymphadenopathy occur
- Rheumatoid factor **negative**
- **Pericarditis and interstitial lung disease** occur

Polyarticular JRA (Juvenile Rheumatoid Arthritis)

- **Most common chronic arthritis** in children is **JRA**
- **Bilateral symmetric fleeting polyarthritis** of small joints is **not always** characteristic of polyarticular JRA (Juvenile Rheumatoid Arthritis).

- Spine, knee, wrist and hip joints may also be involved
- Arthritis with fever, hepatosplenomegaly, lymphadenopathy, toxic look favor diagnosis of rheumatoid factor positive JRA
- Disease onset is **below 16 years** of age
- More common in girls
- Five or more joints affected
- It is not essential for rheumatoid factor to be positive
- Highest risk of **'Chronic Uveitis'** is in ANA seropositive oligoarticular JRA
- **Etanercept** is indicated for reduction of signs and symptoms of moderately to severely active polyarticular-course juvenile rheumatoid arthritis not adequately responsive to disease-modifying antirheumatic drugs.

Fractures in Children

- The **periosteum is extremely strong** in children
- Children's **bones are much more resilient** and less brittle than those of adults
- Bending moments applied to the bone of a child may cause a **Greenstick fracture**, in which there is distraction of the cortex on the convex side and compression of bone on the concave side (**Cortex intact.**)

Ehlers-Danlos Syndrome

Ehlers-Danlos syndrome (EDS) consists of a **group of disorders of connective tissue** characterized by:

- **Joint hypermobility plus fragility and laxity of the skin**
- These conditions are characterized by abnormalities in collagen genes resulting in the **production of abnormal collagen and consequent tissue fragility**
- EDS has **soft, hyperextensible skin, 'cigarette paper' scars, easy bruising and marked hypermobility**. EDS type II is similar to type I but less severe
- Also seen is serious involvement with a **high incidence of rupture of the arteries, the colon or the pregnant uterus**. Management of EDS consists of patient education and support, with genetic counseling for the more severe forms.

Osteogenesis Imperfecta

OI is also called brittle bone disease or **'Lobstein syndrome'**

- Basic defect is in **collagen type 1**
- It is transmitted either as AD or AR Inheritance
- **Type 1 OI** is the **most common type**

- **OI is inherited autosomal dominant trait mostly**
- **'Blue sclera'** is present in several types of OI but not all
- **Saturn ring, arcus juvenilis, hypermetropia and retinal detachment**
- The sclera is **normal** in some types of OI
- Feature of OI is **generalized osteopenia** with recurrent fractures and skeletal deformity. Fracture healing, however, is normal. Fracture in utero may be seen
- Laxity of joint ligaments leads to **hypermobility**

Most common site of acute osteomyelitis in infants: Hip

Most common site of acute osteomyelitis in children: Femur

Acute Pyogenic Arthritis (SEPTIC)

- Joint infection with pyogenic organisms occurs as a result of **hematogenous seeding of the joint,** extension of adjacent osteomyelitis or penetrating wounds of the joint
- Hematogenous pyarthrosis is most commonly observed in children under the age of 5 years
- ***S. aureus* is the most common etiologic agent**, followed by *Hemophilus influenzae, Streptococcus, Gonococcus*, and *Pneumococcus*
- Acute pyarthrosis is **almost always monarticular**
- Patients with immune deficiency may present with multiple joint involvement
- **The hip joint** is the most frequently involved

• A male presents with triad of lytic bony lesions on skull, diabetes Insipidus and exomphalos	**Hand-Schullerchristian disease**
• An infant presents with failure to thrive, pancytopenia. Bones are brittle and fracture easily. Defect is found in osteoclasts	**Infantile osteopetrosis**
• A two-year-old presents with multiple fractures in different stages of healing brought by overconcerned parents	**Battered baby syndrome**
• A six-year-old with b/l symmetrical fractures and blue sclera. Bones are osteopenic and brittle	**Osteogenesis imperfecta**

Sexual precocity in girls with polyostotic fibrous dysplasia and cutaneous pigmentation constitutes **'McCune-Albright syndrome'.** Fibrous dysplasia
McCune-Albright syndrome represents a phenotypic spectrum of disorders caused by **activating mutations in the GNAS1 gene**

Duchenee Muscular Dystrophy

- In Duchenee muscular dystrophy, inheritance **is X-LINKED Recessive**
- Disease of sarcolemmal proteins
- Defect lies in **dystrophin gene** and results in abscenced of dystrophin protein
- Onset is typically below **5 years of age**
- Proximal limb muscles are involved and **pseudohypertrophy** of these muscles occurs
- Patient on standing tries to climb on himself**. (Gower's sign)**
- Characteristic pathological features are:

Necrosis of muscle fibers
Muscle fibers of varying size
Fibrosis
Fatty infiltration

The **less severe** form is the **Becker's dystrophy. Features are:**
- Less common
- Less severe
- Not absence but decreased and altered dystrophin protein
- Later onset
- Cardiac involvement is rare
- May have normal life span
- CPK levels are diagnostic

Floppy Baby Syndrome is caused by

- **Werrding-Hoffman's disease**
- **Central core disease**

- **Mitochondrial myopathies**
- **Down's syndrome**
- **Ehler-Danlos syndrome**
- **Clostridium botulinum**

Slipped Capital Femoral Epiphysis (SCFE)

- **It is displacement of 'Proximal Femoral Epiphysis'**
- **Common in children (obese) in 2nd decade**
- **Pain is the initial and most common complaint**
- **'Epiphysis' slips 'downwards and posteriorly'**
- **Limping is the associated feature**
- **Flexion, abduction and medial rotation are limited**
- **Diagnosis is by: Trethowan's sign, Capener's sign**
- **Trendelenburg's sign may be positive**

Perthe's Disease

- **It is a chronic disease with ischemia of upper end of femur causing 'avascular necrosis.'**
- **Osteochondritis of femoral head**
- **Boys are affected more**
- **Not obese usually**
- **Pain is the initial and most common complaint**
- **Limping is the associated feature**

Ewing's Sarcoma

- **Affects children <15 years usually**
- **Diaphysial tumor**
- **Onion skin lesions on X-ray**
- **Translocation (t11:22)**
- **Mimics osteomyelitis**
- **PAS positive material (glycogen) found**
- **Most radiosensitive bone tumor**

Remember Most Common Causes

• Fungal ball in lung cavity	• **Aspergillosis**
• Bronchiolitis in children	• **Respiratory Syncytial virus**
• Croup	• **Parainfluenza virus**
• Viral pneumonia in adults/children	• **Influenza/Resp syncytial virus**
• **Tropical** hemoptysis	• ***Paragonimus westermanii***
• Meningitis in less than 2 months old	• ***E Coli*, Beta Hemolytic Streptococci**
• Meningitis in 2 months to 12 years	• ***H. Influenzae***
• Meningitis after 12 years	• ***Meningococccus***
• Meningitis in recurrent CSF leaks	• **Streptococcus pneumonia**

• **Endemic** hematuria	• *Schistosoma haemotobium*
• Infection in burns	• *Pseudomonas*
• Bockhart's impetigo	• *Staphylococcus*
• Parotitis	• *Staphylococcus*
• Boil	• *Staphylococcus*

Buzz Phrases

- Cherry-red spot on macula **'without'** hepatosplenomegaly: **Tay-Sachs disease**
- Cherry-red spot on macula **'with'** hepatosplenomegaly: **Niemann-Pick's disease**
- **Bronze skin: Hemochromatosis**
- **Heliotrope rash: Dermatomyositis**
- **Salty tasting infant: Cystic fibrosis**
- **Honey ingestion: Infant botulism**
- **Currant jelly stool: Intussusception**
- **Currant jelly sputum: Klebsiella Pneumoniae**

Clinical Cases Frequently Asked

- **A child presents with:**
  - **Hepatosplenomegaly**
  - **Abdominal distension**
  - **Jaundice, anemia and adrenal calcification**

Wolman's disease

- **A 7-year-old girl with:**
  - Nonproductive cough
  - Mild stridor for 3 months' duration
  - Patient is improving but suddenly developed wheeze-productive cough, mild fever and hyperlucency on CXR and PFT shows obstructive curve
  - Diagnosis is:

Bronchiolitis obliterans

- A **term male baby** weighing 3.5 kg, born of uncomplicated pregnancy, developed **respiratory distress at birth**
  - **Not responding to surfactant, echofinding revealed nothing abnormal**
  - **X-ray showed ground glass appearance and culture is negative**
  - **Apgars are 4 and 5 at 1 and 5 minutes respectively**
  - **History of one-month female sibling died before**
  - The diagnosis is:

Neonatal pulmonary alveolar proteinosis

An infant with:

- Cleft lip
- Cleft palate
- Polydactyly
- **Microcephaly with holoprosencephaly**
- **Ectodermal scalp defect,** is suffering from:

Trisomy 13

- A 3-year-old boy
  - With normal developmental milestones with delayed speech and difficulty in communication and concentration.

- He is not making friends
- Most probable diagnosis is:

Autism

- **A 3-year-old boy presents with**
  - **Fever; dysuria and gross hematuria**
  - Physical examination shows a **prominent suprapubic area which is dull on percussion**
  - **Urinalysis reveals red blood cells but no proteinuria**

Most likely diagnosis is:

Posterior urethral valves

- **An 8-day-old breastfed baby presents with:**
  - **Vomiting, poor feeding and loose stools**
  - On examination, the heart rate is 190/minute, blood pressure 50/30 mm Hg, respiratory rate 72 breaths/minute and capillary refill time 4 seconds
  - Investigations show hemoglobin level of 15 g/dl, Na 120 mEq/l, K 6.8 mEq/l, bicarbonate 15 mEq/l, urea 30 mg/dl and creatinine 0.6 mg/dl. The most likely diagnosis is:

Acute tubular necrosis

- A male infant presented with:
  - **Distension of abdomen shortly after birth with passing of less meconium**
  - Subsequently a full-thickness biopsy of the rectum was performed. The rectal biopsy shows **lack of ganglion cells. Likely diagnosis is:**

Hirshspring's disease

- A **2-year-old boy** has **vitamin D-resistant rickets**. His investigations revealed:
  - Serum Calcium–9 mg/dl
  - Phosphate–2.4 mg/dl
  - Alkaline phosphatase–1041 IU
  - Normal intact parathyroid hormone and bicarbonate–22 mEq/L

The most probable diagnosis is:

Hypophosphatemic rickets

- **A 3-month-old male** infant developed otitis media, for which he was given a course of **Cotrimoxazole**. A few days later:
  - He developed **extensive peeling of the skin;**
  - **There were no mucosal lesions and the baby was not toxic**

The most likely diagnosis is:

Staphylococcal scalded skin syndrome

- **A two-year-old girl child** is brought to the outpatient department (OPD) with features of:
  - **Hand-wringing stereotype movements**
  - **Impaired language and communication development**
  - **Breath-holding spells**
    - Poor social skills and deceleration of head growth after 6 months of age

The most likely diagnosis is:

Rett's syndrome

- **An 11-month-old boy**, weighing 3 kg
  - Has **polyuria, polydipsia and delayed motor milestones**
  - Blood investigations show creatinine of 0.5 mg/dl, potassium 3 mEq/l, sodium 125 mEq/l, chloride 88 mEq/l, calcium 8.8 mg/dl, pH 7.46 and bircarbonate 26 mEq/l
  - Ultrasonography shows **medullary nephrocalcinosis**

The most likely diagnosis is:

Barter's syndrome

- **A 13-year-old boy** is referred for **evaluation of nocturnal enuresis** and **short stature.**

His blood pressure is normal

- The hemoglobin level is 8 g/dl
- Urea 112 mg/dl
- Creatinine 6 mg/dl
- Sodium 119 mEq/dl
- Potassium 4 mEq/l
- Calcium 7 mg/dl
- Phosphate 6 mg/dl and alkaline phosphatase 300 U/l
- Urinalysis shows trace proteinuria with hyaline casts; no red and white cells are seen
- Ultrasound shows bilateral small kidneys and the micturating cystourethrogram is normal. The most likely diagnosis is:

Nephronophthisis

- An **infant** presents with:
  - **Hypotonia and**
  - **Hyporeflexia**
  - **During his intrauterine period, there were polyhydramnios and decreased fetal movements**

Most probable diagnosis is:

Spinal muscular atrophy

- **12-year-old** presented with
  - **Gross hematuria with 80%**
  - **Dysmorphic RBCs 2 days after an attack of upper respiratory tract infection.** Diagnosis is:

IgA nephropathy

- **A neonate** presents with
  - **Jaundice and clay: colored stools**
  - **Liver biopsy shows giant cells.** Diagnosis is:

Neonatal hepatitis with extrahepatic biliary atresia

- **An 8-year-old child** presents with:
  - Lethargy
  - **Multiple epiphyseal breaks**
  - **Wormian bones with growth retardation** and
  - Mental retardation. Diagnosis is:

Hypothyroidism

- **An 8-year-old female child** following URTI developed:
  - **Maculopapular rash** on the jaw spreading onto the trunk which **cleared on the 3rd day** without desquamation and
  - **Tender postauricular and suboccipital lymphadenopathy**

The diagnosis is:

Rubella

- A **month-old-HIV positive child following URTI:**
  - **Developed sudden onset of breathlessness**
  - The chest X-ray shows **hyperinflation**
  - **The O_2 saturation was greater than 90%.** The diagnosis most likely is:

Brochiolitis

Important 'Pediatric' Syndromes

- **Lowe's syndrome:** Hypophosphatemic rickets + aminoaciduria + CNS and eye defects
- **Potter's syndrome:** Pulmonary hypoplasia + renal hypoplasia + ear deformities
- **Cat eye syndrome:** Partial trisomy 22
- **Floppy baby syndrome:** Due to clostridium botulinum
- **Dandy-Walker syndrome:** Due to obstruction of Foramina of Luschka and Megendie

- **McLeod syndrome:** Unilateral pseudoemphysema occurring in childhood
- **William's syndrome:** Infantile hypercalcemia
- **Caudal regression syndrome:** Seen in diabetics

Timothy Syndrome

- **It is a multisystem disorder** characterized by cardiac, hand/foot, facial, and neuro developmental features
- The two forms are type 1 (classic) and type 2, a rare form caused by mutations in an isoform of the same gene
- **Cardiac findings** include a **rate-corrected QT interval of between 480 ms and 700 ms and congenital heart defects (patent ductus arteriosus, patent foramen ovale, ventricular septal defect, tetralogy of Fallot, hypertrophic cardiomyopathy)**
- **Hand/foot findings** are unilateral or bilateral cutaneous **syndactyly variably involving fingers two (index), three (middle), four (ring), and five (little) and bilateral cutaneous syndactyly of toes two and three**
- **Facial findings** include **flat nasal bridge, low-set ears, thin upper lip, and round face**. Neuropsychiatric involvement includes **global developmental delays and autism spectrum disorders**. Ventricular tachyarrhythmia is the leading cause of death, followed by infection and complications of intractable hypoglycemia
- **Diagnosis/testing:** Timothy syndrome is diagnosed by clinical features and by the presence of one of the three known mutations in **CACNA1C,** the gene encoding the CaV1.2 calcium channel. **Molecular genetic testing is available on a clinical basis.**

Landau-Kleffner Syndrome

- **It is a childhood disorder.** A major feature of LKS is the **gradual or sudden loss of the ability to understand and use spoken language**
- All children with LKS have **abnormal electrical brain waves** that can be documented by an electroencephalogram (EEG), a recording of the electric activity of the brain
- Approximately 80 percent of the children with LKS have **one or more epileptic seizures that usually occur at night**. Behavioral disorders such as hyperactivity, aggressiveness and depression can also accompany this disorder
- LKS occurs most frequently in normally developing children who are between 3 and 7 years of age. For no apparent reason, these children begin having trouble understanding what is said to them. Doctors often refer to this problem as **auditory agnosia or 'word deafness'**. The auditory agnosia may occur slowly or very quickly. Parents often think that the child is developing a hearing problem or has become suddenly deaf. **Hearing tests, however, show normal hearing. Children may also appear to be autistic or developmentally delayed**
- The inability to understand language eventually affects the child's spoken language which may progress to a complete loss of the ability to speak (mutism)
- Children who have learned to read and write before the onset of auditory agnosia can often continue communicating through written language.

Fetal Alcohol Syndrome

Remember the features:

- **Microcephaly**
- **Retarded growth**
- **Maxillary hyperplasia (imp)**
- **Small eyes**
- **Mental retardation**
- **Cardiac malformation**
- **Hyperkinetic movements**

'Gray Baby' Syndrome

- It is a disorder that occurs in newborns who have either received **chloramphenicol** immediately after birth or whose mothers have received the medication close to the delivery date
- Symptoms typically appear in the following order: **Abdominal distention with or without emesis, progressive pallid cyanosis, and vasomotor collapse**, frequently accompanied by irregular respiration

- Death can occur as early as a few hours after onset of signs and symptoms
- Other symptoms may include: **Loose, greenish stools, a refusal to suck, ashen color (implied by the name gray baby syndrome) and lactic acidosis.**

Wiskott-Aldrich Syndrome

- It is an **X-linked recessive immunodeficiency** disease characterized by the **triad of thrombocytopenia (hemorrhage may be the presenting complaint), eczema, and recurrent infections** (often respiratory)
- The children have **defects in both T- and B-cell function**, and are vulnerable to pyogenic bacteria, viruses, fungi, and *Pneumocystis carinii*
- These patients have severe disease, and formerly often dies by the age of 15
- Survivors past age 10 have a 10% incidence of cancer, particularly **lymphoma and acute lymphoblastic leukemia**
- Modern treatment consists of splenectomy, **continuous antibiotic therapy, IV immunoglobulin, and bone marrow transplantation.**

Kallmann's Syndrome

- It is an isolated gonadotropin deficiency or familial hypogonadotropic hypogonadism and can present with primary amenorrhea
- Primary amenorrhea is defined as the absence of menses in a female by the age of 16
- Associated findings in Kallmann's syndrome may include **anosmia or hyposmia, color blindness, and cleft lip or cleft palate**. These findings are attributable to the fact that during embryogenesis, the GnRH neurons originally develop in the epithelium of the olfactory placode and normally migrate into the hypothalamus
- Physical examination may **reveal absent to minimal breast development**. Treatment of the patient with Kallmann's syndrome is with exogenous estrogen and progestin replacement therapy. If pregnancy is desired, ovulation induction can be brought about with the pulsatile administration of exogenous GnRH.

Caudal Regression Syndrome

- It is a rare disorder characterized by abnormal development of the lower spine end of the developing fetus
- A wide range of abnormalities may occur including partial absence of the tailbone end of the spine causing no apparent symptoms, to extensive abnormalities of the lower vertebrae, pelvis, and spine
- Neurological impairment as well as inability to control urination and bowel movements (incontinence) may occur in severe cases.

CHARGE Syndrome

Includes

- **Colobomas**
- **Heart defects**
- **Atresia, (choanal)**
- **Retardation**
- **Genitourinary abnormalities**
- **Ear anomalies**

The etiology of the CHARGE syndrome is unknown, but it may involve altered morphogenesis during the second trimester of pregnancy. It is not genetically transmitted and is not associated with a teratogenic effect of any substance.

Constriction Band Syndrome

- This condition occurs sporadically and is alternatively known as **Streeter's dysplasia** or **amniotic band syndrome**
- The etiology remains uncertain but **constriction by intrauterine amniotic bands** remains a hypothesis as well as localized failures of formation. Bands can be multiple and are asymmetric
- Structures proximal to the band are normal but distally they may be deformed or even amputated
- Tight bands can cause severe distal edema and vascular compromise with urgent 'Z'-plasty release required in the neonatal period.

Sturge-Weber Syndrome

- **Facial nevus flames** (usually in the distribution of **1st branch of trigeminal nerve**)
- **Contralateral focal seizures**
- **Calcification (rail-road track)** of the cortex and subcortical structures
- **Glaucoma on the same side** as skin lesions
- **Mental retardation** due to cerebral atrophy

Segawa Syndrome

Segawa syndrome, also called **dopa-responsive dystonia**, is an **inherited disease that can cause physical rigidity and developmental delay**. There are two forms—mild and severe.

In the mild form, symptoms typically begin in childhood. Children develop **jerky movements that quickly progress to physical rigidity**. These children show **spastic movements, and make very little voluntary movement**. If untreated, children with Segawa syndrome may have **expressionless faces, drooping eyelids, tongue tremors, and drooling problems.** They will show both mental and physical developmental delays. Some children with Segawa syndrome show a **'diurnal' pattern, meaning their symptoms are more or less severe on alternate days.**

The severe form of the disease will appear in infancy, **usually before six months of age**. Affected infants have **delayed motor skills, weakness in the chest and abdomen, rigidity in the arms and legs, and problems with movement**. These children will eventually have **learning disabilities, problems with speech, and behavioral/psychological problems**. In addition, some people with the disease have problems with their **autonomic nervous system**, which regulates unconscious functions, such as body temperature regulation, digestion, blood sugar level, and blood pressure. Treatment of the severe form of the disease is often less successful

Segawa syndrome is caused by a **deficiency in an enzyme called tyrosine hydroxylase**. Without it, the amino acid tyrosine cannot properly be converted to dopamine, a key neurotransmitter in the brain. Dopamine is important for many functions, including muscle control and cognition.

USMLE Case Scenario

A 3-day-old infant presents to the emergency department with vomiting, lethargy, hypotonia, and jaundice. Physical examination reveals hepatomegaly and neurologic depression. A full sepsis evaluation is undertaken and the Gram stain of the cerebrospinal fluid reveals gram-negative organisms of the following. The best additional laboratory test to obtain is:

1. Erythrocyte galactose-1-phosphate
2. RBC transketolase
3. Tyrosinase levels
4. Thyroid profile

Ans. 1. Erythrocyte galactose-1-phosphate

USMLE Case Scenario

Clinical feature of microphthalmos, hypertelorism, colobomas, mental retardation, microcephaly are seen in Cat's Eye Syndrome, which involves:

1. Chromosome 11
2. Chromosome 22
3. Chromosome 3
4. Chromosome 13

Ans. 2. Chromosome 22

USMLE Case Scenario

Fetal alcohol syndrome is:

1. Mental retardation, macrocephaly, macrophthalmia, midfacial hyperplasia and cardiac defects
2. Mental retardation, microcephaly, microphthalmia, midfacial hyperplasia and cardiac defects
3. Mental retardation, macrocephaly, microphthalmia, midfacial hyperplasia and cardiac defects
4. Mental retardation, microcephaly, microphthalmia, midfacial hypoplasia and cardiac defects

Ans. 4. Mental retardation, microcephaly, microphthalmia, midfacial hypoplasia and cardiac defects

USMLE Case Scenario

An inborn error in amino acid metabolism with congenital cataract and systemic manifestation of mental retardation, dwarfism, osteomalacia, muscular hypotonia, frontal prominence are a feature of:

1. Alkaptonuria
2. Phenylketonuria
3. Lowe's syndrome
4. Cystinuria

Ans. 3. Lowe's syndrome (oculocerebrorenal) syndrome

USMLE Case Scenario

Discrete maculopapular lesions that become confluent as they spread from 'head to toe' associated with cough, conjunctivitis, coryza and spots in oral cavity are a feature of:

1. Rubella
2. Pox
3. CMV
4. EBV
5. HSV
6. Measles
7. Rabies
8. Erythema infectiousum

Ans. 6. Measles

Typical presentation of measles, which is caused by a paramyxovirus

USMLE Case Scenario

IgA deficiency recurrent respiratory and gastrointestinal infections are common. IgA levels are always low and levels of IgG subclass 2 may be low. Treatment involves:

1. Immunoglobulins in low dose
2. Immunoglobulins in high dose
3. Immunoglobulins with azathioprine
4. No immunoglobulins

Ans. 4. No immunoglobulins

Do not give immunoglobulins, which may cause anaphylaxis due to development of anti-IgA antibodies.

USMLE Case Scenario

Chediak-Higashi syndrome is usually an autosomal recessive disorder characterized by giant granules in neutrophils, infections, and often oculocutaneous albinism. It is caused by a defect in:

1. Microtubule polymerization
2. Lysozome overactivity
3. Mitochondrial dysfunction
4. Peroxisome dysfunction

Ans. 1. Microtubule polymerization

USMLE Case Scenario

A 33-year-old female brings her newborn child to a pediatrician. The child is seen to have a flat, salmon-colored lesion on his glabella. On crying, the lesion becomes darker. The most likely diagnosis is:

1. Cafe au lait spots
2. Erythema toxicum
3. Cavernous hemangioma
4. Salmon patch

Ans. 4. Salmon patch

USMLE Case Scenario

A newborn is seen to have amastia, radial nerve aplasia and aplasia of pectoralis muscle. The child is most likely to have:

1. Waardenburg syndrome
2. Patau's syndrome
3. Poland syndrome
4. Edward syndrome

Ans. 3. Poland syndrome

USMLE Case Scenario

A two-month-old boy is brought by her mother to a pediatrician with projectile vomiting for the last three days. The child is found to have eczematous rash and has a peculiar musty odor. The doctor advices the mother that there is a chance that the baby might have mental retardation as well. Most likely diagnosis is:

1. Cystinuria
2. Alkaptonuria
3. Fragile X syndrome
4. Phenylketonuria

Ans. 4. Phenylketonuria

USMLE Case Scenario

A male infant has initial Apgar scores of 5 and 6 at 1 and 5 minutes following birth by normal vaginal delivery at 30 weeks gestation. However, increasing respiratory distress in the next hour requires intubation and positive pressure ventilation. Two months later, the infant is finally taken off the ventilator, but still does not oxygenate normally. Which of the following diseases has this infant most likely developed?

1. Bronchial asthma
2. Bronchiectasis
3. Tracheoesophageal fistula
4. Bronchopulmonary dysplasia

Ans. 4. Bronchopulmonary dysplasia

The BPD is a complication of the treatment for neonatal respiratory distress. The positive pressure ventilation with the higher FIO2's and the prolonged intubation contribute.

USMLE Case Scenario

An infant presents with jaundice, hypoglycemia, hepatosplenomegaly. He has poor weight gain. He has been adviced galactose-free diet. The infant is at risk for sepsis particularly by:

1. *Streptococcus*
2. *Staphylococcus*
3. *E. coli*
4. *Klebsiella*
5. *Pseudomonas*
6. *H. influenza*

Ans. 3. *E. coli*

USMLE Case Scenario

A 32-weeks gestation infant is seen to develop tachypnea and nasal flaring. An immediate CXR shows hazy lungs with a reticular glandular pattern with air bronchogram. Most likely the child suffers from:

1. Transient tachypnea of newborn
2. Diaphragmatic hernia
3. Persistent fetal circulation
4. Surfactant deficiency
5. Meconium aspiration

Ans. 4. Surfactant deficiency

USMLE Case Scenario

Periventricular calcifications are seen in a premature along with decreased size of head. The child is jaundiced and physical examination reveals hepatosplenomegaly. Most likely TORCH infection is:

1. HSV
2. CMV
3. Toxoplasmosis
4. Rubella

Ans. 2. CMV

USMLE Case Scenario

An ophthalmologist notices chorioretinitis and cataract in a child with a decreased head size. CT scan reveals cortical atrophy. Cutaneous scars and maldevelopment of a limb are noted on general physical examination. Most likely cause is:

1. HSV
2. CMV
3. Toxoplasmosis
4. Varicella

Ans. 4. Varicella

USMLE Case Scenario

In VACTERL, anomalies are seen as V–Vertebral anomalies, A-Anal anomalies, C-Cardiovascular anomalies, T-Tracheal anomalies, E-Esophageal anomalies, R-------, L-Limb anomalies. R stands for:

1. Retinal anomalies
2. Renal anomalies
3. Regional anomalies
4. Right pectoral deformities

Ans. 2. Renal anomalies

USMLE Case Scenario

A 4-year-old boy is seen by a pediatrician in an Ilinos pediatric unit. The boy is weak with decreased muscle tone and hair, which is sparse. Previously a dermatologist had treated him for dermatitis, which is generalized. The boy is seen to be edematous. The most likely diagnosis is:

1. Iron deficiency
2. Protein malnutrition
3. Caloric malnutrition
4. Protein caloric malnutrition

Ans. 4. Protein caloric malnutrition (Kwashiorkor)

USMLE Case Scenario

A 3-year-old child is seen to have a large tongue. Ultrasound shows a large pancreas and a large kidney. At birth, he had a large fontanella and feeding problems. Currently he is having a low blood sugar. Most likely cause is:

1. Glucose 6 phosphate deficiency
2. Hers disease
3. Wilms tumor
4. Beckwith-Weidemann Syndrome

Ans. 4. Beckwith Wiedemann Syndrome

USMLE Case Scenario

Defect in ataxia telangiectasia gene is present on:

1. Short arm of chromosome 1
2. Long arm of chromosome 1
3. Short arm of chromosome 11
4. Long arm of chromosome 11

Ans. 4. Long arm of chromosome 11

USMLE Case Scenario

In Leopard Syndrome, O is:

1. Ocular hypotelorism
2. Ocular hypertelorism
3. Oculogyric crisis
4. Oculomotor palsy

Ans. 1. Ocular hypotelorism

USMLE Case Scenario

Pterygium coli is a feature of:

1. Down's syndrome
2. Klinefelter's syndrome
3. Edwards' syndrome
4. Patau syndrome
5. Turner syndrome
6. Waardenburg syndrome
7. Eagle-Barrett syndrome

Ans. 5. Turner syndrome

USMLE Case Scenario

USG scan of a pregnant female reveals absence of kidneys on both sides in a fetus at 30th week. Most likely cause can be:

1. Poland syndrome
2. Potter syndrome
3. Prune belly syndrome
4. Patau syndrome

Ans. 2. Potter syndrome

USMLE Case Scenario

A pediatrician examines an infant. An infant is found to have poor suckling, floppy and is with poor head control. On making repeated ocular muscle movements, his eyes seem to get tired and he cannot make further ocular movements. An associated anomaly can be:

1. Mydriasis
2. Miosis
3. Proptosis
4. Ptosis

Ans. 4. Ptosis. Condition is MG

USMLE Case Scenario

Wilson's disease is also called hepatolenticular degeneration. Correct statement about Wilson's disease is:

1. Autosomal recessive disease involving sympathetic ganglia with high serum copper and ceruloplasmin levels
2. Autosomal dominant disease involving basal ganglia with high serum copper and ceruloplasmin levels
3. Autosomal recessive disease involving basal ganglia with low serum copper and high ceruloplasmin levels
4. Autosomal recessive disease involving basal ganglia with low serum copper and ceruloplasmin levels

Ans. 4. Autosomal recessive disease involving basal ganglia with low serum copper and ceruloplasmin levels

USMLE Case Scenario

Dancing eyes and dancing feet may be a feature of:

1. Wilms' tumor
2. Pheochromocytoma
3. Embryonal rhabdomyosarcoma
4. Neuroblastoma

Ans. 4. Neuroblastoma

USMLE Case Scenario

A 2-year-old child is brought to a pediatrician for extensive bruising and recurrent epistaxis. The disease occurs in an X-linked recessive manner and Factor IX replacement is effective in treatment. Most probably the disease is:

1. von Willebrand disease
2. Hemophilia A
3. ITP
4. TTP
5. Scurvy
6. Christmas disease

Ans. 6. Christmas disease (i.e. Hemophilia B)

USMLE Case Scenario

Thrombocytopenia is not a feature of:

1. TAR syndrome
2. Wiskott-Aldrich syndrome
3. DiGeorge syndrome
4. Kasabach/Merrit syndrome

Ans. 3. DiGeorge syndrome

USMLE Case Scenario

Diamond-Blackfan syndrome is:

1. Congenital, aplastic anemia often with low MCV
2. Congenital pure red blood cell anemia often with elevated MCV
3. Accquired I thrombocytopenia often with elevated MCV
4. Acquired pure red blood cell anemia often with low MCV

Ans. 2. Congenital pure red blood cell anemia often with elevated MCV

USMLE Case Scenario

A 2-year-old boy who had developmental dysplasia hip at birth is brought to a pediatric clinic with a small-sized foot. The foot is medially rotated with medial rotation of the heel. The child as such is having:

1. Talipes equinovalgus
2. Pes cavus
3. Pes planus
4. Talipes equinovarus

Ans. 4. Talipes equinovarus (clubfoot)

USMLE Case Scenario

A 15-year-old overactive boy has localized swelling and tenderness in his upper shin near the tibial tubercle.
He says that pain gets exaggerated on exertion and is relieved at rest. Radiograph reveals a soft tissue swelling at the site. Rest of skeletal survey is normal. The said disease is a:

1. Benign tumor
2. Malignant tumor
3. Bursitis
4. Apophysitis
5. Synovitis

Ans. 4. Apophysitis (Remember Osgood-Schlatter disease)

USMLE Case Scenario

A 5-year-old child is seen by a pediatrician. The child has severe pain in his knee. He walks with a limp and is febrile. The hip is tender, warm and swollen. The most likely diagnosis is:

1. Streptococcal osteomyelitis of knee
2. Staphylococcal osteomyelitis of knee

3. Syphlitic arthritis of knee
4. Osteoarthritis of knee
5. Congenital dislocation of hip
6. Slipped capital femoral epiphysis
7. Septic arthritis of hip

Ans. 7. Septic arthritis of hip (Remember hip pain is referred to knee)

USMLE Case Scenario

A 3-month-old child from a far off area presents with cough which is paroxysmal in nature. There is no whoop. Facial petechea and subconjunctival hemorrhage are seen. His mother says that the child has not been immunized till date. Blood investigations reveal absolute lymphocytosis. Most likely diagnosis is infection by:

1. *Streptococcus*
2. *Staphylococcus*
3. *Mycoplasma*
4. *Yersinia*
5. *Influenza virus*
6. *Bordetella*
7. *H. influenzae*
8. *Measles virus*
9. *Mycobacterium*
10. *Mycoplasma*

Ans. 1. *Streptococcus*

USMLE Case Scenario

A boy is brought to you with unilateral conjunctivitis, preauricular lymphadenopathy and cervical lymphadenopathy. The doctor confirms the disease as perinaud occuloglandular syndrome. The causative agent is:

1. *Streptococcus*
2. *Staphylococcus*
3. *Mycoplasma*
4. *Yersinia*
5. *Influenza virus*
6. *Bordetella*
7. *H. influenzae*
8. *Bartonella*
9. *Mycobacterium*
10. *Mycoplasma*

Ans. 6. *Bordetella*

USMLE Case Scenario

A DNA virus is found to be a causative agent for a child who presents with red cheeks followed by appearance of a lacy rash in trunk and proximal extremities with sparing of palms and soles. The said infection is:

1. Herpes
2. Measles
3. Mumps
4. *Erythema infectiosum*
5. *Erythema induratum*
6. *Exanthem subitum*

Ans. 4. *Erythema infectiosum*

USMLE Case Scenario

A 12-month-old infant presents with rash after the onset of fever. The rash is red-colored begining in trunk and spreads to neck and proximal extremities. The said infection is:

1. Exanthem subitum caused by HHV 5
2. Exanthem subitum caused by HHV 6
3. Exanthem subitum caused by HHV 7
4. Exanthem subitum caused by HHV 8

Ans. 2. Exanthem subitum caused by HHV 6

USMLE Case Scenario

A 22-year-old male medical student reports to emergency because of fever and severe headache. He says that he developed a rose-colored rash in his ankles which was maculopapular initially and was present on palms as well as soles which responds to tetracycline. He came back from Virginia after he was camping along with his friends. None of his friends is affected in a similar way. Most likely the causative agent is a:

1. Bacteria
2. Virus
3. Fungus
4. Rickettsia

Ans. 4. Rickettsia (Rocky mountain spotted fever)

USMLE Case Scenario

Miliary sudamina, Pastia lines, Sandpaper texture and Strawberry tongue are a feature of infection by:

1. *Staphylococcus*
2. Streptococci
3. Pneumococci
4. Meningococci
5. Gonococci

Ans. 2. Streptococci, Scarlet fever

USMLE Case Scenario

A 3-year-old child presents with painful enlargement of salivary glands and fever and is at a high-risk of developing pancreatitis, orchitis and meningoencephalitis. Erythema is also present along Stensen's duct. The most likely causative agent is:

1. Retrovirus
2. Paramyxovirus
3. Rhabdovirus
4. Herpesvirus
5. Togavirus

Ans. 2. Paramyxovirus

USMLE Case Scenario

A 12-year-old boy from south-west Texas is brought with fever, intense headache, chest pain and an erythematous patch on his shin. DNA probe reveals a fungal origin of the disease. He responds to Amphotericin dramatically. Most likely cause is:

1. Histoplasmosis
2. Candidiasis
3. Cryptococciosis
4. Coccidioidomycosis

Ans. 4. Coccidioidomycosis

USMLE Case Scenario

Dennie's lines and Morgan fold in a child are a feature of:
1. Polymyositis
2. Dermatomyositis
3. Mixed connective tissue disease
4. Sjögren's syndrome
5. SLE
6. Rheumatoid arthritis
7. Atopy
8. Contact dermatitis

Ans. 7. Atopy

USMLE Case Scenario

The abnormal gene in Bruton's X-Linked agammaglobulinemia is:
1. q 22 on short arm of chromosome X
2. q 22 on long arm of chromosome X
3. q 11 on short arm of chromosome X
4. q 11 on long arm of chromosome X

Ans. 2. q 22 on long arm of chromosome X

USMLE Case Scenario

A four-week-old infant with hypertelorism, low set ears, fish mouth and micrognathia presents with recurrent seizures. The infant is fed well. A pansystolic murmur suggesting VSD is auscultated by a cardiologist. Serum concentration of IgA is decreased. Most likely cause is:
1. Trisomy
2. Monosomy
3. Microdeletion
4. Mosaicism
5. Translocation

Ans. 3. Microdeletion

USMLE Case Scenario

A nine-months-old infant is brought with infection of his ear. His mother says that the infant previously had pneumonia along with six episodes of infection till date. On examination, an eczematous rash is noticed by a dermatologist. The skin is studded with minute petechia. Serum levels of IgG are normal but IgM levels are low. The most likely diagnosis is:
1. IgA deficiency
2. Bruton's X-linked agammaglobinemia
3. Severe combined immunodeficiency
4. Ataxia telangiectasia
5. Friedrich's ataxia
6. Wiskott-Aldrich syndrome

Ans. 6. Wiskott-Aldrich syndrome

USMLE Case Scenario

CHARGE syndrome is:
1. Cataract, Heart disease, Atresia (esophageal), Retarded growth, Genital anomalies, Ear anomalies
2. Cataract, Heart disease, Atresia (intestinal), Retarded growth, Genital anomalies, Ear anomalies
3. Coloboma, Heart disease, Atresia (rectal), Retarded growth, Genital anomalies, Ear anomalies
4. Coloboma, Heart disease, Atresia (choanal), Retarded growth, Genital anomalies, Ear anomalies

Ans. 4. Coloboma, Heart disease, Atresia (choanal), Retarded growth, Genital anomalies, Ear anomalies

USMLE Case Scenario

Foramen cecum is related to:

1. Branchial cleft cyst
2. Cystic hygroma
3. Thyroglossal cyst
4. Sternomastoid tumor

Ans. 3. Thyroglossal cyst

USMLE Case Scenario

Most common site for a foreign body in a child less than one year is:

1. Larynx
2. Trachea
3. Carina
4. Right bronchus
5. Left bronchus

Ans. 1. Larynx

In older than one year: right bronchus

USMLE Case Scenario

A physician in an emergency notices a three-year-old child drooling with expiratory stridor. His respiratory rate is 45/minute and temperature of 104 °F. His neck is hyperextended. His voice is muffled. The most likely causative organism is:

1. Group A beta hemolytic streptococci
2. H. influenzae type A
3. H. influenzae type B
4. H. influenzae type C

Ans. 3. H. Influenzae type B

USMLE Case Scenario

A term newborn presents with bilious vomiting shortly after birth. Her abdomen is distended slightly, and facial features are characteristic of Down's syndrome. She has passed a normal meconium stool. The pregnancy was complicated by polyhydramnios. Of the following, the MOST likely diagnosis is:

1. Duodenal atresia
2. Hirschsprung's disease
3. Meconium ileus
4. Midgut volvulus
5. Pyloric stenosis

Ans. 1. Duodenal atresia

USMLE Case Scenario

Which of the following constellations of features BEST describes the fetal alcohol syndrome?

1. Palmar crease, brushfield spots, decreased IQ
2. Cataract, deafness, PDA
3. Sacral agenesis, TGA, large baby
4. Microcephaly, developmental delay and short palpebral fissures
5. Short stature, webbed neck, pulmonic stenosis
6. Cerebral calcification, jaundice, hepatomegaly

Ans. 4. Microcephaly, developmental delay and short palpebral fissures

USMLE Case Scenario

A lateral CXR shows Thumb Print Sign. It is usually seen in:

1. Pharyngitis
2. Laryngitis
3. Epiglottitis
4. Bronchitis
5. Laryngeotracheobronchitis

Ans. 3. Epiglottitis

USMLE Case Scenario

Bronchiolitis is:

1. Upper respiratory tract infection in infants involving small airways of lower respiratory tract
2. Lower respiratory tract infection in infants involving large airways of lower respiratory tract
3. Lower respiratory tract infection in infants involving large airways of lower respiratory tract
4. Lower respiratory tract infection in infants involving small airways of upper respiratory tract
5. Lower respiratory tract infection in infants involving small airways of lower respiratory tract

Ans. 5. Lower respiratory tract infection in infants involving small airways of lower respiratory tract

USMLE Case Scenario

Nasal polyps, Rectal prolapse and Malabsorption are most often associated with:

1. Bronchiolitis
2. Pertussis
3. Asthma
4. Cystic fibrosis

Ans. 2. Pertussis

USMLE Case Scenario

Apical heave suggests:

1. Left atrial enlargement
2. Right atrial enlargement
3. Left ventricular enlargement
4. Right ventricular enlargement

Ans. 3. Left ventricular enlargement

USMLE Case Scenario

A 5-year-old boy has a temperature of 102 °F. He is well fed. Physical examination is normal. On examination by a cardiologist, a systolic murmur is heard at left lower sternal border. The grade of murmur is 2/6. The examination suggests that the boy has:

1. Mitral stenosis
2. Mitral regurgitation
3. Aortic stenosis
4. Aortic regurgitation
5. ASD
6. VSD
7. No significant cardiac disease

Ans. 7. No significant cardiac disease. Innocent murmurs. Further high temperature

USMLE Case Scenario

Association with heart disease is not seen in:

1. Down's syndrome
2. Marfan's syndrome
3. Noonan's syndrome
4. DiGeorge's syndrome
5. Cri du chat syndrome

Ans. 5. Cri du chat syndrome

USMLE Case Scenario

A 4-month-old weak boy is seen by a cardiologist. Physical examination reveals a thrill and a harsh grade 4/6 pansystolic murmur at left lower sternal border. ECG suggests LVH. Most likely cause is:

1. Ostium primum ASD
2. Ostium secondum ASD
3. VSD
4. PDA
5. TAPV

Ans. 3. VSD

USMLE Case Scenario

A 3-year-old girl is brought to you. Her pulse is 100 beats per minute, bounding in nature with wide pulse pressure. Her history suggests that she was born premature. Auscultation reveals a murmur occurring both during systole as well as diastole. CXR reveals an enlarged heart size with prominent pulmonary vascular markings. She eventually dies of heart failure. Most likely she was suffering from:

1. A defect in atrial septum
2. A defect in ventricular septum
3. Failure of closure of ductus arteriosus
4. Failure of closure of ductus venosum

Ans. 3. Failure of closure of ductus arteriosus, PDA

USMLE Case Scenario

A radiologist on angiography notices dilatations in the right and left coronary artery of a four-year-old boy. The boy was febrile and his blood investigations revealed thrombocytosis. The parents of the boy were told to administer aspirin to the patient who raised concern over the development of Reye's syndrome. The doctor still insisted on treating the boy with aspirin along with other medications. Most likely the impression of the disease the boy is suffering from is:

1. Takayasu's disease
2. Polyarteritis nodosa
3. Giant cell arteritis
4. Wegener's granulomatosis
5. Occuloglandular syndrome
6. Marfan's syndrome
7. Mucocutaneous lymph node syndrome

Ans. 7. Mucocutaneous lymph node syndrome

USMLE Case Scenario

Feature of Kawasaki disease is:

1. Unilateral, purulent conjunctival infection
2. Unilateral, nonpurulent conjunctival infection
3. Bilateral purulent conjunctival infection
4. Bilateral nonpurulent conjunctival infection

Ans. 4. Bilateral nonpurulent conjunctival infection

USMLE Case Scenario

Hereditary nephritis is:

1. X-linked dominant
2. X-linked recessive
3. Autosomal dominant
4. Autosomal recessive

Ans. 1. X-linked dominant (Alport's syndrome)

USMLE Case Scenario

A two-month-old infant with large tongue, large fontanelle's is seen by a genetic specialist. The infant is a female with decreased muscle tone and umbilical hernia. Hair is coarse and brittle. The history is insignificant except for an icterus at the time of birth for about three weeks. The most likely cause is:

1. Down's syndrome because of Mosaicism
2. Down's syndrome because of translocation
3. Congenital hypothyroidism because of thyroid dysgenesis
4. Fragile X syndrome
5. Amyloidosis

Ans. 3. Congenital hypothyroidism because of thyroid dysgenesis

USMLE Case Scenario

A 10-year-old boy underwent an USG which showed an enlarged spleen and presence of cholelithiasis. He was adviced hematological check-up which showed Hb=6.5 gms/dl and MCV=60. The boy can have an associated feature as:

1. Maxillary hypoplasia with normocytic normochromic RBC
2. Maxillary hypoplasia with microcytic hypochromic RBC
3. Maxillary hyperplasia with normocytic normochromic RBC
4. Maxillary hyperplasia with microcytic hypochromic RBC

Ans. 4. Maxillary hyperplasia with microcytic hypochromic RBC

USMLE Case Scenario

A special pediatric hematology department receives a twenty-two-month old who has Microcephaly, Microphthalmia. Skeletal survey reveals absent radii and thumbs. Blood investigations reveal aplastic anemia. The doctor informs that the child is at risk for developing AML. The boy is most likely suffering from:

1. Simple aplastic anemia
2. Myelofibrosis
3. Myelosclerosis
4. Congenital pure red cell aplasia
5. Down's syndrome
6. TAR syndrome
7. Fanconi's anemia

Ans. 7. Fanconi's anemia

USMLE Case Scenario

Branchial cleft cysts are remnants of the:

1. First and second branchial pouches
2. Third and fourth branchial pouches
3. Fourth and fifth branchial pouches
4. Fifth and sixth branchial pouches

Ans. 1. First and second branchial pouches

Branchial cleft cysts, sinuses and fistulas are remnants of the first and second branchial pouches.

USMLE Case Scenario

A 35-year-old nonhypertensive patient presents with the sudden onset of an excruciating headache, complains of a stiff neck and photophobia with transient loss of consciousness and third nerve palsy. An angiography reveals a sac-like dilatations in anterior circulation at circle of Willis. The disease may be usually associated with:

1. Osteomas
2. Hemangiomas
3. Rhabdomyosarcomas
4. Myxomas
5. Umbilical adenomas
6. Cherry red spots
7. Cysts in kidney

Ans. 7. Cysts in kidney

USMLE Case Scenario

Tumor originating from Rathke's pouch is:

1. Meningioma
2. Pinealoma
3. Ependymoma
4. Medulloblastoma
5. Craniopharyngiomas

Ans. 5. Craniopharyngiomas

Craniopharyngiomas are cystic tumors with areas of calcification and originate in the epithelial remnants of Rathke's pouch. These usually benign tumors are found in the sellar and suprasellar regions and lead to compression of the pituitary, optic tracts, and third ventricle.

USMLE Case Scenario

In a 77-year-old man, the onset of irregular respirations, bradycardia and finally increased blood pressure with increasing intracranial pressure (ICP) is termed as:

1. The Beck's triad
2. The Cushing's response
3. The Charcot's triad
4. The Hutchinson's triad

Ans. 2. The Cushing's response

USMLE Case Scenario

The Glasgow coma scale was developed to enable an initial assessment of the severity of head trauma. It measures the level of consciousness using three parameters. The score is the sum of the highest number achieved in each category. The fully oriented and alert patient will receive a maximum score of 15. Points in GCS are given as:

1. Verbal response (6 points), motor response (4 points) and eye opening (5 points)
2. Verbal response (5 points), motor response (5 points) and eye opening (5 points)
3. Verbal response (6 points), motor response (6 points) and eye opening (3 points)
4. Verbal response (5 points), motor response (6 points) and eye opening (4 points)

Ans. 4. Verbal response (5 points), motor response (6 points) and eye opening (4 points)

USMLE Case Scenario

Orange-yellow tonsillar hyperplasia due to the cholesterol ester deposition is seen with:

1. Gaucher's disease
2. Nieman-Pick's disease
3. Tay-Sach's-disease
4. I-cell disease
5. Fabry's disease
6. Tangier's disease

Ans: 6. Tangier's disease

USMLE Case Scenario

In the twin-to-twin transfusion syndrome:

1. Hydramnios does not occur
2. Hydramnios can develop in either twin but is more frequent in the recipient because of circulatory overload
3. Hydramnios can develop in either twin but is more frequent in the donor because of circulatory overload
4. Hydramnios can develop in either twin but is equally frequent in both twins

Ans. 2. Hydramnios can develop in either twin but is more frequent in the recipient because of circulatory overload

USMLE Case Scenario

After playing rugby, a boy has a swollen knee bilaterally. He was known to have hemophilia B. Replacement of which of the following is indicated for treatment:

1. Factor C
2. Factor S
3. Factor VII
4. Factor VIII
5. Factor IX
6. Factor XII
7. Fibrinogen

Ans. 5. Factor IX

Hemophilia B is similar to hemophilia A, but is due to X-linked deficiency of blood-clotting factor IX rather than VIII.

USMLE Case Scenario

A 14-year-old boy from Illinois is brought by his parents to a physician. He presents with a three-month history of recurrent headache. Neurologic examination is unremarkable except for bitemporal deficits in his visual field. X-ray and MRI of the head are performed. X-ray films show calcifications in the suprasellar region, while MRI images reveal a multicystic tumor displacing the optic chiasm. Most likely lesion is:

1. Craniopharyngioma
2. Meningioma
3. Ependymoma
4. Cysticercosis
5. Astrocytoma
6. Pituitary microadenoma

Ans. 1. Craniopharyngioma

It is a histologically benign epithelial tumor of odontogenic origin. Located in the suprasellar compartment, extending variably onto the sella, hypothalamus, and optic chiasm. Heavy calcifications, unilocular or multilocular cysts, and a viscous yellow fluid content are the classic features that allow the diagnosis on radiologic and gross examination.

USMLE Case Scenario

A 7-year-old boy has multiple yellow, crusted erosions below the nares and on the cheeks, chin and upper extremities. The rest of the examination is normal. Which of the following is the most appropriate treatment for this condition?

1. Oral acyclovir
2. Silver sulfadiazine
3. Griseofulvin
4. Cephalexin
5. Topical ketoconazole
6. Topical hydrocortisone

Ans. 4. Cephalexin drug of choice for impetigo is oral cephalexin. Cloxacillin, dicloxacillin and azithromycin are good alternatives.

USMLE Case Scenario

A 2-month-old infant born to a mother who was taking lithium for BPD was noted at birth to have an upper left sternal border ejection murmur. The infant at that time was not cyanotic, but slowly developed cyanosis over the next two months. ECG shows right axis deviation and right ventricular hypertrophy. A chest X-ray film showed a small heart with a concave main pulmonary artery segment and diminished pulmonary blood flow. Most likely diagnosis is:

1. Ebstein's anomaly
2. PDA
3. Hypoplastic left ventricle
4. Coarctation of aorta
5. Atrial septal defect
6. Tetralogy of Fallot
7. Transposition of the great arteries

Ans. 6. Tetralogy of Fallot

This is tetralogy of Fallot, in which severe obstruction of right ventricular outflow and a ventricular septal defect allow unoxygenated blood to pass from the right side of the heart to the left. In severe cases, cyanosis presents at birth; in milder cases (such as this baby has), it develops more slowly. The upper left sternal border ejection murmur is due to right ventricle outflow obstruction.

USMLE Case Scenario

A woman over 45 years of age from North America has hypertension, proteinuria, and features suggestive of hyperthyroidism. She has an enlarged-for-dates uterus and has had intermittent bleeding in the first two trimesters. Grossly her lesions appear as small, clear clusters of grape-like vesicles, the passage of which confirms the diagnosis of H mole. A tissue sample would show:

1. No villi
2. Villi without hydropic changes and no vessels
3. Villi with hydropic changes and no vessels
4. Villi with hydropic changes and plenty of vessels

Ans. 3. Villi with hydropic changes and no vessels

USMLE Case Scenario

Fetal hydrops occurs as a result of excessive and prolonged hemolysis due to isoimmunization. Characteristics of fetal hydrops include abnormal fluid in two or more sites, such as the thorax, abdomen and skin. The placenta in fetal hydrops is:

1. Pale, enlarged and boggy
2. Pale, smaller and shrunken
3. Erythematous, enlarged and boggy
4. Erythematous, small and shrunken

Ans. 3. Erythematous, enlarged and boggy

USMLE Case Scenario

The therapeutic range of serum magnesium to prevent seizures is:

1. 4–7 mg/dl
2. 10–12 mg/dl
3. 15–20 mg/dl
4. 25–30 mg/dl

Ans. 1. 4–7 mg/dl

USMLE Case Scenario

At levels between 8 and 12 mg/dl, patellar reflexes are lost. At 10 to 12 mg/dl, somnolence and slurred speech commonly occur. Muscle paralysis and respiratory difficulty occur at 15 to 17 mg/dl and cardiac arrest occurs at levels greater than 30 mg/dl.

1. Appendicitis in pregnancy is easy to diagnose and has lesser mortality
2. Appendicitis in pregnancy is easy to diagnose but has more mortality
3. Appendicitis in pregnancy is difficult to diagnose but has lesser mortality
4. Appendicitis in pregnancy is difficult to diagnose and has more mortality

Ans. 4. Appendicitis in pregnancy is difficult to diagnose and has more mortality

The diagnosis is very difficult in pregnancy because leukocytosis, nausea and vomiting are common in pregnancy and the upward displacement of the appendix by the uterus may cause appendicitis to simulate cholecystitis, pyelonephritis and gastritis. Surgery is necessary even if the diagnosis is not certain. Delays in surgery due to difficulty in diagnosis as the appendix moves up are probably the cause of increasing maternal mortality with increasing gestational age.

USMLE Case Scenario

HELLP syndrome is:

1. Hepatitis, elevated liver enzymes, low plasma albumin
2. Hepatitis, elevated liver enzymes, low platelets
3. Hemolysis, elevated liver enzymes, low platelets
4. Hemolysis, elevated liver enzymes, low plasma albumin

Ans. 3. Hemolysis, elevated liver enzymes, low platelets

USMLE Case Scenario

A 3-year-old child has severe difficulty walking. Neurological examination documents ataxia and mental retardation. The neurologist notes the presence of multiple telangiectasias involving the face. The child also has a history of multiple respiratory tract infections. Diagnosis is:

1. Friedreich's ataxia
2. Ataxia telangiectasia
3. Hemorrhagic telangiectasia
4. ALS
5. Anterior spinal artery syndrome
6. Guillain-Barre syndrome

Ans. 2. Ataxia telangiectasia

USMLE Case Scenario

Chronic granulomatous disease is usually an X-linked recessive disorder that affects males because of a defect in the activity of:

1. Reduced nicotinamide adenine dinucleotide (NAD) oxidase
2. Reduced nicotinamide adenine dinucleotide phosphate (NADPH) oxidase
3. Reduced nicotinamide adenine dinucleotide (NAD) reductase
4. Reduced nicotinamide adenine dinucleotide phosphate (NADPH) reductase

Ans. 2. Reduced nicotinamide adenine dinucleotide phosphate (NADPH) oxidase

USMLE Case Scenario

A tall patient with arachnodactyly, hyperextensible joints, mitral valve prolapse, dislocation of the lens of the eye and a high risk for thoracic aortic dissection is most likely having:

1. Syphilis
2. Osteogenesis imperfecta
3. Galactosemia
4. Homocystinuria
5. Menkes disease

Ans. 4. Homocystinuria

USMLE Case Scenario

Congenital deafness may result from abnormal development of the membranous labyrinth and/or bony labyrinth, as well as from abnormalities of the auditory ossicles. Recessive inheritance is the most common cause of congenital deafness, but a virus infection near the end of the embryonic period is a major environmental factor known to cause abnormal development of the spiral organ and defective hearing. Most likely virus to cause such a defect would be:

1. Measles
2. EBV
3. Herpes
4. Pox
5. Mumps
6. Rabies
7. Rubella
8. CMV

Ans. 7. Rubella

USMLE Case Scenario

A 6-year-old boy brought by his mother presented with easy fatiguability, malaise and lethargy of eight months' duration. He is anorexic and had lost four kg in weight. On examination he was thin, anxious and anemic. There was mild, bilateral, cervical lymphadenopathy and moderate splenomegaly. On investigation, his hemoglobin (70 g/l) and platelet count (67 × 109/l) were low, but the white-cell count was high (27 × 109/l). The blood film showed that most leucocytes were blasts; the red cells were normochromic and normocytic. Bone marrow examination showed an overgrowth of primitive white cells with diminished numbers of normal erythroid and myeloid precursors. Most likely diagnosis is:

1. Mononucleosis
2. Leukemoid reaction
3. Aplastic anemia
4. Malnutrition
5. Acute leukemia
6. Chronic leukemia
7. Hodgkin's disease
8. Nonhodgkin's disease

Ans. 5. Acute leukemia

USMLE Case Scenario

A clinical condition seen in a 24-year-old male from New Orleans is characterized by a facial palsy and is often associated with facial pain and the appearance of vesicles on the eardrum, ear canal and pinna. Vertigo and sensorineural hearing loss (VIII nerve) accompanying it is suggestive of:

1. Down's syndrome
2. Turner's syndrome
3. Bell's palsy
4. Pendred syndrome
5. Ramsay Hunt syndrome
6. Goldenhar's syndrome
7. Alport's syndrome
8. Pierre Robinson syndrome
9. Treacher Collins syndrome

Ans. 5. Ramsay Hunt syndrome

USMLE Case Scenario

An X-linked dominant condition that affects boys more severely than girls and is associated with severe progressive glomerulonephritis and a progressive sensorineural hearing loss suggests:

1. Waardenburg's syndrome
2. Lowe's syndrome
3. Down's syndrome
4. Turner's syndrome

5. Pendred syndrome
6. Goldenhar's syndrome
7. Alport's syndrome
8. Pierrie Robinson syndrome
9. Treacher Collins syndrome

Ans. 7. Alport's syndrome

USMLE Case Scenario

A 7-day-old girl has bruising and gastrointestinal bleeding. Her parents seek advice of the physician. On investigation, laboratory findings include partial thromboplastin time and prothrombin time, greater than 2 minutes; serum bilirubin, 4.9 mg/dl; alanine aminotransferase, 19 mg/dl; platelet count, 335, 550/mm^3; and hemoglobin, 15.3 g/dl. Most likely the cause of bleeding is:

1. Factor IX deficiency
2. Idiopathic thrombocytopenic purpura
3. TTP
4. Hemophilia
5. Liver disease
6. Vitamin K deficiency

Ans. 6. Vitamin K deficiency

It is a hemorrhagic disease of the newborn as a result of vitamin K deficiency. The normal newborn has a moderate deficiency of the vitamin K–dependent coagulation factors. All newborns should receive 0.5-1.0 mg of vitamin K intramuscularly within the first hour after birth.

USMLE Case Scenario

A 48-year-old woman from Holland delivers a 3126 g newborn male. Her pregnancy was normal except that she noted decreased fetal movement compared to her previous pregnancies. She declined an amniocentesis offered by her obstetrician. Physical examination of the newborn reveals an infant with facial features suggestive of Down's syndrome. The infant then has bilious vomiting. An X-ray film showing the kidneys, ureters, and bladder (KUB) is performed, which shows a distended and gas-filled stomach and proximal duodenum and the absence of gas in the distal bowel. Which of the following is the most likely cause of the abdominal signs and symptoms?

1. Duodenal atresia
2. Hirschsprung disease
3. Malrotation
4. Meconium ileus
5. Pyloric stenosis

Ans: 1. Duodenal atresia

Explanation: The 'double bubble' sign is pathognomonic for duodenal atresia, which is a congenital anomaly associated with Down's syndrome. Duodenal atresia is associated with bilious vomiting. Children with Down's syndrome can also have esophageal atresia, imperforate anus, endocardial cushion defects and hypotonia.

USMLE Case Scenario

A 14-year-old boy from Chicago has a small tumor in the wall of the left lateral ventricle. A biopsy of this tumor is consistent with pathologic diagnosis of subependymal giant cell astrocytoma. Which of the following lesions may also be present in this patient?

1. Cafe–au–lait spots
2. Renal angiomyolipomas
3. Sesamoid bones
4. Hemangioblastoma
5. Wickham's striae
6. Lisch nodules
7. Cancers of genital tract
8. Schwannoma of the 8th cranial nerve

Ans. 2. Renal angiomyolipomas. Tuberous sclerosis
It manifests with multiple hamartomatous lesions in the skin, CNS and visceral organs. Cortical tubers are malformed (Hamartomatous) nodules of the cortex, probably resulting from faulty cortical development. Other lesions include shagreen patches and ash-leaf spots on the skin, cardiac myomas and renal angiomyolipomas.

USMLE Case Scenario

Atresia (blockage) of this canal results from failure of the meatal plug to canalize. Usually the deep part of the meatus is open but the superficial part is blocked by bone or fibrous tissue. Most cases are associated with the:

1. First arch syndrome
2. Second arch syndrome
3. Third arch syndrome
4. Fifth arch syndrome

Ans. 1. First arch syndrome

USMLE Case Scenario

A 5-month-old infant is seen by a pediatrician. He has been exclusively fed a commercially available infant formula. Upon introduction of fruit juices, however, the child develops jaundice, hepatomegaly, vomiting, lethargy, irritability and seizures. Tests for urine-reducing substances are positive. Which of the following is likely to explain this child's condition?

1. Alkaptonuria
2. Galactosemia
3. Fructosemia
4. A1-antitrypsin
5. Glucose-6-phosphatase deficiency

Ans. 3. Fructosemia

USMLE Case Scenario

A genotypic male (XY) is born with feminized external genitalia. The testes are retained within the abdominal cavity and the internal reproductive tracts exhibit the normal male phenotype. Which of the following could account for this abnormal development?

1. Complete androgen resistance
2. 5a-reductase deficiency
3. 17a-hydroxylase deficiency
4. Sertoli-only
5. Testicular dysgenesis

Ans. 2. 5a-reductase deficiency
In utero differentiation of the Wolffian ducts into the normal male phenotypic internal reproductive tract requires testosterone, but not dihydrotestosterone. On the other hand, differentiation of the indifferent external genital slit into the penis, prostate, and scrotum does require dihydrotestosterone. A congenital absence of 5a-reductase in these tissues will result in feminization. If left untreated, the affected individuals are generally phenotypic females until puberty, at which time increased amounts of testosterone result in virilization ('penis-at-twelve' syndrome).

USMLE Case Scenario

A 4-year-old boy is brought to the emergency department after the acute onset of headache, vomiting, nuchal rigidity and impaired mental status. MRI reveals a posterior fossa tumor that fills the 4th ventricle. Surgery is immediately started, and intraoperative consultation leads to a 'frozen section' diagnosis of medulloblastoma. Which of the following pathologic mechanisms most likely accounts for this child's clinical presentation?

1. Chronic hemorrhage into the 4th ventricle
2. Alteration of medullary function
3. Increased intracranial pressure
4. Infiltration of the cerebellum by the neoplasm
5. Spread of tumor to the subdural space

Ans. 3. Increased intracranial pressure

Any tumor 'filling the 4th ventricle' blocks the circulation of cerebrospinal fluid (CSF). This blockage leads to increased intracranial pressure, which manifests with nausea, vomiting, headache, nuchal rigidity, and mental status changes. If surgery is not performed promptly, cerebellar tonsillar herniation and rapid death will ensue. In children, medulloblastoma and ependymoma are the most frequent neoplasms presenting in this manner.

USMLE Case Scenario

A child is brought with drowsiness, decreased deep tendon reflexes and seizures. On examination, the child has a line on gums. There is history of constipation. Which will be the most appropriate drug that should be used in this child?

1. EDTA
2. DMSA
3. BAL
4. Penicillamine
5. Penicillin
6. Ampicillin

Ans. 1. EDTA

USMLE Case Scenario

Chronic salicyclism is manifested by headache, dizziness, ringing in the ears (tinnitus), difficulty in hearing, mental confusion, drowsiness, nausea, vomiting, and diarrhea. The CNS changes may progress to convulsions and coma. The drug implicated is:

1. Penicillin
2. Quinine
3. Metoclopramide
4. Cisplatin
5. Paracetamol
6. Aspirin

Ans. 6. Aspirin

USMLE Case Scenario

Cat eye syndrome is:

1. Partial trisomy 18
2. Partial trisomy 13
3. Partial trisomy 21
4. Partial trisomy 22
5. Partial trisomy 20

Ans. 4. Partial trisomy 22

USMLE Case Scenario

A newborn born to a couple (a Japanese husband and an American wife) appears normal at birth, but develops mild vomiting and diarrhea accompanied by jaundice and hepatomegaly within the first few weeks of life. Within five months, the baby has obvious difficulty in vision as per mother which was diagnosed as cataract. By one year of age, he has developed mental retardation. Which of the following is the most likely diagnosis?

1. Fructose intolerance
2. Measles
3. Toxoplasmosis
4. Cystic fibrosis
5. Galactosemia
6. McArdle's disease
7. von Gierke's disease
8. Wilson's disease
9. Rubella

Ans. 5. Galactosemia

USMLE Case Scenario

Which of the following malformations in a newborn is specific for maternal insulin-dependent diabetes mellitus?

1. Transposition of great arteries
2. Caudal regression
3. Holoprosencephaly
4. Meningomyelocele

Ans. 2. Caudal regression

USMLE Case Scenario

A newborn presented with bloated abdomen shortly after birth with passing of less meconium. A full thickness biopsy of the rectum was carried out. Which one of the following rectal biopsy findings is most likely to be present?

1. Fibrosis of submucosa
2. Hyalinization of the muscular coat
3. Thickened muscularis propria
4. Lack of ganglion cells

Ans. 4. Lack of ganglion cells

USMLE Case Scenario

The most common etiological agent for acute bronchiolitis in infancy is:

1. Influenza virus
2. Parainfluenza virus
3. Rhinovirus
4. Respiratory syncytial virus

Ans. 4. Respiratory syncytial virus

USMLE Case Scenario

A 1-month-old boy is referred for failure to thrive. On examination, he shows feature of congestive failure. The femoral pulses are feeble as compared to branchial pulses. The most likely clinical diagnosis is:

1. Congenital aortic stenosis
2. Coarctation of aorta
3. Patent ductus arteriosus
4. Congenital aortoiliac disease

Ans. 2. Coarctation of aorta

USMLE Case Scenario

A specialist is called to the newborn nursery when a male infant born at term is found to have bilateral colobomas, choanal atresia, ear anomalies, and cryptorchidism. There is no history of maternal drug or alcohol abuse during pregnancy. There is no family history of similar congenital defects. Which of the following is the most appropriate initial diagnostic test to exclude any associated abnormalities?

1. Barium swallow
2. Echocardiography
3. Fiberoptic bronchoscopy
4. Renal ultrasonography
5. Skeletal survey

Ans. 2. Echocardiography

The infant in this question likely has the CHARGE syndrome

USMLE Case Scenario

A 7-year-old boy is brought to the clinic for a lifetime history of bedwetting. He has otherwise been completely healthy and has met all development milestones. His parents deny a history of trauma and the history is not consistent with abuse. The patient has been wetting every night but not during the daytime. He has no incontinence. Which of the following is the most appropriate next step in his evaluation?

1. Intravenous pyelogram
2. Renal ultrasound
3. 24-hour urine collection
4. Urinalysis
5. CT of pelvis

Ans. 4. Urinalysis

Given the fact that this patient has had a lifelong history of bedwetting, the initial evaluation will include a urinalysis to rule out infection or bleeding. No neurologic dysfunction exists in this case.

USMLE Case Scenario

A male infant born at term is found to have bilateral colobomas, choanal atresia, ear anomalies, and cryptorchidism. There is no history maternal drug or alcohol abuse during pregnancy. There is no family history of similar congenital defects. It is an example of:

1. Leopard syndrome
2. LAMB syndrome
3. Name syndrome
4. CHARGE syndrome
5. Vacterl syndrome

Ans. 4: CHARGE syndrome

The infant likely has the CHARGE syndrome, which includes colobomas, heart defects, choanal atresia, retardation, genitourinary abnormalities, and ear anomalies.

USMLE Case Scenario

A 17-year-old girl comes to the physician because she has not yet had a menstrual period. She also complains of a lack of breast development. Past medical history is significant for loss of smell and color blindness. Past surgical history is significant for a cleft palate that was repaired in childhood. She takes no medications and has no allergies to medications. Examination is significant for absent breast development, and a hypoestrogenic vulva and vagina. Urine hCG is negative. Which of the following is the most likely diagnosis?

1. Anorexia nervosa
2. Kallmann's syndrome
3. Polycystic ovarian syndrome
4. Pregnancy
5. Testicular feminization syndrome

Ans. 2. Kallamann's syndrome

USMLE Case Scenario

A 7-year-old girl develops fever, conjunctivitis, photophobia, and cough. Her pediatrician notes white spots on a bright red background on the girl's buccal mucosa. Within days, a rash begins around the hairline, then spreads to the trunk and extremities. Most likely diagnosis is:

1. Measles
2. Rabies
3. Mumps
4. Varicella
5. Poxvirus infection

Ans. 1. Measles

USMLE Case Scenario

A 4-year-old child has a history of a blue patch over eyelids, which disappeared at the age of 1 year. The diagnosis is:

1. Strawberry angioma
2. Salmon patch
3. Cavernous hemangioma
4. Port-Wine stain

Ans. 2. Salmon patch

USMLE Case Scenario

A 10-day-old male pseudohermaphrodite child with 46 XY karyotype presents with BP of 110/80 mm Hg. Most likely enzyme deficiency is:

1. 21 hydroxylase
2. 17 hydroxylase
3. 11 hydroxylase
4. 3-beta hydroxylase

Ans. 2. 17 hydroxylase

USMLE Case Scenario

A 16-year-old boy is brought to the emergency department because of sudden onset of headache, fever, vomiting, and a skin rash. His family had spent their vacation camping in North Carolina and just returned the previous day. During their 10-day stay, they had experienced multiple insect bites and removed several ticks from all family members. The boy had started complaining of a headache that morning and developed a high fever by noon. He vomited several times in the following few hours. Early in the afternoon, his mother noticed that a rose-colored rash had developed around his ankles. The boy is in moderate distress. His temperature is 39.0 °C (102.2 °F), pulse is 110/min and respirations are 24/min. He has multiple erythematous macules on his lower legs and hands, and rare petechiae interspersed between them. His mucosae are dry. Which of the following is the most likely diagnosis?

1. Erythema migrans
2. Henoch-Schönlein purpura
3. Erythema multiforme
4. Scarlet fever
5. Rocky mountain spotted fever

Ans. 5. Rocky mountain spotted fever

USMLE Case Scenario

A toddler is brought by overconcerned parents to the emergency department by his parents with burns on both of his thighs and buttocks. The child is hydrated. On examination of the burn areas, the areas are moist and painful to touch. The parents assert that the child accidentally pulled a kettle with hot water while playing. Which of the following is the most important step in management?

1. Early excision and grafting of the burned areas
2. Prompt administration of fluid resuscitation
3. Take parents into custody for neglect
4. Referral to the proper authorities for suspected child abuse
5. Discharge the boy after treatment immediately
6. Counsel the parents not to repeat the negligence on their part

Ans. 4. Referral to the proper authorities for suspected child abuse

Scalding burns in children should always raise the possibility of child abuse. Referral to the proper authorities for suspected child abuse is the most appropriate thing.

USMLE Case Scenario

A one-month-old infant is brought by his parents to a pediatrician. The infant was born at term. On auscultating the chest of the infant, a continuous murmur at the upper left sternal border is heard. The peripheral pulses in all extremities are full and show widened pulse pressure. Most likely diagnosis is:

1. Patent ductus arteriosus
2. Pulmonic stenosis
3. Persistent truncus arteriosus
4. VSD
5. TOF
6. Coarctation of the aorta

Ans. 1. Patent ductus arteriosus

This is patent ductus arteriosus which is a failure of closure of the duct between the pulmonary artery and the aorta. Feature of murmur suggests PDA.

USMLE Case Scenario

Which of the following intrauterine infections is associated with limb reduction defects and scarring of skin:

1. Varicella virus
2. Herpes virus
3. Rubella
4. Parvovirus

Ans. 1. Varicella virus

USMLE Case Scenario

Which of the following agents is likely to cause cerebral calcification and hydrocephalus in a newborn whose mother has history of taking spiramycin but was not compliant with therapy:

1. Rubella
2. Toxoplasmosis
3. CMV
4. Herpes

Ans. 2. Toxoplasmosis

USMLE Case Scenario

Which of the following is a marker for neural tube defects:

1. ↑Phosphatidyl esterase
2. ↑Pseudocholinesterase
3. ↑Acetylcholinesterase
4. ↑Butyrylcholinesterase
5. ↓Phosphatidyl esterase
6. ↓Pseudocholinesterase
7. ↓Acetylcholinesterase
8. ↓Butyrylcholinesterase

Ans. 3. ↑Acetylcholinesterase

USMLE Case Scenario

A child presents with massive hepatomegaly and hypoglycemia. There is no improvement in blood glucose on administration of Glucagon. The probable diagnosis is:

1. von Gierke's disease
2. McArdle's disease
3. Cori's disease
4. Forbe's disease

Ans. 1. von Gierke's disease

USMLE Case Scenario

A 7½-months-old child with cough, mild stridor is started on oral antibiotics. The child showed initial improvement but later developed wheeze, productive cough, and mild fever. X–ray shows hyperlucency and PFT shows an obstructive curve. The most probable diagnosis is:

1. Bronchiolitis obliterans
2. Postviral syndrome
3. Pulmonary alveolar microlithiasis
4. Follicular bronchitis

Ans. 1. Bronchiolitis obliterans

USMLE Case Scenario

A male born at term after an uncomplicated pregnancy, labor and delivery develops severe respiratory distress within a few hours of birth. Results of routine culture were negative. The chest roentgenogram reveals a normal heart shadow and fine reticulonodular infiltrates radiating from the hilum. ECHO findings reveal no abnormality. Family history reveals similar clinical course and death of a male and female sibling at 1 month and 2 months of age respectively. The most likely diagnosis is:

1. Neonatal Alveolar Proteinosis
2. Total Anomalous Pulmonary Venous Circulation (TAPVC)
3. Meconium Aspiration Syndrome
4. Diffuse Herpes Simplex Infection

Ans. 1. Neonatal Alveolar Proteinosis

USMLE Case Scenario

A diabetic mother gives birth to a baby who dies in the first week of life. Autopsy reveals a severe cardiac malformation. Which of the following is the most likely diagnosis?

1. Atrial septal defect
2. Holt-Oram syndrome
3. TAR syndrome
4. Coarctation of the aorta
5. Eisenmenger's syndrome
6. Lutembacher's syndrome
7. Tetralogy of Fallot
8. Transposition of the great arteries
9. Ebstein's anomaly
10. Pentalogy of Fallot

Ans. 8. Transposition of the great arteries

USMLE Case Scenario

A 3½-year-old boy is brought to the hospital in Chicago after the acute onset of headache, vomiting and nuchal rigidity. He has impaired mental status. MRI reveals a posterior fossa tumor that fills the 4th ventricle. Surgery is immediately started, and intraoperative consultation leads to a 'frozen section' diagnosis of medulloblastoma. Which of the following pathologic mechanisms most likely accounts for this child's clinical presentation?

1. Hemorrhage into the 4th ventricle
2. Increased intracranial pressure
3. Decreased intracranial pressure
4. Increased blood pressure
5. Infiltration of the cerebellar vermis by the neoplasm
6. Spread of tumor to the subarachnoid space
7. Altered metabolic response

Ans. 3. Decreased intracranial pressure

USMLE Case Scenario

The leukotriene receptor antagonist used in bronchial asthma is:

1. Zafirlukast
2. Zileuton
3. Ketotifen
4. Omalizumab

Ans. 1. Zafirlukast

USMLE Case Scenario

A newborn has congenital heart failure, which is not improving on treatment. He has bulging anterior fontanelles with a bruit on auscultation. On transfontanelle USG, a hypoechoic midline mass is seen with dilated lateral ventricles. Most probable diagnosis is:

1. Vein of Galen malformation
2. Arachnoid cyst
3. Medulloblastoma
4. Encephalocele

Ans. 1. Vein of Galen malformation

USMLE Case Scenario

A child has Microcephaly, Blue eyes, Fair skin, and Mental retardation-Ferric chloride test is positive. What is the likely diagnosis?

1. Phenylketonuria (PKU)
2. Homocystinuria
3. Tyrosinosis
4. Alkaptonuria

Ans. 1. Phenylketonuria (PKU)

USMLE Case Scenario

Cholangitis is the term used for acute inflammation of the wall of bile ducts, almost always caused by bacterial infection of the normally sterile lumen. It can result from any lesion obstructing bile flow, most commonly choledocholithiasis, and also from surgical reconstruction of the biliary tree. Uncommon causes include tumors, indwelling stents or catheters, acute pancreatitis, and benign strictures. Bacteria most likely enter the biliary tract through the sphincter of Oddi, rather than by the hematogenous route. Ascending cholangitis refers to the propensity of bacteria, once within the biliary tree, to infect intrahepatic biliary ducts. The usual pathogens are:

1. *E.coli, Klebsiella*
2. *Clostridium, Clonorchis sinensis*
3. *Opisthorchis viverrini, Klebsiella*
4. *Clostridium, Pseudomonas*

Ans. 1. *E.coli, Klebsiella*

USMLE Case Scenario

A five-day-old, full-term male infant was severely cyanotic at birth. Prostaglandin E was administered initially and later ballooned atrial septosomy was done which showed improvement in oxygenation. The most likely diagnosis of this infant is:

1. Tetralogy of Fallot
2. Transposition of great vessels
3. Truncus Arteriosus
4. Tricuspid Atresia

Ans. 2. Transposition of great vessels

USMLE Case Scenario

A physician diagnoses a boy with Duchenne muscular dystrophy. Which of the following signs is most consistent with Duchenne muscular dystrophy:

1. Wrist drop
2. Foot drop
3. Gower's sign
4. Festinant gait
5. Waddling gait
6. Positive Babinski sign

Ans. 3. Gower's sign

The Gower's sign is very characteristic of Duchenne muscular dystrophy. It is considered positive if the patient uses his hands to 'walk' up the legs when going from a prone to an upright sitting position because he does not have enough proximal muscle power to get up in a normal fashion.

USMLE Case Scenario

A 7½-year-old boy is brought by his parents because of bedwetting. He was born as a normal child, has been completely healthy and has met all development milestones. The boy has been wetting every night but not during the daytime. He has no incontinence. Appropriate next step in the evaluation of this boy would be:

1. Intravenous pyelogram
1. Ultrasound
2. 24-hour urine collection
3. Urinalysis
4. CT of pelvis
5. Immediate MRI skull

Ans. 4. Urinalysis

The initial evaluation will include a urinalysis to rule out infection or bleeding. No neurologic dysfunction exists in this case.

USMLE Case Scenario

In which of the following a 'Coeur en sabot' shape of the heart is seen:

1. Tricuspid atresia
2. Ventricular septal defect
3. Transposition of great arteries
4. Tetralogy of Fallot

Ans. 4. Tetralogy of Fallot

USMLE Case Scenario

A 4-month-old presents with cholestasis. Biopsy shows inflammation and fibrosing stricture of the hepatic or common bile ducts; inflammation of major intrahepatic bile ducts, with progressive destruction of the intrahepatic biliary tree, marked bile ductular proliferation, portal tract edema and fibrosis, and parenchymal cholestasis; and periportal fibrosis and cirrhosis. Most likely cause is:

1. Cystic fibrosis
2. Hepatitis
3. Biliary Atresia
4. Childhood Cirrhosis

Ans. 3. Biliary Atresia

USMLE Case Scenario

In a newborn, it is found that the main pancreatic duct (Wirsung) is very short and drains only a small portion of the head of the gland, while the bulk of the pancreas (from the dorsal pancreatic primordium) drains through the minor sphincter. The relative stenosis caused by the bulk of the pancreatic secretions passing through the minor sphincter predisposes such individuals to chronic pancreatitis. The condition is:

1. Annular pancreas
2. Pancreas divisum
3. Agenesis of pancreas
4. Ectopic pancreas

Ans. 2. Pancreas divisum

USMLE Case Scenario

A 10-month-old child presents with two weeks' history of fever, vomiting and alteration of sensorium Cranial CT scan reveals basal exudates and hydrocephalus. The most likely etiological agent is:

1. *Mycobacterium tuberculosis*
2. *Cryptococcus neoformans*
3. *Listera monocytogenes*
4. *Streptococcus pneumoniae*
5. *Bordetella*
6. *Meningococcus*

Ans. 1. *Mycobacterium tuberculosis*

USMLE Case Scenario

A 25-year-old woman had premature rupture of membranes and delivered a male child who became lethargic and apneic on the 1st day of birth and went into shock. The mother had a previous history of abortion 1 year back. On vaginal swab culture, growth of β-hemolytic colonies on blood agar was found. On staining these were found to be gram-positive cocci. Which of the following is the most likely etiological agent?

1. *Streptococcus pyogenes*
2. *Streptococcus agalactiae*
3. *Peptostreptococci*
4. *Enterococcus faecium*

Ans. 2. *Streptococcus agalactiae*

USMLE Case Scenario

A 5-year-old boy is detected to be HBsAg positive on two separate occasions during a screening program for hepatitis B. He is otherwise asymptomatic. Child was given three doses of recombinant hepatitis B vaccine at the age of 1 year. His mother was treated for chronic hepatitis B infection around the same time. The next relevant step for further investigating the child would be to:

1. Obtain HBeAg and anti-HBe levels
2. Obtain anti-HBs levels
3. Repeat HBsAg
4. Repeat another course of Hepatitis B vaccine

Ans. 2. Obtain anti-HBs levels

USMLE Case Scenario

Hypophosphatemic rickets is a condition causing abnormal regulation of vitamin D_3 metabolism and defects in renal tubular phosphate transport. Symptoms include growth retardation, osteomalacia, and rickets. It is an:

1. X-linked recessive condition
2. X-linked dominant condition
3. Autosomal dominant condition
4. Autosomal codominant condition

Ans. 2. X-linked dominant condition

USMLE Case Scenario

A 2-year-old boy was admitted to a pediatric hospital with a 7-day history of high fever, lymphadenopathy, conjunctivitis and an erythematous exfoliative rash affecting his trunk and extremities. On the basis of the characteristic clinical picture, a clinical diagnosis of Kawasaki's disease (also known as acute mucocutaneous lymph node syndrome). It is best described as:

1. An acute vasculitic disorder of infants affecting medium-and large-sized blood vessels made
2. A chronic non vasculitic disorder of infants affecting small-and medium-sized blood vessels made
3. A chronic non vasculitic disorder of infants affecting medium-and large-sized blood vessels made

Ans. 1. An acute vasculitic disorder of infants affecting medium-and large-sized blood vessels made

USMLE Case Scenario

A 2-year-old boy was admitted to a pediatric hospital with a 7-day history of high fever, lymphadenopathy, conjunctivitis and an erythematous exfoliative rash affecting his trunk and extremities. On the basis of the characteristic clinical picture, a clinical diagnosis of Kawasaki's disease was done. Since untreated or delayed treatment of Kawasaki's disease is associated with the development of coronary artery aneurysms, urgent treatment is:

1. With high-dose IVIg only
2. With high-dose IVIg in conjunction with paracetamol
3. With high-dose IVIg in conjunction with cyclosporine
4. With high-dose IVIg in conjunction with cycloserine
5. With high-dose IVIg in conjunction with aspirin

Ans. 5. With high-dose IVIg in conjunction with aspirin

USMLE Case Scenario

A child is born with a single functional allele of a tumor suppressor gene. At the age of five, the remaining normal allele is lost through a point mutation. As a result, the ability to inhibit cell cycle progression until the cell is ready to divide is lost. Which of the following neoplasms is most likely to arise via this mechanism?

1. Infiltrating ductal carcinoma of breast
2. Small cell anaplastic carcinoma of the lung
3. Retinoblastoma of eye
4. Cerebral astrocytoma
5. Chronic myeloid leukemia

Ans. 3. Retinoblastoma of eye

USMLE Case Scenario

An 8-year-old boy had abdominal pain, fever with bloody diarrhea for 18 months. His height is 100 cms and weight is 14.5 kg. Stool culture was negative for known enteropathogens. The sigmoidoscopy was normal. During the same period, child had an episode of renal colic and passed urinary gravel. The mantoux test was 5 x 5 mm. The most probable diagnosis is:

1. Ulcerative colitis
2. Crohn's disease
3. Intestinal tuberculosis
4. Strongyloidosis

Ans. 2. Crohn's disease

USMLE Case Scenario

An infant presents with history of seizures and skin rashes. Investigations show metabolic acidosis, increased blood ketone levels. This child is likely to be suffering from:

1. Propionic acidemia
2. Urea cyclic disorder
3. Phenylketonuria
4. Multiple carboxylase deficiency

Ans. 4. Multiple carboxylase deficiency

USMLE Case Scenario

In a family, the father has widely spaced eyes, increased facial hair and deafness. One of the three children has deafness with similar facial features. The mother is normal. Which one of the following is the most likely pattern of inheritance in this case?

1. Autosomal dominant
2. Autosomal recessive
3. X-linked dominant
4. X-linked recessive

Ans. 1. Autosomal dominant

USMLE Case Scenario

Webbing of neck, increased carrying angle, low posterior hair line and short fourth metacarpal are characteristics of:

1. Klinefelter syndrome
1. Turner syndrome
2. Cri du chat syndrome
3. Noonan syndrome
4. Down's syndrome

Ans. 2. Turner syndrome

USMLE Case Scenario

A 10-year-old boy has a fractured neck of femur. Biochemical evaluation revealed Hb 11.5 gm/dL and ESR 18 mm 1st hr. Serum calcium 12.8 mg/dl, serum phosphorus 2.3 mg/dl, alkaline phosphate 28 KA units and blood urea 32 mg/dl. Which of the following is the most probable diagnosis in his case?

1. Nutritional rickets
1. Renal rickets
2. Hyperparathyroidism
3. Skeletal dysplasia
4. Hypoparathyroidism

Ans. 3. Hyperparathyroidism

USMLE Case Scenario

A 5-year-old child from Ilinois presents with history of fever off and on for the past 2 weeks and petechial spots all over the body and increasing pallor for the past 1 month. Examination reveals splenomegaly of 2 cms below costal margin. The most likely diagnosis is:

1. Acute leukemia
1. Idiopathic thrombocytopenic purpura
2. Hypersplenism
3. Aplastic anemia
4. Lymphoma

Ans. A. Acute leukemia

USMLE Case Scenario

An 8-year-old child suffering from recurrent attacks of polyurea since childhood presents to the pediatrics OPD. On examination, the child is short-statured, vitals and BP are normal. Serum Creatinine – 6 mg%, HCO_3 – 16 meq, Na –134, K^+ 4.2. On USG, bilateral small kidneys are seen. Diagnosis is:

1. Reflux Nephropathy
1. Nephronophthisis
2. Polycystic kidney disease
3. Medullary cystic kidney disease

Ans. 2. Nephronophthisis

USMLE Case Scenario

A month-old HIV-positive child following URTI developed sudden onset of breathlessness. The chest X-ray shows hyperinflation. The O_2 saturation was greater than 90%. The treatment of choice is:

1. Cotrimoxazole
1. Ribavarin
2. IV ganciclovir
3. Nebulized acyclovir

Ans. 2. Ribavarin

USMLE Case Scenario

A four-month-old infant is brought to a physician because of increased lethargy and irritability. The father of the infant says that the child rolled off the bed and fell on the cemented floor. According to the father, the child has been previously healthy and is up-to-date on his vaccinations. He has been meeting his development milestones. While in the office, patient develops a seizure. Initial examination shows tense fontanellae and bruises on limbs. Which of the following is the next appropriate step?

1. Give immediate antipyretic
2. Give per rectal diazepam
3. Give IV midazolam
4. Get a CT scan head done
5. Perform a retinoscopic examination
6. Perform a lumbar puncture

Ans. 5. Perform a retinoscopic examination

Perform a retinoscopic examination. The child's history indicates shaken baby syndrome, in which the symptoms may not correlate with the physical findings. The child's fontanelles are full, indicative of increased intracranial pressure. A retinoscopic examination with blurred fundi is suggestive of increased pressure.

USMLE Case Scenario

An 8-year-old female child following URTI developed maculopapular rash on the jaw spreading onto the trunk which cleared on the 3rd day without desquamation and tender postauricular and suboccipital lymphadenopathy. The diagnosis is:

1. Kawasaki disease
2. Erythema infectiosum
3. Rubella
4. Measles

Ans. 3. Rubella

USMLE Case Scenario

An 8-year-old child presents with lethargy, multiple epiphyseal breaks, Wormian bones with growth retardation and mental retardation Diagnosis is?

1. Rickets
2. Hypothyroidism
3. Scurvy
4. Hypoparathyroidism

Ans. 2. Hypothyroidism

USMLE Case Scenario

A child presents with hepatosplenomegaly, abdominal distension, jaundice, anemia and adrenal calcification. Which of the following is the diagnosis?

1. Adrenal hemorrhage
2. Wolman's disease
3. Pheochromocytoma
4. Addison's disease

Ans. 2. Wolman's disease

USMLE Case Scenario

An infant with cleft lip, cleft palate, polydactly, microcephaly with holoprosencephaly, ectodermal scalp defect is suffering from:

1. Trisomy 21
2. Trisomy 18
3. Trisomy 13
4. Turner

Ans. 3. Trisomy 13

USMLE Case Scenario

Which vaccine is contraindicated in a child with history of convulsions?

1. DPT
2. Measles
3. Typhoid
4. BCG

Ans. 1. DPT

USMLE Case Scenario

A 16-month-old is taken to the emergency room after falling while learning to walk. The toddler has an enlarging, swollen bruise on his forehead, which is now over 5 cm across. The parents say that the bruise is noticeably larger than it was when they entered the emergency room an hour earlier. Clotting studies on the blood sample show a prolonged PTT and a normal PT and low levels of factor VIII. Which of the following is the most likely diagnosis?

1. Disseminated intravascular coagulation
2. Hemophilia A
3. Hemophilia B
4. Hyperhomocysteinemia
5. von Willebrand disease

Ans. 2. Hemophilia A

Hemophilia is an X-linked clotting disorder that occurs in two forms: hemophilia A due to deficient factor VIII and hemophilia B due to deficient factor IX. Some individuals with hemophilia have levels of these factors that are 5% of normal or even higher, and have relatively mild disease, only requiring replacement therapy during surgical procedures or other situations in which significant bleeding might occur. In contrast, individuals with factor levels less than 1% of normal have severe bleeding problems throughout life that usually become apparent (as in this case) by 18 months of age. In these individuals, excessive bleeding into joints and tissues may cause crippling musculoskeletal disorders.

USMLE Case Scenario

A 3.5 kg term male baby, born of uncomplicated pregnancy, developed, respiratory distress at birth, not responding to surfactant, ECHO finding revealed nothing abnormal, X-ray showed ground glass appearance and culture negative. Apgars 4 and 5 at 1 and 5 minutes. History of one-month female sibling died before. What is the diagnosis?

1. TAPVC
2. Meconium aspiration
3. Neonatal pulmonary alveolar proteinosis
4. Diffuse herpes simplex infection

Ans. 3. Neonatal pulmonary alveolar proteinosis

USMLE Case Scenario

A 3-year-old boy with normal developmental milestones has a problem of delayed speech and difficulty in communication and concentration. He is not making friends. Most probable diagnosis is:

1. Autism
2. ADHD
3. Mental retardation
4. Specific learning disability

Ans. 1. Autism

USMLE Case Scenario

A 3-month-old child has moderate fever and nonproductive cough and mild dyspnea. After course of mild antibiotic, the condition of the child improved transiently but he again develops high fever, productive cough and increased respiratory distress. Chest X-ray shows hyperlucency and PFT shows obstructive pattern. Most probable diagnosis is:

1. Alveolar microlithiasis
2. Postviral syndrome
3. Follicular bronchitis
4. Bronchiolitis obliterans

Ans. 4. Bronchiolitis obliterans

USMLE Case Scenario

Single gene defect causing multiple unrelated problems is:

1. Pleiotropism
2. Pseudodominance
3. Penetrance
4. Anticipation

Ans. 1. Pleiotropism

USMLE Case Scenario

An 8-day-old breastfed baby presents with vomiting, poor feeding and loose stools. On examination, the heart rate is 190/minute, blood pressure 50/30 mm Hg, respiratory rate 72 breaths/minute and capillary refill time of 4 seconds. Investigations show hemoglobin level of 15 g/dl, Na 120 mEq/l, K 6.8 mEq/l, bicarbonate 15 mEq/l, urea 30 mg/dl and creatinine 0.6 mg/dl. The most likely diagnosis is:

1. Congenital adrenal hyperplasia
2. Acute tubular necrosis
3. Congenital hypertrophic pyloric stenosis
4. Renal tubular acidosis

Ans. 2. Acute tubular necrosis

USMLE Case Scenario

A neonate is being investigated for jaundice. A liver biopsy shows features of a 'Giant cell/Neonatal hepatitis'. Which one of the following conditions usually results in this case?

1. Congenital hepatic fibrosis
2. Hemochromatosis
3. Alpha-1-antitrypsin deficiency
4. Glycogen storage disease Type 1

Ans. 3. Alpha-1-antitrypsin deficiency

USMLE Case Scenario

A 2-month-old girl has failure to thrive, polyuria and medullary nephrocalcinosis affecting both the kidneys. Investigations show blood pH 7.48, bicarbonate 25 mEq/l, potassium 2 mEq/l, sodium 126 mEq/l and chloride 88 mEq/l. The most likely diagnosis is:

1. Distal renal tubular acidosis
2. Primary hyperaldosteronism
3. Bartter's syndrome
4. Pseudohypoaldosteronism

Ans. 3. Bartter's syndrome

USMLE Case Scenario

A 2-year-old child comes with discharge, seborrheic dermatitis, polyuria and hepatosplenomegaly. Which of the following is the most likely diagnosis:

1. Leukemia
2. Lymphoma
3. Langerhan's cell histiocytosis
4. Germ cell tumor

Ans. 3. Langerhan's cell histiocytosis

USMLE Case Scenario

A 3-month-old male infant developed otitis media for which he was given a course of cotrimoxazole. A few days later, he developed extensive peeling of the skin; there were no mucosal lesions and the baby was not toxic. The most likely diagnosis is:

1. Toxic epidermal necrolysis
2. Staphylococcal scalded skin syndrome
3. Stevens-johnson syndrome
4. Infantile pemphigus

Ans. 2. Staphylococcal scalded skin syndrome

USMLE Case Scenario

A child with pyoderma becomes toxic and presents with respiratory distress. His chest radiograph shows patchy areas of consolidation and multiple bilateral thin-walled air-containing cysts. The most likely etiological agent in this case is:

1. *Mycobacterium tuberculosis*
2. *Staphylococcus aureus*
3. *Mycobacterium avium intracellulare*
4. *Pneumocystis carinii*

Ans. 2. Staphylococcus aureus

USMLE Case Scenario

A 2-year-old girl-child is brought to the outpatient with features of handwringing stereotype movements, impaired language and communication development, breath-holding spells, poor social skills and deceleration of head growth after 6 months of age. The most likely diagnosis is:

1. Asperger's syndrome
2. Rett's syndrome
3. Fragile X syndrome
4. Collard syndrome

Ans. 2. Rett's syndrome

USMLE Case Scenario

Posterior iliac horns are seen in:

1. Fisher's syndrome
2. Crouzon syndrome
3. Nail patella syndrome
4. Pierre Robin syndrome

Ans. 3. Nail patella syndrome

USMLE Case Scenario

A 10-year-old child presented with headache, vomiting, gait instability and diplopia. On examination, he had papilloedema and gait ataxia. The most probable diagnosis is:

1. Hydrocephalus
2. Brainstem tumor
3. Suprasellar tumor
4. Midline posterior fossa tumor

Ans. 4. Midline posterior fossa tumor

USMLE Case Scenario

The metabolic derangement in congenital pyloric stenosis is:

1. Hypochloremic alkalosis
2. Hyperchloremic alkalosis
3. Hyperchloremic acidosis
4. Hypochloremic acidosis

Ans. 1. Hypochloremic alkalosis

USMLE Case Scenario

Hair on end appearance is seen in:

1. Thalassemia
2. Scurvy
3. Rickets
4. Hemochromatosis

Ans. 1. Thalassemia

USMLE Case Scenario

Egg on side appearance is seen in:

1. TOF
2. TAPVC
3. Uncorrected TGA
4. Truncus arteriosus

Ans. 3. Uncorrected TGA

USMLE Case Scenario

Snowman appearance on X-ray is seen's in which cardiac pathology:

1. Fallot's tetrology
2. TAPVC
3. TGA
4. Ebstein's anomaly

Ans. 2. TAPVC

USMLE Case Scenario

A 40-year-old female patient presented with recurrent headaches. MRI showd an extra-aixal, dural-based and enhancing lesion. The most likely diagnosis is:

1. Meningioma
2. Glioma
3. Schwannoma
4. Pituitary adenoma

Ans. 1. Meningioma

USMLE Case Scenario

Which of the following is the most common cause of a mixed cystic and solid suprasellar mass seen on cranial MR scan of a 10-year-old child?

1. Pituitary adenoma
2. Craniopharyngioma
3. Optic chiasmal glioma
4. Germinoma

Ans. 2. Craniopharyngioma

USMLE Case Scenario

A 7-year-old boy from Kansas is brought to the emergency department. His parents assert that over the past 3 days, he has become progressively ill with generalized fatigue and mid-abdominal pain that have become steadily worse. On examination, he has a maculopapular rash on both of his thighs.
The rash does not blanch and some lesions near the ankles look petechial.
His temperature is (103.4°F). He has dark stool, which is positive for occult blood.
The physician determines that the boy is dehydrated.
Which of the following is the most likely diagnosis?

1. Pancreatitis
2. Rocky mountain spotted fever
3. Nephrotic syndrome
4. Henöch-Schönlein purpura

Ans: 4. Henöch-Schönlein purpura
Henöch-Scholein Purpura (HSP) is the most likely diagnosis. This boy has abdominal pain with guaiac-positive stools, but also has a prominent rash, mostly on his lower extremities. Other characteristic findings of HSP include hematuria and joint pains. The illness may follow an upper respiratory infection or strep throat.

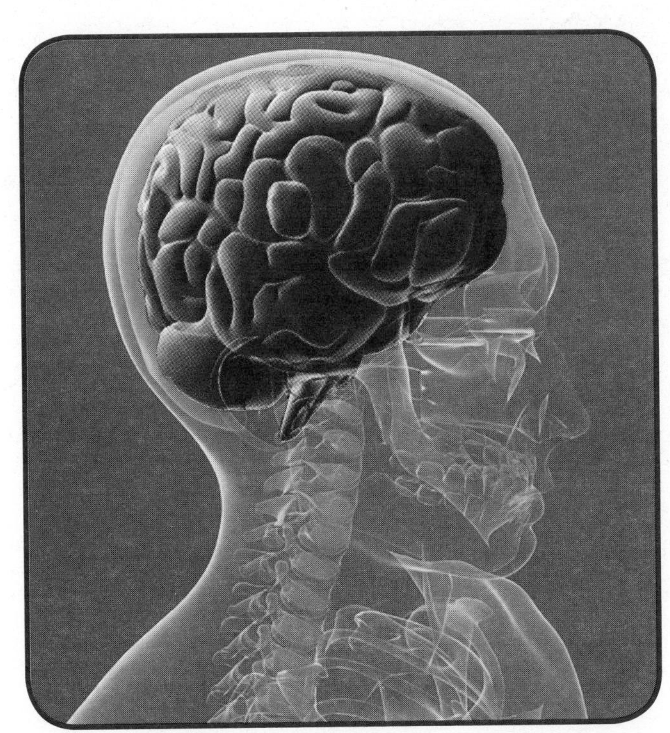

PSYCHIATRY

Psychiatry 3

Basics of Psychiatry

Father of 'Modern' Psychiatry: Johan Weyer
Frued: Freud was an **Austrian: Born in 1856. (1856-1939)**

Freuds Contributions Include

- **Founder of Psychoanalysis**
- **Defense Mechanism**
- **Free association**
  - **Concepts of**
  - **Libido**
  - **Repression**
  - **Transference**
  - **Regression**
  - **Sublimation**
- **Concepts of**
  - **Id**
  - **Ego**
  - **Superego**
- **Oedipus complex**
- **Analysis of Properties of Cocaine**

Basic Terminology Commonly Asked

• **Agnosia**	• **Inability to recognize a specific sensory stimuli**
• **Apraxia**	• **Inability to perform purposive movement**
• **Alexia**	• **Inability to read**
• **Acalculia**	• **Inability to perform arithmetic calculation**
• **Agraphia**	• **Inability to write**
• **Anosmia**	• **Inability to smell**
• **Prospaganosia**	• **Inability to identify a familiar face**
• **Alexithymia**	• **Inability to recognize and describe feelings**

- **Id:** Drives instincts present at birth
- **Ego:** Defense mechanisms, judgment, relation to reality, object relationships, developed after birth
- **Works on reality principle**
- **Superego:** Conscience formed during latency period

Psychiatric Terminology Commonly asked

• Deja vu	• Sensation of feeling of familiarity • Seen in temporal lobe epilepsy • Normal person psychosis
• Jamias vu	• Sensation of feeling of unfamiliarity
• Neologisms	• Idiosyncratically formed new words which cannot be easily understood
• Flight of ideas	• Rapid speech with rapid change in ideas
• Verbigeration	• Senseless repetition of same words over and over again

Neurotransmitters and Their Imbalance Causes

• ↑DA levels	• Schizophrenia
• ↓Ach	• Dementia
• ↑NA	• Mania, Anxiety
• ↓5HT, NA	• OCD
• ↓GABA	• Epilepsy
• ↓Serotonin	• Depression

USMLE Case Scenario

A 41-year-old woman presented with a history of aches and pains all over the body and generalized weakness for four years. She cannot sleep because of the illness and has lost her appetite as well. She has lack of interest in work and does not like to meet friends and relatives. She denies feelings of sadness. Her most likely diagnosis is related to:

1. ↑Serotinin
2. ↓Serotonin
3. ↑Noradrenaline
4. ↓Acetylcholine
5. ↓GABA

Ans: 2. ↓Serotonin

Psychological and Neuropsychological Diagnostic Tests Used in Psychiatry

Category of Test	Test
• Intelligence	• Wechsler Adult Intelligence Scale-revised • Wechsler Intelligence Scale for Children-revised • Wechsler Preschool and Primary Scale of Intelligence
• Achievement	• Wide-Range Achievement Test • Peabody Individual Achievement Test
• Personality (used to identify personality characteristics and psychopathology)	• Minnesota Multiphasic Personality Inventory • Rorschach Test • Sentence Completion Test • Thematic Apperception Test
• Neuropsychological	• Halstead-Reitan Battery • Luria-Nebraska Neuropsychological Battery • Bender Visual-Motor Gestalt Test

COGNITIVE DISORDERS

Functions disturbed in 'Organic Brain Syndrome'

- Consciousness
- Orientation
- Abstract thinking
- Recent memory
- Intelligence

Delirium

- Acute onset
- Memory registration and retention impaired
- Clouding of consciousness
- Disorientation in time, place, person
- Attention and concentration disturbed
- Hallucinations common
- Disturbed sleep wake pattern
- Marked diurnal variation (IMP)

Dementia

- Chronic onset usually
- There is **no disturbance of consciousness**
- There is **cognitive impairment**
- **Impaired judgment**
- **Personality alteration**
- **Impaired memory**
- Attention and concentration undisturbed
- Hallucinations **uncommon**
- Diurnal variation **absent**

- **Retrograde Amnesia** is characterized by an **inability to remember events prior to the onset of disease**, with preservation of the ability to form new memories
- **Anterograde Amnesia** is characterized by an **inability to register and form lasting memories of new or present events.**
- **Proactive Inhibition** is when **something newly learned interferes with previously iearned information.** New material inhibits old material
- **Retroactive Inhibition** is when **previously learned material interferes with the ability to acquire new information.** Old material inhibits new material
- **Transient Global Amnesia** is characterized by **confusion and impairment of recent memory.** It often occurs in elderly people and resolves without sequelaie

Causes of 'Reversible' Dementias

- Hypothyroidism
- **Hypoparathyroidism**
- **Hyperparathyroidism**
- Thiamine deficiency (Wernicke's encephalopathy)

- Vitamin B12 deficiency
- Drug intoxication
- Normal Pressure Hydrocephalus

Causes of 'Irreversible' Dementias

- Alzheimers Dementia **(MC CAUSE)**
- Picks disease
- Huntingtons disease
- Multi infarct dementia
- Leucoencephalopathies
- Vasculitis

Alzheimer's Disease

- **Cortical** Dementia **not Subcortical Dementia**
- Causes **brain atrophy** in advanced cases
- Progressive dementia
- Atrophy usually involves **frontal, temporal and parietal** lobes
- **Nucleus Basalis of Meynert** is effected
  - **Aphasia**
  - **Amnesia**
  - **Agnosia**
  - **Acalculia**
  - **Alexia are features**

There is reduction in **acetylcholine** concentration

Associations with

Down's syndrome, APP (Amyloid precursor Protein gene on Chromosome 21)

APO E gene

- **Presinilin 1** on Chromosome 14
- **Presinilin 2** on chromosome 1
- **Treatment is by**
- **Tacrine**
- **Donepezil**
- **Memantine**
  - **Neurofibrillary tangles** are intracytoplasmic filamentous inclusions found in Alzheimer's disease and, to alesser extent, in normal aging brains
  - **Granulovacuolar degeneration**
  - **Hirano Bodies:** They are Specific protein deposits associated with **AGE (**Advance Glycosylation End products**)** localized within soma of neurons
  - **Amyloid Plaques:** They represent fragmented accumulations of proteins which are normally broken down but accumulate in Alzheimer's disease
  - **Alzheimer's Cells (Special cells)**
  - **Neurofibrillary tangles** are insoluble twisted fibrils composed of **Tau proteins**

Pseudodementia

- It is seen in **depression**
- Severely depressed individuals may appear demented, a phenomenon called **pseudodementia**
- Unlike cortical dementias, **memory and language are usually intact** when carefully tested in depressed persons

- The patients may feel confused and are unable to accomplish routine tasks
- Vegetative symptoms are common, such as insomnia, lack of energy, poor appetite and concern with bowel function
- The psychosocial milieu may suggest prominent reasons for depression
- The patients respond to antidepressant treatment

Cortical Dementia	Subcortical Dementia
• Site affected: **Cortex**	• Site affected: subcortex
• **Severe** memory loss	• Mild – moderate memory loss
• **Aphasia, Amnesia, Agnosia, Acalculia, Dyslexia**	• Dysarthia, dystonia, chorea, rigidity, tremor, ataxia
– **Alzheimer's dementia**	– **Parkinsonism**
	– **Huntingtons chorea**
	– **Wilson's disease**

Pervasive Developmental Disorders

- Pervasive developmental disorders are characterized by the **'failure to acquire or the early loss of social skills and language'**, resulting in life long problems in social and occupational functioning
- These disorders include:
  - **Autistic disorder**
  - **Asperger disorder**
  - **Rett disorder**
  - **Childhood disintegrative disorder**

Autism

- Autism is characterized by onset of symptoms **before 3 years of age**
- **Difficulty in concentration and communication** is typical
- Lesion in frontal lobe, temporal lobe, cerebellum
- **Delayed speech and Language development** (absence of babbling, presence of echolalia)
- **Problems in forming social relationships in early childhood. (Aloofness, absent social smile, lack of eye to eye contact)**
- **Males** are more affected in autism
- **Features:**
  - **Stereotyped movements**
  - **Poor speech**
  - **Lack of social interaction**

Some autistic children develop well developed isolated skills atypically such as remote memory, calculating abilities and musical abilities. This atypical presentation is called as **'Idiot savant syndrome'**

Children develop

- Mental retardation
- Epilepsy
- EEG abnormalities

Differential Diagnosis

Asperger's syndrome is a different entity

Characterized by autism **without any delay in language or cognitive development**

Better Prognosis

Retts Syndrome is mostly common in girls with **deceleration of head growth between five months and 30 months**

Stereotyped movements with **hand clapping and head wringing** are characteristic

Remember: Conduct Disorder

Conduct disorder is a **childhood/adolescent disorder** defined as a **pattern of behavior in which the basic rights of others are violated** with three or more of the following present in the past 12 months:

- Destruction of property
- **Cruelty to animals and people**
- **Deceitfulness or theft**
- **Serious violations of rules**
- **It causes clinically significant impairment in social functioning**

Attention Deficit Hyperactivity Disorder (ADHD)

- **Attention deficit hyperactivity disorder**
- Requires the **presence of six symptoms of inattention for at least 6 months to a degree that is maladaptive and six symptoms of hyperactivity/impulsivity that cause social impairment**
- Symptoms are present in two or more settings (e.g. home and school) and some of the symptoms are **present before age**
- The symptoms are not due to a general medical condition or other mental disorder
- ADHD (Attention Deficient Hyperkinetic Disorder) occurs before **seven years of age**. It is characterized by
  - **Poor attention span or Easy Distractibility**
  - **Hyperactivity**
  - **And Impulsivity ADHD is more common in males**
- ADHD is more common in school going children
- **Methyl phenidate is used in treatment**
- **Atomoxetine is used for treatment**

USMLE Case Scenario

A 7-year-old boy from California is referred by his Science teacher for psychiatric evaluation. The teachers has noticed that, in the past year, he has been unable to sustain attention in class, and has been indulging in excessive talking to his friends during class. He is forgetful and losses things easily. He is not attentitive to what is told to him. Most likely diagnosis is:
Ans. Attention deficit/hyperactivity disorder (ADHD)

Attention deficit/hyperactivity disorder (ADHD) is characterized by impulsivity, hyperactivity, and inattention lasting at least 6 months. To make the diagnosis, the disorder must have started before age 7 and six signs each of inattention and impulsivity/hyperactivity need to be present.

In children, bipolar disorder often presents as extremely irritable and explosive mood, with poor psychosocial functioning, decreased sleep, talkativeness, racing thoughts, and high energy.

Conduct disorder is diagnosed when the child has had symptoms of aggression toward people and animals, destruction of property, deceitfulness or theft, and serious violation of rules. One symptom needs to last at least 6 months, even though the symptoms may have been present intermittently for a year.

Post-traumatic stress disorder develops following trauma, and the child usually has symptoms of hypervigilance, increased arousal avoidance and autonomic reactivity.

Rett syndrome belongs to the pervasive developmental disorders mostly seen in girls. The child has normal development through the first 5 months of life. During the second year, however, she develops multiple deficits, including decreased head growth, decreased hand skills, social impairment and impaired gait and trunk movements.

Intermittent Explosive Disorder

- It is diagnosed in adults only after several episodes of **failure to resist aggressive impulses that lead to assaults or destruction of property**
- The **degree of episodes is not proportionate to precipitating stressor**
- The disorder is not due to any other mental disorder or general medical condition

Oppositional Defiant Disorder

Oppositional defiant disorder is a pattern of **negativistic and defiant behavior lasting at least 6 months** with four or more of the following:

- **Loss of temper**
- **Arguments with adults**
- **Defying rules**
- **Deliberately annoying other people**
- **Blaming others for own faults**
- **Presence of vindictive behavior**
- **Presence of anger and resentment**

- **Conduct disorder** is a childhood/adolescent disorder defined as a pattern of behavior in which the basic rights of others are violated with three or more of the following present in the past 12 months: destruction of property, cruelty to animals and people, deceitfulness or theft, and serious violations of rules. It causes clinically significant impairment in social functioning and it is reserved for patients younger than 18
- **Attention deficit/hyperactivity disorder** requires the presence of six symptoms of inattention for at least 6 months to a degree that is maladaptive and six symptoms of hyperactivity/impulsivity that cause social impairment. Symptoms are present in two or more settings (e.g. home and school), and some of the symptoms are present before age 7. The symptoms are not due to a general medical condition or other mental disorder
- **Intermittent explosive disorder** is diagnosed in adults only after several episodes of failure to resist aggressive impulses that lead to assaults or destruction of property. The degree of episodes is not proportionate to precipitating stressor. The disorder is not due to any other mental disorder or general medical condition
- **Oppositional defiant disorder** is a pattern of negativistic and defiant behavior lasting at least 6 months with four or more of the following: loss of temper, arguments with adults, defying rules, deliberately annoying other people, blaming others for own faults, presence of vindictive behavior, presence of anger and resentment

Never forget to differentiate between

Illusion	Hallucination	Delusion	Depersonalization	Derealization
Misinterpretation of stimuli arising from external object	Perception **without** stimuli	False unshakable belief **not amenable to** reasoning	An alteration in perception **to self**	An alteration in perception **to external world**

Delusion

Delusion is a **false unshakable belief**
Delusion is a disorder of **thought**

- **Capgras syndrome** is delusion of doubles
- **Othello syndrome** is delusion involving infidelity of spouse
- **Delusion of Dysmorphobia** is body parts appearing ugly
- **Nihilistic delusion** is seen in **depression**
- 'The female in a delusional state that the attractive person is in love with her. This is **De Clerambaults Syndrome or erotomanic delusion** that a person of **high status is in love with her.'**
- **Delusion of Reference :** Misinterpretation that events in the outside world are having direct personal relationship

Hallucination

Disorder	Most Common Delusion
Depression	• Nihilistic delusion
Mania	• Delusions of grandeur
Schizophrenia	• Paranoid delusions • Delusions of reference

- Hallucination is **false perception** without external stimulus
- Disorder of **perception**
- **'Auditory' hallucinations** are a feature of **nonorganic disorders**
- **'Visual hallucinations'** are a feature of **organic psychiatric disorders**
- Hallucinations are **involuntary**
- It is viewed as sensory perception and occurs **in inner subjective space**
- **Not dependent on will of observer**
- **'Tactile' hallucinations** are seen in cocaine abuse
- **'Hypnagogic' hallucinations** when one goes to sleep
- **'Hypnopompic' hallucinations** are ones when one wakes from sleep
- **Formed visual hallucinations are seen in temporal lobe lesion**

Neurotic disorders
- Insight **present**
- Reality testing is **intact**

Psycotic disorder
- Insight **absent**
- Reality testing is **not intact**
- Presence of delusions and hallucinations

SCHIZOPHRENIA

First Rank Symptoms in Schizophrenia

Hallucinations

Delusional perception

Thought Alienation phenomenon
- Thought withdrawal
- Thought insertion
- Thought broadcasting

Passivity phenomenon
- Made feelings
- Made impulses
- Made acts
- Somatic passivity

Bleuler's Criterion for Schizophrenia

- **Ambivalence**
- **Autism**
- **Affect disturbance**
- **Association disturbance**

- **Commonest type: Paranoid** Schizophrenia
- **Early onset and bad prognosis: Hebephrenic** Schizophrenia
- **Late onset, best prognosis: Catatonic** Schizophrenia
- **Worst prognosis: Simple** Schizophrenia

- Most common hallucination in Schizophrenia is **Auditory hallucination**
- Ist symptom to go with treatment is **Auditory hallucination**
- Ist symptom to reappear after resistance to drugs is **Auditory hallucination**

- **Amphetamines** cause paranoid Schizophrenia
  - Mutism
  - Rigidity
  - Waxy flexibility
  - Mannerism
  - Grimacing
  - Verbigeration are a feature of **Catatonic schizophrenia**
- **Senseless giggling and mirror gazing** are seen in **Hebephrenic schizophrenia**
- **Dramatic self mutilation** in schizophrenia is called **von Gogh Syndrome**

- **'Brief psycotic disorder':** one day to one month duration of psycosis
- **'Schizeniform disorder'**< 6 months
- **'Schizophrenia':** > 6 months
- **Disorder of thought and perception**

Schizophrenia is a heterogeneous syndrome characterized by **perturbations of language, perception, thinking, social activity, affect, and volition**

Patients may present with

- **'Positive symptoms'** (such as conceptual disorganization, delusions, or hallucinations) or
- **'Negative symptoms'** (loss of function, anhedonia, decreased emotional expression, impaired concentration and diminished social engagement) and must have **'at least two of these for a 1-month period'** and continuous signs for **'at least 6 months'** to meet formal diagnostic criteria
- 'Negative' symptoms predominate in **one-third of the schizophrenic population** and are associated with a **poor long-term outcome** and a **poor response to drug treatment**

- **Catatonic-type** describes patients whose clinical presentation is dominated by profound changes in motor activity, negativism and echolalia or echopraxia
- **Paranoid-type** describes patients who have a prominent preoccupation with a specific delusional system and who otherwise do not qualify as having disorganized-type disease
- **Disorganized-type** in which disorganized speech and behavior are accompanied by a **superficial or silly affect**
- **Residual-type disease**, negative symptomatology exists in the absence of delusions, hallucinations, or motor disturbance

- The diagnosis of **'Schizophreniform disorder'** is reserved for patients who meet the symptom requirements but not the duration requirements for schizophrenia
- The diagnosis of 'Schizo**affective** **disorder**' is used for those whose symptoms of schizophrenia are independent of associated periods of mood disturbance
- About **10% of schizophrenic patients commit suicide**

Epidemiologic surveys identify three principal risk factors for schizophrenia:

- **Genetic susceptibility**
- **Early developmental insults and**
- **Winter birth**

Neuroimaging Structural and Functional Abnormalities

- **Enlargement of the lateral and third ventricles with associated cortical atrophy and sulcal enlargement**
- **Volumetric reductions in the amygdala, hippocampus, right prefrontal cortex, and thalamus**
- **Altered asymmetry of the planum temporale**
- **Decreases in neuronal metabolism in the thalamus and prefrontal cortex**

- **'The Dopamine Hypothesis of Schizophrenia'** is based on the fact that agents that diminish dopaminergic activity have beneficial effects in reducing the acute symptoms and signs of psychosis, specifically agitation, anxiety and hallucinations
- **TREATMENT: Antipsychotic agents** remain the cornerstone of acute and maintenance treatment of schizophrenia and are effective in the treatment of hallucinations, delusions, and thought disorders, regardless of etiology
- **Older agents, such as chlorpromazine and thioridazine, are more sedating and anticholinergic and more likely to cause orthostatic hypotension, while higher potency antipsychotics, such as haloperidol, perphenazine and thiothixene, carry a higher risk of inducing extrapyramidal side effects**

- **Acute onset**
- **Late onset**
- **Short duration**
- **Female**
- **Fatty physique**
- **Family history of Mood disorder**
- **Presence of stressor**
- **Positive symptom predominance**
- **Catatonic type**
- **Good Social Support**
- **Normal CT scan of head**

'Good Prognostic Factors' of Schizophrenia are

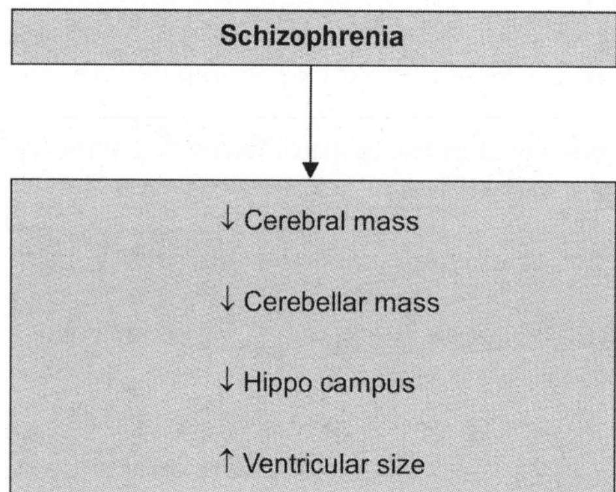

Catatonic Schizophrenia

- **Mutism: Absence of speech**
- **Rigidity seen**
- **Waxy flexibility: Parts of body in uncomfortable position for a long period of time**
- **Defect of conation**
- **Stupor**
- **Negativism**
- **Echolalia: Repetition of phrases/words**
- **Echopraxia**
- **Mannerism and grimacing**
- **Automatic obedience**
- **Ambitendency**
- **Verbigeration: Incomprehensible speech**
- **Cataplexy not catalepsy**

Personality Disorders

- **Are pervasive, fixed, inappropriate patterns of relating to others that cause social and occupational impairment**
- **Have limited insight**
- **Do not have frank psychosis**

The DSM-IV classifies Personality disorders into

- **Cluster A**
- **Cluster B**
- **Cluster C**

Cluster A: Fear Social Relationships

- **Paranoid:** Distrustful, Suspicious, attributes responsibility for own problems to others
- **Schizoid:** Long standing pattern of social withdrawal without psychosis
- **Schizotypal:** Magical thinking, odd thought patterns and odd behavior

Cluster B : Emotional, inconsistent or dramatic

- **Histrionic:** Emotional, extrovert, sexually provocative
- **Narcissistic:** Pompous, with sense of special entitlement, lacks empathy for others
- **Antisocial:** Refuses to confirm to social norms shows no concern for others
- **Borderline:** Erratic, unstable mood, feelings of aloneness

Cluster C : Fearful or anxious

- **Avoidant:** Timid, sensitive to rejection, socially withdrawn
- **Obsessive Compulsive:** Perfectionistic, orderly, stubborn, feelings of imperfection
- **Dependent:** Allows other people to make descisions and poor self-confidence

USMLE Case Scenario

Personality Disorder	Clinical Scenario
• **Paranoid**	• A 42-year-old lecturer in history says that she was fired from her job because she **worked too hard** and made her Head of Department look lazy. She says that when the same thing happened in a previous job, she filed a **lawsuit** against that company
• **Schizoid**	• On a OPD visit the parents of a 22-year-old man say that they are concerned about him because he has **no friends** and spends most of his time hiking in the woods. You examine him and find that he is content with his **solitary life**
• **Schizotypal**	• An oddly dressed 30-year-old woman says that she likes to walk in the woods because the **animals communicate with her.** She says that she never goes out after 6 PM however, because they are 'dangerous hours'. She has few friends
• **Histrionic**	• A 23-year-old man comes to your office dressed in **yellow color** and a cap lined with red satin. He reports that his mild **sore throat felt like 'a hot poker'** when he swallowed and says that he feels so warm that he must have a **fever of at least 106°**
• **Narcissistic**	• A 33-year-old man basically a student with **poor economic and academic career** asks you to that he is the **richest man on earth** and that he is the **most learnt person around**. He says that he is 'better' than your other patients
• **Antisocial**	• A 30-year-old man says that he had **set fire to the school he studied.** He has often been unemployed and has been arrested for stealing and robbery several times
• **Borderline**	• A 20-year-old graduate tells you that because she was afraid to be alone again, she **tried to commit suicide** after a man with whom she had two dates did not call her again. After your interview, she tells you that all of the other doctors she has seen were horrible and that you are the only doctor who has ever understood her problem

Personality Disorder	Clinical Scenario
• **Avoidant**	• A 30-year-old woman who works as a tutor lives with her elderly mother and rarely socializes. She reports that when coworkers ask her to join them for dinner, she refuses because she is afraid that they **will not like her**
• **Obsessive-compulsive**	• A 33-year-old man reports that each night he **washes his hands at least 6 times after dinner. He checks his door at least 7 times before going to sleep** and checks the night lamp frequently
• **Dependent**	• A 28-year-old woman says that **her brother accompanies her everytime** she leaves her home and on her marriage would take him along with her to her new house and she says that she **cannot decide anything of her own** and everyday decisions her brother decides for her

USMLE Case Scenario

A 17-year-old girl was brought to the psychiatric emergency after she slashed her wrists in an attempt to commit suicide. On enquiry her father revealed that she had made several such attempts of wrist slashing in the past, mostly in response to trivial fights in her house. Further she had marked fluctuations in her mood with a pervasive pattern of unstable interpersonal relationship. The most probable diagnosis is:

1. Dependant disorder
2. Borderline personality disorder
3. Major depression
4. Histrionic personality disorder
5. Adjustment disorder

Ans: 2. Borderline personality disorder

Adjustment Disorders

Adjustment disorder	Normal grief	Acute stress disorder	Post-traumatic stress disorder. (PTSD)
Emotional symptoms that **start within 3 months and end within 6 months** of exposure to a stressor.	Expected strong emotional response usually sadness after a loss	Pshycological symptoms **lasting 2 days – 4 weeks/ within a month** after stressor	Psycological symptoms lasting > **4 weeks** after stressor

USMLE Case Scenario

Three years back a woman suffered during an earthquake and she was successfully saved. After recovery she has nightmares about the episode and she also gets up in the night and feels terrified. The most probable diagnosis is:

1. Major depression
2. Post-traumatic stress disorder
3. Mania
4. Schizophrenia

Ans: 2. Post-traumatic stress disorder

Comparison between Normal Grief (Bereavement) and Abnormal Grief (Depression)

Normal Grief	Abnormal Grief
• A 55-year-old woman whose husband died 3 months in a major car accident ago appears well groomed and reports that although she often **feels sad, she enjoys spending time with her children**	• A 62-year-old woman whose husband died 4 months ago appears dirty, has **lost 10 kg and refuses interact with friends and family**

Kubler-Ross's death and <u>dying sequence</u> is a stepwise process with 5 identified stages

The order in which these stages appear is the following

- Denial

- Anger
- Bargaining
- Sadness
- Acceptance

Somatoform Disorders

'Somatoform disorders are characterized by **physical symptoms without a sufficient organic cause.** A person who has a somatoform disorder is not malingering and not delusional but truly believes that he or she has a physical problem.'

The five major DSM-IV classifications of somatoform disorders are:

- **Somatization disorder**
- **Conversion disorder**
- **Hypochondriasis**
- **Body dysmorphic features**
- **Pain disorder**
- **Undifferentiated somatoform disorders**

Somatization Disorder

- Patients with **multiple somatic complaints that cannot be explained by a known medical condition.** The somatoform disorders include a variety of conditions that differ in terms of the specific symptoms that are present and in whether or not the symptoms are intentionally produced
- In somatization disorder the **patient presents with multiple physical complaints referable to different organ systems**
- Onset is usually before age 30, and the disorder is persistent
- Formal diagnostic criteria require the recording of
  - **At least four pain**
  - **Two gastrointestinal**
  - **One sexual**
  - **One pseudoneurologic symptom**
- Patients with somatization disorder often present with **dramatic complaints, but the complaints are inconsistent**
- Symptoms of comorbid anxiety and mood disorder are common and may be the result of drug interactions due to regimens initiated independently by different physicians
- Patients with somatization disorder may be **impulsive and demanding and frequently qualify for a formal comorbid psychiatric diagnosis**

Conversion Disorder

- Here symptoms focus on deficits that **involve voluntary motor or sensory function and on psychological factors** that initiate or exacerbate the medical presentation
- Like somatization disorder, the **deficit is not intentionally produced or simulated,** as is the case in factitious disorder (malingering)
- Deficit is proceeded by conflicts/stressors
- Deficit cannot be fully explained by medical condition or substance use
- Deficit can cause significant distress/impairment
- **La Belle Indifference** is noted
- **Primary and secondary gain are associated**

Hypochondriasis

- Here the essential feature is a **belief of serious medical illness that persists despite reassurance and appropriate medical evaluation**
- Abnormal preoccupation with normal body function

- Belief is **persistent** even after normal reports
- Patients with **hypochondriasis** have a history of poor relationships with physicians stemming from their sense that they have been evaluated and treated inappropriately or inadequately
- Fear or belief is **not a delusion**

Munchausen's Syndrome

- The patient **consciously and voluntarily produces physical symptoms of illness**
- It is reserved for individuals with **particularly dramatic, chronic, or severe factitious illness**
- A variety of signs, symptoms and diseases have been either simulated or caused by factitious behavior the most common including **chronic diarrhea, fever of unknown origin, intestinal bleeding or hematuria, seizures and hypoglycemia**
- Sole purpose is to obtain medical attention
- **Pseudologia fantastica** is a feature
- **Grid abdomen with multiple scars** is a feature
- Patients are **manipulative, convincing liars** and have superficial knowledge of medical terminology

USMLE Case Scenario

A 40-year-old male from Texas is admitted with complaints of abdominal pain and headache. General physical examination revealed six scars on the abdomen from previous surgeries. He seems to maintain a sick role and seeks attention from the nurses. He demands multiple diagnostic tests including a liver biopsy. The treating team failed to diagnose any major physical illness in the patient. His mental status examination did not reveal any major psychopathology. One of the treating staff recognized him to have appeared in several other hospital with abdominal pain and some other vague complaints. He is most likely suffering from:

1. Schizophrenia
2. Malingering
3. Somatization disorder
4. Factitious disorder
5. Conversion disorder

Ans. 4. Factitious disorder

Munchausen Syndrome by Proxy

Munchausen syndrome by proxy is also called **fabricated, fictitious or falsified illness.** This form of abuse results from the **production or presentation of false illness in the child by an adult, usually a parent.** Related behaviors include mothering to death, doctor shopping, overanxious parents

- The syndrome requires a parent who exhibits the behavior **('the perpetrator')** and **assumes the sick role by proxy, a child who is dependent and unable to prevent the deception and a doctor who is deceived into accepting the child as ill**
- The **parent positively gains attention** and care for themselves as the **'good' parent of a sick child,** as well as status with friends and family, and **continual social, professional and most of all personal gratification.** Other **rewards may be financial, through disability allowance, social through relationships with health care staff**, but these are not essential parts of the syndrome. Addiction to hospitals has been described. Additional gains may be acquired, e.g. through the media, active participation in parent support groups and from the legal process if cases go to court. Harm results from the betrayal of trust by the adult of the **Features:**
  - **Excessively heavy case notes** are a characteristic feature
  - **Frequent admission to hospital**
  - **Attendance at several clinics for a variety of complaints**
  - **Symptoms and signs are produced which do not resolve**
  - **There is constant production of new, varied symptoms** and signs
  - The child's **clinical appearance is not consistent with the description of his symptoms**
  - **The parents' response to the serious clinical picture, which they communicate of their child is inappropriate**
  - **There is ever-increasing pressure by the parents to discover what is wrong** a plea for investigations, enthusiasm for admission
  - **Progress of the clinical condition is not as expected or diagnosis** does not fit a typical pattern

- **In somatoform disorders,** the patient does not intentionally create symptoms (unconscious process)
- **In factitious disorders,** patients intentionally create an illness or symptoms (e.g. they inject insulin to create hypoglycemia) and subject themselves to procedures in order to assume the role of a patient (no financial or other secondary gain)
- **In malingering**, patients intentionally create their illness for secondary gain (e.g. money, release from work or jail).

Chronic Fatigue Syndrome (CFS)

- (CFS) is the current name for a disorder characterized by **debilitating fatigue and several associated physical, constitutional, and neuropsychological complaints**
- **Chronic mononucleosis, chronic Epstein-Barr virus infection, and postviral fatigue syndrome** may have had what is now called chronic fatigue syndrome
- Common in **women**
- Mild to moderate depression is present in half to two-thirds of patients
- Typically, CFS arises suddenly in a previously active individual. An otherwise unremarkable flulike illness or some other acute stress leaves unbearable exhaustion in its wake. Other symptoms, such as headache, sore throat tender lymph nodes, muscle and joint aches, and frequent feverishness, lead to the belief that an infection persists, and medical attention is sought. Over several weeks, despite reassurances that nothing serious is wrong, the symptoms persist and other features of the syndrome become evident ¾ disturbed sleep, difficulty in concentration, and depression
- Ultimately, isolation, frustration, and pathetic resignation can mark the protracted course of illness
- Practical advice should be given regarding lifestyle

Disorder	Clinical Scenario
Somatization Disorder	• A 36-year-old woman with a 16 years history of vague and chronic physical complaints. She says that she has always been in pain and has pain in abdomen, chest, legs, etc. sick but that her doctors have not been able to identify her problem
Conversion Disorder	• A 22-year-old female experiences a sudden loss of vision, after a fight with her husband but appears unconcerned ('la belle indifference'). She reports that the onset of her blindness, she saw her child going to the street
Hypochondriasis	• A 48-year-old man says that he has been 'ill' for most of his life. He has attended multiple doctors but is angry with most of them because they ultimately referred him to mental health clinicians. He now fears that he has pancreatic cancer reports are normal. Many of his previous 'illnesses' also seem to be amplified responses to normal physical sensations
Body dysmorphic disorder	• A 22-year-old woman seeks plastic surgery for her nose which is normal. She rarely meets her friends

EATING DISORDERS

Anorexia Nervosa

Anorexia nervosa typically begins in mid to late **adolescence**

The disorder occasionally develops in **early puberty,** before menarche, but seldom begins after age 40

Despite being **underweight,** patients with **anorexia nervosa** rarely complain of hunger or fatigue and often exercise extensively

Further weight loss is viewed by the patient as a fulfilling accomplishment, while weight gain is seen as a personal failure

Physical Features

- Amenorrhea is a feature
- Patients with **anorexia nervosa** typically have few physical complaints but may note **cold intolerance and constipation**
- Vital signs may **reveal bradycardia, hypotension and hypothermia**
- Soft, downy hair growth (lanugo) sometimes occurs, especially on the back and alopecia may be seen
- **Salivary gland enlargement** which is associated with starvation as well as with binge eating and vomiting may make the face appear surprisingly full in contrast to the marked general wasting.

- **Acrocyanosis of the digits** is common, and **peripheral edema** can be seen in the absence of hypoalbuminemia, particularly when the patient begins to regain weight
- Some patients who consume large amounts of vegetables containing vitamin A develop a yellow tint to the skin **(hypercarotenemia),** which is especially notable on the palms

Laboratory Abnormalities

- **Mild normochromic, normocytic anemia** is frequent, as is mild to moderate leukopenia, with a disproportionate reduction of polymorphonuclear leukocytes
- **Dehydration** may result in slightly increased levels of blood urea nitrogen and creatinine
- **Serum liver enzyme levels** may increase, especially during the early phases of refeeding. The level of serum proteins is usually normal
- **Hypokalemic alkalosis** suggests self-induced vomiting or the use of diuretics
- **Hyponatremia is common** and may result from excess fluid intake and disturbances in the secretion of antidiuretic hormone

Endocrine Abnormalities

Amenorrhea is hypothalamic in origin and reflects diminished production of gonadotropin releasing hormone (GnRH)

Anorexia Nervosa is characterized by

- **Low estrogen**
- **Low FSH**
- **Low LH**
- **Low normal thyroxine**
- **Low blood sugar**
- **Increased cortisol**

Cardiac output is reduced, and congestive heart failure occasionally occurs during rapid refeeding

The electrocardiogram usually shows:

- **Sinus bradycardia**
- **Reduced QRS voltage**
- **Nonspecific ST-T-wave abnormalities**
- Some patients develop a **prolonged QT_c interval**, which may predispose to serious arrhythmias

Anorexia	Bulimia
Binge eating is **uncommon**	Common
Weight loss **common**	Mostly normal
Amenorrhea in **100%**	In 50%
Skin changes **common**	Rare
Antisocial behavior **rare**	Common
Restrict food intake	Self induced vomiting

Bulimia Nervosa

It is a condition characterized by recurrent episodes of binge eating followed by a compensatory behavior to prevent weight gain (vomiting, exercise, laxative abuse). Other features include stealing (food), alcohol and drug abuse, self-mutilation and depression. The individuals are usually at or slightly over the normal weight for their height, sexual activity is normal or increased and they continue to menstruate. Clinical findings that are caused by recurrent vomiting include dental caries, periodontal disease and pharyngeal lacerations and nail changes. Metabolic alkalosis and hypokalemia are also present. Complications include aspiration and rupture of the esophagus or stomach

USMLE Case Scenario

A young lady presented with repeated episodes of excessive eating followed by purging by use of laxatives, which is the most appropriate diagnosis?

1. Bulimia nervosa
2. Anorexia
3. Binge eating disorder
4. Psychogenic vomiting

Ans.1. Bulimia nervosa

Postpartum Psychiatric Diseases

• **Postpartum blues**	• Within 1st week	• Mood lability, Tearfulness, insomnias, anxiety
• **Postpartum depression**	• Within 2–3 months	• Depressed mood, excess anxiety, insomnia
• **Postpartum phycosis**	• Within 2–4 weeks	• Agitation, decreased mood, delusions, depression, disorganized behavior

Postpartum blues are **self limited**
Postpartum depression is **moderate**
Postpartum Psychosis is **severe**

- Postpartum Psychosis (PPP) occurs within **2–4 weeks of child birth**
- However most cases occur within 3–4 weeks of child birth
- PPP is the **most severe** of postpartum mood disorder
- PPP is the **rarest** of mood disorder
- Incidence 1–2 women/thousand women giving birth
- PPP has **5%** suicide rate and **4%** Infanticide rate

Signs of PPP

- Hallucinations
- Delusions
- Illogical thoughts
- Insomnia
- Refusal to eat
- Anxiety
- Agitation

Increased Risk In

- Positive family history of pshychosis
- Bipolar disorder
- Schizophrenia

Treatment should be immediate: Antipsychotics, Antidepressants or Antianxiety drugs

Impulse Control Disorders

• **Kleptomania**	Irresistible desire to steal articles
• **Pyromania**	Irresistible desire to set things on fire
• **Multilomania**	Irresistible desire to mutilate animals
• **Dipsomania**	Irresistible desire for alcohol drinks

• **Trichotillomania**	Need to pull out hair
• **Pathological gambling**	Overwhelming need to gamble
• **Intermittent explosive Disorder**	Patient loses self contol and attacks other persons without adequate cause

Sleep Enuresis

- It is another parasomnia that occurs **during slow-wave sleep (stage IV)** in the young
- **Before age 5 or 6, nocturnal enuresis should probably be considered a normal feature** of development
- The condition usually **improves spontaneously at puberty**
- Persistence of enuresis into adolescence or adulthood may reflect a variety of underlying conditions
- In older patients with enuresis a distinction must be made **between primary and secondary enuresis**, the latter being defined as bedwetting in patients who have been fully continent for 6 to 12 months
- **Treatment of primary enuresis is reserved for patients of appropriate age (older than 5 or 6 years) and consists of bladder training exercises and behavioral therapy.** Urologic abnormalities are more common in primary enuresis and must be assessed by urologic examination
- Important causes of secondary enuresis include emotional disturbances
  - **Urinary tract infections or malformations**
  - **Caudaequina lesions**
  - **Epilepsy**
  - **Sleep apnea**
  - **Certain medications**

Symptomatic pharmacotherapy is usually accomplished with

- **Intranasal desmopressin**
- **Oral oxybutynin chloride or**
- **Imipramine**

PHOBIA

Phobic Disorders

- **Marked and persistent fear of objects or situations, exposure to which results in an immediate anxiety reaction**
- The patient avoids the phobic stimulus, and this avoidance usually impairs occupational or social functioning
- Panic attacks may be triggered by the phobic stimulus or may emerge spontaneously during the course of the illness
- Unlike patients with other anxiety disorders, individuals with phobias experience anxiety only in specific situations

'Extended Definition' of Agoraphobia Includes

- **Fear of open spaces**
- **Fear of public places**
- **Fear of crowded places**
- **Fear of any place from where there is no easy escape to a safe place**
- Agoraphobia is associated with **panic disorders. Exposure therapy** in the form of graded exposure and flooding is done along with **cognitive behavioral therapy** as a form of treatment

Cognitive behavioral therapy is the best therapy for phobia

SSRI are effective in phobia

Drugs used:

- Anxiolytic drugs
- TCA
- SSRI
- MAO inhibitors

- **<u>Exposure therapy</u>** a type of behavior therapy is the most commonly used treatment of specific phobia. The therapist usually desensitizes the patient by a gradual exposure to the phobic stimulus. Relaxation and breathing control are important parts of the treatment
- **<u>Hypnosis</u>** is used to enhance the therapist's suggestions that the phobic object is not dangerous. At times, self-hypnosis can be taught so that the patient uses it as a method of relaxation when confronted with the phobic stimulus
- **<u>Insight-oriented psychotherapy</u>** was initially used to treat phobias, but analyzing unconscious conflicts did not resolve phobic symptoms. It does help the patient understand the origins of the phobia and how to deal with anxiety-provoking stimuli
- **<u>Medication</u>** is used in the treatment of a specific phobia only if it is associated with panic attacks and generalized anxiety. The pharmacologic treatment is then directed toward the panic attacks
- **<u>Supportive therapy</u>** may be used in helping the patient actively confront the phobic stimulus during treatment. It is usually used in addition to an ongoing treatment

Remember Other Phobias

- **Acrophobia: Fear of heights**
- **Claustrophobia: Fear of closed spaces**
- **Sitophobia: Fear of eating**
- **Alogophobia: Fear of pain**
- **Xenophobia: Fear of strangers**
- **Thanatophobia: Fear of strangers**
- **Zoophobia: Fear of animals**

Panic Disorder

It is defined by the **<u>'presence of recurrent and unpredictable panic attacks, which are distinct episodes of intense fear and discomfort associated with a variety of physical symptoms'</u>**, including:

- **Palpitations**
- **Sweating**
- **Trembling**
- **Shortness of breath, chest pain, dizziness**
- **A fear of impending doom or death**
- **Paresthesias, gastrointestinal distress, and feelings of unreality** are also common

Panic attacks have a **sudden onset,** developing within 10 min and usually resolving over the course of an hour and they **occur in an unexpected fashion**

Insight present:

The frequency and severity of panic attacks varies, ranging from once a week to clusters of attacks separated by months of well-being

TREATMENT

- Achievable goals of treatment are to decrease the frequency of panic attacks and to reduce their intensity. The cornerstone of drug therapy is **antidepressant medications**
- The tricyclic antidepressant (TCA) agents imipramine and clomipramine can benefit 75 to 90% of panic disorder patients
- Selective serotonin reuptake inhibitors **(SSRIs)** are equally effective and do not have the adverse effects of TCAs. SSRIs should be started at one-third to one-half of their usual antidepressant dose (**fluoxetine,** sertraline, paroxetine)
- Monoamine oxidase inhibitors **(MAOIs)** are at least as effective as TCAs and may specifically benefit patients who have comorbid features of atypical depression (i.e. hypersomnia and weight gain)
- Because of anticipatory anxiety and the need for immediate relief of panic symptoms, **benzodiazepines are useful early in the course of treatment**
- **Early psychotherapeutic intervention and psychoeducation** aimed at symptom control enhances the effectiveness of drug treatment

Panic Disorder	Generalized Anxiety Disorder
• Presence of recurrent and unpredictable panic attacks, which are **distinct episodes of intense fear and discomfort associated with a variety of physical symptoms**, including palpitations, sweating, trembling, shortness of breath, chest pain, dizziness and a fear of impending doom or death • Paresthesias, gastrointestinal distress, and feelings of unreality are also common • Panic attacks have a **sudden onset, developing within 10 min and usually resolving over the course of an hour and they occur in an unexpected fashion** • The frequency and severity of panic attacks varies, ranging from once a week to clusters of attacks separated by months of well-being • The first attack is usually outside the home • Onset is usually in late adolescence to early adulthood.	• Patients have **persistent, excessive, and/or unrealistic worry** associated with other signs and symptoms, which commonly include muscle tension, impaired concentration, autonomic arousal**, feeling 'on edge' or restless and insomnia** • Onset is usually **before age 20** and a history of childhood fears and social inhibition may be present • Over 80% of patients with GAD **also suffer from major depression, dysthymia, or social phobia** • **Comorbid substance abuse is common** in these patients, particularly alcohol and/or sedative/hypnotic abuse • Patients with GAD **readily admit to worrying excessively over minor matters**, with life-disrupting effects • Unlike in panic disorder, complaints of symptoms such as shortness of breath, palpitations and tachycardia are relatively **rare** • **Treatment** • **Paroxitine** • **Alprazolam** • **Venlafaxine** • **Buspirone**

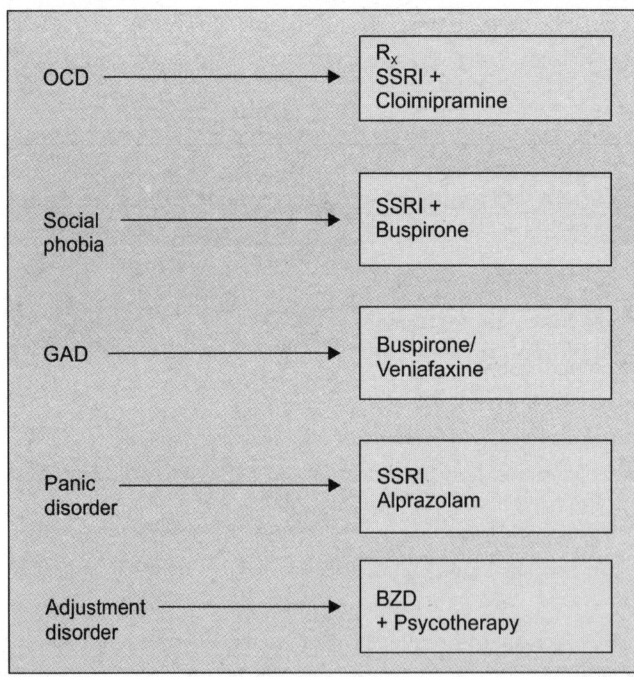

Illnesses that mimic Anxiety disorder
'Differential Diagnosis' to be considered:

- **Hyperthyroidism**
- **Pheochromocytoma**
- **Hypoglycemia**
- **Paroxysmal arrhythmias**
- **Alcohol withdrawal**
- **Temporal lobe epilepsy**

USMLE Case Scenario

A 28-year-old apprehensive patient presented in casualty to a resident with a history of sudden palpitation, sensation of impending doom and constriction in his chest. This lasted for about 10–15 minutes after which he become all right the diagnosis is likely to be:

1. Phobia
2. Personality disorder
3. Generalized anxiety disorder
4. Panic attack

Ans. 4. Panic attack

Defense mechanisms

- Are **unconscious mental techniques used by ego to keep conflicts out of awareness, reduce anxiety and maintain persons self-esteem and sense of safety and equilibrium**
- Although defense mechanisms protect the person, if used excessively, neurotic symptoms can occur

The defense mechanisms used are:

Isolation of effect

- Does not experience or express emotions associated with stressful event, **e.g. a man whose father dies in a road traffic accident describes the circumstances of his death dispassionately**

Rationalization

- Gives reasonable explanation for unacceptable feelings, **e.g. a candidate not passing MD/MS entrance examinations says that passing was not good for me anyway**

Undoing

- Attempting to reverse past actions with present actions, **e.g. a man diagnosed with lung cancer as a result of smoking buys books on nutrition, stop smoking**

Reaction formation

- Denying unacceptable feelings and adopting opposite attitudes and behavior, **e.g. a man who is angry with his friend compliments his shirt**

USMLE Case Scenario

A 34-year-old woman who was previously lethargic comes to a psychiatric unit with her husband who says that she 'worries too much.' On questioning her she admits that, over the past 8 months, She has difficulties falling asleep, partly because of worrisome thoughts. In the past month, she has had ten episodes of irritability, frequent episodes of shortness of breath, and restlessness and has been unable to go to work or do anything at home. Her physical examination and laboratory tests, as well as her electrocardiogram are unremarkable. The most likely diagnosis: Generalized Anxiety Disorder

Generalized Anxiety Disorder

It is defined as unrealistic worry about life events for a period longer than 6 months, during which time a person is worried most days. It also includes at least six symptoms of the following types:

- **Easy fatigability**
- **Difficulties falling asleep**
- **Restlessness**
- **Difficulties concentrating**
- **Irritability**
- **Muscle tension**

The symptoms are not due to other psychiatric or medical conditions and they cause significant impairment in everyday functioning

Anhedonia is a Disorder of 'Affect'

- Affect is feeling or emotion
- Conation is action or motor behavior
- Cognition is thought
- **Cognitive dysfunctions are:**
  - Overgeneralization
  - Selective abstraction
  - Catastophization

Major Depression

- Major depression is defined as **depressed mood on daily basis for a minimum duration of two weeks**
- Markedly diminished interest or pleasure in all/almost all activities most of the day, nearly everyday
- Significant weight loss/weight gain
- Insomnia/hypersomnia nearly everyday
- Psychomotor retardation/agitation nearly everyday
- Fatigue/loss of energy nearly everyday
- Feeling of worthlessness nearly everyday
- Diminished ability to think, concentrate or indecisiveness nearly everyday
- Recurrent thoughts of death, suicidal ideation

- **Anhedonia** (Greek a without hedone, pleasure): It is an inability to experience pleasure from normally pleasurable life events such as eating, exercise, and social or sexual interaction
- Anhedonia is recognized as one of the key symptoms of the mood disorder depression according to both the Diagnostic and Statistical Manual of Mental Disorders Fourth Edition (DSM IV) and the International Statistical Classification of Diseases and Related Health Problems (ICD)
- Anhedonia is also seen in **schizophrenia and schizoaffective disorder**

Depression

- Depression is the **MC Pshyciatric disorder in India**
- Depression involves **middle aged females mostly**
- Depression is associated with:
  - **Post MI**
  - **Postpartum**
  - **AIDS**
  - **Myxedema**

Neurotransmitter involved: serotonin and norepinephrine

MC cause for suicide is depression

MC type of post purpureal pshycosis is depression

In children anhedonia **(loss of enthusiasm and interest in play, socializing, school activities, loss of pleasure and boredom are manifestations of depression.)**

- **Nihilistic ideas are seen in depression**
- Dysthymic disorder consists of a pattern of chronic (at least 2 years), ongoing, mild depressive symptoms that are less severe and less disabling than those found in major **depression**; the two conditions are sometimes difficult to separate, however, and can occur together **('double depression')**

- A seasonal pattern of **depression**, called **seasonal affective disorder**, may manifest with onset and remission of episodes at predictable times of the year
- This disorder is more common in women, whose symptoms are anergy, fatigue, weight gain, hypersomnia, and episodic carbohydrate craving. The prevalence increases with distance from the equator, and mood improvement may occur by altering light exposure.

Dysthymia	Involutional melanocholia
• Persistent mood symptoms for > 2 years	Usually in old age
• Mild depression	Delusions of sin, guilt, poverty
	Intense nihilism (obsession with death) with
	Agitation and dejection

Associations of suicide:
- **Depression**
- **Schizophrenia**
- **Substance abuse**

Risk Features for Suicide in Depression

- **Family history**
- **Male sex**
- **45 years of age**
- **Single, unemployed, separated or divorced or widowed, recently bereaved, chronic illness**
- **Conduct disorder in child**
- **Substance abuse**
- **Mood disorder, personality disorder, pshycosis, hypochondriasis**
- **Endogeneous** type of depression
- **Psycotic depression.**

USMLE Case Scenario

A 30-year-old bussiness woman with documented bipolar disorder is brought to the hospital because of extreme feelings of guilt and worthlessness. She has a huge debt of 200, 000 dollars. On further questioning, she reveals that she bought a poison earlier in the day because it would be easier for everyone if she 'wasn't here anymore.' She plans to poison herself 'and do what needs to be done.' Next step in management would be: Admitted to the hospital.

Point to Remember

Any patient with serious suicidal thoughts, suicidal intent, and a plan, must be hospitalized, against her will, if necessary. The patient expressed a desire to die, she bought a poison and developed a believable plan. She needs to be hospitalized for her own safety. Patients with bipolar disorder have a lifetime suicide rate of 10–15%.

Bipolar Disorder Types

Bipolar I: Having one or more manic episodes with depression
Bipolar II: Having episodes of major depression and Hypomania rather than mania
Mania alone is a bipolar disorder but not depression alone

Bipolar Disorder

It is characterized by unpredictable swings in mood from **mania** (or hypomania) to depression

Some patients suffer only from recurrent attacks of **mania**, which in its pure form is associated with:

- **Increased psychomotor activity**
- **Excessive social extroversion**
- **Decreased need for sleep**
- **Impulsivity and impairment in judgment**
- **Expansive, grandiose**
- **Sometimes irritable mood**

In severe **mania**, patients may experience delusions and paranoid thinking indistinguishable from schizophrenia. Half of patients with bipolar disorder present with a mixture of psychomotor agitation and activation with dysphoria, anxiety, and irritability. It may be difficult to distinguish mixed **mania** from agitated depression

In bipolar II disorder the full criteria for **mania** are lacking and the requisite recurrent depressions are separated by periods of mild activation and increased energy (hypomania)

Chromosome 18 is involved

Cyclothymic Disorder

- There are **numerous hypomanic periods, usually of relatively short duration, alternating with clusters of depressive symptoms that fail, either in severity or duration, to meet the criteria of major depression**
- The mood fluctuations are chronic and should be **present for at least 2 years** before the diagnosis is made.

Mania

Abnormally and persistently elevated, expansive or irritable mood lasting for at least one week

- Inflated self-esteem, grandiosity
- Decreased sleep
- Flight of ideas
- Distractibility
- Increase in goal directed activity
- Excessive involvement in pleasurable activities
- More talkative

USMLE Case Scenario

A 22-year-old male from Texas old male suffers from decreased sleep, increased sexual activity, excitement and spending excessive money for last 8 days. The diagnosis is:

1.Confusion
2. Mania
3. Hyperactivity
4. Loss of memory

Ans. 2. Mania

Alcohol and Psychiatry

Wernicke's Encephalopathy is **Global confusion, Ophthalmoplegia and ataxia. Involves mammilary bodies**

Korsakoff's Psychosis (alcohol-induced persisting amnestic disorder)

Korsakoff's syndrome presents as **profound and persistent anterograde amnesia** (inability to learn new material) and a milder retrograde amnesia. and confabulation (IMPAIRMENT) About 1% of alcoholics develop **cerebellar degeneration**, a syndrome of **progressive unsteady stance and gait often accompanied by mild nystagmus.** Atrophy of the cerebellar vermis is seen on brain computed tomography and magnetic resonance imaging scans, but the cerebrospinal fluid is usually normal

Alcoholics can show severe **cognitive problems and impairment in recent and remote memory for weeks to months after an alcoholic binge.** Increased size of the brain ventricles and cerebral sulci are seen in 50% or more of chronic alcoholics, but these changes are often reversible, returning toward normal after a year or more of abstinence

Permanent CNS impairment (alcohol-induced persisting dementia) can develop and accounts for up to 20% of chronically demented patients

IN ALCOHOLIC PARANOIA, hallucinations are seen

Finally, almost every psychiatric syndrome can be seen temporarily during heavy drinking or subsequent withdrawal. These include intense sadness lasting for days to weeks in the midst of heavy drinking in 40% of alcoholics, which is classified as an alcohol-induced mood disorder in the Fourth Diagnostic and Statistical Manual of the American Psychiatric Association (DSM-IV); severe anxiety in 10 to 30% of alcoholics, often beginning during alcohol withdrawal and which can persist for many months after cessation of drinking **(alcohol-induced anxiety disorder);** and auditory hallucinations and/or paranoid delusions in the absence of any obvious signs of withdrawal, a state now called **alcohol-induced psychotic disorder** and reported at sometime in 1 to 10% of alcoholics

CAGE questionare is used in alcoholism.

Marchiafava-Bignami Disease: A rare demyelination of the corpus callosum that occurs in chronic alcoholics, predominantly males. Patients become agitated and confused and show progressive dementia with frontal release signs.

Alcoholic Withdrawal

- **Hangover**
- **Visual or tactile hallucinations**
- **Alcoholic hallucinosis:** Hallucinations usually auditory
- **Alcoholic seizures (Rum Fits):**
  - Multiple seizures occurring during absistence usually 12–48 hours after heavy drink
- **Delerium tremens:**
  - Occurs within 5 days of abstinence
  - Clouding of consciousness
  - Disorientation, anxiety, perceptual defect
  - Hallucinations
  - Autonomic disturbance
  - Agitation, insomnia
  - Mc symptom of withdrawal
  - **Chlordiazepoxide is used for treatment.**

Chronic use Causes

- **Wernickes encephalopathy:** Global confusion+ ophthalmoplegia+ Ataxia
- **Korsakoff's Psychosis:** Confabulations+ Amnesia
- **Marchiafava Bignami syndrome:** Ataxia+Dysarthia+Epilepsy+Hallucinations+Disorientation
- **Alcoholic black out: Amnesia of events during drinking.**

Differentiate Between

Alcohol withdrawal	Opioid withdrawal	Cocaine withdrawal
• Hangover	• Yawning	• Hypersomnia/insomnia
• Hallucinations/illusions	• Insomnia, dusphoric mood	• Vivid unpleasant dreams

Alcohol withdrawal	Opioid withdrawal	Cocaine withdrawal
• Hyperactivity • Insomnia • Seizures • Symptoms appear commonly on 2nd day	• ↑BP, RR, Temp • Pupillary dilation	• ↑appetite

Substance	Feature
• Alcohol	• **Morbid Jealousy**
• Cocaine	• **Magnus symptom**
• Cannabis **(absent withdrawal symptoms)**	• **Amotivational syndrome, Run Amok**
• LSD **(absent withdrawal symptoms)**	• **Flashbacks/Bad Trips (Loss of self-control)**
• Amphetamine	• **Paranoid features**

Specific Drug Abuses

- **LSD abuse:**
- **Features:**
  - Profuse perspiration
  - Blurred vision
  - Tachycardia
  - Dilated pupils
  - Bad trips
  - Flashbacks
- **Phencyclidine (Angel dust):**
- **Features**
  - Hypertension
  - Hyperthermia
  - Nystagmus
  - Euphoria
  - Amnesia
- **Marijuana:**
- **Features**
  - Alteration in memory
  - Sensory perception
  - Time perception
  - Psychotic symptoms

- Tolerance **does not** develop with Cocaine
  - **Magnus phenomenon** or
  - **Cocaine bugs** or
  - **Tactile hallucinations** are a feature of cocaine intoxication

- Treatment is not required in withdrawal of LSD
- **Flashbacks or bad trips** are seen in LSD

- Most common substance of abuse in India is cannabis
- Physical dependence is not seen with cannabis.

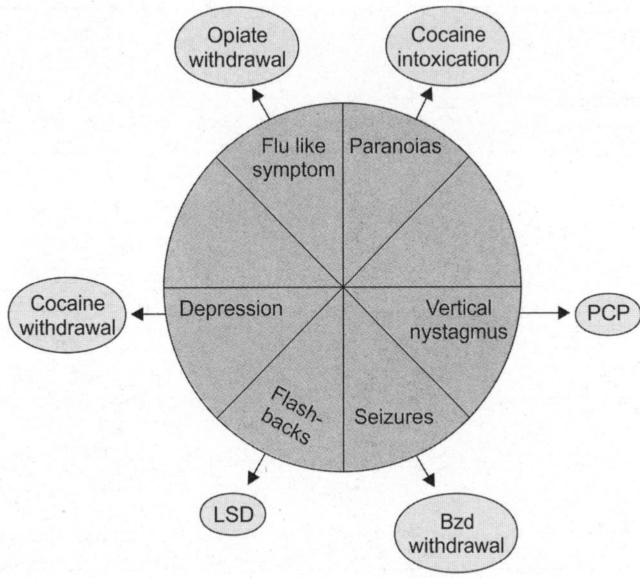

Drugs used

• **Methadone**	• Used in opioid dependent for short-term and long-term detoxification.
• **Naloxone**	• Used in opioid overdose treatment (DOC)
• **Naltrexone** • **Toipromate**	• Used in opioid dependent for rapid detoxification and maintenance therapy to prevent relapse • Used to decrease craving and prevent relapse in heavy alcohol drinking • Alcohol dependence
• **Nalmifene (iv)**	• Used in opioid dependent for rapid detoxification and maintenance therapy
• **Chlordiazepoxide and Diazepam**	• Used in alcohol withdrawal
• **Methadone and clonidine**	• Used in opium withdrawal

Sleep

REM sleep
NREM sleep

Neurotransmitters in Sleep

- ↑Serotonin
- ↑acetylcholine
- ↑Dopamine

Beta waves: seen in active mental concentration.		
Alpha waves: seen when person relaxes with eyes closed.		
Stage 1:	**Theta waves**	**Lightest phase**
Stage 2:	**Sleep spindles and K complexes**	**Largest percentage of sleep**
Stage 3 and 4: Delta (slow wave sleep) Deepest phase		
REM sleep: • Saw tooth • **↑BP**		

- **↑RR**
- **↑PR**
- **Absence of sk. Muscle movement**
- **Alpha rhythm**

Events in REM Sleep

Nightmares

Nocturnal penile trumescene

Events in NREM

- **Night terrors**
- Nocturnal enuresis
- Bruxism
- Sleepwalking (somnambulism)
- Sleep talking (somniloquy)

Narcolepsy

Narcolepsy is both a **disorder of the ability to sustain wakefulness voluntarily and a disorder of REM sleep regulation**

The classic **'narcolepsy tetrad'** consists of **excessive daytime somnolence plus three specific symptoms related to an intrusion of REM sleep characteristics** (e.g. muscle atonia, vivid dream imagery) into the transition between wakefulness and sleep:

- **Sudden weakness or loss of muscle tone without loss of consciousness, often elicited by emotion (cataplexy)**
- **Hallucinations at sleep onset (hypnogogic hallucinations) or upon awakening (hypnopompic hallucinations) and**
- **Muscular paralysis upon awakening (sleep paralysis).**

SLEEP APNEA SYNDROMES

Respiratory dysfunction during sleep is a common, serious cause of excessive daytime somnolence as well as of disturbed nocturnal sleep

These episodes may be due to either an occlusion of the airway **(obstructive sleep apnea)**, absence of respiratory effort **(central sleep apnea)**, or a combination of these factors **(mixed sleep apnea)**

SLEEPWALKING (SOMNAMBULISM)

Patients affected by this disorder **carry-out automatic motor activities that range from simple to complex.** Individuals may **leave the bed, walk, urinate inappropriately, eat, or exit from the house while remaining only partially aware.** Full arousal may be difficult, and some patients may respond to attempted awakening with agitation or even violence. Sleepwalking arises from **stage 3 or 4 NREM sleep**

SLEEP TERRORS

This disorder, also called **pavornocturnus,** occurs primarily in young children during the first several hours after sleep onset, **in stages 3 and 4 of NREM sleep**

The child **suddenly screams, exhibiting autonomic arousal with sweating, tachycardia, and hyperventilation**

The individual **may be difficult to arouse and rarely recalls the episode on awakening in the morning**

In contrast, **nightmares (dream anxiety attacks)** occur during REM sleep and **cause full arousal, with intact memory for the unpleasant episode**

DOC is Diazepam

SLEEP BRUXISM

Bruxism is an **involuntary, forceful grinding of teeth during sleep** that affects 10 to 20% of the population. The patient is usually unaware of the problem

SLEEP ENURESIS

Bedwetting, like sleepwalking and night terrors, is another parasomnia that occurs during slow-wave sleep in the young

Before age 5 or 6, nocturnal enuresis should probably be considered a normal feature of development.

Miscellaneous Parasomnias

Other clinical entities fulfill the definition of a parasomnia in that they occur selectively during sleep and are associated with some degree of sleep disruption. Examples include:

- **Jactatio capitis nocturna (nocturnal headbanging)**
- **Sleep talking**
- **Nocturnal paroxysmal dystonia**
- **Nocturnal leg cramps**

Rapid Time Zone Change (JET LAG) Syndrome

- People experience **transmeridian air travel annually, which is often associated with excessive daytime sleepiness, sleep onset insomnia,** and frequent arousals from sleep, particularly in the latter half of the night
- Gastrointestinal discomfort is common
- The syndrome is transient, typically lasting 2 to 14 depending on the number of time zones crossed, the direction of travel and the traveler's age and phase-shifting capacity.

Shift Work Sleep Disorder

People work at night, either on a permanent or rotating schedule. Leading to both sleep loss and misalignment of their circadian rhythms with respect to their sleep wake cycle.

- Chronic shift workers have higher rates of cardiac, gastrointestinal and reproductive disorders
- Studies of regular night-shift workers indicate that the circadian timing system usually fails to adapt successfully to such inverted schedules. This leads to a misalignment between the desired work-rest schedule and the output of the pacemaker and in disturbed daytime sleep
- Consequent sleep deprivation, increased length of time awake prior to work, and misalignment of circadian phase produce decreased alertness and performance, increased reaction time, and increased risk of performance lapses, thereby resulting in greater safety hazards among night workers and other sleep-deprived individuals.

Dissociative Disorders

- Dissociative amnesia
- Dissociative fugue
- Dissociative identity disorder
- Depersonalization disorder

Dissociative Amnesia

A navy officer cannot recall an unfortunate event of fire on his ship in which 45 sailors lost life

- MC type
- Sudden inability to recall important personal information
- Patchy impairment of personal memory
- Patient is aware of amnesia.

Dissociative Fugue

A doctor in California for 5 years has no memory of coming and living in California

- **Feature is wandering away from home**
- Purposeful new identity with complete amnesia for earlier life
- Not aware of amnesia

Dissociative Identity Disorder

A female is shown her previous photograph and she has no recollection of same as to who's photograph it is

- Person is dominated by two or more personalities
- One personality is not aware of existence of other

Depersonalization

A female says that she is outside of herself watching her life in a movie. She knows that she is really living her life

- An alteration in perception or experience of self to the extent that persons sense of his/her own reality is lost
- It is detachment from self, social situation or environment. (Derealization)

Ganser's Syndrome

- **Hysterical Pseudodementia**
- Feature is **'approximate answers'**
- **Answer is wrong** but **person understands the nature of question asked**
- Hallucinations and apparent clouding of consciousness is a feature.

Newer Concepts

• **Holiday heart syndrome**	**Atrial or ventricular arrhythmia** after taking a binge of alcohol with no other evidence of heart disease.
• **van Gogh syndrome**	**Self mutilation in schizophrenia.**
• **Othello syndrome**	A psychosis in which **jealousy involving spouse** is noticed.
• **Clerambault's syndrome**	**Erotomania** in which usually a female has got a conviction that a person of higher status is in love with her.
• **Capgras syndrome**	Patient sees a familiar person as a stranger. **Delusion of doubles.**
• **Cotard's syndrome**	**Delusion that one has lost everything** (possessions, strength and even organ such as heart). Thinks that his bowels are rotting and he will never pass tools again.
• **Gilles de la tourette syndrome**	Multiple motor ticks.
• **Kleine Levin syndrome**	**Hypersomnia, Hyperphagia and Hyper sexuality** **Amygdala involved**
• **Pickwickian syndrome**	Sleep apnea seen in obese persons associated with Hypersomnia.
• **Gelineau's syndrome**	**Narcolepsy with Hypersomnia**
• **Stockholm syndrome**	**Feelings of captives towards capitor**

Lithium

- Lithium acts by interfering with cell membrane ion transport and excitability, **adenylatecyclase activation, neurotransmitter (norepinephrine) release and Na^+, K^+-ATPase activity**
- Lithium is not bound to plasma proteins
- Therapeutic serum levels are **0.6 to 1.2 mmol/l**
- **Liver is not affected in lithium toxicity.**

Clinical Toxicity

Effects begin 1 to 4 hour after acute ingestion

Gastrointestinal effects include nausea, vomiting and diarrhea

Polyuria is the commonest symptom

Neuromuscular effects include weakness, confusion, ataxia, tremors, fasciculations, myoclonus, choreoathetosis, coma and seizures

Cardiovascular effects include arrhythmias and hypotension

Hyperthermia can occur

Leukocytosis, hyperglycemia, albuminuria, glycosuria, nephrogenic diabetes insipidus, and a falsely elevated serum chloride level (due to interference by lithium with its assays) resulting in a low anion-gap may be present

ECG changes include sinus tachycardia or bradycardia, flattened or inverted T waves, AV block, and a prolonged QT interval

Hypothyroidism is seen

Prolonged or permanent **encephalopathy and movement disorders** can occur in patients with severe poisoning

Diagnosis: A serum level must be requested specifically

Contraindicated in pregnancy

Causes CVS defects

- Drugs used in MDP: Lithium, Valproate, Carbamezapine, Levothyroxine
- DOC in Rapid Cycling MDP: Lithium + Levothyroxine
- DOC for acute mania: Lithium
- DOC for Prophylaxis of mania: Lithium

USMLE Case Scenario

A patient is brought to the casualty in the state of altered sensorium. He was on lithium for affective disorder and has suffered through an attack of epileptic fits. On examination he has tremors increased DTR's and incontinence of urine. He has also undergone an episode of severe gastroenteritis 2 days ago. The serum lithium was found to be 1.95 m moles/l. The cause of **her conditon is:**
Lithium Toxicity

Drugs Causing Depression

- Oral Contraceptives
- Methyldopa
- Reserpine
- Bromocriptine

List of TCA'S

- Amitriptyline
- Amoxapine
- Cloimipramine
- Desipramine
- Doxepin

Tetracyclic Antidepressants (Second Generation)

- Lofepramine
- Maprotiline
- Mianserin

SSRI'S are

- Fluoxetine
- Fluvoxamine
- Paroxetine
- Sertaline
- Citalopram

Safest Antidepressants in Cardiac Disease are the SSRI

- **Less anticholinergic**
- **Less sedation and**
- **Less cardiovascular side effects**
- Sertaline is a SSRI and the antidepressant of choice in cardiac disease

Remember in any case (Serotonin Involving Drugs)

- **Buspirone: $5HT_{1A}$ agonist**
- **Sumitriptan: $5HT_{1D}$ agonist**
- **Olanzapine: $5HT_{2A}$ antagonist**
- **Ondansetron: $5H_{T3}$ antagonist**
- **Cyproheptadine: $5HT_{2A}$ antagonist**

Azapirones

- **Buspirone**
- **Gepirone**
- **Ipsapirone**

Buspirone: 5 HT_{1A} receptor agonist

- **Nonsedating**
- **No tolerance**
- **No physical dependence**

ECT

Used in:

- **Major severe depression**
- **Delusional depression**
- **Severe psychosis**
- **Severe catatonia**
- **Absolute contraindication is: Raised ICT**
- **Mc side effect in Direct ECT is T4-T8 spine #**
- **Mc side effect of Modified ECT is retrograde amnesia**
- **Antegrade amnesia also occurs but with ↓ frequency**
- **ECT ↓IOT (intraoccular pressure)**

Disulfiram Inhibits

- **Aldehyde dehydrogenase**
- **Alcohol dehydrogenase**
- **Dopamine β hydroxylase**
- **Cytochrome P450 enzymes**

Drugs in Psychiatry Acting on

- **Bupropion** inhibits dopamine and has modest effect on Norepinephrine
- **Buspirone** affects serotonin pathway not Bupropion
- **Mirtazapine** stimulates Serotonin and NE release
- **Duloxetine** is a serotonin –NE reuptake inhibitor SNRI
- **Trazodone** acts as a serotonin receptor antagonist and alpha 1 blocker
- **Amitriptyline** inhibits serotonin and NE reuptake equally.

Antipsychotics

Antipsychotics act as **dopamine D2 receptor antagonists**, blocking dopaminergic transmission in the mesolimbic pathways. Conventional antipsychotics are associated with problematic extrapyramidal side-effects which has led to the development of **atypical antipsychotics such as clozapine.**

- **Extrapyramidal side-effects**
- **Parkinsonism**
- **Acute dystonia (e.g. torticollis, oculogyric crisis)**
- **Akathisia (severe restlessness)**
- **Tardive dyskinesia** (late onset of choreoathetoid movements, abnormal, involuntary, may occur in 40% of patients, may be irreversible, most common is chewing and pouting of jaw.

Other Side-effects

- **Antimuscarinic: dry mouth, blurred vision, urinary retention, constipation**
- **Sedation, weight gain**
- **Raised prolactin: galactorrhea**
- **Neuroleptic malignant syndrome: pyrexia, muscle stiffness**
- **Reduced seizure threshold (greater with atypicals)**
- **Antipsychotics are not addictive**

Cognitive Behavioral Therapy

- Cognitive behavioral therapy (or cognitive behavior therapy, CBT) is a **psychotherapeutic approach that aims to influence dysfunctional emotions, behaviors and cognitions through a goal-oriented, systematic procedure**
- CBT can be seen as an umbrella term for a number of psychological techniques that share a theoretical basis in behavioristic learning theory and cognitive psychology
- Cognitive Behavioral therapy is based on **learning theory/operant conditioning**
- Here patients symptoms are relieved by **altering behavior and thinking pattern**
- Strategy: Weekly, for as long as 25 weeks, the patient is helped to identify distorted and negative thoughts about self and replace them with positive and self assuring thoughts
- **Flooding** is a type of Behavioral therapy
- **Proven concepts are:**
  - **Contemplation**
  - **Precontemplation**
  - **Consolidation**

CBT is used for

- **Mild to moderate depression**
- **Somatoform disorders**
- **Eating disorders**
- **Phobia**
- **Systemic desensitization is done for phobia**

USMLE Case Scenario

The drug which is used for long-term maintenance in opioid addiction:

1. Naloxone
2. Nalorphine
3. Butorphanol

4. Methadone
5. Propranolol

Ans. 4. Methadone

USMLE Case Scenario

Naltrexone is used in opioid addiction:

1. To treat withdrawal symptoms
2. To treat overdose of opioids
3. Prevent relapse
4. Has addiction potential

Ans. 3. Prevent relapse

USMLE Case Scenario

The following is a typical antipsychotic:

1. Thioridazine
2. Clozapine
3. Olanzapine
4. Resperidone

Ans. 1. Thioridazine

USMLE Case Scenario

A 19-year-old boy suffering from chronic schizophrenia is put on Haloperidol in the dose of 20 mg/day. A week after the initiation of medication, the patient shows restlessness, fidgety, irritability and cannot sit at one place. The most appropriate treatment strategy is:

1. Increase in the dose of Haloperidol
2. Addition of anticholinergic drug
3. Addition of beta blocker
4. Adding another antipsychotic drug

Ans. 3. Addition of beta blocker

USMLE Case Scenario

A 42-year-old male with a past history of a manic episode presents with an illness of 1-month duration characterized by depressed mood, anhedonia and profound psychomotor retardation. The most appropriate management strategy is prescribing a combination of:

1. Antipsychotics and antidepressants
2. Antidepressants and mood stabilizers
3. Antipsychotics and mood stabilizers
4. Antidepressants and benzodiazepines

Ans. 2. Antidepressants and mood stabilizers

Cataplexy

- Cataplexy is 'sudden and transient episode of **loss of muscle tone, often triggered by emotions'**
- It is a rare disease, but frequently affects people who have narcolepsy, a disorder whose principal signs are EDS (Excessive Daytime Sleepiness), sleep attacks, sleep paralysis, hypnagogic hallucinations and disturbed night-time sleep
- The term cataplexy originates from the Greek 'kata', meaning down, and plexis, meaning a stroke or seizure
- Cataplexy manifests itself as **muscular weakness** which may range from a barely perceptible slackening of the facial muscles to the dropping of the jaw or head, weakness at the knees, or a total collapse
- Usually the speech is slurred, vision is impaired (double vision, inability to focus), but hearing and awareness remain normal. These attacks are triggered by strong emotions such as exhilaration, anger, fear, surprise, orgasm, awe, embarrassment and laughter.

Cataplexy may be partial or complete, affecting a range of muscle groups, from those controlling facial features to (less commonly) those controlling the entire body

Arm weakness

- **Sagging jaw**
- **Drooping head**
- **Slumping of the shoulders**
- **Slurred speech**
- **Generalized weakness**
- **Knee buckling**

Adjustment Disorder

- It is the commonest group of psychiatric disorders as most patients **do not fulfill the criterion for depression**
- Precipitants of Adjustment disorder are: **Terminal illness**, new marriage, separation, divorce, death of companion, natural disaster
- Symptoms vary from anxiousness, depressive or mixed
- It starts within **3 months.** Depression is common in
  - **AIDS**
  - **Postsurgery**
  - **Post MI**
  - **Postpartum**
  - **Myxedema**

Cancer patients have highest fear for relapse of disease **(Damocles syndrome)**

Restless Legs Syndrome

'Crawling or creeping dysthesia within calves, feet or upper extremities with irresistible urge to move limbs is Restless legs syndrome.'(RLS)

RLS is aggravated by:

- Sleep deprivation
- Caffeine
- Pregnancy
- Iron deficiency
- Renal failure

RLS responds to **Levodopa, dopamine agonists (Bromocriptine, pergolide). Narcotics, benzodiazepines and anticonvulsants** are also useful

Neurolept malignant syndrome

Caused by Phenothiazines, Haloperidol, Prochloroperazine, Metoclopramide

Features: Lead pipe rigidity, Extrapyramidal effects, Hyperthermia

Treatment: Removal of offender, L**evadopa, amantidine, Benzodiazepines**

Serotonin syndrome

Causes: **SSRI, MAO inhibitors, Serotogenic medications**

Malignant Hyperthermia

Causes: **Halothane, Succinylcholine**

Features: ↑ Temperature,↑ Muscle metabolism,↑ Sr Pottasium

'Obsessive-Compulsive' Disorder

It is characterized by **obsessive thoughts and compulsive behaviors that impair everyday functioning.** Serotonin is implicated

Obsessive-compulsive disorder describes patients with recurrent thoughts or impulses

(Obsessions) and/or recurrent behaviors or actions (compulsions) that cause marked dysfunction in their occupational and/ or interpersonal lives. It is not the same as obsessive-compulsive personality disorder. Look for washing rituals (washing of hands repeatedly in a day) and/or checking rituals (checking to see if the window is locked repeatedly per day).

- Preoccupied with details, rules, list, order organization or schedules
- **Shows perfectionism**
  - **Repetitive thoughts or images**
  - **Rigidity**
  - **Stubbornness**
- **Fears of contamination and germs are common,** as are **handwashing, counting behaviors and having to check and recheck** such actions as whether a door is locked
- Patients often **conceal their symptoms**, usually because they are embarrassed by the content of their thoughts or the nature of their actions
- Obsession is **ego alien** (conscious about disorder)
- OCD usually has a **gradual onset, beginning in early adulthood**
- OCD has a prevalence **of 2–3% worldwide**
- OCD is characterized by **obsessive thoughts** and **compulsive behaviors** that impair everyday function
- ALL cases of OCD take-up greater than **I hour**
- Group a streptococcal infections are associated with **OCD**
- Childhood onset is not rare and the disorder has a waxing and wanning course
- The Anatomy of OCD is thought to involve **frontal subcortical neural circuit involving orbital frontal cortex, caudate nucleus and globuspallidus**
- **Defense mechanism used is: undoing, rationalization, displacement Clomimipramine,**
- **Fluoxetine and (DOC)**
- **Fluvoxamine** are used for treatment of OCD
- **Behavioral therapy** is effective in the treatment as well
- **Exposure and response prevention.**

Remember the Terms

- **Confabulation** is defined as the unconscious filling of gaps in memory by imagined or untrue experiences that the patient believes are true, even though they are not based on facts. It is associated with organic pathology.
- **Magical thinking** is a form of thinking in which thoughts, words, or actions assume power, such as causing or preventing events. It is typical for the preoperational phase of thinking in children.
- **Ideas of influence** constitute a type of delusion in which a person believes that he or she is being controlled by another person or external force.
- **Ideas of reference** are delusions in which a person has a false belief that others (including people on TV or radio) are talking about him or her. In a broader sense the behavior of others refers to one self, other persons, or objects that have special significance and meaning.
- **Clang associations** are disorders of thought in which the associations of words are similar in sound but not in meaning. Words have no logical connection, but there may be rhyming.
- **Noesis** refers to the feeling of revelation in which a person experiences illumination associated with a sense of being chosen as a leader.
- **Obsessions** are pathologically persistent intrusive thoughts or impulses that cannot be eliminated from consciousness by logical effort and thus cause anxiety. The person is aware that they are not imposed from the outside but are a product of his or her own mind.
- **Concrete thinking** is described as literal thinking that shows a lack of understanding of the nuances of meaning. These individuals lack the ability to use metaphors.
- **Abstract thinking** refers to the ability to appreciate nuances of meaning and the ability to use metaphors and hypotheses appropriately.
- **Blocking** is a disturbance in thought form, characterized by an abrupt interruption in the train of thought before the thought is finished. After a pause, the person is unable to recall what was being said.

USMLE Case Scenario

A 78-year-old woman who was a housewife previously is complaining to her doctor about her problems. She reports that her neighbor from 33 years ago called her and is now harassing her by controlling her blood pressure, movements, and thoughts by a remote control device. They have stolen that device from FBI an Intellegence agency. This patient most likely has Ideas of influence constitute a type of delusion in which a person believes that he or she is being controlled by another person or external force.

USMLE Case Scenario

A 88-year-old patient is seen in the psychiatry ward of New Yorks Main City Hospital by a medical student. To assess the patient's cognitive functions, the student asks the patient what the proverb 'Honesty is the best policy' means. The patient answers that honest people are always rich. The type of thinking is this patient is exhibiting is:
Concrete thinking
It is described as literal thinking that shows a lack of understanding of the nuances of meaning. These individuals lack the ability to use metaphors.

USMLE Case Scenario

An Intern is interviewing a 78-year-old man. He has been talking to him for last 45 minutes and got very little information. Everytime the intern asks a question, the patient starts talking and goes into unnecessary details, eventually answering the question but only after he had told his story to the medical student. This patient's speech is an example of: Circumstantiality Refers to speech that is delayed from reaching the point, characterized by overinclusion of details. Eventually, it does get to the original goal.

Sexual Disorders and Psychiatry

Telephone Scatologia

Gaining sexual pleasure from making telephone calls to unsuspecting women and engaging them in sexual conversations

Sexual aversion disorder

Aversion to and Avoidance of sexual activity

Hypoactive sexual disorder

Decrease interest in sexual activity.

Sexual Perversions Include

• **Sadism**	Infliction of pain to partner is mode of pleasure
• **Machoism**	Infliction of pain to self is mode of pleasure Associated with sexual asphyxia (autoerotic hanging)
• **Fetichism**	Sexual gratification by contact with clothes/parts of opposite sex
• **Exhibitionism**	Exhibition of genitalia
• **Transvestism**	Desire to be identified with opposite sex
• **Voyeurism**	Desire to watch sexual intercourse
• **Frotteurism**	Sexual gratification by rubbing genitals with others
• **Tribadism** • **Lesbianism** • **Female homosexuality**	Women-women sex

• **Sodomy** • **Gerantophilia** • **Paedestry**	Anal sex Anal sex with adult Anal sex with a child. If a boy **(catamite)**
• **Incest**	Sexual Intercourse with close relative
• **Bestality**	Sex with **lower** animal

Excessive sexual desire in male: Satyriasis
Excessive sexual desire in female: Nymphomania
Trans sexualism is change to opposite sex by surgery

Gilles De la Tourette's Syndrome

- Gilles de la **Tourette's syndrome** consists of chronic **multiple motor and phonic tics** that have no known cause
- There is an autosomal dominant mode of inheritance with variable penetrance that is gender related
- Boys are affected much more commonly than girls
- The first signs consist of single or multiple motor tics in 80% of cases and of phonic tics in 20%
- Motor tics commonly affect the face and may consist of **repetitive sniffing, winking, blinking, elevation of the eyelids, eye closure, pursing of the lips, or facial twitching**
  - Patients eventually develop several different motor and phonic tics, the latter frequently taking the form of **grunts, barks, hisses, sighs, throat-clearing, coughing**, and verbal utterances that may involve
  - **Coprolalia (involuntary and inappropriate swearing or obscene speech)**
  - **Echolalia (involuntary repetition of the phrases of others)**
  - **Palilalia (repetition of words or phrases)**
  - The tics may change in location, severity, complexity and character with time; **are worsened by emotional stress; and can be suppressed voluntarily for short periods**
  - In some cases, **tics are complex (such as jumping up in the air) or involve repetitive self-mutilating activities (such as nail-biting, hair-pulling, or lip-biting)**
- Tics that involve **repetitive sensory phenomena**, such as pressure, tickle, or thermal sensations, also occur
- Many patients have associated behavioral abnormalities, especially **obsessive-compulsive disorder and attention deficit hyperactivity disorder**
- **Clonidine** alleviates motor and phonic tics in some children, possibly by reducing activity in noradrenergic neurons of the locus coeruleus
- **Haloperidol** has been used as DOC.

Erectile Dysfunction (ED)

Penile tumescence leading to erection depends on the increased flow of blood into the lacunar network after complete relaxation of the arteries and corporal smooth muscle. Subsequent compression of the trabecular smooth muscle against the fibroelastic tunica albuginea causes a passive closure of the emissary veins and accumulation of blood in the corpora. In the presence of a full erection and a competent valve mechanism, the corpora become noncompressible cylinders from which blood does not escape

Nitric oxide, which induces vascular relaxation, promotes erection and is opposed by endothelin-1 (ET-1), which mediates vascular contraction

Diabetic, atherosclerotic and drug-related causes account for > 80% of cases of ED in older men

Vasculogenic: The most frequent organic cause of ED is a disturbance of blood flow to and from the penis

Diabetic ED occurs in 35 to 75% of men with diabetes mellitus. Pathologic mechanisms are primarily related to diabetes-associated vascular and neurologic complications

Psychogenic the most common causes of psychogenic ED

Performance anxiety, depression, relationship conflict, loss of attraction, **sexual** inhibition, conflicts over **sexual** preference, **sexual** abuse in childhood and fear of pregnancy or sexually transmitted disease. Almost all patients with ED, even when it has a clear-cut organic basis, develop a psychogenic component as a reaction to ED.

Medication-Related

- **Thiazide diuretics and beta blockers**
- **Calcium channel blockers and angiotensin-converting enzyme inhibitors are less frequently cited. Estrogens**
- **GnRH agonists**
- **H_2 antagonists**
- **Spironolactone**
- **Antidepressant and antipsychotic agents particularly neuroleptics, tricyclics and SSRIs Digoxin**
- **Sildenafil** is the only approved and effective oral agent for the treatment of ED
- **Vacuum Constriction Devices** are a reasonable treatment alternative for select patients who cannot take sildenafil or do not desire other interventions
- **Intraurethral Alprostadil** If a patient fails to respond to oral agents, a reasonable next choice is intraurethral or self-injection or vasoactive substances. Intraurethral prostaglandin E_1 (alprostadil)
- **Intracavernosal Self-Injection**
- **Surgery** A less frequently used form of therapy for ED involves the surgical implantation of a semi-rigid or inflatable penile prosthesis

Important Points

Counsel patients about injury risk and prevention

- All physicians, regardless of specialty, have the opportunity to intervene with the 'host.' It is standard practice during history taking for physicians to inquire about tobacco and alcohol use, sexual practices, and exercise habits of adult patients, and to counsel parents about specific risks at different stages of child development. There are known risks for injury and protective strategies that patients can use to lower the risk of injury for themselves and their families
- **Identify and refer abused patients.** Family violence is a serious and underdiagnosed problem in American society. Abused patients include children, battered spouses and/or partners, elders, and those raped and sexually abused by those with whom they have a personal or intimate relationship. Hospitals, clinics, and doctors' offices may provide the first opportunity for abused patients, particularly adult women, to acknowledge the abuse, receive support, find protection, and break the cycle of violence
- **Emphasize rehabilitation and community follow-up.** Tertiary prevention involves minimizing functional disability, a consequence of serious injury. Physicians can help their patients return to productive lives by ensuring that patients receive appropriate physical and occupational therapy and that they have access to community services after discharge.

Remember

Even if a seriously ill patient refuses treatment on religious grounds ⟶ Do not treat

If life of a child is at risk but risk is not immediate ⟶ court takes gaurdainship

Consent is taken from

Girl herself : if she is married at 17 years
Guardian : if she is pregnant at 17 years
Girl herself : if she is 17 years old, living on her own and taking care of herself

As a doctor remember

- Do not abandon patient
- Competent patients have right to refuse treatment
- Patients need to be detained if they harm themselves or others

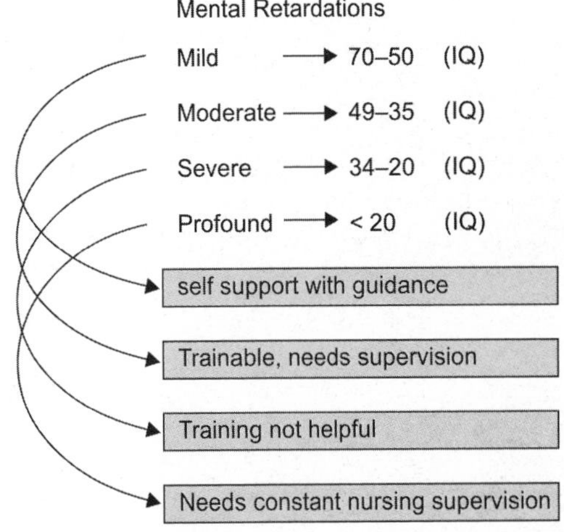

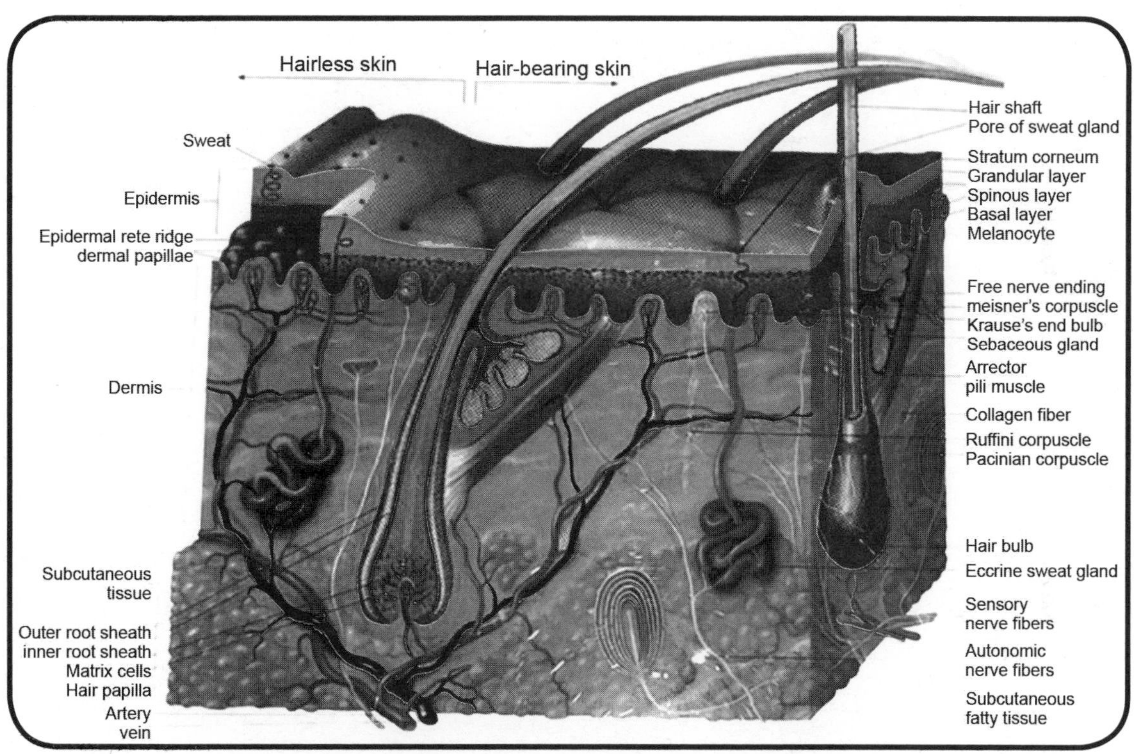
Hairless skin
Hair-bearing skin
Sweat
Epidermis
Epidermal rete ridge
dermal papillae
Dermis
Subcutaneous
tissue
Outer root sheath
inner root sheath
Matrix cells
Hair papilla
Artery
vein
Hair shaft
Pore of sweat gland
Stratum corneum
Grandular layer
Spinous layer
Basal layer
Melanocyte
Free nerve ending
meisner's corpuscle
Krause's end bulb
Sebaceous gland
Arrector
pili muscle
Collagen fiber
Ruffini corpuscle
Pacinian corpuscle
Hair bulb
Eccrine sweat gland
Sensory
nerve fibers
Autonomic
nerve fibers
Subcutaneous
fatty tissue

DERMATOLOGY

Dermatology 4

Primary Skin Lesions

• **Macule:** A flat, colored lesion, < 2 cm in diameter, not raised above the surface of the surrounding skin. A 'freckle,' or ephelid, is a prototype pigmented macule.
• **Patch:** A large (> 2 cm), flat lesion with a color different from the surrounding skin. This differs from a macule only in size.
• **Papule:** A small, solid lesion, < 1 cm in diameter, raised above the surface of the surrounding skin and hence palpable (e.g. a closed comedone, or whitehead, in acne).
• **Nodule:** A larger (1–5 cm), firm lesion raised above the surface of the surrounding skin.
• **Tumor:** A solid, raised growth > 5 cm in diameter.
• **Plaque:** A large (> 1 cm), flat-topped, raised lesion; edges may either be distinct (e.g. in psoriasis) or gradually blend with surrounding skin (e.g. in eczematous dermatitis)
• **Vesicle:** A small, fluid-filled lesion, <1 cm in diameter, raised above the plane of surrounding skin. Fluid is often visible, and the lesions are often translucent.
• **Pustule:** A vesicle filled with leukocytes. Note: The presence of pustules does not necessarily signify the existence of an infection.
• **Bulla:** A fluid-filled, raised, often translucent lesion > 1 cm in diameter.
• **Cyst:** A soft, raised, encapsulated lesion filled with semisolid or liquid contents.
• **Wheal:** A raised, erythematous papule or plaque, usually representing short-lived dermal edema.
• **Telangiectasia:** Dilated, superficial blood vessels.

Basics of Dermatology

Important Questions asked as definition
• **Acanthosis**: Increase in thickness of prickle cell layer.
• **Acantholysis**: Loss of coherence between epidermal cells. Seen in **Pemphigus**
• **Corps Grains**: Acantholytic, Dyskeratotic, Basophilic cells with rounded nuclei and perinuclear halo. Seen in Dariers disease
• **Dyskeratosis**: Abnormal development of epidermal cells. (Feature of Premalignant lesions)
• **Hyperkeratosis**: Increased thickness of **Stratum Corneum**
• **Para keratoses**: Presence of immature nucleated cells in **Stratum Corneum**

Dermatological Conditions Effecting newborn/Infants (NEWER CONCEPTS)

Erythema Toxicum Neonatorum

- This is a transient condition of unknown etiology occurring in up to **70% of neonates**
- The onset is from birth to 14 days but most cases start between day 1 and day 4
- The commonest lesions are **erythematous macules and papules** but in some cases pustules appear
- Lesions occur anywhere on the body surface **except palms and soles** but with a **predilection for face and trunk**. In cases present at birth, lesions are more acrally distributed and are often pustular
- **A peripheral blood eosinophilia is present** and smears from pustules demonstrate sheets of eosinophils. The condition usually resolves in 2 to 3 days but, rarely, may persist for several weeks
- Recognition of this entity is important to avoid unnecessary investigations of serious neonatal infections

Transient Neonatal Pustular Dermatosis

- This is a benign condition in which **superficial pustules are present at birth**
- The **pustules rupture within 24 hour**, developing a brown crust that separates after a few days to leave normal skin or a hyperpigmented macule in dark-skinned individuals
- Lesions occur mainly on chin, upper anterior trunk, lower back and buttocks. They are asymptomatic and the infant is otherwise well. Lesions are sterile on culture enabling differentiation from important neonatal infections. If hyperpigmented macules occur, they resolve over 3 to 4 months

Acropustulosis of Infancy

- This is a **benign condition** of unknown etiology occurring in otherwise healthy infants
- The onset is usually in the **neonatal period** but may be delayed for some months
- **Recurrent crops of papules** which quickly evolve into 2 to 4 mm vesicopustules occur, most commonly on the palms and soles and dorsa of hands and feet
- Initially each crop takes 1 to 2 weeks to settle and new crops occur every 2 to 3 weeks. As time goes on the crops occur less frequently and the episodes are less severe and of shorter duration
- **Lesions are pruritic** but are accompanied by no systemic symptoms. The condition finally resolves by 2 to 3 years.

MILIA

- These **represent retention cysts of the pilosebaceous follicles**
- They occur in approximately **50% of neonates** as firm pearly white 1 to 2 mm papules particularly on the face
- They usually **disappear by 4 weeks of age**
- **Epstein's pearls** are epidermal cysts on the palate present in the majority of newborns
- Persistent milia maybe a marker for certain syndromes including
  - Bazex's syndrome
  - Orofaciodigital syndrome type I and
  - Marie–Unna hypotrichosis

SCABIES IS A FREQUENTLY ASKED TOPIC

Remember

- Causative agent: **Sarcoptes scabiei**
- Type of disease: **Water washed**
- **IP: 4 Weeks**
- MC complaint: **Itching**, Itching is **worst at night** with **other members of similar complaint.**
- Lesion: Papule, vesicle or burrow
- Pathogonomic lesion: **Burrow**
- **Burrow** lies in **stratum Corneum**
- MC Site: **Interdigital space**

- MC Site **in infants**: Scalp, face
- Most **severe** form: Norwegian scabies
- DOC: **Permethrin** followed by GBHC (gamma benzene hexa chloride)
- DOC in Pregnancy: Permethrin cream
- Drug used **'orally'**: **Ivermectin**

Scabies

An infestation caused by the mite **Sarcoptes scabiei**, and the treatment of choice is permethrin cream application overnight, repeated once in 7 days.

All family members and caretakers of the child should be treated. Bedlinens and clothes should be laundered in hot water, or dry cleaned if laundering is not feasible.

Ivermectin in a **single oral dose** is used to treat scabies in immunocompromised individuals who have overwhelming infestation that would not respond to standard topical therapy. It is not recommended for use in ordinary scabies.

Lindane cream should not be used in small infants because of its potential for neurotoxicity. It is relatively safe for use in adults, but permethrin cream has an established safety record that makes it the treatment of choice today.

It is very important to treat all family members and caretakers simultaneously for the same reason.

Precipitated sulfur in petroleum was often used to treat scabies in infants and pregnant women but has become rather obsolete, as permethrin cream has proven.

Pediculosis

- Caused by **lice**
- Lays down eggs called **nits**
- **Pediculosis capitis head**
- **Pediculosis corporis body (Vagabonds disease)**
- **Pediculosis pubis pubic region**
- **Maculae cerulea** are a feature
- **Permethrin** is drug of choice.

Scarlet fever

- Caused by **Group A β Hemolytic streptococci**
- Common in **children**
- Balanchable erythema
- **Circumoral pallor** with malar flush
  - **Sand paper skin**
  - **Pastias lines**
  - **Red strawberry tongue.**

Psoriasis

Most important topic in Dermatology * (DETAILED)

- **'Chronic inflammatory skin disorder'** clinically characterized by **erythematous, sharply demarcated papules and rounded plaques, covered by 'silvery micaceous scale'**
- The skin lesions of **psoriasis** are variably **pruritic**
- Traumatized areas often develop lesions of **psoriasis (Koebner or isomorphic phenomenon)**
- Additionally, factors that may exacerbate **psoriasis** including **infections, stress, and medications (lithium, beta blockers, and antimalarials)**.

- **The most common variety of psoriasis** is called **'plaque type.'** Patients with plaque-type **psoriasis** will have stable, slowly growing plaques, which remain basically unchanged for long periods of time
- The most common areas for plaque **psoriasis** to occur are the **'extensors'** elbows, knees, gluteal cleft, and the scalp. Involvement tends to be symmetric
- **'Inverse psoriasis'** affects the intertriginous regions including the axilla, groin, submammary region, and navel, it also tends to affect the scalp, palms, and soles
- Eruptive **psoriasis (Guttate psoriasis) is most common in children and young adults.** It develops acutely in individuals without **psoriasis** or in those with chronic plaque **psoriasis.** Patients present with many small erythematous, scaling papules, frequently after upper respiratory tract infection with α-hemolytic streptococci
- About half of all patients with **psoriasis** have **fingernail involvement**, appearing as **punctuate pitting, nail thickening, or subungual hyperkeratosis**
- About 5 to 10 % of patients with **psoriasis** have associated joint complaints and these are most often found in patients with fingernail involvement
- Although some have the coincident occurrence of classic rheumatoid arthritis many have joint disease that falls into one of three types associated with psoriasis: **(1) asymmetric inflammatory arthritis most commonly involving the distal and proximal interphalangeal joints and less commonly the knees, hips, ankles and wrists; (2) a seronegative rheumatoid arthritis-like disease; a significant portion of these patients go onto develop a severe destructive arthritis; or (3) disease limited to the spine (psoriatic spondylitis)**
- Psoriasis has been linked to **HLA-Cw6** and, to a lesser extent, to **HLA-DR7**.

In nut shell remember

Well demarcated, Erythematous, **scaly lesions**
More common on **extensor aspect**
Scalp involvement is **common**
Facial and mucosal involvement less common
Traumatized lesions develop Psoriatic lesion (**Koebners Phenomenon)**
Signs Positive:

- **Auspitz sign**
- **Candle grease sign**
- **Grattage test**

Nail Changes

- **Thimble pitting**
- **Nail plate thickening**
- **Subungual hyperkeratosis**
- **Oncholysis**
- **Oil spots**
- **Brownish discoloration**

Histopathology

Hyperkeratoses
Parakeratosis
Orthokeratosis
Micro Munro abscesses in stratum Corneum
Suprapapillary thinning

Also Remember

- Turnover time in Psoriasis is **4 days only** instead of 28 days
- Psoriatic involvement on flexor aspects is called **Inverse Psoriasis**
- **Burkleys Membrane is seen in** Psoriasis
- **Arthritis mutilans is** severe but rare form of Psoriatic arthritis
  - **Treatment of choice for Psoriasis is PUVA therapy**
  - Treatment of choice for **Psoriatic arthopathy** is **Methotrexate**
  - **Retinoids** are the drugs of choice for **Psoriasis in AIDS, Pustular Psoriasis, Psoriatic Erythoderma**
  - In **pregnancy** safest drug for pustular Psoriasis is **Prednisolone**
- **Lithium, NSAIDS, Beta blockers, Antimalarials** cause **deterioration** of disease
- **Auspitz sign**: Rubbing of skin leading to removal of scales leads to pinpoint bleeding is**. It is seen in Psoriasis**
- **Grattage sign** is other sign in Psoriasis which is scratching of skin with glass slide accentuates scale formation. **Seen in Psoriasis**
- On continuous scratching a glistening white membrane appears called **Burkleys membrane. Seen in Psoriasis**
- **von Zumbusch phenomenon:** Combination **of 'Erythroderma plus sterile pustular psoriasis'.**

USMLE Case Scenario

A Pathologist describes a lesion in which there is thinning of the epidermal cell layer overlying the tips of dermal papillae (suprapapillary plates) and blood vessels within the papillae are dilated and tortuous. These vessels bleed readily when the scale is removed, giving rise to multiple punctate bleeding points. This sign is called as:

1. Trousseas sign
2. Chovestks sign
3. Grey Turner sign
4. Auspitz sign
5. Troises sign

Ans. 4. Auspitz sign

Pemphigus

- Uncommon autoimmune skin disorder characterized by **blistering and erosions involving the mucous membranes and skin.** The autoimmune attack is on the junctions between epithelial cells in the epidermis. The blisters occur high in the epithelium and can rupture easily, producing painful erosions. **Nikolsky's sign**, in which rubbing of apparently unaffected skin causes a separation of the outer layers, is a helpful diagnostic clue
- Pemphigus tends to begin in the mouth, where rapid rupture of the blisters may lead to the impression that the initial lesion is an ulcer rather than a blister
- **Biopsy with immunofluorescence studies** can demonstrate blister formation high in the epithelium that is accompanied by **IgG deposition** on epithelial cell surfaces.

There are three types of pemphigus which vary in severity: pemphigus vulgaris, pemphigus foliaceus, and paraneoplastic pemphigus.

- It occurs when antibodies attack Desmoglein 3
- **Antibodies against intercellular substance**
- **Autoimmune disease**
- **Intradermal acantholytic bullae present**
- **Intradermal acantholytic bullae present with oral mucosal lesions**
- **Acantholysis is seen in epidermis**
- **Mucus membrane lesions seen**
- **Pemphigus Foliaceus** is the **least severe** of the three varieties
- Desmoglein 1, the protein that is destroyed by the autoantibody, is only found in the top dry layer of the skin
- Pemphigus foliaceus (PF) is characterized by crusty sores that often begin on the scalp, and may move to the chest, back, and face
- **Mouth sores do not occur. It is not as painful as pemphigus vulgaris,** and is often mis-diagnosed as dermatitis or eczema.

- The **<u>least common and most severe type</u>** of pemphigus is Paraneoplastic **pemphigus** (PNP)
- This disorder is a complication of cancer, **usually** lymphoma **and** Castleman's disease. It may precede the diagnosis of the tumor
- Painful sores appear on the mouth, lips, and the esophagus
- In this variety of pemphigus, the disease process **often involves the lungs, causing** Bronchiolitis obliterans (constrictive bronchiolitis)
- Complete removal and/or cure of the tumor may improve the skin disease, but lung damage is generally irreversible.

Hailey-Hailey Disease

- **Also called <u>Familial Benign Pemphigus</u>**
- **It is an inherited (genetic) skin disease**
- **Not an autoimmune disease**
- **No subepidermal blistering**
- **It is therefore not considered part of the Pemphigus group of diseases**

Definitive diagnosis requires examination of a **skin biopsy**.

- The pathologist looks for an **intraepidermal vesicle** caused by the breaking apart of epidermal cells **(acantholysis)**
- Thus, the superficial (upper) portion of the epidermis sloughs off, leaving the bottom layer of cells on the 'floor' of the blister. This bottom layer of cells is said to have a **'tombstone appearance'**
- Definitive diagnosis also requires the demonstration of **anti-desmoglein autoantibodies** by **direct immunofluorescence on the skin biopsy.** These antibodies appear as IgG deposits along the desmosomes between epidermal cells, a pattern reminiscent of **chicken wire**. Anti-desmoglein antibodies can also be detected in a blood sample using the ELISA technique
- A high titre of **c-ANCA** (cellular Anti Neutrophil Cytoplasmic Antibody) is an important feature of the disease.

Treatment

If not treated, pemphigus can be fatal due to overwhelming infection of the sores

The most common treatment is the administration of **oral steroids**, especially prednisone. The side effects of cortico-steroids may require the use of so-called steroid-sparing or adjuvant drugs. The immuno-suppressant (Mycophenolic acid) is among those being used:

Intravenous gamma globulin (IVIG) may be useful in severe cases, especially paraneoplastic pemphigus.

Mild cases sometimes respond to the application of topical steroids.

Recently, **Rituximab, an anti-CD20 antibody**, was found to improve otherwise untreatable severe cases of Pemphigus vulgaris.

If skin lesions do become infected, **antibiotic** may be prescribed.

Pemphigus Erythematosus

- Also known as **Senear-Usher syndrome**
- It is an **overlap syndrome**
- It has erythematous, scaly plaques in a lupus-like butterfly distribution on the face as well as involving the scalp, back, chest, and intertriginous areas
- Sunlight may exacerbate the disease.

Pemphigus	Pemphigoid
• Common in age group 40–60 years	• Common greater **60 years**
• Nikolskys sign **present**	• Nikolskys sign **absent**
• **Intraepidermal** bullae • **Flaccid** bullae	• **Subepidermal** bullae • **Tense** bullae
• Mucosal involvement **common**	• Mucosal involvement **uncommon**
• Acantholysis **present**	• Acantholysis **absent**

A 46-year-old female presents to Dermatology clinic with painful oral ulcers. Physical examination demonstrates widespread erosions of her mucous membranes. Dermatological examination reveals a friable mucosa. Biopsy of perilesional mucosa demonstrates acantholysis; direct immunofluorescence demonstrates an intraepidermal band of IgG and C3. The most likely diagnosis is: Pemphigus vulgaris.

An 88 year old elderly patient from Carolina complains to a dermatologist of sores in the oral cavity and on the skin. These lesions have developed over about a month. Physical examination demonstrates three painful erosions on the oral mucosa and tongue. Raw areas with crusting on the skin is seen on the face and trunk. The patient states that the skin lesions had started as blisters that had quickly broken. While the involved areas were painful, no itchiness had been experienced. Careful examination of the edge of the skin lesions demonstrates a few flaccid bullae. Rubbing of the skin near an affected area easily detaches the superficial part of the epidermis from the underlying skin. No target-like lesions are seen. The most likely diagnosis is:

PEMPHIGUS VULGARIS

USMLE Case Scenario

Bullous pemphigoid is an autoimmune disease in which the characteristic finding is linear deposition of IgG antibodies and complement in the basement membrane zone. Reactivity also occurs in the basal cell-basement membrane attachment plaques (hemidesmosomes), where most of the bullous pemphigoid antigen (BPAG) is located. Early lesions show a perivascular infiltrate of lymphocytes and variable numbers of eosinophils, occasional neutrophils, superficial dermal edema, and associated basal cell layer vacuolization. Bullous pemphigoid is characterized by a:

1. Epidermal, nonacantholytic blister
2. Epidermal, acantholytic blister
3. Subepidermal, acantholytic blister
4. Subepidermal, nonacantholytic blister

Ans. 4. Subepidermal, nonacantholytic blister

Lichen Planus

- **Flat toppled** papules with white lacy markings on mucosa **(Wickham's striae)**
- Associated with **Hepatitis C**
- **'Civatte bodies' seen**
- **'Basal cell degeneration' seen**
- **'Max Josephs' space seen**

Pityriasis Rosacea (PR)

- Pityriasis Rosacea (PR) is **a papulosquamous** eruption of unknown etiology
- First feature invariably is development of annular or oval erythematous scaly lesion
- **(Herald patch)** followed by appearance of smaller lesions in few weeks

Lesions are:

- Oval with long axis parallel to skin folds. **(Christmas tree appearance)**
- Usually on trunk and have **Cigarette paper consistency**
- **Collarette of scales**
- **Pruritic**

Multiple, erythematous, annular lesions with 'collarette of scales' predominantly on 'trunks' is diagnostic of Ptyriasis Rosacea.

Oral Hairy Leukoplakia

- Oral hairy leukoplakia (OHL) is a disease of the **mucosa.**
- The Epstein-Barr virus (EBV), a **ubiquitous herpesvirus.**
- Many cases have been reported in **heart, kidney, and bone marrow transplant recipients** and patients with **hematological malignancies.**

- This pathology is associated with **Epstein-Barr virus (EBV)** and occurs mostly in people with HIV, **both immunocompromised and immunocompetent**, albeit it can affect patients who are HIV negative.
- Unilateral or bilateral nonpainful white lesions can be seen on the margins, dorsal or ventral surfaces of the tongue, or on buccal mucosa. The lesions may vary in appearance from smooth, flat, small lesions to irregular **'hairy' or 'feathery'** lesions with **prominent folds or projections.**
- Lesions are adherent, and only the most superficial layers can be removed by scraping. There is no associated erythema or edema of the surrounding tissue. Hairy leukoplakia may also involve dorsal and ventral tongue surfaces, the buccal mucosa, or the gingiva. On the ventral tongue, buccal mucosa, or gingiva, the lesion may be flat and smooth, lacking the characteristic 'hairy' appearance.

TINEA

- A dermatophyte is **a parasitic fungus** (mycosis) that infects the skin
- The term embraces the imperfect fungi of the genera **Epidermophyton, Microsporum and Trichophyton**
- Dermatophytes (name based on the Greek for **'skin plants'**) are a common label for a group of three types of Fungus that commonly causes skin disease in animals and humans
- They are **anamorphic** (asexual or imperfect)
- Dermatophytes cause infections of the **skin, hair and nails** due to their ability to obtain nutrients from Keratinized material. **(Superficial)**
- The organisms colonize **the keratin tissues** and inflammation is caused by host response to metabolic by-products
- They are usually **restricted to the nonliving cornified layer of the epidermis** because of their inability to Penetrate viable tissue of an immunocompetent host. Invasion does elicit a host response ranging from mild to severe
- Acid proteinases, elastase, keratinases, and other proteinases reportedly act as virulence factors.

Types of Dermatophyte Infections

Athlete's foot or tinea pedis

- Contrary to the name, it does not affect just athletes. Tinea pedis affect men more than women
- Frequently affects the webs between the toes first, before spreading to the sole of the foot in a 'moccasin' pattern

Presents with severe itching and hyperhidrosis.

Jock itch or tinea cruris

- Frequently, the feet are also involved. The theory is that the feet get infected first from contact with the ground
- The fungus spores are carried to the groin from scratching, from putting on underclothing or pants

Frequently extend from the groin to the perianal skin and gluteal cleft.

Ringworm of the body or tinea corpora

Facial ringworm or tinea faciei

Can be misdiagnosed for other conditions like psoriasis, discoid lupus, etc. Can be aggravated by treatment with topical steroid or immunosuppressive cream.

Blackdot ringworm or tinea capitis

- Infected hair shafts are broken off just at the base, leaving a black dot just under the surface of the skin

Scraping these residual black dots will yield the best diagnostic scrapings for microscopic exam. Numerous green arthrospores will be seen under the microscope inside the stubbles of broken hair shafts at 400x

Tinea capitis cannot be treated topically, and must be treated systemically with antifungals.

Ringworm of the hands or tinea manuum

- In most cases of tinea manuum, only one hand is involved

Frequently both feet are involved concurrently, thus the saying 'one hand, two feet'.

Ringworm of the nail, Onychomycosis, or tinea unguium Affects nail plate.

Treatment

- **Tinea corpora (body), tinea manus (hands), tinea cruris (groin), tinea pedis (foot) and tinea facie (face)** can be treated topically
- **Tinea unguium (nails)** usually will require oral treatment with terbinafine, itraconizole, or griseofulvin
- Griseofulvin is usually not as effective as terbinafine or itraconizole
- **Tinea capitis (scalp)** must be treated orally, as the medication must be present deep in the hair follicles toeradicate the fungus. **Usually griseofulvin** is given orally for 2 to 3 months
- Clinically dosage up to twice the recommended dose might be used due to relative resistance of some strains of dermatophytes
- Tinea pedis is usually treated with topical medicines, like ketoconazole or terbinafine, and pills, or with medicines that contains miconazole, clotrimazole, or tolnaftate. Antibiotics may be necessary to treat secondary bacterial infections that occur in addition to the fungus (for example, from scratching)

Dermatophytes are filamentous fungi that infect only superficial keratinized tissue skin, hair and nail.

They are of three types

1. **Tri**chophyton infect hair, skin and nail
2. Microsporum infect hair and skin
3. Epidermophyton infect skin and nails

Tinea Causes

- Tinea capitis: Ringworm of **scalp**
- Tinea circinata: Ringworm of **glabrous skin**
- Tinea barbae: Ringworm of **beard**
- Tinea pedis/Trichophyton rubrum: **Athletes foot**
- Tinea cruris: **Dhobi itch or Jock itch**
- Tinea unguium: **Ringworm of nails**

Remember: 'Tinea In cognito' is extensive ringworm infection with atypical appearance due to steroid misuse.

Malasezia Furfur

- Causes **Tinea Versicolor** (**Versatile colors**)
- **Scaly, Hypopigmented macules** appearing on trunk and shoulders
- Head and lower limbs are spared usually
- Short Hyphae and round spores (**Sphagetti and meat balls**) appearance on KOH is seen
- Tinea versicolor is a common, benign, superficial cutaneous fungal infection usually characterized by **Hypopigmented or hyperpigmented macules** and patches on the chest and the back. In patients with a predisposition, the condition may chronically recur
- The fungal infection is localized to the **stratum corneum**
- **Ketocanozole and itracanazole** as systemic therapy are useful
- **Griseofulvin is ineffective**

- Tinea versicolor is caused by the dimorphic, lipophilic organism, Malassezia furfur, M furfur is now the accepted name for the organism. 'Pityrosporon orbiculare, Pityrosporon ovale, and Malassezia ovalis' are synonyms for M furfur.
- M furfur is a member of normal human cutaneous flora.
- The involved skin regions are usually the trunk, the back, the abdomen, and the proximal extremities. The face, the scalp, and the genitalia are less commonly involved.

- The color of each lesion varies from almost white to reddish brown or fawn colored.
- Patients often complain that the involved skin lesions fail to tan in the summer.
- Occasionally, a patient also complains of mild pruritus.
- Greater than 20% of patients report a positive family history of the condition. This subset of patients records a higher rate of recurrence and longer duration of disease.

Acne Vulgaris

- Acne vulgaris affects the majority of adolescents and hormonal influences, abnormal keratinization of pilosebaceous units and colonization by bacteria (Propionibacterium acnes) are important pathogenetic elements
- Acne vulgaris is a self-limited disorder primarily of **teenagers and young adults, Involves pilosebacious glands**
- The permissive factor for the expression of the disease in adolescence is the **increase in sebum** release by sebaceous glands after puberty
- Small cysts, called **comedones,** form in hair follicles due to **blockage of the follicular orifice** by retention of sebum and keratinous material
- The activity of lipophilic yeast **(*Pityrosporum orbiculare*)** and bacteria **(*Proprionobacterium acnes*)** within the comedones releases free fatty acids from sebum, causes inflammation within the cyst, and results in rupture of the cyst wall. The clinical hallmark of acne vulgaris is the **comedone**, which may be **closed (whitehead)** or **open (blackhead)**.Comedones are usually accompanied by inflammatory lesions: papules, pustules, or nodules
- The **most common location** for acne is the **face**, but involvement of the chest and back is not uncommon
- Systemic medications such as **lithium, isoniazid, halogens, phenytoin, and phenobarbital** may **produce acneiform eruptions**

Treatment

- **Minimal to moderate, pauci-inflammatory disease** may respond adequately to **local therapy alone**
- **Topical agents such as retinoic acid, benzoyl peroxide, or salicylic acid** may alter the pattern of epidermal desquamation, preventing the formation of comedones and aiding in the resolution of preexisting cysts. Topical antibacterial agents such as **benzoyl peroxide, azelaic acid, topical erythromycin (with or without zinc), clindamycin, or tetracycline are also useful adjuncts to therapy**
- **Patients with moderate to severe acne** with a prominent inflammatory component will benefit from the addition of systemic therapy. **Oral tetracyclines or erythromycin** in doses of 250 to 1000 mg/d will decrease follicular colonization with some of the lipophilic organisms
- **Severe nodulocystic acne** not responsive to oral antibiotics, hormonal therapy, or topical therapy may be treated with the **synthetic retinoid isotretinoin.**

Acne vulgaris affects the **majority of adolescents. Hormonal influences, abnormal keratinization of pilosebaceous units and colonization by bacteria** (*Propionibacterium acnes*) are important pathogenetic elements

Treatment of acne depends on the severity of the condition

Topical application of **comedolytic agents such as retinoids** (tretinoin, adapalene, and the new yeast-derived agent azaleic acid) is effective for mild to moderate forms of noninflammatory acne, characterized by open comedones. Daily application of these compounds will result in improvement within several weeks after starting treatment. Mild skin irritation and scaling may be minimized by starting with low-concentration creams and then progressively increasing the concentration. Another side effect of retinoids is increased photosensitivity. The patient must be instructed to avoid prolonged exposure to the sun and to use a sunscreen.

Acne Rosacea

- Acne rosacea is an **inflammatory disorder** predominantly affecting the **central face**
- It is seen almost exclusively in **adults,**
- Rosacea is seen more often in **women,** but those most severely affected are men
- It is characterized by the presence of
  - **Erythema,**
  - **Telangiectases, and**
  - **Superficial pustules**

Rosacea only rarely involves the chest or back

- There is a relationship between the tendency for **pronounced facial flushing** and the subsequent development of acne rosacea. Often, individuals with rosacea initially demonstrate a pronounced flushing reaction. This may be in **response to heat, emotional stimuli, alcohol, hot drinks, or spicy foods**
- Rosacea of **'glandular form'** of very long standing may lead to connective tissue overgrowth, particularly of the nose **(rhinophyma)**
- Rhinophyma is also called as **Potato nose**

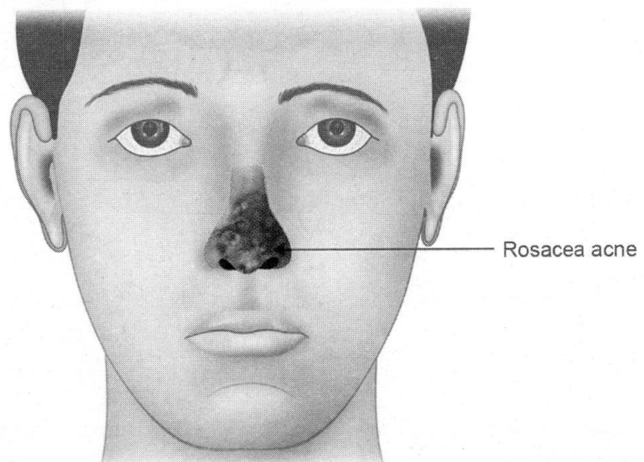

TREATMENT

Acne rosacea can generally be treated effectively with **oral tetracycline** in doses ranging from 250 to 1000 mg/d. **Topical metronidazole or sodium sulfacetamide** has also been shown to be effective. In addition, the use of low-potency, **nonfluorinated topical glucocorticoids,** particularly **after cool soaks,** is helpful in alleviating facial erythema.

New Drugs for Acne

Adapalene: Tretinoin like drug binding directly to nuclear retinoic acid receptor and modulates keratinization and differentiation of follicular epithelial cells.

Tazoretene is a synthetic retinoid used in psoriasis and acne vulgaris as well.

Nadifloxacin is used in inflamed acne and folliculitis

Dapsone gel is used as 5% aqeous gel base for acne vulgaris

Erythrasma

- Erythrasma is a **chronic superficial infection of intertriginous areas**
- Organism causing erythrasma is **Corynebacterium Minutissimum**
- Erythrasma produces **coral red fluorescence** under wood light secondary to production of porphyrins
- Erythrasma is more common in blacks
- Typical lesion is well demarcated, reddish brown macule with wrinkled appearance of skin
- Inner thighs, crural region, scrotum and toe webs are commonly involved.

Corynebacterium Minutissimum

It is a part of normal skin flora

- It is lipophilic
- Gram-positive
- Aerobic

- Catalase positive
- Nonspore forming diphtheroid

It ferments

- Glucose
- Dextrose
- Sucrose
- Maltose and
- Mannitol

Atopic Dermatitis

- Atopic dermatitis (AD) is the cutaneous expression of the **atopic state, characterized by a family history of asthma, hay fever, or dermatitis**
- **Also termed as ITCH DISEASE**
- The infantile pattern is characterized by **weeping inflammatory patches** and **crusted plaques** that occur on the **face (MC)**, neck, extensor surfaces, and groin
- The **childhood and adolescent pattern** is marked by dermatitis of flexural skin, particularly in the **antecubital** and popliteal fossae
- **Pruritus** is a prominent characteristic of AD and many of the cutaneous findings in affected patients are secondary to rubbing and scratching
- Other cutaneous stigmata of AD are **perioral pallor**, an extra fold of skin beneath the lower eyelid **(Dennie's line), increased palmar markings**, and increased incidence of cutaneous infections, particularly with *Staphylococcus aureus*
- Atopic individuals often have **dry itchy skin, abnormalities in cutaneous vascular responses**, and, in some instances, **elevations in serum IgE**
- **Biopsy is the best test**
- **'Berloque dermatitis'** is due to contact with **Cosmetics**
- **Excoriation, Lichenification, Hyperlinear palms** are seen.

Contact Dermatitis

- Contact dermatitis is an inflammatory process in skin caused by an exogenous agent or agents that directly or indirectly injure the skin
- This injury may be caused by an inherent characteristic of a compound **irritant contact dermatitis (ICD).** An example of ICD would be dermatitis induced by a concentrated acid or base. Agents that cause allergic contact dermatitis (ACD) induce an antigen-specific immune response. The clinical lesions of contact dermatitis may be acute (wet and edematous) or chronic (dry, thickened and scaly), depending on the persistence of the insult
- The most common presentation of contact dermatitis is hand **eczema** and it is frequently related to occupational exposures

ICD

- **It is generally strictly demarcated and often localized to areas of thin skin** (eyelids, intertriginous areas) or to areas where the irritant was occluded
- Lesions may range from **minimal skin erythema to areas of marked edema, vesicles, and ulcers**
- **Chronic low-grade irritant dermatitis** is the **most common type** of ICD and
- The most common area of involvement is the **hands**
- The most common irritants encountered are **chronic wet work, soaps, and detergents**. Treatment should be directed to avoidance of irritants and use of protective gloves or clothing

ACD

- It is a manifestation of **delayed type hypersensitivity mediated** by memory **T lymphocytes** in the skin
- The most common cause of ACD is **exposure to plants**, specifically to members of the family **Anacardiaceae;** including the genera *Toxicodendron, Anacardium, Gluta, Mangifera*, and *Semecarpus*
- **Poison ivy, poison oak and poison sumac** are members of the genus *Toxicodendron* and cause an allergic reaction marked by erythema, vesiculation and severe pruritus
- The eruption is **often linear**, corresponding to areas where plants have touched the skin.

Patch Tests

Patch testing is used to validate a diagnosis of allergic contact sensitization and to identify the causative allergen. Because the entire skin of sensitized humans is allergic, the test reproduces the dermatitis in one small area where the allergen is applied, usually on the back. The suspected allergen is applied to the skin, occluded, and left in place 48 hours. A positive test reproduces an eczematous response at the test site from 48 hours up to a week later. The latter is a delayed hypersensitivity reaction. Considerable experience is required to accurately perform and interpret patch tests. Photopatch testing is performed to detect photocontact allergy. Suspected photoallergens are placed on the skin in two sets. One set of allergens is irradiated with appropriate wavelengths of light after the patches are in place on the skin 24 hours; the second set of the same photoallergens is kept covered to serve as controls. Photoallergens cause an erythematous reaction that is evident 24 hours after exposure to light.

Nummular Eczema

- Nummular **eczema** is characterized by circular or oval **'coinlike' lesions**
- Initially, this eruption consists of small edematous papules that become crusted and scaly. The most common locations are on the **trunk or the extensor surfaces** of the extremities, particularly on the pretibial areas or dorsum of the hands
- It occurs more frequently in **men** and is most commonly seen in middle age.

Hand Eczema

Hand **eczema** is a **very common, chronic skin disorder**

It represents a **large proportion** of occupation-associated skin disease

It may be associated with other cutaneous disorders such as atopic dermatitis or may occur by itself

It may present with **dryness and cracking of the skin of the hands** as well as with variable amounts of erythema and edema. Often, the dermatitis will begin under rings where water and irritants are trapped

A variant of hand dermatitis, **dyshidrotic eczema**, presents with multiple, intensely pruritic, small papules and vesicles occurring on the thenar and hypothenar eminences and the sides of the fingers.

Lichen Simplex Chronicus

- Lichen simplex chronicus may represent the **end stage of a variety of pruritic and eczematous disorders**
- It consists of a **well-circumscribed plaque or plaques with lichenified or thickened skin due to chronic scratching or rubbing**
- Common areas involved include the **posterior nuchal region, dorsum of the feet, or ankles**
- Treatment of lichen simplex chronicus centers around breaking the cycle of chronic itching and scratching, which often occur during sleep
- **High-potency topical glucocorticoids are helpful** in alleviating pruritus in most cases, but in recalcitrant cases, application of topical glucocorticoids under occlusion or intralesional injection of glucocorticoids may be required.

Asteatotic Eczema

- Asteatotic **eczema**, also known as **xerotic eczema or 'winter itch,'** is a mildly inflammatory variant of dermatitis that develops most commonly on the **lower legs of elderly individuals** during **dry times of year**
- Fine cracks, with or without erythema, characteristically develop on the anterior surface of the lower extremities. Pruritus is variable
- Asteatotic **eczema** responds well to avoidance of irritants, rehydration of the skin, and application of topical emollients.

Stasis Dermatitis and Stasis Ulceration

- Stasis dermatitis develops on the **lower extremities** secondary to **venous incompetence and chronic edema**
- Early findings in stasis dermatitis consist of **mild erythema and scaling** associated with pruritus. The typical initial site of involvement is the **medial aspect of the ankle**, often over a distended vein
- As the disorder progresses, the dermatitis becomes progressively **pigmented**, due to chronic erythrocyte extravasation leading to cutaneous **hemosiderin deposition**.

- Chronic stasis dermatitis is often associated with **dermal fibrosis** that is recognized clinically as **brawny edema of the skin**
- Stasis dermatitis is often complicated by **secondary infection** and contact dermatitis
- Severe stasis dermatitis may precede the development of **stasis ulcers.**

Tumors Affecting Skin

Basal Cell Carcinoma BCC is a malignancy arising from epidermal basal cells

- The **most common type** is **noduloulcerative** BCC, which begins as a small, **pearly nodule**, often with small telangiectatic vessels on its surface
- The nodule grows slowly and may undergo central ulceration
- Lymphatic spread does not occur
- Various amounts of melanin may be present in the tumor; tumors with a heavier accumulation are referred to as pigmented BCC.

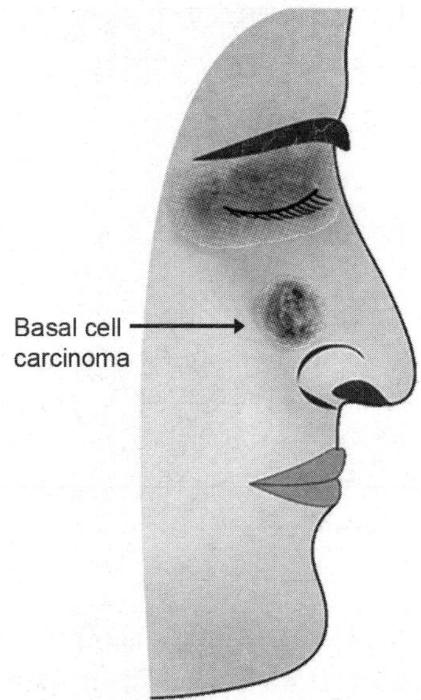

Squamous Cell Carcinoma: Primary cutaneous SCC is a malignant neoplasm of **keratinizing epidermal cells.**

Unlike BCC, which has a very low metastatic potential, SCC can **metastasize and grow rapidly.** The clinical features of SCC vary widely.

Predisposition to SCC

- **Actinic keratosis**
- **Bowens disease**
- **Lichen planus**
- **DLE**

Commonly, SCC appears as an **ulcerated nodule or superficial erosion on the skin or lower lip, but it may present as a verrucous papule or plaque.**

Unlike BCC, overlying telangiectasias are uncommon.

The margins of this tumor may be ill-defined, and fixation to underlying structures may occur. Cutaneous SCC may develop anywhere on the body, but it usually arises on sun-damaged skin.

Keratoacanthoma

- Typically appears as a dome-shaped papule with a central keratotic crater, Expands rapidly, and commonly regresses without therapy
- This lesion can be difficult to differentiate from SCC.

Melanomas

Originate from melanocytes, pigment cells normally present in the epidermis and sometimes in the dermis.

The individuals **most susceptible** to development of melanoma are:

- Those with fair complexions, red or blonde hair, blue eyes and freckles and who tan poorly and sunburn easily.
- Family history of melanoma
- The presence of a clinically atypical mole (dysplastic nevus)
- A giant congenital melanocytic nevus, or a small to medium-sized congenital melanocytic nevus the presence of a higher than average number of ordinary melanocytic nevi; and immunosuppression. Melanoma is relatively rare in heavily pigmented people

Melanomas often **express cell-surface antigens** that may be recognized by host immune cells, e.g. **Melanoma antigens (MAGEs) and Tyrosinase**

The presence of **'microscopic satellites'** is also predictive of microscopic metastases to the regional lymph nodes.

An alternative prognostic scheme for clinical stages I and II melanoma, proposed by **Clark,** is based on the anatomic level of invasion in the skin. **(Clarks Level)**

- **Level I** is intraepidermal (in situ)
- **Level II** penetrates the papillary dermis
- **Level III** spans the papillary dermis
- **Level IV** penetrates the reticular dermis
- **Level V** penetrates into the subcutaneous fat

- Melanomas may spread by the **lymphatic channels or the bloodstream**
- The earliest metastases are often to regional lymph nodes
- Most common site for Malignant melanoma is **skin** (90%)
- Cutaneous melanoma arises from **epidermal melanocytes**
- **Junctional melanoma** predisposes to MM
- Maybe **familial**

Early detection of melanoma may be facilitated by applying the **'ABCD rules'**:

- A asymmetry, benign lesions are usually symmetric
- B border irregularity, most nevi have clear-cut borders
- C color variegation, benign lesions usually have uniform light or dark pigment
- D diameter > 6 mm (the size of a pencil eraser).

- **Lentigo maligna** is the **least common type**
- It is also known as **Hutchinson's** freckle
- **Face** is the most common site involved by it
- **Superficial spreading is the most common type**
- It may occur at any site on body
- **Nodular Melanoma** is the **most malignant type**
- It is common in younger age group
- **Acral lentigous** occurs on **palms and soles especially**
- **Amelanotic** has the **worst prognosis**

- **'Clark's level' is classification based on level of 'invasion into skin'**
- **'Breslows staging'** is based on **thickness of invasion**
- **No's of MM (Malignant Melanoma)**
- <u>**No**</u> incisional biopsy

- **No** induration
- **No** role of radiotherapy
- Not known usually before puberty

Adnexal Tumors

Adnexal Or Appendageal tumors arise from **cutaneous appendages**

They may serve as **markers for internal malignancies**

They are mostly in the form of solitary or multiple nodules/papules

- **Eccrine porcoma is seen on p alms and soles**
- **Cylindroma or turban tumor is seen on forehead and scalp**
- **Syringomas are seen in vicinity of lower eyelids**
- **Trichoepitheliomas and trichilemmoma arise from hair follicles and are seen on face, scalp, neck and upper trunk**
- **Sebaceous adenoma arises from sebaceous glands**

Pyogenic granuloma

- **Total misnomer**
- **Neither' infectious' nor 'Granulomatous.'**
- Also called as **lobular capillary hemangioma**
- Usually occurs in **children**, young adults
- Called as Pregnancy **(pregnancy tumor)** or **Granuloma Gravidarum**
- This lesion most commonly develops at a site of previous injury, and is best considered a variation of granulation tissue formation. The name is a misnomer, since the lesion is neither related to bacterial infection nor a true granuloma. Microscopically, proliferating blood vessels in an immature fibrous stroma are seen. The lesions can occasionally be confused with dysplastic nevi or malignant melanoma, but are completely benign. Treatment is with surgical excision, curettage, or electrodesiccation.

Cutaneous T cell Lymphoma: Mycosis Fungoides

- It is an **indolent** lymphoma
- **Mc skin lymphoma**
- **Erythroderma + circulating tumor cells with mycosis fungoides = Sezary syndrome**
- Presence of **Sezary cells**
- **Pautriers microabscesses** seen
- **Presents with diffuse erythroderma**

Actinic Keratosis

- Actinic keratosis (AK)
- It is a **UV light-induced lesion of the skin** that may progress to invasive **squamous cell carcinoma**
- **Most common lesion with malignant potential** to arise on the skin
- Actinic keratoses arise on **fair-skinned people** in areas of **long-term sun exposure**, such as the face, ears, bald scalp, forearms, and backs of the hands
- They may occur on any area that is **repeatedly exposed to the sun**, such as the back, the chest, and the legs
- **Long-term UV light exposure** is implicated as the cause from both epidemiologic observations and molecular analysis of tumor cells
- Clinically, actinic keratoses range from **barely perceptible** rough spots of skin to elevated, hyperkeratotic plaques **several centimeters** in diameter.

- Most often, they appear as
- **Multiple discrete, flat or elevated, keratotic lesions**
- Lesions typically have an **erythematous base covered by scale (hyperkeratosis)**
- They are usually 3 to 10 mm in diameter and gradually enlarge into broader, more elevated lesions
- Overtime, actinic keratoses may develop into invasive squamous cell.

Medical Eponyms

• **Turban tumor:**	• **Cylindroma**
• **Marjolins ulcer:**	• **Squamous cell cancer**
• **Molluscum sebaceum:**	• **Keratocanthoma**
• **Cocks Peculiar tumor:**	• **Infected sebaceous cyst**
• **Brooks tumor:**	• **Tumor of hair follicles**

Dermatitis Herpetiformis

- (DH) is an
  - Intensely **pruritic**
  - **Papulovesicular skin disease** characterized by lesions **symmetrically distributed**
  - Over **extensor surfaces** (i.e. elbows, knees, buttocks, back, scalp, and posterior neck)
  - **Pruritus is prominent,** patients may present with excoriations and crusted papules
- Patients have an associated, usually subclinical, **gluten-sensitive enteropathy**
- More than 90% express the **HLA-B8/DRw3 and HLA-DQw2** haplotypes
- Biopsy of early lesional skin reveals **neutrophil-rich infiltrates within dermal papillae**. Neutrophils, fibrin, edema, and microvesicle formation at these sites are characteristic of early disease. Older lesions may demonstrate nonspecific features of a subepidermal bulla or an excoriated papule
- Direct immunofluorescence microscopy of normal-appearing perilesional skin demonstrate **granular deposits of IgA** (with or without complement components) in the papillary dermis and along the epidermal basement membrane zone
- Drug of choice **Dapsone (D for D).**

Acanthosis Nigricans

1. Acanthosis nigricans is a skin condition characterized by '**<u>dark, thick, velvety skin in body folds and creases</u>**'
2. Most often, acanthosis nigricans affects '**armpits, groin and neck**.' Sometimes the lips, palms orsoles of the feet are affected as well
3. **'Slow progression'**. The skin changes appear slowly, sometimes over months or years
4. **Possible itching.** 'Rarely,' the affected areas itch
5. Acanthosis nigricans is often associated with conditions that increase insulin level, such as **type2 diabetes** or being **overweight.** If insulin level is too high, the extra insulin may trigger activity in skin cells. This may cause the characteristic skin changes
6. In some cases, acanthosis nigricans is inherited. Certain **medications** —such as '**human growth hormone, oral contraceptives and large doses of niacin'** — can contribute to the condition

Other hormone problems, endocrine disorders or tumors may play a role as well.

- **The posterior neck** is the most commonly affected site **<u>in children</u>**
- **The vulva** is the most commonly affected site in <u>females</u> who are hyperandrogenic and obese
- **'Acrochordons' (skin tags)** are often found in and around the affected areas
- The most common cause of Acanthosis nigricans is **insulin resistance, which leads to increased circulating insulin levels. Insulin spillover into the skin results in its abnormal growth, and the stimulation of color producing cells (melanocytes)**.

- The most common cause of Acanthosis nigricans is **Type 2 diabetes mellitus followed by obesity or endocrinopathies, such as hypothyroidism or hyperthyroidism, acromegaly, polycystic ovary disease, insulin-resistant diabetes, or Cushing's disease**
- Other causes of Acanthosis nigricans are **familial, drug-induced, and idiopathic** as mentioned.

In the context of a malignant disease, Acanthosis nigricans is a paraneoplastic syndrome and is then commonly referred to as **'Acanthosis nigricans maligna'**

Involvement of mucous membranes is <u>rare</u> and suggests a coexisting malignant condition

When seen in individuals **older than age 40**, this disorder is commonly associated with an internal malignancy, usually:

- **Adenocarcinoma of lungs**
- **Cancers of GI tract**
- **Uterine cancers**
- **Cancers of prostate**
- **Cancers of breast**
- **Cancers of ovary**

Skin Disorders Associated with Thyroid Disease

Skin manifestations of hypothyroidism

- Dry (anhydrosis), cold, yellowish skin
- Non-pitting edema (e.g. hands, face)
- Dry, coarse scalp hair, loss of lateral aspect of eyebrows
- Eczema
- Xanthomata

Skin manifestations of hyperthyroidism

- Pretibial myxedema: erythematous, edematous lesions above the lateral malleoli
- Thyroid acropachy: clubbing
- Scalp hair thinning
- Increased sweating
- Pruritus can occur in both hyper- and hypothyroidism

Dermatologic Manifestations of HIV Infection

Dermatologic problems occur in about **90% of patients with HIV infection**. From the macular, roseola-like rash seen with the acute seroconversion syndrome to extensive end-stage <u>KS</u>, cutaneous manifestations of HIV disease can be seen throughout the course of HIV infection

- **Seborrheic dermatitis**. In HIV-infected patients, seborrheic dermatitis may be **aggravated by concomitant infection with Pityrosporum, a yeast like fungus**
- **Eosinophilic pustular folliculitis. It presents as multiple, urticarial perifollicular papules that may coalesce into plaquelike lesions**. Patients with HIV infection have also been reported to develop a severe form of **Norwegian scabies** with hyperkeratotic psoriasiform lesions
- **Psoriasis and ichthyosis**, Preexisting psoriasis may become guttate in appearance and more refractory to treatment in the setting of HIV infection
- **Reactivation herpes zoster (shingles)**. Acyclovir or famciclovir is the treatment of choice. Foscarnet is of value in patients with acyclovir-resistant virus
- **Infection with herpes simplex virus** in HIV-infected individuals is associated with **recurrent oro labial, genital, and perianal lesions as part of recurrent reactivation syndromes**
- Diffuse skin eruptions due to **Molluscum contagiosum** may be seen in patients with advanced HIV infection. These flesh-colored, umbilicated lesions may be treated with local therapy
- **Condyloma acuminatum** lesions may be more severe and more widely distributed in patients with low CD4+ T cell counts.

- The skin of patients with HIV infection is often a '**Target Organ' for drug reactions**
- Although most skin reactions are mild and not necessarily an indication to discontinue therapy, patients may have particularly severe cutaneous reactions, including **Erythroderma and Stevens-Johnson syndrome,** as a reaction to drugs, particularly sulfa drugs, the nonnucleoside reverse transcriptase inhibitors, abacavir, and amprenavir
- Similarly, patients with HIV infection are often **quite 'photosensitive' and 'burn easily'** following exposure to sunlight or as a side effect of radiation therapy.

Dermatological Changes in Diabetes

- **Protracted wound healing and skin ulcerations**. Diabetic dermopathy, sometimes termed **pigmented pretibial papules, or 'diabetic skin spots**,' begins as an erythematous area and evolves into an area of circular hyperpigmentation. These lesions result from minor mechanical trauma in the pretibial region and are more common in elderly men with DM. Bullous diseases (shallow ulcerations or erosions in the pretibial region) are also seen
- **Necrobiosis lipoidica diabeticorum** is a rare disorder of DM that predominantly affects young women with type 1 DM, neuropathy, and retinopathy. It usually begins in the pretibial region as an erythematous plaque or papules that gradually enlarge, darken, and develop irregular margins, with atrophic centers and central ulceration. They may be painful
- **Acanthosis nigricans** (hyperpigmented velvety plaques seen on the neck or extensor surfaces) is sometimes a feature of severe insulin resistance and accompanying diabetes
- Generalized or localized **Granuloma annulare** (erythematous plaques on the extremities or trunk) and scleredema (areas of skin thickening on the back or neck at the site of previous superficial infections) are more common in the diabetic population
- **Lipoatrophy and lipohypertrophy** can occur at insulin injection sites but are unusual with the use of human insulin. Xerosis and pruritus are common and are relieved by skin moisturizers.

Dermatological Changes in Syphilis

Early Congenital syphilis

- **Snuffles or rhinitis** is the early feature
- **Vesico bullous** lesions (not found in any other variety of syphilis)
- **Snail track ulcers** on oral mucosa

Late Congenital Syphilis

- **Hutchinsons triad** (Hutchinson's teeth +8 th Cranial nerve deafness+ Interstitial Keratitis)
- Moon's molars and **maldevelopment of the maxilla resulting in 'bulldog' facies**
- **Saddle nose**
- **Sabre Tibia**
- **Mulberry Molars**
- **Rhagades** (*The infant may fail to thrive and have a characteristic 'old man' look, with fissured lesions around the mouth (rhagades) and a mucopurulent or blood-stained nasal discharge causing snuffles.*)
- **Frontal bossing of Parrot**
- **Periostitis Higoumenakis sign**

Dermatological changes in secondary syphilis:

- **Cutaneous rashes** usually appear within 6 to 12 weeks after infection. The lesions may be transitory or may persist for months. In untreated patients they frequently heal, but fresh ones may appear within weeks or months. (MC Manifestation)
- Over 80% of patients have **mucocutaneous lesions**
- Generalized enlargement of the **lymph nodes**
- Lesions of the eyes **(uveitis)**
- **Moth eaten alopecia**
- Bones **(periostitis)** and joints
- **Meninges**
- **Kidney (glomerulitis)**
- Mild **constitutional symptoms** of malaise, headache, anorexia, nausea, aching pains in the bones and fatigability are often present, as well as fever, anemia, jaundice, albuminuria, and neck stiffness.

DERMATOLOGICAL CHANGES IN LEPROSY

Tuberculoid Leprosy

- The initial lesion of tuberculoid leprosy is often a **hypopigmented macule** that is sharply demarcated and hypoesthetic
- Infective form
- Fully developed lesions are **densely anesthetic** and **devoid of the normal skin organs** (sweat glands and hair follicles)
- Patients eventually have one or more **asymmetrically distributed, hypopigmented, anesthetic, nonpruritic, well defined macules, often with an erythematous or raised border**
- Tuberculoid leprosy patients may also have **asymmetric enlargement of one or a few peripheral nerves**
- Although any peripheral nerve may be enlarged (including small digital and supraclavicular nerves), those most commonly affected are the **ulnar, posterior auricular, peroneal and post tibial nerves**, with associated hypesthesia and myopathy
- At times, tuberculoid leprosy may present with **only nerve-trunk involvement** with no skin lesions; in such cases it is termed ***neural leprosy***
- In TT leprosy the **epidermis** may be involved histologically
- On hematoxylin and eosin staining, TT and BT lesions appear as well defined **noncaseating granulomas** with many lymphocytes and Langhans' giant cells
- In tuberculoid leprosy, T cells breach the perineurium, and destruction of Schwann cells and axons may be evident, resulting in fibrosis of the epineurium, replacement of the endoneurium with epithelial granulomas and occasionally caseous necrosis
- AFB are generally absent or few in number
- Invasion and destruction of nerves in the dermis by T cells are pathognomonic for leprosy.

Lepromatous Leprosy

- Lepromatous Leprosy at the **more severe** end of the leprosy spectrum is lepromatous disease, which encompasses the LL and BL forms
- The initial skin lesions of lepromatous leprosy are skin-colored or slightly erythematous papules or nodules. In time, individual lesions grow in diameter up to 2 cm; new papules and nodules then appear and may coalesce
- Patients later present with **symmetrically distributed skin nodules**, raised plaques, or diffuse dermal infiltration which, when on the face, results in **leonine facies**
- Late manifestations include loss of eyebrows eyelashes, pendulous earlobes, and dry scaling skin, particularly on the feet
- **Gynacomastia, madriosis, collapse of nasal bridge**
- Dermatopathology in lepromatous leprosy is **confined to the dermis** and particularly affects the dermal appendages
- Histologically, the dermis characteristically contains highly vacuolated cells **(foam cells) and fewer or absent noncaseating granuloma**
- The dermis in lepromatous leprosy contains **few lymphocytes and giant cells, and granulomas are absent**
- In LL leprosy, **bacilli are numerous in the skin** (as many as 10^9/g), where they are often found in **large clumps (*globi*)**, and in peripheral nerves, where they initially invade Schwann cells, resulting in foamy degenerative myelination and axonal degeneration and later in Wallerian degeneration.

- Leprosy is also called as **Hansen's Disease**
- **Virchow's cells seen**
- The sensation to be lost earliest in Leprosy is **Touch**
- **Rifampicin** is the drug **most rapidly acting** and **most potent** against Leprosy bacillus
- **Dapsone is the 'drug of choice'. Dose is '1–2 mg/kg'. Half life is '24 hours'**
- **Ist line drugs are: rifampicin, dapsone, clofazamine**
- **DOC in neuritis is STEROIDS**
- **Nerve abscess treated by incision and drainage**

- Leprosy bacillus is a **gram-positive, acid fast bacillus**
- **Lepra cells** are also called as **foamy cells** are actually Histiocytes within which globi are found
- Generation time of lepra bacillus is **12 days**
- Only source of infection is the **patient**.

- Incubation period of leprosy is **2–5 years**
- Most common nerve involved is **ulnar nerve** followed by postauricular nerve
- **Schwann cells** are involved first of all
- CNS, ovaries, lungs are **'not commonly' involved** in leprosy.

Lepra reactions

Type 1 reaction is also called as 'Downgrading' or 'reversal' reaction

- It occurs in **Borderline Leprosy**
- It is type **'IV delayed Hypersensitivity reaction'**
- Signs of inflammation in previous lesions, Neuritis and fever are characteristic. **(Ulnar nerve is most commonly affected)**

Treatment:

- **Continue antileprotics**
- **Use Analgesics**
- **Corticosteroids** are the 'drug of choice'
- **Unresponsive to thalidomide**

Type II reaction **is also called as 'Erythema Nodosum Leprosum'**

- It occurs in **Lepromatous Leprosy**
- It is type **'III Hypersensitivity reaction'**

Treatment:

- **Corticosteroids** are the initially used drugs
- **Thalidomide is effective**

Lepromin test is positive in patients having cell mediated immunity

- Cell mediated immunity is present in Tuberculosis. Hence Lepromin test is positive. As the spectrum of leprosy passes from tuberculoid to lepromatous type the Lepromin test gets weaker
- Lepromin test is **not a diagnostic test**
- Lepromin test is **a prognostic test**
- Positive test suggests good prognosis
- Negative test suggests poor prognosis
- Lepromin test is negative in most children in first 6 months of life
- BCG vaccination may convert Lepra reaction from negative to positive

Lepromin Test has Two Reactions

- **Early Fernandez** in 24 to 48 hours with erythema and Induration
- **Late mitsuda** in 4 weeks with indurated skin nodule
- **Indicates strong immunity**

DERMATOLOGICAL CHANGES IN LUPUS

Cutaneous Lupus is an important topic nowadays. Important features are

- Cutaneous lupus presents as a **malar or butterfly** rash
- The rash is **photosensitive, fixed and erythematous** over cheeks and bridge of the nose
- Scarring is **absent**
- **Loss of scalp hair** (alopecia) can be present
- **Exposure to sunlight precipitates DLE**
- Discoid Lupus Erythematosus (DLE) **occurs in 20% of cases of SLE**
- Lesions have **central scarring and atrophy** with loss of appendages

- **'Follicular plugging**'and'**Telengiactasis'** are characteristic of DLE. (Discoid **lupus** erythematosus (DLE) is characterized by discrete lesions, most often on the face, scalp, or external ears. The lesions are erythematous papules or plaques with a thick, adherent scale that occludes hair follicles (follicular plugging). When the scale is removed, its underside will show small excrescences that correlate with the openings of hair follicles and is termed a **'carpet tack'** appearance)
- Lesions occur in **face, scalp and sun exposed** areas of the body
- Only **5%** patients with DLE develop SLE
- When SLE lesions are in the form of urticaria, bullae, erythema multiformae, Lichen planus, the condition called **'Lupus Profondus.'**

Important Points about Subacute Lupus Erythomatosus

- **Subacute lupus** is a distinct subset with '**recurrent, Extensive**' dermatitis'
- **Erythema** of nasal and malar regions occurs
- Arthritis and Fatigue being **common** manifestations
- CNS and Renal involvement is **rare**
- Deposits of Ig and C occur in '**Dermoepidermal 'junction** in less than 50% patients and is **'not specific'**. Most patients have antibodies to **Ro (SS-A) or to (ss) DNA.**

Skin Disease Due To NTM

Swimming-Pool and Fish-Tank Granuloma

Between 1 week and 2 months (usually 2 to 3 weeks) after contact with contaminated tropical fish tanks, swimming pools, or saltwater fish, a small violet nodule or pustule may appear at a site of minor trauma

This lesion may evolve to form a crusted ulcer or small abscess or may remain warty. Lesions are multiple and disseminated on occasion particularly, but not exclusively, in immunosuppressed patients

The causative organism is **M marinum**. The patient's clinical history, combined with the isolation of M marinum after biopsy and culture, establishes the diagnosis

Buruli Ulcer

In many tropical areas throughout the world**, M ulcerans** may cause an itching nodule on the arms or legs, which then breaks down to form a shallow ulcer of variable.

Erythroderma

Erythroderma is the term used when the **majority of the skin surface is erythematous** (red in color)

There may be associated scale, erosions, or pustules as well as shedding of the hair and nails. Potential systemic manifestations include fever, chills, hypothermia, reactive lymphadenopathy, peripheral edema, hypoalbuminemia and high-output cardiac failure. The major etiologies of erythroderma are:

1. **Cutaneous diseases such as psoriasis and dermatitis**
2. **Drugs**
3. **Systemic diseases and**
4. **Idiopathic.**

Alopecia

- The two major forms of alopecia are **scarring and nonscarring**
- **In scarring alopecia** there is associated fibrosis, inflammation, and loss of hair follicles
- **In nonscarring alopecia** the hair shafts are gone, but the hair follicles are preserved, explaining the reversible nature of nonscarring alopecia
- The most common causes of **nonscarring alopecia** include:
  - **Telogen effluvium,**
  - **Androgenetic alopecia,**
  - **Alopecia areata,**

- Tinea capitis, and
- Traumatic alopecia

- Exposure to various drugs can also cause diffuse hair loss, usually by inducing a telogen effluvium. An exception is the anagen effluvium observed with antimitotic agents such as daunorubicin. Alopecia is a side effect of the following drugs:
  - **Warfarin**
  - **Heparin**
  - **Propylthiouracil**
  - **Carbimazole**
  - **Vitamin A, isotretinoin, acetretin**
  - **Lithium**
  - **Beta blockers**
  - **Colchicine and amphetamines**
- Less commonly, nonscarring alopecia is associated with lupus erythematosus and secondary syphilis
- **Scarring alopecia** is more frequently the result of a primary cutaneous disorder such as
  - **Lichen planus,**
  - **Folliculitis decalvans,**
  - **Cutaneous lupus, or**
  - **Linear scleroderma (morphea)** than it is a sign of systemic disease
  - Less common causes of scarring alopecia include sarcoidosis

Alopecia aereta:

- It is autoimmune
- Exclamation hair mark present

Alopecia Aerata

- Initial lesion is well circumscribed, totally bald, smooth patch
- **Autoimmune in origin**
- Scalp is the usual first site to be infected
- Stumps in alopecia aerata form **exclamation mark**
- It is the broken part of hair (Paler and narrower)
- **Pitting of nails is an associated feature**
- **Testosterone is contraindicated**
- **Minoxidil is used in treatment.**

Scarring alopecia	Nonscarring alopecia
• Lichen planus	• Thyroid disorders (Hyper/ Hypo)
• Leprosy	• Ectodermal dysplasia
• Lupus vulgaris	• Mineral deficiencies
• Linear scleroderma	• Drugs
• Lupus erythematosus	

USMLE Case Scenario

A 44-year-old woman presents to a dermatology Clinic. She has lost most of the hair on her body, including scalp, eye brows, eye lashes, axilla and groin hair and the fine hairs on her body and extremities. She most likely has a variant of which of the following?

1. Alopecia areata
2. Androgenic alopecia
3. Cutaneous lupus erythematosus
4. Lichen planus
5. Trichotillomania

Ans. 1. Alopecia areata

Pemphigoid Gestationis

- Pemphigoid gestationis (PG), also known as **herpes gestationis**, is a rare, nonviral, subepidermal blistering disease of pregnancy and the puerperium
- PG may begin **during any trimester of pregnancy** or present shortly after delivery
- Lesions are usually distributed over the **abdomen, trunk, and extremities; mucous membrane lesions are rare**
- Skin lesions in these patients may be quite polymorphic and consist of erythematous urticarial papules and plaques, vesiculopapules, and/or frank bullae
- Lesions are almost always **very pruritic**. Severe exacerbations of PG frequently occur after delivery, typically within 24 to 48 h
- PG tends to **recur in subsequent pregnancies**, often beginning earlier during such gestations. Occasionally, infants of affected mothers demonstrate transient skin lesions.

Pyoderma Gangrenosum

The border of the ulcers has a characteristic appearance of an undermined necrotic bluish edge and a peripheral erythematous halo

Most commonly found on the lower extremities, they can arise anywhere on the surface of the body, including sites of trauma **(pathergy)**

An estimated 30 to 50% of cases are **idiopathic**, and the most common associated disorders are:

- **Ulcerative colitis and Crohn's disease**
- **Chronic active hepatitis**
- **Seropositive rheumatoid arthritis**
- **Acute and chronic granulocytic leukemia**
- **Polycythemia vera, and**
- **Myeloma**

Important Points about Dermatomyositis

- **Dermato + Myositis**: Involves skin and muscles usually
- **Females** are more commonly affected
- Features are '**rash and muscle weakness**'.

- Eyelids with edema **(Helitrope rash)**
- Erythema of knuckles with scaly eruption (**Gottron rash)**
- Neck and anterior chest **(V sign)**
- Back and shoulder **(Shawl sign)**

'Proximal' muscle weakness with loss of fine motor movements is seen

Dermatomyositis can be associated with malignancy in **10–20% cases**

Periungual telangiectasia may be prominent, and a lacy or reticulated erythema may be associated with fine scaling on the extensor surfaces of the thighs and upper arms. Other patients, particularly those with long-standing disease, develop areas of **hypopigmentation, hyperpigmentation, mild atrophy, and telangiectasia known as poikiloderma vasculare atrophicans.**

Note

• MYCOSIS CELL:	• T lymphocyte
• LE CELL:	• Neutrophil
• LEPRA CELL:	• Plasma cell
• TZANCK CELL:	• Modified keratinocyte
• VIRCHOW'S CELL:	• Leprosy
• MAJOCCHI'S GRANULOMA:	• Tinea rubrum
• PALISADING GRANULOMA:	• Granuloma annulare
• GRANULOMA INGUINALE:	• Calymmatobacterium granulomatosis

Associations never to be forgotten

- **Pseudomonas** in **' Hot-tub folliculitis'**
- **Pseudomonas** in **'Ecthyma gangrenosum'**
- **HSV (Herpes simplex virus)** on the head and neck of young wrestlers **'Herpes gladiatorum'**
- **HSV Eczema**
- **HSV (Herpes simplex virus)** on the digits of health care workers **'Herpetic whitlow'**
- **'Impetigo contagiosa'** is caused by **Strep Pyogenes**
- **'Bullous impetigo'** is due to S aureus
- **'Swimmer's itch'** in skin surface is exposed to water infested with freshwater avian **schistosomes.**
- '**Bacillary angiomatosis'** by **Bartonella henselae.**
- **'Verruca peruana'** is caused by **Bartonella bacilliformis**
- **Human papillomavirus** may cause singular warts **'verruca vulgaris'**
- **Human papillomavirus** with warts in the anogenital area **'condylomata acuminata'**
- **Mycobacterium leprae** may be associated with cutaneous ulcerations in patients with lepromatous leprosy related to **'Lucio's phenomenon'**
- **'Erysipelas** is due to **Strep Pyogenes**
- **'Cellulitis'** may be caused by indigenous flora colonizing the skin and appendages by **S aureus and S pyogenes**
- **'Necrotizing fasciitis'**, formerly called streptococcal gangrene, may be associated with **group A Streptococcus or mixed aerobic-anaerobic bacteria** or may occur as part of gas gangrene caused by Clostridium perfringens.

USMLE Case Scenario

An infant presents with a superficial cellulitis of the skin with marked lymphatic involvement, caused by beta-hemolytic group A streptococci beginning with an area of redness and enlarges to form the typical tense, painful, bright red, shiny, brawny infiltrated plaque with a well demarcated, distinct, and slightly raised border. Most likely the diagnosis is:

1. Botromycosis
2. Gangrene
3. Rodent ulcer
4. Varicose ulcer
5. SSSS
6. Erysipelas

Ans. 6. Erysipelas

Impetigo Contagiosa

A **staphylococcal, streptococcal, or combined infection** characterized by discrete, thin-walled vesicles that rapidly become pustular and then rupture. Impetigo occurs more frequently on the exposed parts of the body-the face, hands, neck, and extremities-although it may appear at sites of friction as well. Over 50% of cases are due to ***Staphylococcus aureus*, with the remainder being due to *Streptococcus pyogenes* or acombination of the two bacteria**. Group B streptococci are associated with newborn impetigo. Impetigo is most commonly seen in early childhood and during hot, humid summers in temperate climates.

Erysipelas

A **superficial cellulitis of the skin with marked lymphatic involvement**, caused by **beta-hemolytic group A streptococci**. Erysipelas most commonly occurs in infants, very young children, and the elderly. In most cases, the organism gains access by direct inoculation through a break in the skin, but infrequently, hematogenous infection may occur. It begins with an area of redness and enlarges to form the typical tense, painful, bright red, shiny, brawny infiltrated plaque with a well demarcated, distinct, and slightly raised border (as opposed to deepercellulitis, which has no distinct border and is flush with surrounding skin).

Bartonella Henselae

It is the pathogen of **cat-scratch disease**, which is a very common cause of chronic **lymphadenitis in children**. It typically presents as an enlarging nontender lymph node, often located in the cervical, axillary, or inguinal regions. After being scratched by a kitten, a papule develops at the scratch site. Affected lymph nodes draining the involved area become enlarged in 2 weeks. Other symptoms include low-grade fever, malaise, fatigue and nonspecific body aches. The diagnosis of cat-scratch disease is best made by a serological test, such as an indirect fluorescence antibody test for antibodies to *B henselae*. Usually, treatment is necessary only in severe systemic infection.

Collodion baby: Babies are borne with shiny, transparent membrane which peels off after a week or so, the peel looking like collodion

Harlequin fetus: Child is borne encased in a thick, abnormal fissured hyperkeratotic skin, abnormality of keratin synthesis

Café au lait spots:

- **Smooth** (Coast of California): Neourofibromatosis
- **Irregular** (Coast of Maine): Mc Cune Albright Syndrome

Cutaneous Manifestations of Medically Important Diseases

- **Tuberous sclerosis:** The earliest cutaneous sign is an **ash leaf spot** plus **adenoma sebaceum** (multiple angiofibromas of the face), **ungual and gingival fibromas**, fibrous plaques of the forehead, and connective tissue nevi **(shagreen patches)**
- **Sarcoidosis: Lupus pernio** is a particular type of sarcoidosis that involves the tip of the **nose and the earlobes**, with lesions that are violaceous in color rather than red-brown
- **Osler-Rendu-Weber disease:** In **Hereditary Hemorrhagic Telangiectasia:** The lesions (Telengeiectasis) usually appear during adulthood and are most commonly seen on the mucous membranes, face, and distal extremities, including under the nails
- **Antiphospholipid syndrome: Livideo reticularis:** The majority of cases are secondary to venous hypertension, and disorders of hypercoagulability, e.g. the antiphospholipid syndrome
- **Disseminated gonococcal infection:** (**Arthritis-dermatitis syndrome**), a small number of **papules and vesicopustules with central purpura** or hemorrhagic necrosis are found over the joints of the distal extremities. Additional symptoms include arthralgias, tenosynovitis, and fever
- **Urticaria pigmentosa**: A generalized distribution of red-brown macules and papules is seen in the form of mastocytosis known as **urticaria pigmentosa** Each lesion represents a collection of **mast cells in the dermis**, with hyperpigmentation of the overlying epidermis. Stimuli such as rubbing cause these mast cells to degranulate, and this leads to the formation of localized urticaria **(Darier's sign)**
- ***Amyloidosis*:** The cutaneous lesions associated with primary systemic amyloidosis are **pink in color** and translucent. As a result, petechiae and purpura develop in clinically normal skin as well as in lesional skin following minor trauma, hence the term '**pinch purpura.**' Amyloid deposits are also seen in the striated muscle of the tongue and result in macroglossia. (Pinch purpura is diagnostic of **primary systemic amyloidosis**)
- **Sweet's syndrome** is characterized by red to **red-brown plaques** and **nodules** that are frequently painful and occur primarily on the head, neck, and upper extremities. The patients also **have fever, neutrophilia, and a dense dermal infiltrate of neutrophils in the lesions**
- **Fabry's disease: Multiple angiokeratomas** are seen in Fabry's disease, an X-linked recessive lysosomal storage disease that is due to a deficiency of galactosidase A. The lesions are red to red-blue in color and can be quite small in size (1 to 3 mm), with the most common location being the lower trunk.

USMLE Case Scenario

A 6-year-old male is brought to the pediatric unit with a recent onset of a rash, urticaria, and a fever of 102 degrees F. Physical examination reveals mild lymphadenopathy. The patient's past medical history is unremarkable except that he just finished a 6 day course of cefaclor suspension for treatment of URTI. The patient most likely has: Serum sickness

Serum Sickness

It is a condition commonly caused by hypersensitivity to drugs. It is suggested that the drug acts as a hapten, which binds to plasma proteins. This drug-protein complex is recognized as being foreign to the body and induces the serum sickness. Common signs and symptoms of serum sickness include fever, cutaneous eruptions (morbilliform and/or urticarial), lymphadenopathy, and arthralgias. Erythema multiforme may also appear in severe cases. With respect to cefaclor, the incidence of serum sickness is much higher infants and children than in adults.

Erythema Multiforme

It is a reaction pattern that clinically manifests with 'target' lesions on the palms and soles in milder cases, whereas more severe forms have mucosal blisters and a widespread vesicular/bullous skin eruption. 'Target' lesions are characteristic for erythema multiforme and consist of a dusky red center with or without a central vesicle surrounded by an erythematous halo. Erythema multiforme is most commonly seen after herpes simplex infection, streptococcal pharyngitis, or Mycoplasma pneumonia.

USMLE Case Scenario

A 33-year-old female working as a secretary abruptly develops an intensely itchy rash. Physical examination demonstrates multiple erythematous patches of the distal arms and legs. Some of the patches show central clearing with surrounding erythematous rings. Which of the following is the most likely diagnosis?

1. Erythema nodosum
2. Erythema chronicum migrans
3. Erythema migrans chronicum
4. Erythema multiforme

Ans. 4. Erythema multiforme

Typical Lesions: Never FORGET

Lichen Planus

- Papule
- Plain topped
- Polygonal
- Purple
- Papules
- Wickhams Straie
- Civatte Bodies
- Pterygium of Nails
- Hepatitis C association

Atopic dermatitis:

- White Dermographism
- Dennie Morgan Folds
- Hertoghes sign
- Cataract and Keratoconus

Dermatomyositis:

- Helitrope rash
- Gottrons papules
- Poikiloderma
- Dowlings lines

Ptyriasis Rosea:

- Herald Patch
- Christmas tree pattern
- **Annular collaratte of scales**
- **Mother patch**
- **Self limiting**

Mycosis Fungoides/Cutaneous T cell Lymphoma:

- Sezary Lutner cells
- Pautrier Microabscesses

Tuberous sclerosis:
- Ash leaf spot
- Adenoma sebaceum
- Shagreen patches
- **Infantile spasms**
- **Delayed milestones**

USMLE Case Scenario

The characteristic Nail finding in lichen planus is:
1. Pitting
2. Pterygium
3. Beau's lines
4. Hyperpigmentation of the Nails

Ans.2. Pterygium

Nummular Dermatitis

It is a chronic inflammation of the skin, the etiology of which is still unknown. **'coin-shaped'** or **'discoid'** are seen. Microscopically, the dominant feature is a **localized spongiosis** (corresponding to edema) of the epidermis, which may also contain minute fluid-filled holes that correspond to the tiny vesicles seen clinically in early lesions. Treatment of these patients is problematic, and numerous regimens involving corticosteroids or antibiotics have been recommended, each of which appears to work with some but not all patients.

Diabetic Ulcers

A 76-year-old man has had an indolent, nonhealing ulcer at the heel of the right foot for several weeks. The patient began wearing a new pair of shoes shortly before the ulcer started and noticed a blister as the first anomaly at the site where the ulcer eventually developed. The ulcer is painless, 3.5 cm in diameter, the ulcer base looks dirty, and no granulation tissue. The skin around the ulcer looks normal. The patient has no sensation to pin prick anywhere in that foot. Peripheral pulses are weak but palpable. He is obese and has varicose veins, high cholesterol, and poorly controlled type 2 diabetes mellitus. It is an example of diabetic ulcer.

Diabetic ulcers typically develop at pressure points, and the heel is a favorite location. The patient has evidence of neuropathy, and the correlation with the trauma inflicted by the new shoes is classic.

Hypomelanosis

The differential diagnosis of localized hypomelanosis includes the following primary cutaneous disorders:
- **Idiopathic guttate hypomelanosis**
- **Postinflammatory hypopigmentation**
- **Tinea (pityriasis) versicolor**
- **Vitiligo**
- **Chemical leukoderma**
- **Nevus depigmentosus**
- **Piebaldism**

Disorders of Hyperpigmentation

- **Seborrheic keratoses** are common lesions, but in one clinical setting they are a sign of systemic disease, and that setting is the sudden appearance of multiple lesions, often with an inflammatory base and in association with **acrochordons (skin tags)** and **acanthosis nigricans.** This is termed the **sign of Leser-Trelat** and signifies **an internal malignancy**
- **Acanthosis nigricans** can also be a reflection of an internal malignancy, most commonly of the gastrointestinal tract, and it appears as velvety hyperpigmentation, primarily in flexural areas. In the majority of patients, acanthosis nigricans is associated with obesity, but it may be a reflection of an **endocrinopathy such as acromegaly, Cushing's syndrome, the Stein-Leventhal syndrome, or insulin-resistant diabetes mellitus (type A, type B, and lipoatrophic forms).**

- A proliferation of **melanocytes** results in the following pigmented lesions: **Lentigo, melanocytic nevus, and melanoma**
- **LEOPARD Syndrome:** Lentigines; ECG abnormalities, ocular hypertelorism; pulmonary stenosis and subaortic valvular stenosis; abnormal genitalia (cryptorchidism, hypospadias); retardation of growth; and deafness (sensorineural) syndromes
- The lentigines in patients with **Peutz-Jeghers syndrome** are located primarily around the nose and mouth, on the hands and feet, and within the oral cavity. While the pigmented macules on the face may fade with age, the oral lesions persist
- Lentigines are also seen in association with **cardiac myxomas** and have been described in two syndromes whose findings overlap
- **LAMB (lentigines, atrial myxomas, mucocutaneous myxomas, and blue nevi) syndrome and NAME [nevus, atrial myxoma, myxoid neurofibroma and ephelides (freckles)] syndrome**
- The third type of localized hyperpigmentation is due to a local increase in pigment production, and it includes **ephelides and cafe au lait macules (CALM).** The latter are most commonly associated with two disorders, neurofibromatosis (NF) and McCune-Albright syndrome.
- Localized hyperpigmentation is seen as a side effect of several other systemic medications, including those that produce fixed drug reactions **[phenolphthalein, nonsteroidal anti-inflammatory drugs (NSAIDs), sulfonamides, and barbiturates]** and those that can complex with melanin (antimalarials). **Chloroquine and hydroxychloroquine**
- **Estrogen** in oral contraceptives can induce melasma, symmetric brown patches on the face, especially the cheeks, upper lip, and forehead
- The endocrinopathies that frequently have associated hyperpigmentation include **Addison's disease, Nelson syndrome, and ectopic ACTH syndrome**
- The metabolic causes of hyperpigmentation include **porphyria cutanea tarda (PCT), hemochromatosis, vitamin B12 deficiency, folic acid deficiency, pellagra, malabsorption, and Whipple's disease**
- Of the autoimmune diseases associated with diffuse hyperpigmentation, **biliary cirrhosis and scleroderma** (**Calcinosis cutis)**
- Actual deposits of a particular drug or metal in the skin are seen with **silver (argyria),** where the skin appears blue-gray in color; **gold (chrysiasis),** where the skin has a brown to blue-gray color.

NEWER CONCEPTS

Subcorneal Pustular Dermatosis

- Subcorneal pustular dermatosis is a **rare, benign, chronic, relapsing sterile pustular eruption** involving the flexural aspect of trunk and proximal extremities
- **Palmar, plantar and facial forms** of disease are **rare**
- It commonly affects **females**
- It is a disease of **elderly**
- **IgA** has been found to be associated with this condition
- It is associated with:
  - Paraproteinemias
  - Inflammatory bowel diseases
  - SLE
  - Rheumatoid arthritis
  - Lymphoproliferative disorders
- **'Half- Half blister'** is the **classic lesion** in which purulent fluid accumulates in the lower half of the blister
- **Dapsone is most effective** in the treatment of this disorder and **the 'treatment of choice'.**

Barthelemy's Disease or Acne Scrofulosum

- No need to confuse it with **Acne Vulgaris**
- It is a **Cutaneous form** of TB
- Features are Papulonecrotic lesions of face **(acinitis)** trunk, and hand
- Initially colorless, later bluish, suppuration, pustules, crusting excoriation
- They are transient but recur

Reiter's Syndrome

Mucocutaneous lesions: Small, painless superficial ulcers are commonly seen on the oral mucosa, tongue, and glans penis **(balanitis circinata)**.

Patients may also develop hyperkeratotic skin lesions of the palms and soles and around the nails **(keratoderma blennorrhagica)**
Cardiovascular involvement with **aortitis, aortic insufficiency, and conduction defects** occurs rarely.

PUVA Therapy

Methoxsalen is a **psoralen derivative** with **photosensitizing activity**. Exact mechanism of erythemogenic, melanogenic, and cytotoxic response in the epidermis is unknown, involves **increased tyrosinase activity** in melanin-producing cells, as well as **inhibition of DNA synthesis, cell division, and epidermal turnover.** Successful pigmentation requires the presence of functioning melanocytes. Used in treatment of:

- **Mycosis fungoides**: Photopheresis, using methoxsalen with ultraviolet radiation of white blood cells, is indicated for use with the UVAR System in the palliative treatment of the skin manifestations of mycosis fungoides (also known as cutaneous T-cell lymphoma) in persons who have not been responsive to other forms of treatment
- **Psoriasis**: Indicated in the treatment of severe, refractory, disabling psoriasis that has not responded to other **therapy**
- **Vitiligo** is indicated for repigmentation in the treatment of vitiligo
- **Lichen Planus**

Isotretinoin and Pregnancy

Pregnancy: **Isotretinoin is teratogenic in humans and is contraindicated during pregnancy**
Although not every fetus exposed to **isotretinoin** has been affected, **the risk is high that an infant will have a deformity or abnormality if the pregnancy occurred while the mother was taking isotretinoin, even for a short period of time**
Major human fetal deformities or abnormalities associated with the use of **isotretinoin** include:

- **Central nervous system (CNS) abnormalities, including hydrocephalus, microcephaly, and cranial nerve deficit;**
- **Eye abnormalities, including microphthalmia;**
- **Heart defects;**
- **Parathyroid deficiency;**
- **Skeletal or connective tissue abnormalities**, including absence of terminal phalanges, alterations of the skull and cervical vertebra, and malformations of hip, ankle, and forearm; facial dysmorphia; cleft or high palate; low-set ears, micropinna, and small or absent external auditory canals; meningomyelocele; multiple synostoses; and syndactyly; and
- **Thymus gland abnormality.**

Drugs Causing:

Toxic epidermal necrolysis	Photodermatitis	Hyperpigmentation	Steven Johnson Syndrome
Barbiturates	Sulfonamides	Phenolphthalein, (NSAIDs),	Barbiturates
Phenytoin	OCP	Sulfonamides and Barbiturates	Phenytoin
Phenylbutazone	Tetracyclines	Chloroquine Hydroxychloroquine	Phenylbutazone
Pencillins	Phenothiazines		Pencillins
Sulfonamides	Thiazides		Sulfonamides
NSAIDS	Furosemide		
Allopurinol	Griseofulvin		
	Sulfonylureas		

Dermatological Signs

Frequently asked Dermatological signs

- **Asboe Hansen Sign** (Bulla Spread Sign): **Pemphigus**
- **Carpet Tack sign**: **DLE**

- **Cerebiform Tongue sign**: Pemphigus Vegitans
- **Coup D Lounge sign**: Tinea Versicolor
- **Crowe sign: Axillary freckling in Neurofibromatosis**
- **Fitzpatrick sign**: Dermatofibrosarcoma Protuberans
- **Dubios sign**: **Congenital syphilis**
- **Hertoghes sign**: Loss of lateral 1/3 of eyebrow in **Atopic Dermatitis**
- **Leser Trelat sign**: Appearance of large number of **Seborrheic keratoses**
- **Ollendroff sign**: Tender papule in **Secondary syphilis**
- **Pillow sign**: Patient sees hair on pillow on getting up at morning. **(ALOPECIA)**
- **Shawl sign**: Erythema overback and shoulders in **Dermatomyositis**

Causative organisms of STD (Sexually Transmitted Diseases)

• **Donovaniosis**	• Calymmatobacter granulomatosis
• **LGV (esthiomine)**	• Chlamydia trachomatis
• **Chancroid**	• H ducreyi, Herpes hominis
• **Condyloma acuminate**	• HPV 6, 11, 16, 18
• **Yaws**	• T pertune
• **Pinta**	• T caratenum

Different Types of Erythema

- **Erythema chronicum migrans. Lymes Disease**
- **Erythema Ab Agne**: Reticulate pigmentation due to long-term heat exposure
- **Erythema Gyratum Repens**: Internal malignancies
- **Erythema Nodosum**: Multisystemic disorders, e.g. sarcoidosis
- **Erythema multiforme**: Mucosal involvement with viral, bacterial, rickettsial diseases with target lesions
- **Erythema Induratum**: Bazins Disease
- **Erythema elevatum diutinum** (EED) chronic leukocytoclastic vasculitis, also presents with papules that are red-brown in color. The papules coalesce into plaques on the extensor surfaces of knees, elbows, and the small joints of the hand. Flares of EED have been associated with streptococcal infections.

Different types of Lupus

- **Lupus Vulgaris**: Cutaneous form of **Tuberculosis**
- **Lupus Pernio**: Indurated, shiny, swollen lesions seen in **sarcoidosis**
- **Lupus Profundus**: Lymphocytic infiltration of subcutaneous fat in **DLE.**

Steroids

Low potency steroids	• **Hydrocortisone** • **Betamethasone valerate** • **Clobetasol 17 butyrate**
Medium potency	• **Flucinonide** • **Triamcinolone acetonide 1**
High potency	• **Betamethasone dipropionate** • **Halcinonide** • **Triamiclinolone acetonide**
Highest potency	• **Clobetasol 17 propionate**

Topical steroids are most potent in ointment form.

Different Types of Scales

• **Silvery scales**	**Psoriasis**
• **Cigarette scales**	**Pityriasis Rosacea**
• **Fish scales**	**Ichthyoris**
• **Sand paper**	**Solar keratosis**
• **Yellow greasy scales**	**Seborrheic dermatitis**
• **Furfareous scales**	**Tinea versicolor**
• **Limpet scaling**	**Rieter's disease**

Eponyms

- **'Micro Munro' abscesses**: Degenerated polymorphonuclear leucocytes in horny layer **(stratum corneum)** seen in **Psoriasis**
- **Spongiform Pustules of Kagoj**: Pustules of flattened keratinocytes. Seen in **Psoriasis**
- **Pautrier Microabscesses:** Atypical mononuclear cell collection in epidermis in **Mycosis Fungoides**
- **Grenz Zone**: **Area of uninvolved dermis** between epidermis and dermis in inflammatory neoplastic conditions
- **Max Joseph space** is a feature of **Lichen Planus**

Nails in Dermatology

Important Points about nails

- **Half and half nails**: White proximally, pink distally. Seen in **CRF**
- **Terrys nails**: White nails with pink tip, seen in **cirrhosis**
- **Blue nails**: Chloroquine, Wilsons disease
- **Mees lines: Arsenic poisoning**
- **Onchyolysis: Psoriasis**
- **Koilonychia: Iron deficiency anemia**
- **Yellow nail syndrome**: Seen with pleural effusions, edema
- **Nail Patella Syndrome**: Hypoplastic nails and patella.
- **Muehrcke's nails**: Associated with **hypoalbumenia**
- **Koenens periungal fibroma: tuberous sclerosis**

USMLE Case Scenario

A 87-year-old man is undergoing a general physical examination. The patient was admitted recently with the diagnoses of 'failure to thrive' He has multiple chronic medical conditions, including a history of stroke, coronary artery disease, diabetes, hypertension, hyperlipidemia, and hepatitis C-related cirrhosis. While demonstrating a thorough physical examination, the attending physician points out that the patient's finger nails appear abnormal. The proximal nail beds appear white and pale but have a distal band that is darker and pink. It is an example of:

Terry Nails

Have a **nail bed that is white or light pink** with a distal band measuring 0.5 to 3.0 mm that is pink to brown in color

- This finding is associated with **advancing age and a variety of medical conditions, including type 2 diabetes mellitus, congestive heart failure, chronic renal failure, and cirrhosis**
- In young patients, this finding should prompt one to think of serious underlying pathology
- In elderly patients, the finding is usually incidental.

IMPORTANT DERMATOLOGICAL TESTS

KOH Preparation

A potassium hydroxide (KOH) preparation is performed on scaling skin lesions when a **fungal etiology** is suspected. When the preparation is viewed under the microscope, the **refractile hyphae** will be seen more easily when the light intensity is reduced. This technique can be utilized to:

- **Identify 'hyphae' in dermatophyte infections,**
- **'Pseudohyphae' and 'budding yeast' in Candida infections,**
- **'Fragmented hyphae and spores' in tinea versicolor.**

Diascopy

Diascopy is designed to assess whether a skin lesion will blanch with pressure as, for example, in determining whether a red lesion is hemorrhagic or simply blood-filled. A **hemangioma will blanch with pressure**, whereas a **purpuric lesion caused by necrotizing vasculitis will not**

Diascopy is performed by pressing a microscope slide or magnifying lens against a specified lesion and noting the amount of blanching that occurs. Granulomas often have an **'apple jelly'** appearance on diascopy.

Wood's Light

A Wood's lamp generates **360-nm ultraviolet (or 'black') light** that can be used to aid the evaluation of certain skin disorders

Wood's lamp filter is made of **nickel and silica**

Wood's lamp will **cause erythrasma** (a superficial, intertriginous infection caused by Corynebacterium minutissimum) to show a characteristic **coral red color**

Wounds colonized by Pseudomonas to appear pale blue

Tinea capitis caused by certain dermatophytes such as Microsporum canis or M audouinii exhibits a yellow fluorescence

Pigmented lesions of the epidermis such as freckles are accentuated, **dermal pigment** such as postinflammatory hyperpigmentation fades under a Wood's light

Vitiligo appears totally white under a Wood's lamp, and previously unsuspected areas of involvement often become apparent

A Wood's lamp may also aid in the demonstration of **tinea versicolor** and in recognition of **ash leaf spots** in patients with tuberous sclerosis.

USMLE Case Scenario

A 24-year-old man from Chicag had multiple, small hypopigmented macules on the upper chest and back for the last three months. The macules were circular, arranged around follicles and many had coalesced to form large sheets. The surface of the macules showed fine scaling. He had similar lesions one year ago which subsided with treatment. The most appropriate investigation to confirm the diagnosis is:

1. Potassium hydroxide preparation of scales
2. Slit skin smear from discrete macules
3. Tzanck test
4. Skin biopsy of coalesced macules

Ans. 1. Potassium hydroxide preparation of scales

USMLE Case Scenario

A 62-year-old female with severe bronchial asthma presents with white patches on the inside of the cheeks that can be easily wiped off, leaving a red, bleeding, sore surface. He is currently using beclomethasone and albuterol inhalers for his Asthma: The patient most likely has: Oral candidiasis

Candidiasis may be divided into the following types

- **Oral candidiasis**
- **Perlèche (around mouth)**

- **Candidal vulvovaginitis**
- **Candidal intertrigo**
- **Diaper candidiasis**
- **Perianal candidiasis**
- **Candidal paronychia**
- **Erosio interdigitalis blastomycetica**
- **Chronic mucocutaneous candidiasis**
- **Systemic candidiasis**

Cutaneous Manifestations of SLE

- The **malar ('butterfly') rash** is a photosensitive, fixed erythematous rash, flat or raised, over the cheeks and bridge of the nose, often involving the chin and ears
- **Scarring is absent**; telangiectases may develop
- A more diffuse maculopapular rash, predominant in sun-exposed areas, is also common and usually indicates disease flare
- **Loss of scalp hair** is usually patchy but can be extensive
- Patients with SLE can develop vasculitic skin lesions. These include purpura, subcutaneous nodules, nail fold infarcts, ulcers, vasculitic urticaria, panniculitis and gangrene of digits. Shallow, slightly painful ulcers in the mouth and nose are frequent in patients with SLE
- **Steroids are used in pregnancy for erythematous rashes.**

Tuberculosis of Skin

Lupus vulgaris:

- It is skin TB with **no underlying active focus**
- **MC type of cutaneous TB**
- Form of cutaneous TB common in children and young adults
- Feature **is indurated plaque, annular in shape**
- Heals with scarring Blanching with glass slide (diascopy) reveals grey or green foci (**Apple jelly nodules**)

Scrofulodema:

It is skin TB **secondary** to involvement of underlying structure, e.g. joint, lymph node

Tuberculosis Verrucosa cutis

TB bacillus here is **inoculated into skin** and seen in TB patient, Pathologists, Veterinary surgeons

It is a form of post primary tuberculosis with good resistance

Tuberculosis cutis orifacialis

TB of orifices as **oral cavity, anal canal, urogenital tract**. Other lesions noted are:

- **Acne agminata**
- **Erythema induratum**
- **Erythema nodosum**
- **Rosea like lesions**

- **Tuberculids** is **hypersensitivity reaction to Mycobacterium. Tuberculosis** where evidence of etiology is not definite but shows tubercular granuloma in histology and positive response to antitubercular treatment. Seen in
- **Lichen scrofulosorum**
- **Erythema nodosum**

Dermatological Diseases Caused by Staph Aureus Causes

- **SSSS** (Staphyloccocal scalded skin syndrome)
- **Reiter's disease** (SSSS in newborn)
- **Lyell's disease or TEN** (SSSS in older children)
- **Bullous Impetigo/Impetigo contagiosa**
- **Osteomyelitis**
- **Carbuncles**
- **Furuncles or Boils**
- **Sycosis barbae and Sycosis Nuchae** (Nuchal region)

Basic Terms in Dermatological Pathology

- **Hyperkeratosis:** Hyperplasia of the stratum corneum, often associated with a qualitative abnormality of the keratin Parakeratosis: Mode(s) of keratinization characterized by retention of the nuclei in the stratum corneum; on mucosal membranes, parakeratosis is normal
- **Acanthosis:** Epidermal hyperplasia preferentially involving the stratum spinosum
- **Dyskeratosis:** Abnormal keratinization occurring prematurely within individual cells or groups of cells below the stratum granulosum
- **Acantholysis**: Loss of intercellular connections resulting in lack of cohesion between keratinocytes
- **Papillomatosis:** Hyperplasia of the papillary dermis with elongation and/or widening of the dermal papillae
- **Lentiginous:** Refers to a linear pattern of melanocyte proliferation within the epidermal basal cell layer; lentiginous melanocytic hyperplasia can occur as a reactive change or as part of a neoplasm of melanocytes
- **Spongiosis**: Intercellular edema of the epidermis.

Remember: (Disease Associations)

• **Casals necklace**	Pellagra
• **Iris pearls**	Leprosy
• **Liver spots**	Senility
• **Crocodile skin**	Icthyosis
• **Caynee pepper stippling**	Plasma cell balanitis of Zoon
• **Calcinosis cutis**	Scleroderma
• **Berloque dermatitis**	**Cosmetics**

Repeated NAMES

- Candida albicans — **Yeast like fungi**
- Histoplasma capsulatum — **Darling's disease**
- Aspergillus — **Fungus ball disease**
- Coccoides immitis — **Desert rheumatism**

- Obstruction of **pilosebaceous gland** leads to: Acne vulgaris
- Obstruction of **sweat gland** leads to: Crystalline miliaria
- Obstruction of **Apocrine gland** leads to: Fox Fordyce disease
- Obstruction of **hair root** leads to: Furuncle

USMLE Case Scenario

A 30-year-old man, presented with subcutaneous itchy nodules over the left iliac crest. On examination they are firm, non-tender and mobile. Skin scrapping contains microfilaria and adults worms. Most likely cause is:

1. A duodenale
2. H nana
3. Onchocerca volvulus
4. Tinea
5. Trichomonas
6. Gardenella

Ans. 3. Onchocerca volvulus

USMLE Case Scenario

An adult presents with oval scaly hypopigmented macule over the chest and the back. The diagnosis is:

1. Atopic Eczema
2. Lichen planus
3. Acne
4. Psoriasis
5. Pemphigus
6. Tinea corporis
7. Tinea cruris
8. Pityriasis versicolor

Ans. 8. Pityriasis versicolor

USMLE Case Scenario

A patient presents with scarring Alopecia, thinned nails, hypopigmented macular lesions over trunk and oral mucosa. The diagnosis is:

1. Oral submucosal fibrosis
2. Actinic keratosis
3. Cholinergic urticaria
4. Atopic Eczema
5. Lichen planus
6. Acne
7. Psoriasis
8. Pemphigus
9. Pityriasis versicolor
10. Scabies

Ans. 5. Lichen Planus

USMLE Case Scenario

A child has multiple itchy papular lesions on the genitalia and fingers. Similar lesions are also seen in younger brother. Most possible diagnosis is:

1. Atopic Eczema
2. Lichen planus
3. Acne
4. Psoriasis
5. Pemphigus
6. Pityriasis versicolor
7. Scabies

Ans. 7. Scabies

USMLE Case Scenario

A 27-year-old male had burning micturition and urethral discharge. After 4 weeks he developed joint pains involving both the knees and ankles, redness of the eye and skin lesion. The most probable clinical diagnosis is:

1. Vogt Harada Syndrome
2. Caplan's Syndrome
3. Felty's Syndrome
4. Sjögren's Syndrome
5. Reiter's Syndrome
6. Behçet's Syndrome

Ans. 5. Reiter's Syndrome

USMLE Case Scenario

A child with fever presents with multiple tender erythematous skin lesions. On microscopic examination the skin lesions are seen to have neutrophilic and histiocytic infiltration in the dermis. The diagnosis is:

1. Sweet's syndrome
2. Erythema nodosum
3. Erythema chronicum migrans
4. Cystic fibrosis
5. Lichen planus
6. Erythema migrans chronicum
7. Acne Rosacea
8. Erythema multiforme

Ans.1. Sweet's Syndrome

USMLE Case Scenario

A 45-year-old abruptly develops an intensely itchy rash. Physical examination demonstrates multiple erythematous patches of the distal arms and legs. Some of the patches show central clearing with surrounding erythematous rings. Which of the following is the most likely diagnosis?

1. Erythema nodosum
2. Erythema chronicum migrans
3. Erythema migrans chronicum
4. Erythema multiforme

Ans. 4. Erythema multiforme

USMLE Case Scenario

A 36-year-old mother of two children in Washington presented with a generalized, blistering rash of 4 weeks' duration with her trunk mainly affected. On fine examination, there was extensive blistering and large areas of denuded skin. Ulcers were also present in her mouth. Direct immunofluorescent examination of a biopsy of normal skin taken from a site adjacent to one bulla showed deposition of IgG around the keratinocytes. Most likely diagnosis is:

1. Pemphigoid
2. Lichen planus
3. Tinea versicolor
4. Psoriasis
5. Pemphigus
6. Hailey-Hailey disease

Ans. 5. Pemphigus

USMLE Case Scenario

A 15-year-old boy, presented with a 6 month history of recurrent episodes of swelling of his lips, eyes and tongue. The swellings came on suddenly, grew over a period of 15 to 25 min, and lasted from 10 to 48 hours. Urticaria was absent. Hereditary angioedema is diagnosed. Blood samples taken for complement analysis would show:

1. Both the C3 concentration and C4 level extremely elevated
2. The C3 concentration decreased but the C4 level extremely elevated
3. The C3 concentration and the C4 level normal
4. The C3 concentration unchanged but the C4 level was extremely low

Ans. 4. The C3 concentration unchanged but the C4 level was extremely low

USMLE Case Scenario

A 42-year-old female presents to New York Central Hospital with painful oral ulcers. Physical examination demonstrates widespread erosions of her mucous membranes. Dermatological examination reveals a friable mucosa. Biopsy of perilesional mucosa demonstrates acantholysis; direct immunofluorescence demonstrates an intraepidermal band of IgG and C3. The most likely diagnosis is:

1. Bullous pemphigoid
2. Dermatitis herpetiformis
3. Herpes simplex I
4. Pemphigus vulgaris

Ans. 4. Pemphigus vulgaris

USMLE Case Scenario

Cells similar to fibroblasts are seen growing in a storiform ('pinwheel') pattern. This pattern of cells is characteristic of:

1. Leiomyosarcoma
2. Basal cell carcinoma
3. Keratocanthoma
4. Dermatofibrosarcoma

Ans. 4. Dermatofibrosarcoma

USMLE Case Scenario

A 44-year-old male presents to the dermatologist with pain in the joints along with silvery, scaling plaques on his elbows and knees. The most likely diagnosis is:

1. Acne vulgaris
2. Pemphigus vulgaris
3. Psoriasis vulgaris
4. Pemphigoid

Ans. 3. Psoriasis vulgaris

USMLE Case Scenario

Wickham's striae is seen in:

1. Lichen nitidus
2. Psoriasis
3. Pityriasis rosea
4. Lichen planus
5. Psoriasis
6. SSSS

Ans. 4. Lichen planus

USMLE Case Scenario

A pathologist from Mexico reports the presence of koilocytes in a cervical biopsy from a 22-year-old woman. Which of the following conditions does this patient most likely have?

1. Chlamydia infection
2. Gonococcal infection
3. Herpes simplex virus infection
4. Human papillomavirus infection

Ans. 4. Human papillomavirus infection

USMLE Case Scenario

A 24-year-old man had multiple, small hypopigmented macules on the upper chest and back for the last three months. The macules were circular, arranged around follicles and many had coalesced to form large sheets. The surface of the macules showed fine scaling. He had similar lesions one year ago which subsided with treatment. The most appropriate investigation to confirm the diagnosis is:

1. Potassium hydroxide preparation of scales
2. Slit skin smear from discrete macules
3. Tzanck test
4. Skin biopsy of coalesced macules

Ans. 1. Potassium hydroxide preparation of scales

USMLE Case Scenario

A 88-year-old man on steroids for last 5 years comes to the physician because of a 5-day history of right-sided chest pain. He denies any shortness of breath. Physical examination shows a unilateral, erythematous, maculopapular rash extending from the anterior chest wall around to the back along the sixth intercostal spaces. Most likely presentation would resemble:

1. Dome-shaped papules with central umbilication
2. Expanding annular lesion without central clearing
3. Expanding annular lesion with central clearing
4. Denuded skin all over
5. 'Slapped-cheek' appearance and a lacy reticular rash
6. Vesicles at various stages of evolution

Ans. 6. Vesicles at various stages of evolution

This patient has herpes zoster, which is a reactivation of the Varicella-Zoster Virus (VZV) that was dormant in the dorsal root ganglion.

USMLE Case Scenario

Patch test is done to document:

1. Type I hypersensitivity
2. Delayed type hypersensitivity
3. Autoimmune disease
4. Immunocomplex deposition

Ans. 2. Delayed type hypersensitivity

USMLE Case Scenario

Which of the following shows deposition of IgA in dermal papilla?

1. Dermatitis herpetiformis
2. IgA papillomatosis of childhood
3. Bullous pemphigoid
4. Gestational herpes

Ans. 1. Dermatitis herpetiformis

USMLE Case Scenario

Intraepidermal IgG deposition is seen in:
1. Pemphigus
2. Bullous pemphigoid
3. Herpes genitalis
4. Psoriasis

Ans. 1. Pemphigus

USMLE Case Scenario

A 25-year-old person suffers from B27 associated reactive arthritis, urethritis and conjunctivitis. Which is most likely organism involved in this case?
1. Borrelia burgdorferi
2. Ureaplasma urealyticum
3. Betahemolytic streptococci
4. Streptococcus bovis

Ans. 2. Ureaplasma urealyticum

USMLE Case Scenario

A 35-year-old man presented with decreasing vision and painful swollen knees. He had a six year history of relapsing and remitting mouth ulcers and frequent episodes of genital ulceration. On examination he had retinal vasculitis, few mouth ulcers and synovitis in both knees. Investigations show a raised erythrocyte sedimentation rate at 99 mm/h but a normal blood count and negative tests for rheumatoid factor, antinuclear antibodies, cytomegalovirus and HIV infection. A clinical diagnosis suggests:
1. Reiters syndrome
2. Ankylosing spondylitis
3. Psoriatic arthritis
4. Pseudogout
5. CPPD deposition disease
6. Polymyalgia
7. Behçet's syndrome

Ans. 7. Behçet's syndrome

USMLE Case Scenario

A 34-year-old woman after presented to a medical practitioner with a three and a half-week history of an acute rash which started beneath her watch. Two weeks later, a further patch appeared at the umbilicus. She had previously noted that she could not wear cheap earrings without triggering a rash on her ear lobes. There was no past medical history of note and no personal or family history of atopy. On examination, two patches of dermatitis were seen over the presenting areas. The appearances are suggestive of:
1. Atopic dermatitis
2. Urticaria
3. Angioedema
4. Nonspecific dermatitis
5. Photosensitivity
6. Hay fever
7. Contact dermatitis
8. Idiosyncrasy

Ans. 7. Contact dermatitis

USMLE Case Scenario

Herald patch is seen in:

1. Pityriasis vesicolor
2. Pityriasis alba
3. Pityriasis rosea
4. Pityriasis rubra pilaris
5. Eczema
6. Sweet's Syndrome
7. Psoriasis
8. Dermatitis herpetiformis

Ans. 3. Pityriasis rosea

USMLE Case Scenario

A 44-year-old woman presented with a six month history of erythema and swelling of the periorbital region and papules and plaques on the dorsolateral aspect of forearms and knuckles with ragged cuticles. There was no muscle weakness. The most likely diagnosis is:

1. Dermatomyositis
2. Polymyositis
3. SLE
4. Sjögren's syndrome
5. Rheumatoid arthritis

Ans. 1. Dermatomyositis

USMLE Case Scenario

Keratoderma blennorrhagicum is seen in:

1. Psoriasis
2. Reiter's syndrome
3. Syphilis
4. Disseminated gonococcal infection

Ans. 2. Reiter's syndrome

USMLE Case Scenario

A pathologist describes a lesion where there is marked epidermal thickening (acanthosis), with regular downward elongation of the rete ridges. Increased epidermal cell turnover and lack of maturation results in loss of the stratum granulosum with extensive overlying parakeratotic scale. There is thinning of the epidermal cell layer. Neutrophils form small aggregates within both the spongiotic superficial epidermis (pustules of Kogoj) and the parakeratotic stratum corneum (Munro microabscesses). Most likely lesion is:

1. Lichen planus
2. Solar keratosis
3. Carcinoma in situ skin
4. Psoriasis
5. Pemphigus
6. Pemphigoid

Ans. 4. Psoriasis

USMLE Case Scenario

Erythema multiforme is mediated by:

1. IgE antibodies
2. Nonantigen specific T cells

3. Antigen nonspecific T cells
4. Antigen specific T cells
5. Nonantigen specific B cells
6. Antigen nonspecific B cells
7. Antigen specific B cells

Ans. 4. Antigen specific T cells

There are many specific inflammatory dermatoses; they may be mediated by IgE antibodies (urticaria), antigen specific T cells (eczema, erythema multiforme, and psoriasis), and trauma (lichen simplex chronicus).

USMLE Case Scenario

A 3-year-old child has eczematous dermatitis on extensor surfaces. His mother has a history of Bronchial asthma. Diagnosis should be:

1. Atopic dermatitis
2. Contact dermatitis
3. Seborrheic dermatitis
4. Infantile eczematous dermatitis

Ans. 1. Atopic dermatitis

USMLE Case Scenario

Pemphigus is a rare autoimmune blistering disorder resulting from loss of integrity of normal intercellular attachments within the epidermis and mucosal epithelium. Most individuals who develop pemphigus are middle-aged and older. Pemphigus vulgaris and pemphigus foliaceus are caused by a:

1. Type I hypersensitivity reaction
2. Type II hypersensitivity reaction
3. Type III hypersensitivity reaction
4. Type IV hypersensitivity reaction

Ans. 2. Type II hypersensitivity reaction

USMLE Case Scenario

Max. Joseph's space is a histopathological feature of:

1. Psoriasis vulgaris
2. Lichen planus
3. Pityriasis rosea
4. Parapsoriasis

Ans. 2. Lichen planus

USMLE Case Scenario

Ivermectin in indicated in the treatment of:

1. Syphilis
2. Scabies
3. Tuberculosis
4. Dermatophytosis
5. Psoriasis

Ans. 2. Scabies

USMLE Case Scenario

Darrier's sign is seen in:

1. Darrier's disease
2. Urticaria pigmentosa

3. Pemphigus vulgaris
4. Lichen planus
5. Eryhthema multiforme

Ans. 2. Urticaria pigmentosa

USMLE Case Scenario

Airborne contact dermatitis can be diagnosed by:

1. Skin biopsy
2. Patch test
3. Prick test
4. Estimation of serum IgE levels

Ans. 2. Patch Test

USMLE Case Scenario

Bullous pemphigoid is an autoimmune disease in which the characteristic finding is linear deposition of IgG antibodies and complement in the basement membrane zone. Reactivity also occurs in the basal cell-basement membrane attachment plaques (hemidesmosomes), where most of the bullous pemphigoid antigen (BPAG) is located. Early lesions show a perivascular infiltrate of lymphocytes and variable numbers of eosinophils, occasional neutrophils, superficial dermal edema, and associated basal cell layer vacuolization. Bullous pemphigoid is characterized by a:

Epidermal, nonacantholytic blister

1. Epidermal, acantholytic blister
2. Subepidermal, acantholytic blister
3. Subepidermal, nonacantholytic blister

Ans. 3. Subepidermal, nonacantholytic blister

USMLE Case Scenario

In an 8-day-old child with no history of consanguinity in the parents, the mother reports blisters and bleeding off of the skin at the site of handling and pressure. There was a similar history in the previous child which proved to be fatal. The diagnosis is:

1. Pemphigoid
2. Pemphigus
3. Psoriasis
4. Congenital epidermolysis bullosa
5. Sweet's syndrome

Ans. 4. Congenital epidermolysis bullosa

USMLE Case Scenario

Impetigo is primarily seen in children but can sometimes affect adults. The disease often begins as a single small macule that rapidly evolves into a larger lesion with a 'honey-colored crust'. The disease involves direct contact, usually with:

1. Staphylococcus epidermis, or less commonly Streptococcus pyogenes
2. Staphylococcus aureus, or less commonly Streptococcus pneumonaie
3. Staphylococcus aureus, or less commonly Streptococcus pyogenes
4. Streptococcus or less commonly pseudomonas

Ans. 3. Staphylococcus aureus, or less commonly Streptococcus pyogenes

USMLE Case Scenario

Pautrier's micro-abscess is a histological feature of:

1. Sarcoidosis
2. Tuberculosis

3. Mycosis fungoides
4. Pityriasis lichenoides chronica

Ans. 3. Mycosis fungoides

USMLE Case Scenario

An infant presents with a superficial cellulitis of the skin with marked lymphatic involvement, caused by beta-hemolytic group A streptococci beginning with an area of redness and enlarges to form the typical tense, painful, bright red, shiny, brawny infiltrated plaque with a well demarcated, distinct, and slightly raised border. Most likely the diagnosis is:

1. Botromycosis
2. Gangrene
3. Rodent ulcer
4. Varicose ulcer
5. SSSS
6. Erysipelas

Ans. 6. Erysipelas

USMLE Case Scenario

Lucio phenomenon is a widespread diffuse infiltration of the skin with secondary alopecia of the hair, eyebrows and eyelashes, and generalized sensory loss. The patients are systemically ill with fever, chills, malaise, arthralgias, myalgias, and tender cutaneous lesions that are responsive to steroids but not to thalidomide. Lucio phenomenon is usually associated with:

1. Mycoplasma
2. Chlamydia
3. Mycobacterium avium
4. Mycobacterium africanum
5. Mycobacterium tuberculosis
6. Mycobacterium leprae

Ans. 6. Mycobacterium leprae

USMLE Case Scenario

A 35-year-old presents with a painful ulcer in mouth. She presented to ophthamologist and gynecologist two days back for uveitis and ulcer on genital respectively. The most likely diagnosis is:

1. Herpe's simplex infection
2. Rieter's disease
3. Behçet's disease
4. Sjögren's disease

Ans. 3. Behçet's disease

USMLE Case Scenario

Clear vesicles with red base developing into macules on palms and soles in a patient with Rieter's syndrome are:

1. Pompholyx
2. Keratoderma
3. Circanate balanitis
4. Herpes Zoster

Ans. 2. Keratoderma

USMLE Case Scenario

A 27-year-old male had burning micturition and urethral discharge. After 4 weeks he developed joint pains involving both the knees and ankles, redness of the eye and skin lesion. The most probable clinical diagnosis is:

1. Psoriasis vulgaris

2. Reiter's syndrome
3. Behçet's syndrome
4. Sarcoidosis

Ans. 2. Reiter's syndrome

USMLE Case Scenario

A 88-year-old man has an indolent, nonhealing ulcer at the heel of the right foot for several weeks. He is obese and has varicose veins, high cholesterol, and poorly controlled type 2 diabetes mellitus. The patient began wearing a new pair of shoes shortly before the ulcer started and noticed a blister as the first anomaly at the site where the ulcer eventually developed. The ulcer is 2.6 cm in diameter, the ulcer base looks dirty, and there is hardly any granulation tissue. The skin around the ulcer looks normal. The patient has no sensation to pin prick anywhere in that foot. Peripheral pulses are weak but palpable. Which of the following most accurately characterizes the ulcer?

1. Ischemic ulcer due to arteriosclerosis
2. Ischemic ulcer due to embolization
3. Squamous cell carcinoma
4. Basal cell carcinoma
5. Stasis ulcer due to venous insufficiency
6. Diabetic ulcer

Ans. 6. Diabetic ulcer

USMLE Case Scenario

Which one of the following is the treatment of choice for Dermatitis Herpetiformis?

1. Corticosteroids
2. Dapsone
3. Methotrexate
4. Retinoids

Ans. 2. Dapsone

USMLE Case Scenario

A dermatologist describes lesions which are very common in fair-skinned individuals, are usually less than 1 cm in diameter; tan-brown, red, or skin colored; and have a rough, sandpaper-like consistency, there is a predilection for sun-exposed areas (face, arms, dorsum of the hands), and the lesions accumulate with age and degree of sun exposure. They can infrequently progress to carcinoma in situ as well. Most likely lesion is:

1. Lupus vulgaris
2. Scrofuloderma
3. Actinic keratosis
4. Scarlet fever
5. Hansen's disease
6. Pyogenic granuloma

Ans. 3. Actinic keratosis

USMLE Case Scenario

A 12-year-old boy who visited India and returned to USA after one year had a gradually progressive plaque on a buttock for the last 3 years. The plaque was 15 cm in diameter, annular in shape, with crusting and induration at the periphery and scarring at the center. The most likely diagnosis is:

1. Tinea corporis
2. Granuloma annulare
3. Lupus vulgaris
4. Borderline leprosy

Ans. 3. Lupus vulgaris

USMLE Case Scenario

A 24-year-old man from Chicago had multiple, small hypopigmented macules on the upper chest and back for the last three months. The macules were circular, arranged around follicles and many had coalesced to form large sheets. The surface of the macules showed fine scaling. He had similar lesions one-year-ago which subsided with treatment. The most appropriate investigation to confirm the diagnosis is:

1. Potassium hydroxide preparation of scales
2. Slit skin smear from discrete macules
3. Tzanck test
4. Skin biopsy of coalesced macules

Ans. 1. Potassium hydroxide preparation of scales

USMLE Case Scenario

A 45-year-old male from Indian subcontinent had multiple hypoesthetic mildly erythematous large plaques with elevated margins on trunk and extremities. His ulnar and lateral popliteal nerves on both sides were enlarged. The most probable diagnosis is:

1. Leprosy
2. Polio
3. Tuberculosis
4. Brucellosis
5. Lichen planus

Ans. 1. Leprosy

USMLE Case Scenario

A 24-year-old female from New Texas seeks a dermatologists opinion. She has flaccid bullae in the skin and oral erosions. Histopathology shows intraepidermal acantholytic blister. The most likely diagnosis is:

1. Pemphigoid
2. Erythema multiforme
3. Pemphigus vulgaris
4. Dermatitis herpetiformis

Ans. 3. Pemphigus vulgaris

USMLE Case Scenario

A 45-year-old male with a 10-year history of treatment with steroids has developed multiple grouped vesicular lesions present on the T10 segment dermatome associated with pain. The most likely diagnosis is:

1. Herpes zoster
2. Dermatitis herpetiformis
3. Herpes simplex
4. Scabies

Ans. 1. Herpes zoster

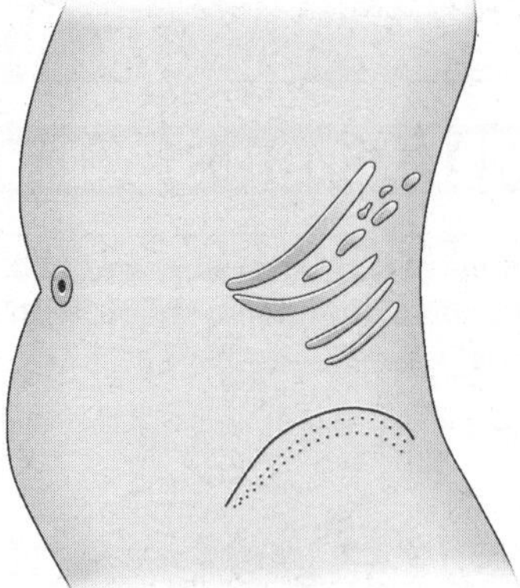

USMLE Case Scenario

Lichen planus shows well developed changes of chronicity: epidermal hyperplasia, hypergranulosis, and hyperkeratosis. Anucleate, necrotic basal cells are seen in the inflamed papillary dermis and are referred to as:

1. Micro munro abscesses
2. Pautrier's abscesses
3. Civatte bodies
4. Torre's bodies

Ans. 3. Civatte bodies

USMLE Case Scenario

Hyperplasia of the papillary dermis with elongation and/or widening of the dermal papillae is known as:

1. Acantholysis
2. Acanthosis
3. Hyperkeratosis
4. Papillomatosis

Ans. 4. Papillomatosis

- Hyperkeratosis: Hyperplasia of the stratum corneum, often associated with a qualitative abnormality of the keratin
- Parakeratosis: Mode (s) of keratinization characterized by retention of the nuclei in the stratum corneum; on mucosal membranes, parakeratosis is normal
- Acanthosis: Epidermal hyperplasia preferentially involving the stratum spinosum
- Dyskeratosis: Abnormal keratinization occurring prematurely within individual cells or groups of cells below the stratum granulosum
- Acantholysis: Loss of intercellular connections resulting in lack of cohesion between keratinocytes
- Papillomatosis: Hyperplasia of the papillary dermis with elongation and/or widening of the dermal papillae
- Lentiginous: Refers to a linear pattern of melanocyte proliferation within the epidermal basal cell layer; lentiginous melanocytic hyperplasia can occur as a reactive change or as part of a neoplasm of melanocytes
- Spongiosis: Intercellular edema of the epidermis.

USMLE Case Scenario

A 45-year-old abruptly develops an intensely itchy rash. Physical examination demonstrates multiple erythematous patches of the distal arms and legs. Some of the patches show central clearing with surrounding erythematous rings. Which of the following is the most likely diagnosis?

1. Erythema nodosum
2. Erythema chronicum migrans
3. Erythema migrans chronicum
4. Erythema multiforme

Ans. 4. Erythema multiforme

USMLE Case Scenario

A 42-year-old female presents to New York Central Hospital with painful oral ulcers. Physical examination demonstrates widespread erosions of her mucous membranes. Dermatological examination reveals a friable mucosa. Biopsy of perilesional mucosa demonstrates acantholysis; direct immunofluorescence demonstrates an intraepidermal band of IgG and C3. The most likely diagnosis is:

1. Bullous pemphigoid
2. Dermatitis herpetiformis
3. Herpes simplex I
4. Pemphigus vulgaris

Ans. 4. Pemphigus vulgaris

USMLE Case Scenario

Cells similar to fibroblasts are seen growing in a storiform ('pinwheel') pattern. This pattern of cells is characteristic of:
1. Leiomyosarcoma
2. Basal cell carcinoma
3. Keratocanthoma
4. Dermatofibrosarcoma

Ans. 4. Dermatofibrosarcoma

USMLE Case Scenario

A 44-year-old male presents to the dermatologist with pain in the joints along with silvery, scaling plaques on his elbows and knees. The most likely diagnosis is:
1. Acne vulgaris
2. Pemphigus vulgaris
3. Psoriasis vulgaris
4. Pemphigoid

Ans. 3. Psoriasis vulgaris

USMLE Case Scenario

A pathologist from Mexico reports the presence of koilocytes in a cervical biopsy from a 22-year-old woman. Which of the following conditions does this patient most likely have?
1. Chlamydia infection
2. Gonococcal infection
3. Herpes simplex virus infection
4. Human papillomavirus infection

Ans. 4. Human papillomavirus infection

USMLE Case Scenario

Some genetically predisposed individuals develop antibodies to dietary gluten (derived from the wheat protein gliadin). The antibodies cross-react with reticulin, a component of the anchoring fibrils that tether the epidermal basement membrane to the superficial dermis. The resultant injury and inflammation produce a subepidermal blister. The antibodies are:
1. IgG antibodies
2. IgA antibodies
3. IgM antibodies
4. IgD antibodies
5. IgE antibodies

Ans. 2. IgA antibodies

USMLE Case Scenario

A 53-year-old female has intense pruritis over bilaterally symmetrical lesions. Patient uses the terms 'coin-shaped' or 'discoid' are used to describe skin lesions. Microscopically, the dominant feature is a localized spongiosis of the epidermis, containing minute fluid-filled holes that correspond to the tiny vesicles seen clinically in early lesions. Patient gets relief with high potency steroids. Most likely diagnosis is:
1. Psoriasis
2. Pompholyx
3. Pemphigus vegetans
4. Nummular Eczema
5. Seborrhea

Ans. 4. Nummular Eczema

USMLE Case Scenario

A pathologist describes a lesion in which there is thinning of the epidermal cell layer overlying the tips of dermal papillae (suprapapillary plates) and blood vessels within the papillae are dilated and tortuous. These vessels bleed readily when the scale is removed, giving rise to multiple punctate bleeding points. This sign is called as:

1. Trousseau's sign
2. Chvosteks sign
3. Grey Turner's sign
4. Auspitz sign
5. Troises sign

Ans. 4. Auspitz sign

USMLE Case Scenario

A 45-year-old man came to see an immunologist who has noted several 1 to 2 cm reddish purple, nodular lesions present on the skin of his right arm which have increased in size and number over the past 3 months. The lesions do not itch and are not painful. He has had a watery diarrhea for the past month. On physical examination, he has generalized lymphadenopathy and oral thrush. Which of the following infections is most likely to be related to the appearance of these skin lesions?

1. *Candida albicans*
2. Human herpesvirus 8
3. Mycobacterium tuberculosis
4. Pseudomonas aeruginosa
5. Pneumocystis jiroveci

Ans. 2. Human herpesvirus 8

USMLE Case Scenario

Lyme disease is caused by Borrelia burgdorferi, presents with a red macule or papule at the site of the tick bite. The initial lesion slowly expands to form a large annular lesion with a red border and central clearing. The lesion is warm, but usually not painful. This initial lesion is called as:

1. Erythema nodosum
2. Erythema gyrum repens
3. Erythema chronicum migrans
4. Erythema multiforme
5. Erythema ab igne

Ans. 3. Erythema chronicum migrans

USMLE Case Scenario

A 25-year-old boy presents to a dermatology clinic with scarring Alopecia, thinned nails, hypopigmented macular lesions over trunk and oral mucosa. The diagnosis is:

1. Psoriasis
2. Leprosy
3. Lichen planus
4. Pemphigus
5. Tuberculosis of skin
6. Lichen nitidus

Ans. 3. Lichen planus

USMLE Case Scenario

Celiac disease has association with:

1. Herpes simplex virus
2. Herpes zoster virus

3. Ramsay hunt syndrome
4. Dermatitis
5. Dermatitis herpetiformis

Ans. 5. Dermatitis herpetiformis

USMLE Case Scenario

The characteristic Nail finding in lichen planus is:

1. Pitting
2. Pterygium
3. Beau's lines
4. Hyperpigmentation of the Nails

Ans. 2. Pterygium

USMLE Case Scenario

A 40-year-old farmer from Rural America with a history of recurrent attacks of porphyria complains of itching when exposes to the sun and maculopapular rash on sun exposed areas, his symptoms are exaggerated in the summer. The diagnosis is:

1. Seborrheic dermatitis
2. Contact dermatitis
3. Psoriasis
4. Porphyria cutanea tarda

Ans. 4. Porphyria cutanea tarda

USMLE Case Scenario

A 44-year-old woman presents to a dermatology clinic. She has lost most of the hair on her body, including scalp, eyebrows, eyelashes, axilla and groin hair, and the fine hairs on her body and extremities. She most likely has a variant of which of the following?

1. Alopecia areata
2. Androgenic alopecia
3. Cutaneous lupus erythematosus
4. Lichen planus
5. Trichotillomania

Ans. 1. Alopecia areata

It is caused by an autoimmune attack on hair follicles.

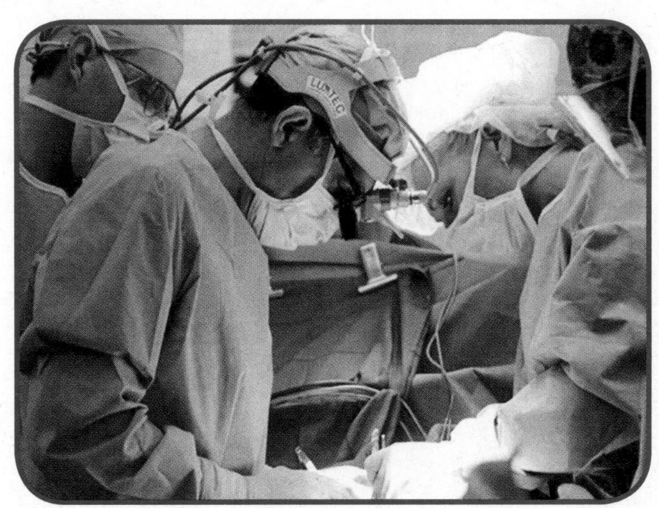

SURGERY

Surgery 5

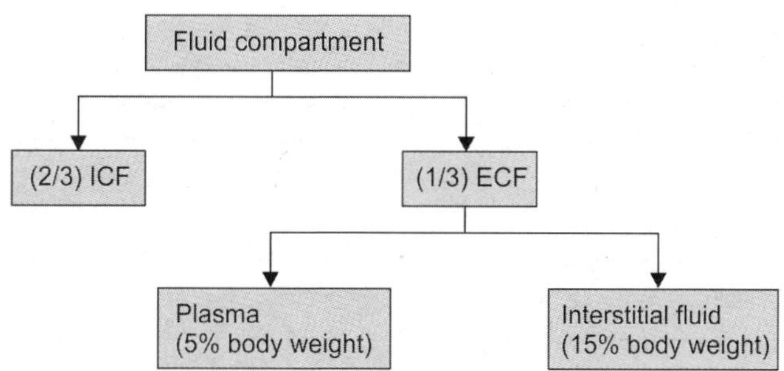

Fluids

- Water constitutes between 50% and 70% of total body weight
- The water of the body is divided into three functional compartments
- **The intracellular water** represents between 30% and 40% of body weight
- **The extracellular water** represents approximately 20% of body weight and is divided between intravascular fluid, or plasma (5% of body weight) and interstitial, or extravascular, extracellular fluid (15% of body weight)
- **Intracellular fluid**. Measurement of intracellular fluid (ICF) is determined indirectly by subtraction of the measured extracellular fluid (ECF) from the measured total body water. The intracellular water is **between 30% and 40% of body weight**, with the largest proportion in the skeletal muscle mass. Because of the smaller muscle mass in the female, the percentage of intracellular water is lower than in the male. The chemical composition of **ICF with potassium and magnesium as the principal cations**, and **phosphates and proteins as the principal anions**
- **Extracellular fluid.** The total ECF volume represents approximately 20% of body weight. The ECF compartment has two major subdivisions. **The plasma volume** is approximately 5% of body weight in the normal adult. **The interstitial, or extravascular, ECF volume**, obtained by subtracting the plasma volume from the measured total ECF volume, accounts for approximately 15% of body weight
- **The interstitial fluid** is further complicated by having a rapidly equilibrating or functional component as well as several more slowly equilibrating, or relatively nonfunctioning, components. The nonfunctioning components include connective tissue water as well as transcellular water, which includes cerebrospinal and joint fluids. This nonfunctional component normally represents only 10% of interstitial fluid volume (1%–2% of body weight) and is not to be confused with the relatively nonfunctional ECF, often called a *third space,* found in burns and soft tissue injuries
- The normal constituents of **ECF are with sodium as the principal cation and chloride and bicarbonate as the principal anions.**

Congenital Vascular Malformations

Hemangioma: Malformation of the developing blood vessels. They commonly appear in the skin but may develop in any organ

Strawberry nevus

- Usually appear at about a week of age and may rapidly enlarge in the first few months of life
- Usually **resolve spontaneously** by intravascular thrombosis
- This process is normally complete by 5 to 7 years of age leaving only a minor blemish or none at all.

Stork mark

- It is a superficial capillary hemangioma which may be seen on the forehead, bridge of the nose and upper eyelids. The lesion is often V-shaped pointing down to the nose and there is a corresponding mark on the nape of the neck
- Capillary hemangiomas are bright red to blue and vary from a few millimeters to several centimeters in diameter; hemangiomas can be level with the surface of the skin or slightly elevated and have an intact overlying epithelium.

Port-wine stain (Nevus flammeus)

- Unlike a strawberry nevus, this is present at birth and may be very disfiguring, as it becomes darker and increasingly nodular with age
- **Persists (P for P)**
- Port-wine stains are vascular malformations on the skin, and most commonly occur on the face. Over time, port-wine stains darken and pose psychological stress to the affected person because of cosmetic reasons. Port-wine stains rarely disappear on their own, and the most effective therapy is pulsed dye laser. Pulsed dye laser reduces the size of most port-wine stains, and in some cases, can eradicate the stain completely. Factors affecting the response to pulsed dye laser include location, timing, and size. Smaller port-wine stains respond better than the bigger ones. The earlier the treatment takes place, the better the response.

Sturge-Weber syndrome

- It is a severe form of port-wine stain on the scalp and face, in the distribution of one of the branches of the **trigeminal nerve**, associated with an underlying vascular anomaly of the arachnoid covering the cerebral hemisphere
- This leads to **epilepsy, hemiplegia and mental retardation.**

Cavernous hemangioma

These may occur alone or in association with a capillary lesion in the overlying skin. They increase in size after birth but usually in proportion to the growth of the infant. Most resolve spontaneously but some persist requiring excision

Grossly, cavernous hemangiomas appear as red-blue, soft, spongy masses 1 to 2 cm in diameter; rare giant forms can affect large subcutaneous areas of the face, extremities, or other body regions. Histologically, the mass is sharply defined but not encapsulated, and it is composed of large, cavernous blood-filled vascular spaces separated by a mild-to-moderate amount of connective tissue stroma. Intravascular thrombosis with associated dystrophic calcification is common.

Kasabach-Merritt syndrome

Hemangiomas associated with a generalized bleeding disorder caused by the trapping of platelets within them which produces a profound **thrombocytopenia.**

Lymphangioma

- Lymphagioma are similar to hemangiomas but involve lymphatics. They may also occur anywhere in the body but, in particular, they may present as a cystic hygroma
- Most commonly arising in the cervical region.

Klippel-Trenaunay Syndrome

- **Congenital AV fistulas**
- **Hemangiomas**
- **Varicose veins**
- **Hypertrophy of limbs**

Other Conditions Related to Vascular System

Vascular Ectasias

- **Vascular ectasias are common lesions characterized by local dilation of pre-existing vessels; they are not true neoplasms**

Spider Telangiectasia

- This **non-neoplastic vascular lesion grossly resembles a spider**; there is a radial, often pulsatile, array of dilated subcutaneous arteries or arterioles (resembling legs) about a central core (resembling a body) that blanches when pressure is applied to its center
- It is commonly seen on the face, neck, or upper chest and is most frequently associated with **hyperestrogenic states, such as pregnancy or cirrhosis.**

Hereditary Hemorrhagic Telangiectasia (Osler-Weber-Rendu Disease)

- In this autosomal dominant disorder, the telangiectasias are malformations composed of dilated capillaries and veins
- Present from birth, they are widely distributed over the skin and oral mucous membranes, as well as in the respiratory, GI, and urinary tracts. Occasionally, these lesions rupture, causing serious epistaxis (nosebleeds), GI bleeding, or hematuria

Hemangiopericytomas

- These are rare tumors derived from pericytes-myofibroblast-like cells that are normally arranged around capillaries and venules
- Hemangiopericytomas can occur as slowly enlarging, painless masses at any anatomic site, but they are most common on the lower extremities (especially the thigh) and in the retroperitoneum
- They consist of numerous branching capillary channels and gaping sinusoidal spaces enclosed within nests of spindle-shaped to round cells. The tumors may recur after excision, and roughly half metastasize, usually hematogenously to lungs, bone, or liver.

Aneurysms

- The most common type of **true aneurysm** is fusiform type
- The most common site of **arterial aneurysm** is Infrarenal part of abdominal aorta
- Popliteal aneurysms are the **most common peripheral aneurysms**
- The most common site for **dissecting aneurysms** is ascending aorta
- MC cause of AAA is A: Abdominal Aortic Aneurysm is atherosclerosis
- **'Cirsoid aneurysms'** are common in superficial temporal artery

Types of Aneurysms

- **Berry aneurysm** occurs in circle of willis
- **Microaneurysms** are seen in diabetes and hypertension
- **Mycotic aneurysms** are seen in **bacterial** infections
- **Aortic dissecting aneurysms** are due to degeneration of tunica media. Occur in Marfan's syndrome and hypertension
- **Syphilitic aneurysms or luetic aneurysms** involve ascending aorta
- **Pseudoaneurysm follows trauma usually.**

Abdominal Aortic Aneurysm (AAA)

- **It is imperative to recognize the potential presence of an abdominal aortic aneurysm (AAA)**
- **The combination of the history of hypertension and smoking, the new back pain, and a pulsatile mass on examination is highly suggestive for abdominal aneurysm**
- **The back pain occurs as the expanding mass compresses structures in the retroperitoneum**
- **It is particularly important to make the diagnosis because large aneurysms (greater than 5 cm in diameter) are associated with a very high risk of rupture and subsequent mortality.**

ARTERIAL DISEASES

Buerger's Disease (Thromboangiitis Obliterans)

Thromboangiitis obliterans (Buerger disease) is a distinctive disease that often leads to vascular insufficiency; it is characterized by segmental, thrombosing acute and **chronic inflammation of medium-sized and small arteries**, principally the tibial and radial arteries, with occasional secondary extension into extremity veins and nerves. Buerger disease is a condition that occurs almost exclusively in **heavy smokers of cigarettes**, usually beginning before age 35.

- Affects **small and medium-sized** arteries
- Affects young
- Affects **smokers**
- Ankle pressure index is low here
  - Coldness and numbness of toes are the first sign
  - **Xanthiol nicotinate** is used for treatment

- **Lumbar sympathetectomy is done**
- **Martorell's sign** is positive.

Raynaud's disease: Affects arterioles. Features are Blanching, Dusky cyanosis, Red engorgement

Raynaud's phenomenon is vasospastic condition of diverse etiology

Leriche's syndrome is due to aortoiliac occlusion

Butcher's thigh is due to injury to femoral artery in femoral triangle.

Thrombotic Obliteration of the Abdominal Aorta and Iliac Arteries (LERICHE'S SYNDROME)

Chronic occlusion of the **aortic bifurcation by thrombosis:** It typically affects men 35 to 60 years of age

Characteristic symptoms of thrombotic occlusion of the terminal aorta include:

- ***Extreme liability to fatigue of both lower limbs, described as a weariness rather than the typical intermittent claudication;***
- ***Symmetrical atrophy of both lower limbs without trophic changes in the skin or nails;***
- ***Pallor of the legs and feet; and***
- ***Inability to maintain a stable erection due to inadequate arterial flow to the penis from hypogastric arterial obstruction, thus reducing the blood flow through the internal pudendal artery and its blood flow to the corpora cavernosa***
  - The physical findings include absence of pulses in the abdominal aorta and in the arteries distally. The occlusion may involve any portion of the abdominal aorta from the renal arteries distally
  - **Surgical management:** Although thromboendarterectomy with direct reconstitution of flow is appropriate in a few patients, the majority of patients with occlusion of the abdominal aorta are managed by bypass grafts from the aorta to the iliac or, more often, the common femoral arteries
  - It may be necessary to perform a thromboendarterectomy distal to the renal arteries to permit a patent lumen for the proximal anastomosis.

Deep Venous Thrombosis

- Most important consequences of this disorder are **'pulmonary embolism'** and the **'syndrome of chronic venous insufficiency'**
- Deep venous thrombosis of the iliac, femoral, or popliteal veins is suggested by **unilateral leg swelling warmth,** and **erythema, pain**
- **Earliest sign is rise in temperature**
- **Occurs less frequently in the upper extremity** than in the lower extremity
  - The noninvasive test used most often to diagnose deep venous thrombosis is **duplex venous ultrasonography**
  - Impedance plethysmography measures changes in venous capacitance during physiologic maneuvers
  - It is much less sensitive for diagnosing deep venous thrombosis of the calves
  - Heparin is used for DVT prophylaxis
  - **Thrombolytic therapy, bandaging arre effective**
  - **Magnetic resonance imaging (MRI)** is another noninvasive means to detect deep vein thrombosis. Its diagnostic accuracy for assessing proximal deep vein thrombosis is similar to that of duplex ultrasonography. It is useful in patients with suspected thrombosis of the superior and inferior venae cavae or pelvic veins.

Signs of DVT

Hoffmann's sign	Forced dorsiflexion of ankle causes pain in calf
Moses' sign	Pain in calf on squeezing calf muscles
Pratt's sign	Lateral squeezing of calf muscles causes pain
Phlegmasia alba dolens	Swollen leg (whitish) with edema and blanching
Phlegmasia cerulea dolens	Painful (blue) leg

Varicose Veins

- *These are* ***dilated, tortuous superficial veins*** *that result from defective structure and function of the valves of the saphenous veins, from intrinsic weakness of the vein wall, from high intraluminal pressure, or, rarely, from arteriovenous fistulas*
- **Primary varicose veins** originate in the superficial system and occur two to three times as frequently in women as in men. Approximately half of patients have a family history of varicose veins
- **Secondary varicose veins** result from deep venous insufficiency and incompetent perforating veins or from deep venous occlusion causing enlargement of superficial veins that are serving as collaterals
- Varicose dilation renders the venous valves incompetent and **leads to stasis, congestion, edema, pain, and thrombosis.** The most disabling sequelae include persistent edema in the extremity and secondary ischemic skin changes including **stasis dermatitis and ulcerations; poor wound healing and superimposed infections can become chronic varicose ulcers.** Notably, embolism from these superficial veins is very rare
- **Duplex imaging is gold standard**
- Varicose veins can **usually be treated with conservative measures**
  - **External compression stockings** provide a counterbalance to the hydrostatic pressure in the veins
  - **Small symptomatic varicose veins can be treated with sclerotherapy,** in which a sclerosing solution is injected into the involved varicose vein and a compression bandage is applied
  - **Ethanolamine oleate is used as sclerosant**
  - **Surgical therapy usually involves extensive ligation and stripping of the greater and lesser saphenous veins**
  - **Brodie Trendelenburg test demonstrates saphenofemoral incompetence**
  - **Ecchymosis is the most common complication of stripping**
  - **Cockett and Dodd's operation is subfascial ligation operation.**

Lymphatic Diseases

Lymphedema congenita	Present at birth
Lymphedemapraecox	Starts at puberty
Lymphedema tarda	Starts at adulthood
Milroy's disease	Congenital lymphedema of familial type

Wounds and Tissue Repair

The types of healing are customarily divided into repair by first, second, or third intention

- **Primary or first intention healing** occurs in closed wounds **in which the edges are approximated**, such as a **clean skin incision** closed with sutures. The incisional defect re-epithelializes rapidly, and matrix deposition seals the defect
- **Second intention healing** occurs when the **wound edges are not apposed**, such as an open punch skin biopsy wound, a deep burn and an infected wound left open to granulate. Granulation tissue fills the wound, and the wound contracts and re-epithelializes
- **Delayed primary or third intention healing** occurs when an **open wound is secondarily closed several days after injury.** Such a wound is initially left open because of gross contamination. A classic example is wound management after removal of a ruptured appendix. After the peritoneum and fascia are closed to prevent evisceration, the skin and subcutaneous tissue are left open and the wound is packed loosely with sterile moist gauze. The wound is closed several days later after the wound contamination has markedly diminished.

A scar is loosely defined as an abnormal, disorganized collection of collagen following wound repair. The collagens are a large group of triple-helix structural matrix proteins

- **Type I collagen** is the major structural component of bones, skin, and tendons
- **Type II** is found predominantly in cartilage
- **Type III** is found in association with Type I, although the ratio varies in different tissues
- **Type IV** is found in **basement membranes** in association with mucopolysaccharides and laminin
- **Type V** is found in the cornea in association with Type III and is important in maintaining transparency.

Clinical Factors that Affect Wound Healing

Nutrition

- Protein depletion impairs wound healing
- Vitamin C (ascorbic acid) deficiency causes scurvy. In patients with this deficiency, wound healing is arrested during fibroplasia
- Vitamin A (retinoic acid) requirements increase during injury. Severely injured patients require supplemental vitamin A to maintain normal serum levels. Vitamin A also partially reverses the impaired healing in chronically steroid-treated patients
- Vitamin B_6 (pyridoxine) deficiency impairs collagen cross-linking
- Vitamin B_1 (thiamine) and vitamin B_2 (riboflavin) deficiencies cause syndromes associated with poor wound repair
- **Vitamin E** has **inhibitory role in wound healing**
- Deficiencies of trace metals such as **zinc, copper and oxygen**
- Anemia, and↓ perfusion
  - **Oxygen** is required for successful inflammation, angiogenesis, epithelialization, and matrix deposition
  - **Anemia**
  - **Diabetes mellitus and obesity**
  - **Corticosteroids, chemotherapy, and radiation therapy**
  - **Infection**

Keloids

- Keloids are made of dense **connective tissue**
- Keloids are best treated by **intrakeloidal injection of triamiclonolone**

Feature	Hypertrophic scar	Keloid
• **Hereditary**	Not familial	May be familial
• **Race**	No predilection	Common in blacks
• **Sex**	No predilection	Common in females
• **Borders**	Confined to wound	Outgrow wound
• **Course**	Subsides	Rarely subsides May turn malignant
	• *Does not extend beyond wound margin* • *Red, raised, tender* • *Remodelling phase* ↑ • *Where tension of skin is more* • *Best scars seen in old people*	Recurrence common **Sternum mc site** **Appears after surgery in a few days** **Best treated by intralesional steroidal application** **Excision and repair are even better**

Wounds

Clean wound	• No violation of mucosa • No inflammation • No drains • No need of any prophylactic antibiotic, **e.g. Varicose Vein Surgery**
Clean contaminated wound	**Elective Herniotomy** • Violation of mucosa but no spillage • Need of prophylactic antibiotic, **e.g. Elective cholecystectomy**

Contaminated wound	• Pre-existing infection • Spillage of viscus contents • Need of prophylactic antibiotic, **e.g. Appendicectomy**

Grafting-related Terms

- **Imbibition:** refers to absorption of nutrients into the graft
- **Inosculation:** donor and recipient capillaries become aligned
- **Revascularization** is completed by connecting vessels into arterioles and venules.

Skin grafts

- Skin grafts are harvested from a donor site and transferred to a recipient site on which they must survive, a process known as take
- All skin grafts initially adhere to the recipient bed by the formation of fibrin. Oxygen and nutrients diffuse by a process known as plasmatic imbibition to keep the graft alive
- New blood vessels then grow from the recipient site and link up with dermal capillaries to re-establish a blood supply, a process known as inosculation
- Thin skin grafts are more likely to survive by imbibition and will revascularize readily and are, therefore, more likely to take than thicker grafts.

Partial-thickness skin grafts (Thiersch graft)

- Consist of **epidermis and a variable thickness of dermis**
- Partial-thickness grafts are used to resurface relatively large areas of skin defect and are particularly useful in burns

Full-thickness grafts (Wolfe's graft)

- Consist of **epidermis and all of the dermis**
- The donor site will not epithelialize and must be closed, usually directly. Full-thickness grafts are most commonly used in repairing defects on the face.

Composite grafts

- **Consist of skin and some underlying tissue** such as fat and cartilage
- Again, donor sites must be closed directly. Composite grafts carry the highest risk of failure

Biologic Dressings

Viable cutaneous allograft is the **biologic dressing of choice**, against which all other available materials must be evaluated. In the operating room using sterile technique, allograft skin is harvested from cadavers free of jaundice, cutaneous malignancy or infection, and viral disease. The harvested grafts are spread on fine-mesh gauze that is thinly impregnated with petrolatum, placed in sterile containers, and then refrigerated for up to 2 weeks. Alternatively, the tissue can be frozen using cryoprotective techniques. If refrigerated, such tissue performs better as a biologic dressing the sooner it is used after harvest.

Cutaneous Allograft

- Prevents wound desiccation
- Promotes maturation of granulation tissue
- Limits bacterial proliferation in the burn wound
- Prevents exudative protein and red blood cell loss
- Decreases wound pain, thereby facilitating movement of involved joints
- Diminishes evaporative water loss from the burn wound surface, thus decreasing heat loss; and serves to protect tendons, vessels, and nerves.

Lyophilized Allograft Skin

- *It has an indefinite shelf life*
- *It is easily reconstituted*
- *It shows less adherence to the wound than viable allograft skin, and*
- *If harvested at too great a thickness, undergoes dermal-epidermal separation after application to the wound with subsequent* desiccation of the exposed dermis.

Cutaneous Xenografts

- *These are less effective as physiologic dressings and allow survival of greater numbers of subgraft bacteria, presumably because such tissue is not vascularized by the host*
- *Such tissues* are not rejected in the true sense of the word but slough following necrosis.

Amnion

- It is a physiologic dressing that is **readily available and inexpensive**
- Since the amniotic tissue will desiccate and spontaneously separate from the wound bed if left exposed, it must be covered with occlusive dressings that preclude continuous observation of the dressing and underlying wound bed
- Amnion, like cutaneous xenografts, is **not vascularized by the host**, and biologic union occurs by ingrowth of granulation tissue.

Swellings of Skin

• Lipoma	• **Universal tumor**
• **Adiposis dolorosa (Dercum's disease)**	• **Multiple lipomata**
• Cavernous hemangioma	• **Arises from veins**
• Plexiform hemangioma	• **Arises from arteries**
• Warts	• **Human papilloma virus**
• Rhinophyma **(Potato nose)**	• **Acne rosacea**
• Cavernous **lymphangioma**	• **Cystic hygroma**
• Sebaceous cyst	• **Wen**
• **Buschke-Lownstein tumor**	• **Massive veneral wart**
• **Marjolin's growth**	• **Squamous cell carcinoma**
• **Bedsore**	• **Trophic ulcer**
• **Pilomatrixoma**	• **Calcifying epithelioma**
• **Pott's puffy tumor**	• Skull osteomyelitis
• **Raspberry tumor**	• Umbilical adenoma

Sebaceous Cyst

- It is also called **Wen**
- It usually lies in dermis
- It is a **retention cyst**
- Its contents are **sebum and keratin**
- Common sites are face and scalp
- They **don't occur on** palm and scalp
- **Cock's peculiar tumor** is a complication

Lipoma

- **Most common site: Trunk**
- **'Slipping margin' sign positive**
- **Pedunculated lipoma is called: lipoma arborscens**

- **Mc type: Subcutaneous**
- **Painful: Neurofibroma**
- **Vascular: Naevo lipoma**

Dercum's disease

- ***Adiposis dolorosa***
- ***Fatty deposits on limbs/trunk with facial sparing***
- ***Rare disease***
- ***Multiple painful lipomas in adult life***

Ulcers of Skin

Ulcers of skin

- **Rodent ulcer:** Basal cell carcinoma
- **Martorell's ulcer:** Hypertensive/Atherosclerotic ulcer
- **Bazin's ulcer:** Erythrocyanoid ulcer
- **Snail-track ulcer:** Syphilitic ulcer

Premalignant Skin Lesions

- **Bowen's disease**
- **Solar keratoses**
- **Radiodermatitis**
- **Marjolin's ulcer**

TUMORS AFFECTING SKIN

Basal Cell Carcinoma

- **Basal Cell Carcinoma (BCC)** is a malignancy arising from epidermal basal cells
- **Also called rodent ulcer**
- Commonest site is face
- The **most common type** is **noduloulcerative** BCC, which begins as a small, **pearly nodule**, often with small telangiectatic vessels on its surface
- The nodule grows slowly and may undergo central ulceration
- Direct spread seen
- Lymphatic spread does not occur
- **Mohs micrographic excision procedure is used for BCC.**

Squamous Cell Carcinoma

Squamous Cell Carcinoma: Primary cutaneous SCC is a malignant neoplasm of **keratinizing epidermal cells**

- **Squamous cell carcinoma *in situ* is characterized by highly atypical cells at all levels of the epidermis, with nuclear crowding and disorganization.**

- **The squamous dyplasia is broad and occupies the full thickness of the epithelium**
- **Invasive squamous cell carcinomas exhibit variable differentiation, ranging from tumors formed by atypical squamous cells arranged in orderly lobules showing large zones of keratinization to neoplasms formed by highly anaplastic, rounded cells with foci of necrosis and only abortive, single-cell keratinization (dyskeratosis)**
- **While morphologic variation is wide, all squamous cell carcinomas share the feature of keratinization**

Unlike BCC, which has a very low metastatic potential, SCC can **metastasize and grow rapidly**. The clinical features of SCC vary widely

  - **Actinic keratosis predisposes to SCC**
  - **Bowen's disease**
  - **Lichen planus**
  - **DLE**

Marjolin's Ulcer

- Squamous cell carcinoma in scar/burn/long-standing ulcer
- Slow-growing
- Less malignant
- Painless without lymphatic spread
- Wide excision is the treatment of choice.

Keratoacanthoma

Keratoacanthoma typically appears as a dome-shaped papule with a central keratotic crater, expands rapidly, and commonly regresses without therapy

This lesion can be difficult to differentiate from SCC

- **Benign**
- **Self-limiting course**
- **Affects elderly men usually**

Melanomas

Melanomas originate from melanocytes, pigment cells normally present in the epidermis and sometimes in the dermis.

An alternative prognostic scheme for clinical stages I and II melanoma, proposed by **Clark**, is based on the anatomic level of invasion in the skin **(Clark's level)**.

- Melanomas may spread by the **lymphatic channels or the bloodstream**
- The earliest metastases are often to regional lymph nodes
- Most common site for malignant melanoma is **skin** (90%)
- Cutaneous melanoma arises from **epidermal melanocytes**
- **Junctional melanoma** predisposes to MM
- It may be **familial**.

Melanomas can develop either de novo or in an existing mole. Sunlight exposure is a significant risk factor and fair-skinned persons are at an increased risk of developing melanoma. The most significant factor for long-term prognosis is the depth of the lesion, since the superficial dermis lies about 1 mm under the skin surface, and penetration to this depth is associated with a much higher incidence of metastasis than is seen with a more superficial location.

Early detection of melanoma may be facilitated by applying the **'ABCD rules'**:

- A–asymmetry, benign lesions are usually symmetric
- B–border irregularity, most nevi have clear-cut borders
- C–color variegation, benign lesions usually have uniform light or dark pigment
- D–diameter > 6 mm (the size of a pencil eraser).

- **Lentigo maligna** is the least common type
- It is also known as Hutchinson's freckle
- Face is the most common site involved by it
- **Superficial spreading is the most common type**
- It may occur at any site on the body

- **Nodular melanoma** is the most malignant type
- It is common in younger age group.

- **Acral lentiginous melanoma** occurs on palms and soles especially

- **Amelanotic melanoma** has the worst prognosis

- **'Clarks level' is the classification based on the level of 'invasion into skin'**
- **'Breslow's staging'** is based on **thickness of invasion**

Nos of MM (Malignant Melanoma)

- **No** incisional biopsy
- **No** induration
- **No** role of radiotherapy
- **Not** known usually before puberty

Soft Tissue Tumors

- **Mc soft tissue tumor in a child is Rhabdomyosarcoma**
- The gross appearance of rhabdomyosarcoma is variable. Some tumors, particularly those arising near the mucosal surfaces of the bladder or vagina, can present as soft, gelatinous, grape like masses, designated sarcoma botryoides. In other cases, they are poorly defined, infiltrating masses. Rhabdomyosarcoma is histologically subclassified into the embryonal, alveolar, and pleomorphic variants
- **The rhabdomyoblast is the diagnostic cell in all types;** it exhibits granular eosinophilic cytoplasm rich in thick and thin filaments. The rhabdomyoblasts may be round or elongated; the latter are known as tadpole or strap cells and may contain cross-striations visible by light microscopy. The diagnosis of rhabdomyosarcoma is based on the demonstration of skeletal muscle differentiation, either in the form of sarcomeres under the electron microscope or by immunohistochemical demonstration of muscle-associated antigens such as **desmin and muscle-specific actin**
  - Mc type: Embryonal rhabdomyosarcoma
  - Resection is the treatment of choice
  - Soft tissue sarcomas mostly spread hematogenously
  - But lymphatic metastasis is seen in embryonal rhabdomyosarcoma
  - Grade of tumor detects prognosis
  - Liposarcoma is the mc retroperitoneal tumor
  - Lymphoma and retroperitoneal sarcoma are mc retroperitoneal malignant lesions.

SALIVARY GLANDS

Pleomorphic Adenoma

- **Mc benign salivary gland tumor**
- **Most common site is superficial lobe**
- **Malignant transformation is uncommon**
- **Treatment is by superficial parotidectomy (Patey's operation)**

Warthin's Tumor

- **Second most common** benign tumor of parotid gland
- Consists of **epithelial+lymphoid elements** (adenolymphoma)
- Common **in males** in 5th-7th decade
- Bilateral in about 10% cases
- Encapsulated
- Shows **Hot Spot** in Tc-Pertechnetate scan
- Superficial parotidectomy is the treatment.

Adenoid Cystic Carcinoma

- Also called **cylindroma/treacherous tumor**
- Mc cancer of minor salivary glands
- Invades **perineural space and lymphatics**
- Treatment is radical parotidectomy

Mucoepidermoid Cancer

- Mc malignant salivary gland tumor
- **Arises from mucinsecreting cells and epidermal cells**
- Mc malignant tumor of parotid
- Mc radiation-induced salivary tumor

Remember

- Most tumors of major salivary glands are **benign**
- Pleomorphic adenoma is the **most common benign salivary gland tumor**
- Most of the **minor** salivary gland tumors are **malignant**
- Most common site of minor salivary gland tumor is **oral cavity**
- Most of salivary gland tumors are **radioresistant**
- **Godwin's tumor** is benign lymphoepithelial tumor of parotid
- **Calculi** are most common in **submandibular duct**
- **Most common organism as a cause of acute parotitis is staph aureus**
- Most common cause of acute parotitis is mumps
- Most of submandibular calculi are **radiopaque**
- **Sialolithiasis refers to stones in salivary ducts**
- **Sialadenosis is noninflammatory swelling affecting salivary glands**
- **Frey's syndrome** (gustatory sweating) occurs after parotid surgery due to involvement of auriculotemporal nerve
- **Sialography is not done in acute infection of salivary glands.**

Breast

- **Modified sweat gland**
- **'Axillary tail of Spence' is prolongation of breast tissue into axilla**
- **'Foramen of LANGER' is the space through which axillary tail passes**
- **'Ligaments of cooper attach breast to superficial fascia**
- **'Mammary ridge' is the embryonic precursor**
- **'Subareolar plexus of Sappy' is a lymphatic plexus**
- **Peau d'orange is lymphatic permeation**
- **Blood supply: Internal mammary artery, lateral thoracic, superior thoracic and acromiothoracic arteries**

Risk Factors for Breast Cancer

- Race: White females
- Age: Elderly
- Family history
- Relatives (true)
- Nonbreastfeeding mothers
- ↑Fatty food intake
- Nulliparity
- BRCA1 and BRCA2 mutations
- Cancer in other breast
- Mammary dysplasia/Atypical hyperplasia/Sclerosing adenosis
- Early menarche
- Late menopause
- Late first pregnancy

- *Mc disorder of breast: Fibroadenosis*
- *Mc tumor of breast: Fibroadenoma*
- *Mc carcinoma of breast: Ductal/Schirrous carcinoma*
- *Mc bilateral tumor, Lobular carcinoma of breast*
- Mc inviolved lymph nodes are axillary group
- *Mc cause of breast discharge: Duct ectasia*
- *Mc cause of bloody discharge: Duct papilloma*
- *Mc site of metastasis of breast ca: Bone*
- *Mc site of breast ca: Upper outer quadrant*
- *FIRST INVESTIGATION FOR BREAST LUMP: FNAC*
- *BEST INVESTIGATION FOR BREAST LUMP: BIOPSY*

Clinical Scesnarios

• *A **16-year-old** female **has firm, rubbery mass** in right breast **moving with palpation***	Fibroadenoma
• *A 16-year-old female has firm, rubbery mass in right breast is **8 cms in** diameter*	Giant fibroadenoma
• *A 30-year-old female has history of **bilateral breast tenderness related to menstrual cycle** with lumps coming and going*	Fibrocystic disease
• *A 30-year-old female has **bloody discharge** from nipple. **No other palpable masses** are seen*	Intraductal papilloma
• *A 30-year-old **lactating mother has red, hot, tender mass** with fever and leukocytosis*	Breast abscess
• *A **55-year-old woman has 3.5 cms hard mass** in her left breast **with ill-defined borders** and **not mobile**. The skin overlying has orange peel appearance*	Breast ca
• *A 60-year-old has **headaches not responding** to medications. She had **undergone modified radical mastectomy** 1 year back*	Brain metastasis from breast ca

Galactocele

- It is a **milk-filled cyst**
- **Round, well-circumscribed**, and **easily movable** within the breast
- Usually occurs **after the cessation of lactation** or when feeding frequency has been curtailed significantly
- **Inspissated milk** within a large lactiferous duct is responsible
- The tumor is usually located in the **central portion of the breast or under the nipple.**

- Needle aspiration produces **thick, creamy material** that may be tinged dark-green or brown. Although it appears purulent, the fluid is sterile
- The treatment is needle aspiration. Withdrawal of thick milky secretion confirms the diagnosis
- Operation is reserved for those cysts that cannot be aspirated or that become superinfected.

Phyllodes Tumor

- **Serocystic disease of Brodie** or **Cystosarcoma Phyllodes**
- Name is **misnomer** as it is rarely cystic or rarely develops into sarcoma
- **Phyllodes: Leaf.** It is a **benign** breast tumor. It is a **stromal** breast tumor
- They present as a **large, massive tumor with uneven bosselated** surface
- They are however mobile and resemble fibroadenoma
- They account for **less than 1%** of all breast neoplasms
- This is predominantly a tumor of **adult women,** with very few examples reported in adolescents
- Patients typically present with **a firm, palpable mass**
- These tumors are **very fast growing**, and can increase in size in just a few weeks
- Occurrence is most common **between the ages of 40 and 50**, prior to menopause
- The common treatment for phyllodes is **wide local excision**. Other than surgery, there is no cure for phyllodes, as chemotherapy and radiation therapy are not effective.

Indicators of Poor Prognosis in Breast Cancer

- ↑PCNA, Ki67 expression
- ↑BCL2 expression
- ↑bax expression
- ↑HER2 expression
- ↑EGFR expression
- ↑p53 expression

Treatment of Breast Cancer

Stage I, II:
- **Breast conserving therapy**
- **MRM + Systemic therapy**

Stage III (operable)
- **MRM + chemotherapy + radiotherapy**

Stage IV
- **Palliative**

Surgeries Commonly Asked

- **QUART: (Quadrenectomy) + axillary block dissection + radiotherapy**
- **Lumpectomy: Rremoval of tumor +2 cm rim of normal breast atleast**
- **Simple mastectomy: Removal of breast + skin**
- **MRM (Patey's): Removal of breast + axillary block dissection**
- **Radical mastectomy: MRM + removal of pectoral muscles + thoracodorsal nerve + artery to latissimus dorsi**
- **Extended radical mastectomy: Radical mastectomy + removal of internal mammary lymph nodes**
- **Had field operation: Cone excision of major duct**

Stage I: Breast conservative therapy/lumpectomy + axillary clearance + radiotherapy
Stage II: Breast conservative therapy/lumpectomy + axillary clearance + radiotherapy
Stage III: Neoadjuvant chemo + MRM + radiotherapy (operable)
Stage IV: Inoperable/IV: Palliative (radiotherapy)/hormonal ablation/chemotherapy

Male Breast Cancer

- Breast cancer occurring in the mammary gland of males is **infrequent,** accounting for no more than 1% of the incidence in women
- It generally occurs at an **older age**
- The average age at diagnosis is **10 years older in men** than in women
- Probably because the breast tissue is scant in men, breast tumors in males **involve the pectoralis major muscle more commonly**
- Delay in diagnosis also must play a role in the more advanced presentation of male breast cancer
- Histologically, tumors of the male breast are most commonly **infiltrating ductal carcinomas** that are similar in appearance to their counterparts in females
- Male breast cancer very often contains **steroid hormone receptors**
- The treatment of carcinoma in the male breast depends on the stage and local extent of the tumor. If the underlying pectoral muscle is involved, radical mastectomy is the procedure of choice. Alternatively, modified radical mastectomy with excision of the involved portion of muscle is adequate treatment
- **For smaller tumors**, which are movable across the chest wall, modified radical mastectomy appears to be the procedure of choice. Because of the local aggressiveness of these tumors, some authors have advocated the use of postoperative radiation therapy
- The presence of nodal metastases appears to have at least the same prognostic power in men as in women.

Risk Factors

- Conditions with **hyperestrogenic** and **hypoandrogenic** states
- **Cirrhosis of liver**
- **Undescended testis**
- **Mumps orchitis**
- **Klinefelter's syndrome**
- **May accompany gynecomastia**
- Most common variety is **infiltrating ductal cancer**
- Presents with **unilateral lump** with majority being **Estrogen receptor positive.**

Aortic Injury

- Widening of superior mediastinum > 8 cms is considered a reliable sign of Aortic injury
- **'PA view'** is better than AP view in this type of injury
- X-ray is used as a **'screening tool' here**
- **'Acceleration or deceleration' injuries** are associated with aortic rupture.

Other Signs

- Obscured aortic knob
- Widened mediastinum
- Deviation of left main stem bronchus
- Obliteration of aorticopulmonary window
- Deviation of nasogastric tube
- Left apical cap
- Opacification of aortopulmonary window
- Left pulmonary Hilar hematoma

Zones in Neck Injury

- Zone I: Sternal notch to cricoid cartilage
- Zone II: Cricoid cartilage to angle of mandible
- Zone III: Angle of mandible to base of skull

- **Whiplash injury** is acute hyperflexion of spine. Especially cervical spine
- **Coup and contrecoup injuries** are a feature of brain
- **Blast injuries** cause damage to lungs and intestines

Blast Injury

- Rupture of tympanic membrane, dislocation of ear ossicles
- Injury to lungs
- Perforation of stomach, gut
- Conjuctival hemorrage in eyes

Thoracic Outlet Syndrome

- Thoracic outlet syndrome, Scalenus anticus syndrome, Cervical rib syndrome, Paget-Schreutter syndrome, Costoclavicular syndrome, Cervical band syndrome, Cervicobrachial myofascial pain syndrome, Brachial plexopathy
- Thoracic outlet syndrome (TOS) is due to compression/irritation of brachial plexus elements **(Neurogenic TOS)** and/or subclavian vessels **(Vascular TOS)** in their passage from the cervical area toward the axilla. The usual site of entrapment is the **interscalene triangle**
- Provocation tests that can suggest the presence of thoracic outlet syndrome include:
  - **Adson's maneuver**
  - **Wright test**
  - **Roos' stress test**

NECK

Dermoid Cysts

- These usually occur at sites of **embryological fusion**
- These may be in the midline
- A dermoid cyst in the neck may be mistaken for a thyroglossal cyst, although **it will not move on swallowing or protrusion of the tongue**
- A common site is the **external angular dermoid cyst in the eyebrow** area at the outer angle of the eye. Occasionally, there may be a dumbbell extension intracranially
- They occur if **ectodermal cells** become buried beneath the skin surface during development
- An **inclusion dermoid cyst** may similarly arise secondary to trauma.

Cystic Hygroma

- Commonly arising in the neck, these **fluid-filled lesions of lymphatic origin, lymphangioma**
- **MC site: Posterior triangle of neck**
- Seen in **Turner's syndrome, trisomies, fetal alcohol syndrome, multiple pterygium syndrome**
- **Brilliantly translucent, positive cough impulse**
- They are either present at birth, sometimes being diagnosed on antenatal ultrasonography, or may appear within the first 2 years or sometimes later
- **Infection l**eads to difficulty with subsequent surgery, which is thus best performed soon after diagnosis.

- **Excision is treatment of choice**
- Aspiration of the cysts and injection of a **streptococcal derivative 'OK432', bleomycin, picibanil** is a treatment that is proving to be an effective alternative to surgery.

Sternomastoid Tumor

- **It is due to infarction of sternomastoid muscle**
- Usually **during delivery**
- Infarcted muscle replaced by fibrosis
- Present **immediately after birth as a 'swelling' with the newborn keeping his/her neck to one side.**

Branchial Cyst

- Remanant of **second branchial cleft**
- Mc site is **upper part of neck** at junction of upper **anterior border** of sternomastoid
- **Wall is made of lymphoid tissue**
- **'NON'-translucent**
- **Complete excision** is treatment of choice.

Ranula (Latin rana = frog)

- This is a **sublingual cyst** which may be small or may fill the **floor of the mouth**
- Extravasation cyst of sublingual glands
- It may be related to a salivary or mucous gland
- It is thin-walled and contains clear viscid fluid. ↑
- Care is required not to **damage the submandibular duct** during its excision and marsupialization is often safer.

Chemodectoma

- **'Potato tumor' or carotid body tumor**
- **'Benign tumor' but rarely metastasizes (unusual combination)**
- **Arises from 'chemoreceptor zone'**
- **Nonchromaffin paraganglioma**
- **Origin from Schwann cells: Association with high altitude. Family history and pheochromocytoma**
- **Biopsy is contraindicated**
- Usually **unilateral**
- **Firm, rubbery, mobile from side to side, slow-growing**
- **Bruit** may be present
- **Angiogram** is diagnostic
- **Good prognosis, rarely metastasizes**
- **Surgical excision** is **'treatment of choice'**

- **Branchial Cyst**
  - ***Arises from 2nd branchial cleft***
  - ***Located usually at anterior border of upper 1/3 of sternomastoid***
  - ***Contains cholesterol crystals***
- **Branchial Fistula**
  - ***Represents persisting in 2nd branchial cleft***
  - ***Located usually at anterior border of lower 1/3 of sternomastoid***

- **Cystic Hygroma**
  - ***Represents lymphatic venous anastomotic failure***
  - ***Located usually in the neck lower in posterior triangle***
  - ***Brilliantly translucent***
- **Cervical Rib**
  - ***Mostly unilateral***
  - ***Mostly on right side***

Surgically Important Thyroid Conditions

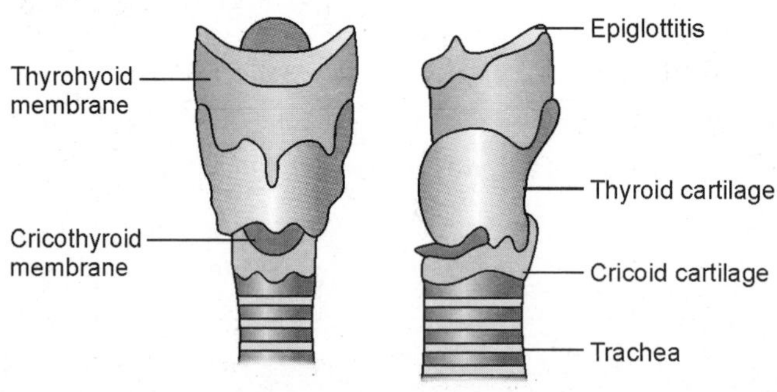

Ectopic thyroid and anomalies of the thyroglossal tract

- Some **residual thyroid tissue** along the course of the thyroglossal tract is not uncommon, and may be lingual, cervical or intrathoracic
- Very rarely the whole gland is ectopic.

Lingual thyroid

- This forms a rounded swelling at the **back of the tongue** at the **foramen cecum** (and it may represent the only thyroid tissue present
- It may cause dysphagia, impairment of speech, respiratory obstruction or hemorrhage
- It is best treated by full replacement with thyroxine when it should get smaller, but excision or ablation with radioiodine is sometimes necessary.

Median (thyroglossal) ectopic thyroid

- This forms a swelling in the **upper part of the neck** and is usually mistaken for a thyroglossal cyst.

Lateral aberrant thyroid

- There is no evidence that aberrant thyroid tissue ever occurs
- 'Normal thyroid tissue' found laterally, separate from the thyroid gland, **must be considered and treated as a metastasis** in a cervical lymph node from an occult thyroid carcinoma, almost **invariably of papillary type**.

Struma ovarii

- It is not ectopic thyroid tissue, but **part of an ovarian teratoma**
- Very rarely, neoplastic change occurs or hyperthyroidism develops.

Thyroglossal Cyst

- This may be present in any part of the **thyroglossal tract**
- MC site is **beneath the hyoid**, in the region of the thyroid cartilage, and above the hyoid bone
- **Occupies the midline**, except in the region of the thyroid cartilage, where the thyroglossal tract is pushed to one side, usually to the left.

- The **swelling moves upwards on protrusion of the tongue as well as on swallowing** because of the attachment of the tract to the foramen cecum

Never to be forgotten:

  - ***Subhyoid***
  - ***Painless***
  - ***Midline***
  - ***Nontransluminant but fluctuant swelling***

A thyroglossal cyst **should be excised (Sistrunk's operation)** because infection is inevitable, owing to the fact that the wall contains nodules of lymphatic tissue which communicate by lymphatics with the lymph nodes of the neck

Thyroglossal Fistula

- Thyroglossal fistula is **never congenital**
- It follows **infection or inadequate removal** of a thyroglossal cyst
- The cutaneous opening of such a fistula is **drawn upwards on protrusion of the tongue**
- A thyroglossal fistula is **lined by columnar epithelium**, discharges mucus, and is the seat of recurrent attacks of inflammation.

(Sistrunk's Operation)

Because the thyroglossal tract is so closely related to the body of the hyoid bone, this central part must be excised, together with the cyst or fistula, or recurrence is certain. When the thyroglossal tract can be traced upwards towards the foramen cecum, it must be excised with the central section of the body of the hyoid bone, and a central core of lingual muscle

USMLE HIGH YIELD

Remember

Most common congenital, cystic, midline neck mass. Thyroglossal duct cysts are benign cysts that can arise anywhere along the embryonic path of descent of the thyroid gland (from the foramen cecum to the level of the thyroid). Thyroglossal duct cysts can become infected, demonstrating rapid enlargement and tenderness, but are otherwise generally nontender and asymptomatic. Treatment is with surgical excision. The Sistrunk procedure, in which the cyst, the middle-third of the hyoid bone, and the thyroglossal duct tract are all excised, is associated with the lowest rate of recurrence.

GRANULOMATOUS THYROIDITIS—SUBACUTE THYROIDITIS

De Quervain's Thyroiditis

- This is due to a **virus infection**
- There is **pain in the neck**, **fever, malaise and a firm, irregular enlargement** of one or both thyroid lobes
- There is a **raised erythrocyte sedimentation rate**
- **Absent thyroid antibodies, uptake of Iodine in the gl and is low**
- The condition is **self-limiting:** Subsequent hypothyroidism is rare
- In 10 percent of cases, the onset is acute, the goiter very painful and tender, and there may be symptoms of hyperthyroidism
- The specific treatment for the acute case with severe pain is to give prednisone

Riedel's Thyroiditis

- Thyroid tissue is **replaced by cellular fibrous tissue** which infiltrates through the capsule into adjacent muscles, paratracheal connective tissue and the carotid sheaths
- It may occur in association with **retroperitoneal and mediastinal fibrosis**
- The goiter may be unilateral or bilateral and is **very hard and fixed**
- The **differential diagnosis from anaplastic carcinoma** can only be made with certainty by biopsy, when a wedge of the isthmus should also be removed to free the trachea
- If unilateral, the other lobe is usually involved later and subsequent **hypothyroidism** is common.

Solitary Thyroid Nodules

- More common in females
- Nodules classified as cold, warm or hot
- Most solitary thyroid nodules are cold
- Most cancers arise in cold nodules
- Risk of cancer in a cold nodule is 10-15%
- **Risk of tumor in a hot nodule is negligible**
- Scintigraphy of minimal use in evaluation of solitary thyroid nodules
- FNAC is the investigation of choice
- Thyroidectomy done (Hemithyroidectomy for solitary nodule)

MEN Syndromes

The multiple endocrine neoplasia (MEN) syndromes are distinct genetic entities that are expressed in several specific patterns of involvement.

MEN 1 is characterized by the concurrence of:

- Parathyroid hyperplasia
- Pancreatic islet cell neoplasms
- Adenomas of the anterior pituitary gland

MEN 2A is characterized by the concurrence of:

- Medullary thyroid carcinoma (MTC)
- Pheochromocytomas, and
- Parathyroid hyperplasia

MEN 2B consists of:

- MTC
- Pheochromocytoma
- Mucosal neuromas, and distinctive marfanoid habitus

These syndromes may occur de novo (especially MEN 2B) and are transmitted as **'autosomal dominant' traits**.

Medullary Carcinoma Thyroid

- MTC constitutes **5% to 10% of all thyroid malignancies**
- Approximately **80% of these represent sporadic cases of MTC**
- **Twenty percent of MTC** cases occur in a **familial setting**, either in association with **MEN 2A or MEN 2B**
- MTC is **usually the first abnormality expressed in both MEN 2A and MEN 2B** and in most patients, MTC is diagnosed either before or concurrently with pheochromocytoma
- The peak incidence of MTC in the setting of MEN 2A or MEN 2B is in the second or third decade of life, compared with the fifth or sixth decade in patients with sporadic MTC
- ***A diffuse premalignant proliferation of C-cells in the thyroid gland of patients with familial MTC has been described and is termed as C-cell hyperplasia.*** *Parafollicular clusters of increased number of C-cells represent the early manifestation of hyperplasia or microinvasive carcinoma that progresses to multifocal MTC*
- *The presence of bilateral MTC or microscopic evidence of C-cell hyperplasia in the areas of thyroid adjacent to macroscopic foci of MTC strongly suggests the presence of familial disease*
- ***MTC appears grossly as a circumscribed, gritty, whitish-tan nodule***
- *Microscopically, it consists of nests or sheets of uniform round or polygonal cells separated by variable amounts of fibrovascular stroma*
- ***Material with the staining properties of amyloid is frequently present in the stroma of MTC***
- *MTC can be* ***diagnosed immunohistochemically by demonstrating calcitonin within the MTC cells.***

- The most important product of MTC cells is **calcitonin**, which is a **sensitive tumor marker for the presence of MTC** whether in preoperative screening or postoperative evaluation
- Patients with clinically evident MTC most commonly present with a **palpable thyroid nodule or multinodular thyroid gland**. Enlarged, firm cervical lymph nodes suggest metastatic disease. Patients with locally **advanced disease may present with hoarseness, dysphagia, respiratory difficulty, or signs of distant metastases (e.g. lung, liver and bone).**

Papillary Carcinoma

- Mc thyroid cancer
- Encapsulated tumor
- Psammoma bodies seen
- **It can be diagnosed by FNAC (contrast follicular type)**
- **Usually multifocal.**

- Follicular type is a variety of papillary cancer
- Hurthle cell is a variety of follicular type
- Anaplastic is a rare type
- Thyroid lymphoma presents as rapidly growing tumor

- ***Thyroid tumor associated with MEN II: Medullary carcinoma***
- ***Thyroid tumor in thyroglossal cyst: Papillary carcinoma***
- ***Thyroid tumor in Hashimoto's thyroiditis: Papillary carcinoma***
- ***Thyroid tumor with best prognosis: Papillary carcinoma***
- ***Thyroid tumor least malignant: Papillary carcinoma***
- ***Thyroid tumor associated with worst prognosis: Anaplastic cancer***
- ***Thyroid tumor rarest: Anaplastic***

Thyroid Lymphoma

- **Seen in Hashimoto's disease**
- **Diffuse large type is a variant**
- **Radiosensitive**
- **Rapidly growing**
- **Radiotherapy + chemotherapy is used for treatment**

Complications of Thyroidectomy

1. Hemorrhage
2. Recurrent laryngeal nerve palsy
3. Superior laryngeal nerve palsy
4. Hypoparathyroidism
5. Hypothyroidism
6. Tracheal collapse
7. Thyroid crisis

- Hypocalcemia does not occur in hemithyroidectomy
- Neck swelling immediately after thyroid operation is usually tension hematoma
- In such cases: open immediately.

Cavernous Sinus Tumors

These are the most common cause of cavernous sinus syndrome. Tumors may be primary or may arise from either local spread or as metastases. Examples of primary tumors include **meningiomas or neurofibromas.** Examples of locally spreading tumors are **nasopharyngeal carcinoma or pituitary tumors**. Metastatic lesions are most often from the breast, prostate, or lung. Radiotherapy may offer transient relief, particularly in nasopharyngeal cancer.

Cavernous Sinus Aneurysms

Unlike intracranial aneurysms in other anatomic locations, carotid-cavernous aneurysms do not involve a major risk of subarachnoid hemorrhage. However, their rupture can result in direct C-C fistulas, which may lead to cerebral hemorrhage. These aneurysms, which are more frequent in the elderly population, **present with an indolent ophthalmoplegia.**

Carotid-Cavernous Fistulas

C-C fistulas are of 2 types: direct and indirect. **Direct fistulas** occur if the carotid artery and cavernous sinus are in continuity. They manifest with **abrupt onset of proptosis, chemosis, visual loss, and ophthalmoplegia**. **Indirect fistulas** occur with communication between the cavernous sinus and the branches of the internal carotid artery, external carotid artery, or both. They have a more insidious presentation than direct fistulas, often with spontaneous resolution. **Trauma or aneurysm rupture is a common cause of carotid-cavernous fistulas.**

Masses in Mediastinum

Anterior Mediastinal Masses	Middle Mediastinal Masses	Posterior Mediastinal Masses
• Thymoma • Lymphoma • Teratoma • Thyroid/parathyroid masses • Lipoma • Hiatal hernia • Retrosternal goiter	• Bronchogenic cysts • Pleura pericardial cysts • Aneurysms • Myxoma • Esophageal lesions • Lipoma	• Neurogenic tumors • Lymphoma • Metastatic germ cell tumor

Mediastinal Emphysema

- Air may enter the mediastinum from the **esophagus, trachea, bronchi, lung, neck, or abdomen,** producing **mediastinal emphysema or pneumomediastinum**
- Can occur from blunt or penetrating trauma, intraluminal injury, such as during endoscopy, as well as barotrauma. Positive-pressure ventilation
- ***Blunt trauma due to compressive forces on the thorax, especially when the glottis is closed and ventilation is being achieved with high pressures (usually in the setting of decreased lung compliance), may cause sufficient pressures at the intra-alveolar region to rupture alveoli***
- Dissection of air along vascular structures into the hilum and mediastinum creates a pneumomediastinum
- Mediastinal emphysema may also be caused by intra-abdominal air dissecting through the diaphragmatic hiatus
- **Spontaneous pneumomediastinum** is usually seen in patients with exacerbation of bronchospastic disease
- The clinical manifestations of this include substernal chest pain, which may radiate into the back and crepitation in the region of the suprasternal notch, chest wall and neck
- With increasing pressure, **the air can dissect into the neck, face, chest, arms, abdomen, and retroperitoneum**
- Frequently, **pneumomediastinum and pneumothorax 'occur simultaneously'**
- *Auscultation over the pericardium demonstrates a characteristic crunching sound that is accentuated during systole and is termed as **'Hamman's sign.'***

Mediastinitis

- **Infection of the mediastinal space**
- It is a **serious and potentially fatal process**

- These factors responsible include *perforation of the esophagus due to instrumentation, foreign bodies, penetrating or, more rarely, blunt trauma, spontaneous esophageal disruption (Boerhaave's syndrome), leakage from an esophageal anastomosis, tracheobronchial perforation, and mediastinal extension from an infectious process originating in the pulmonary parenchyma, pleura, chest wall, vertebrae, great vessels, or neck*
- Mediastinitis is manifested clinically by fever, tachycardia, leukocytosis, and pain that may be localized to the chest, back, or neck, although, in some patients, the clinical course remains indolent for long periods.

Mediastinal Hemorrhage

Mediastinal hemorrhage is most frequently caused by blunt or penetrating trauma, thoracic aortic dissection, rupture of aortic aneurysm, or surgical procedures within the thorax

Spontaneous mediastinal hemorrhage is a recognized entity with predisposing factors related to the following:

(1) complication of a mediastinal mass, of which thymoma, malignant germ cell tumor, parathyroid adenoma, retrosternal thyroid, and teratoma are the most common;

(2) sudden sustained hypertension;

(3) altered hemostasis due to anticoagulant therapy, thrombolytic therapy, uremia, hepatic insufficiency, or hemophilia; and

(4) transient, sharp increases in intrathoracic pressure, which occur during coughing or vomiting, an entity initially described by

Retrosternal pain radiating to the back or neck is common

'Compression of mediastinal structures' (primarily the great veins) develop, *including dyspnea, venous distention, cyanosis, and cervical ecchymosis due to blood dissecting into soft tissue planes*

Sufficient accumulation of blood causes ***mediastinal tamponade*** *manifested by tachycardia, hypotension, reduced urinary output, equalization of right- and left-sided cardiac filling pressures, and diastolic collapse of the right ventricle*

The development of mediastinal tamponade ***is more insidious*** *than pericardial tamponade because of the larger volume of the mediastinum.*

Diagnostic measures include chest films, which may indicate:

- **Superior mediastinal widening**
- **Loss of the normal aortic contour and**
- **Soft tissue density in the anterosuperior mediastinum**

- *MC anterior mediastinal mass: Thymoma*
- *MC middle mediastinal mass: Bronchogenic cyst*
- *MC posterior mediastinal mass: Neurogenic tumor*
- *MC malignant mass of mediastinum: Lymphoma*

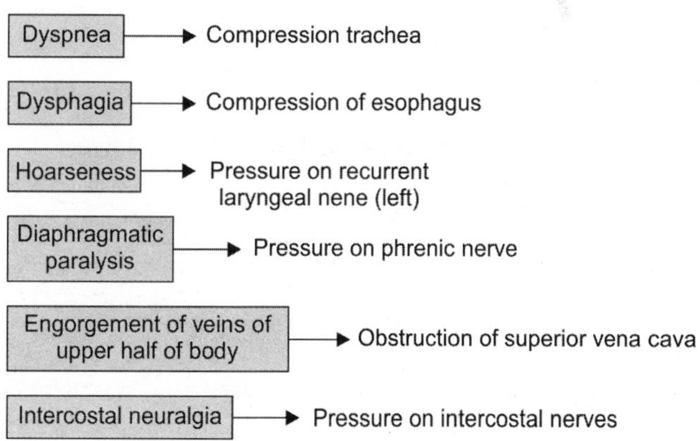

Cardiac Tumors

Primary cardiac tumors are rare and usually require an intensive work-up to pinpoint the diagnosis. Seventy-five percent of primary cardiac tumors are benign and among these, myxoma is the most common. The tumors are usually single; the most common location is the left atrium. They may cause syncopal episodes or even shock and death due to obstruction by a 'ball valve' mechanism.

Most Common Site

• Cancer lip	• **Vermillion border of lower lip**
• Cancer tongue	• **Lateral border**
• Cancer cheek	• **Angle of mouth**
• Nasopharyngeal carcinoma	• **Fossa of Rosenmuller**
• Cancer larynx	• **Glottis**
• **Epulis**	• **Discrete swelling on gums (Mc fibrous epulis)**
• **Radicular/Dental cyst**	• **Arises from normally erupted tooth**
• **Dentigerous cyst**	• **Arises from nonerupted tooth**
• **Adamantinoma**	• **Arises from dental lamina, MC site mandible**

Esophagus

- **25 cms** long
- Upper 1/3: Striated, middle 1/3 mixed. Lower 1/3: smooth muscle
- Constrictions: **15 cms, 25 cms, 40 cms** from incisor teeth
- **Most common site** of impaction is **below cricopharyngeus**
- **No submucosal plexus,** only Auerbach's plexus present
- **No serosa** present
- **Three parts: Cervical, thoracic, abdominal**
- **Arterial supply:** Inferior thyroid artery, branches of aorta and left gastric artery respectively

Esophagitis

Esophagitis

Most common causes are:

- **Reflux esophagitis (mc)**
- Infectious esophagitis
- Eosinophilic esophagitis
- Drug-induced esophagitis
- Radiation esophagitis
- Corrosive esophagitis

Monilial Esophagitis

- Esophagitis due to *Candida albicans* is relatively common in **patients taking steroids, including steroid inhalers for asthma**
- It may present with **dysphagia or odynophagia**
- There may be visible thrush in the throat
- Endoscopy shows numerous **white plaques that cannot be moved**, unlike food residues
- **Biopsies are diagnostic.** In severe cases, a barium swallow may show dramatic mucosal ulceration and irregularity that is surprisingly similar to the appearance of esophageal varices

Acquired Immunodeficiency Syndrome (AIDS) and the Esophagus

- Dysphagia and odynophagia may occur in immune deficiency due to infection with a variety of agents including *Candida*, **herpes simplex virus and cytomegalovirus**
- Similar infections may arise in **immune suppression** due to any other cause.

Crohn's Disease

- The esophagus is **not commonly** affected by Crohn's disease.

- Rarely, it may be the only site of Crohn's disease
- Symptoms are **severe**
- Endoscopy shows **extensive esophagitis**. Biopsies may show only nonspecific inflammation. In severe cases, a barium swallow may show **deep sinuses in the esophagus**
- Crohn's esophagitis **responds poorly to medical treatment** and resection may be required.

Plummer–Vinson Syndrome

- **Also called the Brown Kelly–Patterson syndrome or sideropenic dysphagia**
- Describes young women with koilonychias, iron-deficiency anemia and dysphagia referred high in the neck
- The dysphagia is caused by spasm or a web in the postcricoid area
- The patients have an increased tendency to postcricoid cancer

Schatzki's Ring

- It is a circular submucosal ring in the **distal esophagus** usually at the **squamocolumnar junction**
- Short segment of luminal stenosis.
- The core of the ring consists of variable amounts of **fibrous tissue and cellular infiltrate**
- Most rings are **incidental findings** on barium examination
- Some are associated with **dysphagia for solids which is intermittent** and a **single dilatation is curative.**

Mallory–Weiss syndrome

- Forceful vomiting may produce a **mucosal/submucosal tear at the cardia rather than a full perforation of the esophagus**
- Vomiting occurs against an **open** glottis
- Common in alcoholics
- **Cardia of stomach** and not esophagus is the commonest site
- Diagnosis is by esophagogastroscopy.

Boerhaave's Syndrome

- Forceful vomiting may produce **full perforation of the esophagus** (spontaneous perforation)
- Presents with acute chest pain
- Most serious type of perforation because of the volume of infected material that is released under pressure
- Vomiting occurs against a **closed glottis**. The pressure in the esophagus rapidly increases and the esophagus bursts at its weakest point in the lower third. Mostly follows **heavy bout of drinking alcohol**
- Part above gastroesophagel junction is the commonest site
- Pain in chest and upper abdomen is the mc manifestation. Surgical exploration in the form of **primary repair** is done.

Achalasia Cardia

- Esophegal **motility disorder**
- **Increased difficulty in swallowing for both liquids/solids**
- **Failure of relaxation** of lower esophageal, increased pressure
- **Dysphagia is the presenting symptom**
- Loss of ganglion cells in Auerbach's plexus
- **Bird-beak appearance**
- **Cucumber esophagus**
- **Heller's myotomy** is treatment of choice
- **Pseudoachalasia: Caused by adenocarcinoma of cardia, bronchogenic ca, pancreatic ca.**

USMLE Case Scenario

A 46-year-old nonalcoholic presents to a gastroenterologist with multiple episodes of chest pain, regurgitation of saliva and undigested food. The characteristic appearance of the esophagram shows a tapered 'bird's beak' deformity at the level of the esophagogastric junction. Further manometry yields high resting pressures of the lower esophageal sphincter, which fails to relax. Most likely the disease is: Achalasia of the cardia

Diffuse Esophageal Spasm

- Incoordinate contractions of esophagus
- **'Corkscrew'** appearance on barium swallow
- **Heller's myotomy and partial fundoplication are used as treatment**.

Motility Disorders of Esophagus

Also occur in:
- **Systemic sclerosis**
- **Polymyositis**
- **Dermatomyositis**
- **Mixed CT disorders**

Dysphagia Lusoria

It is dysphagia **secondary to vascular anomalies**:
- Double aortic arch
- Right aortic arch
- Aberrant right subclavian artery
- Abnormal innominate artery
- So diagnosis is by **arteriography**

Zenker's Diverticulum

- **Mc esophegeal diverticulum**
- **In elderly age group usually**
- **Weakness in the posterior hypopharyngeal wall (Killian's triangle)**

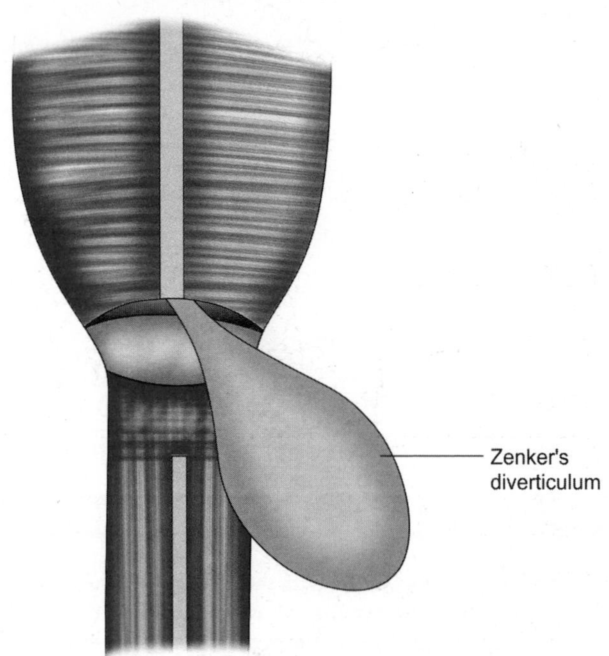

- **Pulsion** diverticulum
- **Intermittent dysphagia, regurgitation, gurgling sound in the neck**
- Causes halitosis, regurgitation of saliva and food, dysphagia or complete obstruction. Symptomatic Zenker's diverticula are treated by **cricopharyngeal myotomy with or without diverticulectomy**
- Very large symptomatic esophageal diverticula are **removed surgically by:**
  - Excision of pouch or cricopharyngeal myotomy
  - Dohlman's procedure

Esophageal Hernias

Type I

- **'Sliding' hernia**
- It is **dislocation of cardia of stomach** into posterior mediastinum and presents with GERD
- MC type
- Lesser complications occur
- Treatment is generally medical for uncomplicated cases
- Treatment is surgical for all complicated cases

Type II

- **'Paraesophegal'** hernia
- Cardia is normal but gastric fundus, colon or small gut is dislocated
- Cardiorespiratory arrest, dysphagia are seen
- Complications are more common and severe
- Treatment is surgical even for uncomplicated cases

Barrett's Esophagus

- **Metaplasia seen**
- Metaplasia of **'squamous epithelium'** to **columnar in esophagus at lower end**
- **Because of prolonged GERD**
- **Intestinal type metaplasia** is the commonest
- Progression to **adenocarcinoma** occurs

Complications:

- **Barrett's ulcer**
- **Stricture**
- **Perforation**
- **Progression to adenocarcinoma occurs**
- **Diagnosis suggested by endoscopy**
- **Diagnosis confirmed by biopsy**

Barrett's esophagus may occur in a small number of patients who have gastroesophageal reflux disease (GERD). This condition is a metaplasia of the normal squamous mucosa of the esophagus to a columnar (glandular) type of epithelium, and is usually seen as a response to repeated acid exposure to the distal esophagus. Tobacco and alcohol use are also thought to contribute to the process. The significance of Barrett's esophagus is that it may lead to the development of low-grade dysplasia, high-grade dysplasia, or esophageal adenocarcinoma.

Esophageal Diverticula

These are epithelial-lined mucosal pouches that protrude from the esophageal lumen. Almost all of them are acquired and occur predominantly in adults.

- **A true diverticulum: Contains all layers of the normal esophageal wall, including mucosa, submucosa, and muscle, whereas a false diverticulum consists primarily of only mucosa and submucosa**
- **Pulsion diverticula arise because elevated intraluminal pressure forces the mucosa and submucosa to herniate through the esophageal musculature; therefore, they are false diverticula.**

Traction diverticula are the result of external inflammatory reaction in adjacent mediastinal lymph nodes that adhere to the esophagus and pull the entire wall toward them as they heal and contract; they are true diverticula.

Pharyngoesophageal Diverticula

- **The pharyngoesophageal diverticulum is the most common esophageal diverticulum, generally occurring in patients between 30 and 50 years of age and, therefore, believed to be acquired**
- **The diverticulum characteristically arises within the inferior pharyngeal constrictor, between the oblique fibers of the thyropharyngeus muscle and the more horizontal fibers of the cricopharyngeus muscle, the upper esophageal sphincter (UES).**
- **The transition in the direction of these muscle fibers (Killian's triangle) represents a point of potential weakness in the posterior pharynx and is the site of formation of the pharyngoesophageal diverticulum**
- **Pharyngoesophageal diverticula are usually associated with complaints of cervical dysphagia, effortless regurgitation of undigested particles of food or pills sometimes consumed hours earlier, a gurgling sensation in the neck on swallowing, choking, and recurrent aspiration**
- **A barium esophagogram establishes the diagnosis**
- **Surgical therapy in symptomatic patients is indicated in most cases, regardless of the size of the pouch and, it is hoped, before complications occur.**

Esophageal Varices

- Important site for communication between the intra-abdominal splanchnic circulation and the systemic venous circulation is through the esophagus
- The increased pressure in the esophageal plexus produces dilated tortuous vessels called varices. Persons with cirrhosis develop varices so that varices are present in approximately two-thirds of all cirrhotic patients
- Varices appear as tortuous dilated veins lying primarily within the submucosa of the distal esophagus and proximal stomach.

Intramural Hematoma

- Emetogenic injury, particularly in patients with **bleeding abnormalities**, can cause bleeding between the mucosal and muscle layers of the esophagus
- The patients develop sudden dysphagia
- The diagnosis is made by barium swallow and computed tomography
- Resolution is usually spontaneous.

Foreign Bodies

- Foreign bodies may lodge in the cervical esophagus
- Impaction of a bolus of food, particularly a piece of meat or bread, may occur when the esophageal lumen is narrowed due to stricture, carcinoma, or a lower esophageal ring (nonprogressive dysphagia)
- Acute impaction causes a complete inability to swallow and severe chest pain
- Both foreign bodies and food boluses may be removed endoscopically.

Esophageal Cancer

Predisposing factors for esophageal cancer

- **Excess alcohol**

- **Cigarette smoking**
- **Ingested (nitrates, fungal toxins in pickles)**
- **Smoked opiates**
- **Hot tea**
- **Corrosives**
- **Radiation strictures**
- **Chronic achlasia**
- **Caustic ingestion**
- **External beam irradiation**
- **Diverticulae**
- **Plummer-Vinson syndrome**
- **Tylosis**
- **Molybdenum, Zinc and Vitamin A deficiency**
- **Celiac sprue**
- **Barrett's esophagus**

Features: Progressive dysphagia (mc) weight loss, weakness, anemia, hoarseness

Esophagoscopy is the diagnosis of choice.

- **Mc type** of esophageal cancer: Squamous cell ca
- **Mc site** of esophageal cancer: Lower end
- Mc site of adenocarcinoma: Lower end
- Mc site of squamous cell ca: Middle 1
- Chemotherapy has limited role and **cisplatin, bleomycin and 5 fluorouracil** are used.

Esophagectomies

- Cervical esophagus: **Transhiatal** esophagectomy
- Upper thoraxic: **Transincisional/Transhiatal** esophagectomy
- Mid thoraxic: **Transincisional/Ivor Lewis surgery**
- Lower thoraxic: **Ivor-lewis surgery**

Abdomen

The abdominal wall is composed of nine layers.

From outward in, they are:

(1) Skin
(2) Subcutaneous tissue
(3) Superficial fascia (Scarpa's fascia)
(4) External abdominal oblique muscle
(5) Internal abdominal oblique muscle
(6) Transversus abdominis muscle
(7) Transversalis fascia
(8) Extraperitoneal adipose and areolar tissue
(9) Peritoneum

Omphalitis

- This is infection of the umbilicus
- Results from poor hygiene and is treated with appropriate cleansing and local care to the umbilicus
- However, in the neonatal period, omphalitis may result from bacterial infection and may potentially be associated with serious sequelae, such as portal vein thrombosis.

Rectus Sheath Hematoma

- Extravasation of blood into the rectus sheath.
- It is usually the result of trauma.
- Patients with rectus sheath hematomas most often give a history of receiving anticoagulant drugs for various conditions.
- When the hematoma develops, it ordinarily occurs at the level of the semicircular line of Douglas, where the inferior epigastric artery enters the rectus sheath.
- Patients complain of an acute illness, with abdominal pain over the hematoma, nausea, and vomiting. Frequently, a tender mass is palpable. Operation is indicated only if more serious conditions cannot otherwise be excluded.

Desmoid Tumors

- These are benign fibrous tumors that arise from the musculoaponeurotic abdominal wall.
- These tumors are histologically benign but frequently are locally invasive and are prone to recurrence after local excision.
- They present as firm, subcutaneous masses that grow slowly. They should be widely excised to prevent local recurrence. They do not have a propensity toward metastasis.

STOMACH: MOST DISTENSIBLE/DILATED PART OF DIGESTIVE TRACT

Arterial Supply

Left gastric artery	**Branch of celiac trunk**
Right gastric artery	**Branch of common hepatic artery**
Left gastroepiploic artery	**Branch of gastroduodenal artery**
Right gastroepiploic artery	**Branch of splenic artery**

Celiac Trunk

- **LEFT GASTRIC ARTERY**→ esophageal branch, gastric branch
- **COMMON HEPATIC ARTERY**→ right hepatic, left hepatic, gastroduodenal artery → supraduodenal, right gastroepiploic, superior pancreaticoduodenal artery
- **SPLENIC ARTERY**→ short gastric, left gastroepiploic, pancreatic branches

'Congenital' Hypertrophic Pyloric Stenosis on USG

- Common in males
- Presents about 4 weeks after birth
- Nonbilious vomiting is a feature
- Weight loss with hypochloremic alkalosis is a feature
- Halstead's procedure is done
- Isotonic normal saline is the fluid of choice

Pyloric Mass Best Felt During Feeding

- **Target sign:** Hypoechoic ring and hypertrophied pyloric muscle
- Pyloric muscle wall **thickness 3 mm**
- Pyloric volume greater than **1.4 cm^3**
- Pyloric length greater than **1.2 cm**
- **Cervix sign:** Indentation of muscle mass on fluid-filled antrum on long scan
- **Antral nipple sign:** Redundant pyloric canal mucosa protruding into gastric antrum

Chronic Gastritis

It is defined as the presence of chronic inflammatory changes in the mucosa leading eventually to mucosal atrophy and epithelial metaplasia.

Classification of Gastritis

- **Type A:** Autoimmune gastritis—Associated with pernicious anemia. Body of the stomach is usually affected
- **Type B:** Environmental gastritis—Results from dietary or intraluminal factors, specially *Helicobacter* pylori. Usually localized in the antrum. In severe cases, the inflammation spreads to the proximal part of the stomach
- **Type C:** Chemical gastritis—Associated with ingestion of nonsteroidal anti-inflammatory drugs or bile influx.

MC BENIGN NEOPLASM IS LEIOMYOMA

Gastric Cancer

- More than 90% of gastric tumors are **carcinomas**
- Lymphomas, carcinoids and stromal tumors are **relatively infrequent**
- The two main types of gastric adenocarcinomas are the **intestinal and diffuse types**
- Macroscopic patterns of both types may be exophytic, flat or depressed, or excavating
- **Intestinal type of adenocarcinoma *is associated with chronic gastritis caused by H. pylori infection,*** with gastric atrophy and intestinal metaplasia; composed of malignant cells forming intestinal glands
- **Diffuse type of adenocarcinoma *is not associated with H. pylori infection; composed of gastric type of mucous cells*** (signet ring cells) that permeate the mucosa without forming glands.

Adenocarcinoma Most Common

Antrum Most Common Site

- ***Helicobacter*** seems to be principally associated with **carcinoma of the body and distal stomach** rather than the proximal stomach
- As ***Helicobacter*** is associated with gastritis, gastric atrophy and intestinal **pernicious anemia and gastric atrophy** are at increased risk, as are those with gastric polyps metaplasia
- **Peptic ulcer surgery**, particularly those who have had drainage procedures such as **Billroth II or Polya gastrectomy, gastroenterostomy or pyloroplasty**
- **Excessive salt intake, deficiency of antioxidants**
- **Exposure to N-nitroso compounds**
- **Type A blood group**
- **Family history**
- **Li-Fraumeni syndrome, HNPCC, FAP, Peutz-Jeghers syndrome**

Features

- *Earliest symptom is **vague postprandial heaviness***
- *Features: weight loss, (MC), ascites, jaundice*
- *Enlarged lt. **Supraclavicular node (Virchow's node) 'Troisier's' sign***
- ***Sister Mary Joseph's nodule** around the umbilicus*
- *Secondaries in ovary **(Krukenberg's tumor)***
- *Peritoneal implants in pelvis **(Blumer's shelf)***
- ***'Trousseau's' sign and DVT (both Troiser's and Trousseau's sign)***
- Best diagnosis is by: 'ENDOSCOPY WITH BIOPSY'

Complications After Gastric Surgeries

- **Duodenal fistula (blow-out)**
- **Recurrent ulceration**
- **Gastrojejunocolic fistula**

- **Dumping syndromes**
- **Osteomalacia/osteoporosis**
- **Anemia**
- **Intestinal obstruction**
- **Carcinoma**

'Early' gastric cancer

- Primary lesion confined to **mucosa and submucosa**
- **Excellent prognosis**

'Advanced' cancer

- It is extension **below submucosa into muscle (Muscularis)**

Gastric Lymphoma

- Most common in the **sixth decade**
- The common symptoms being **pain, weight loss and bleeding**
- Acute presentations of gastric lymphoma such as hematemesis, perforation or obstruction are not common
- Primary gastric lymphomas are **B-cell-derived**, the tumor arising from the **mucosa-associated lymphoid tissue (MALT)**
- Primary gastric lymphoma remains in the stomach for a prolonged period before involving the lymph nodes
- Diagnosis is by **endoscopic biopsy**
- Infection with ***H. pylori,*** increases the risk for gastric lymphoma in general and MALT lymphomas in particular
- Microscopically, the vast majority of gastric lymphoid tumors are **non-Hodgkin's lymphomas of B-cell origin**; Hodgkin's disease involving the stomach is extremely uncommon
- Radiotherapy plus chemotherapy is used for treatment
- Bleeding, perforation and residual disease warrant surgery

- **MALT lymphomas are present at extranodal sites**
- **MALT lymphomas are predisposed by *H. pylori***
- **MALT lymphomas are sensitive to chemotherapy.**

Acute Gastric Dilatation

- This condition usually occurs in association with some form of ileus which is not treated by nasogastric suction
- **The stomach, which may also be atonic, dilates enormously**
- Often the patient vomits, is also dehydrated and has electrolyte disturbances
- Failure to treat this condition can result in a sudden massive vomit with aspiration into the lungs
- The **treatment is nasogastric suction, fluid replacement** and treatment of the underlying condition.
- Surgery is not advocated.

Trichobezoar and Phytobezoar

Trichobezoar (hair balls)

- These are unusual and are virtually exclusively found in **female psychiatric patients**, often young
- It is caused by the pathological **ingestion of hair which remains undigested** in the stomach
- The hair ball can **lead to ulceration and gastrointestinal bleeding, perforation or obstruction**
- The diagnosis is made easily at **endoscopy** or, indeed, from a plain radiograph
- Treatment consists of **removal of the bezoar** which may require open surgical treatment

Phytobezoar

- **These are made of the 'vegetable matter'** and found principally in patients who have gastric stasis.

Volvulus of the Stomach

- **Rotation of the stomach** usually occurs around the axis and between its two fixed points, i.e. the cardia and the pylorus.

- Rotation can occur in the **horizontal (organoaxial) 'most common'** or vertical (mesenterioaxial) direction
- This condition is usually associated with **paraesophageal herniation**
- The transverse **colon moves upwards to lie under the left diaphragm**, thus taking the stomach with it, and the stomach and colon may both enter the chest through the eventration of the diaphragm
- The condition is **commonly chronic**, the patient presenting with difficulty in eating. An acute presentation with ischemia may occur.

Ulcers

These are defined as a break in the mucosal surface >5 mm in size, with depth to the submucosa.

Duodenal ulcer	Gastric ulcer
• **More** common	• Less common
• More associated with ***H. pylori***	• Associated with ***H. pylori***
• **Early age** of onset	• Later age of onset
• Occurs most often in the **first portion of duodenum**, with ~90% located within 3 cm of the pylorus	• Occurs most often in the lesser curvature
• **Less chances of malignancy**	• More chances of malignancy
• **No loss** of weight	• Loss of weight
• Tenderness usually ***in R. Hypochondrium***	• Tenderness usually midline
• Night pain **common**	• Night pain uncommon

- **Curling's ulcer: GI ulcers in severe burns**
- **Cushing's ulcer: GI ulcers in head injury**

• ***MC site of gastric ulcer***	• Lesser curvature
• ***MC site of duodenal ulcer***	• Duodenal cap
• ***MC site of carcinoma stomach***	• Antrum
• ***MC site of Zollinger-Ellison syndrome***	• Pancreas

Malignant Gastric Ulcer

- Ulcer ≥ 2.5 cms
- Ulcer within a mass
- Folds that don't radiate from ulcer margin

Perforated Peptic Ulcer

- It is the **second most common complication** of peptic ulcer
- Usually located anteriorly
- *Duodenal ulcer perforation is more common in younger*
- *Gastric ulcer perforation is more common in older*
- *Gastroduodenal artery bleeds in duodenal ulcer*
- Free gas under diaphragm is indicative
- Treatment is by: Nasogastric suction, acid suppression, broad-spectrum antibiotics are used
- Exploratory laparotomy

Surgical treatment of duodenal ulcers:

- **Highly selective vagotomy (Least chance of diarrhea/dumping syndrome)**
- **Selective vagotomy and drainage**

- **Truncal vagotomy and drainage**
- **Truncal vagotomy and anterectomy (lowest chance of recurrence)**

Surgical treatment of gastric ulcers:

- **Distal gastrectomy**
- **Vagotomy, pyloroplasty and ulcer excision**

Dumping Syndrome

Dumping syndrome consists of a series of vasomotor and gastrointestinal signs and symptoms and occurs in patients who have undergone vagotomy and drainage (especially Billroth procedures)

Early Dumping

- Takes place **15 to 30 min** after meals
- Consists of crampy abdominal discomfort, nausea, diarrhea, belching, tachycardia, palpitations, diaphoresis, light-headedness and, rarely, syncope
- Cause: **Rapid emptying of hyperosmolar gastric contents** into the small intestine
- Fluid shift into the gut lumen with plasma volume contraction and acute intestinal distention
- Release of vasoactive gastrointestinal hormones (vasoactive intestinal polypeptide, neurotensin, motilin)

Late Dumping

- Typically occurs **90 min to 3 h** after meals
- **Vasomotor symptoms** (light-headedness, diaphoresis, palpitations, tachycardia, and syncope) predominate during this phase
- This component of **dumping** is thought to be **secondary to hypoglycemia** from excessive insulin release
- *Dumping **syndrome** is most noticeable after **meals rich in simple carbohydrates** (especially sucrose) and **high osmolarity***
- *Ingestion of **large amounts of fluids** may also contribute*
- *Up to **50% of postvagotomy and drainage patients** will experience **dumping syndrome** to some degree*
- *Signs and symptoms **often improve with time***
- ***Dietary modification** is the cornerstone of therapy for patients with **dumping syndrome***
- ***Small, multiple (six) meals devoid of simple carbohydrates** coupled with elimination of liquids during meals is important*
- ***Antidiarrheals and anticholinergic agents** are complimentary to diet*

*The somatostatin analogue **octreotide** has been successful in diet-refractory cases.*

Short Bowel Syndrome

Clinical problems that often occur following resection of varying lengths of small intestine

Features

- **Diarrhea and/or steatorrhea**
- **Increase in renal calcium oxalate calculi** is observed in patients with a small intestinal resection with an intact colon and is due to an increase in oxalate absorption by the large intestine, with subsequent hyperoxaluria
- **Gastric hypersecretion** of acid

Treatment

- Diet should be **low-fat, high-carbohydrate** to minimize the diarrhea proton pump inhibitor may be helpful
- **Fat-soluble vitamins**, folate, cobalamin, calcium, iron, magnesium, and zinc are the most critical factors to monitor on a regular basis
- If these approaches are not successful, **TPN r**epresents an established therapy that can be maintained for many years
- **Intestinal transplantation** is beginning to become established as a possible approach for individuals with extensive intestinal resection who cannot be maintained without TPN.

Bacterial Overgrowth Syndrome or Stagnant Bowel Syndrome

- **Diarrhea, steatorrhea, and macrocytic anemia** whose common feature is the proliferation of colon-type bacteria within the small intestine
- Due to **stasis caused by:**
  - **Impaired peristalsis (i.e. functional stasis)**
  - **Changes in intestinal anatomy (i.e. anatomic stasis)**
  - **Direct communication between the small and large intestine**
- Presence of increased amounts of a colonic-type bacterial flora, such **as *E. coli* or Bacteroides**, in the small intestine
- **Macrocytic anemia** is due to cobalamin, not folate, deficiency
- **Steatorrhea** is due to impaired micelle formation as a consequence of a reduced intraduodenal concentration of bile acids and the presence of unconjugated bile acids
- Best established by a **Schilling test** which should be abnormal following the administration of 58 co-labeled cobalamin, with or without the administration of intrinsic factor
- **Following the administration of tetracycline for 5 days, the Schilling test will become normal, confirming the diagnosis of bacterial overgrowth.**

Healthy Differences Between Two Unhealthy Diseases

Ulcerative Colitis	**Crohn's disease**
• Involves rectum always	• Involves ileum mostly
• May cause '**pancolitis**' • **Diffuse involvement**	• Nondiffuse involvement • Called **'regional enteritis'**
• Retrograde spread to ileum is **backwash ileitis**	
• Disease of continuity	• Skip lesions
• Pseudopolyps present	• Pseudopolyps absent
• Limited to mucosa and submucosa	• Transmural inflammation
• Noncaseasting granulomas not seen	• Noncaseating granulomas seen
• Creeping fat not seen • Crypt abscess	• Creeping fat seen • Crypt abcess also seen
• Strictures, ulcerations, fistula less frequent	• Strictures, ulcerations, fistula frequent
• Toxic megacolon occurs	• Rare
• Malignant transformation +++ • Malignant transformation + • Malignant transformation from dysplastic sites • **Takes 10 years to develop** • **Common in younger patients** • Associations of UC: – **Pyoderma gangreonosum** – **Erythema nodosum**	• Malignant transformation +

'Pseudomembranous' Enterocolitis

A 14-year-old girl presents to the GI Clinic with the complain of watery diarrhea tinged with blood. Her medications are topical benzoyl peroxide and oral clindamycin for acne vulgaris. Physical examination reveals a slightly distended abdomen that is diffusely tender.

Surgery in UC

There are several well-identified complications that require urgent **operation for survival**. These include:

- ***Massive, unrelenting hemorrhage***
- ***Toxic megacolon with impending or frank perforation***
- ***Fulminating acute ulcerative colitis that is unresponsive to steroid therapy***
- ***Obstruction from stricture***
- ***Suspicion or demonstration of colonic cancer***

The largest number of colectomies for ulcerative colitis are performed for less dramatic indications, as the disease enters an intractable chronic phase and becomes both a physical and a social burden to the patient

For Hemorrage/Bleeding: Prompt surgical intervention is indicated after hemodynamic stabilization. More than 50% of patients with acute colonic bleeding have toxic megacolon. So one should be suspicious of the coexistence of the two complications. Uncontrollable hemorrhage from the entire colorectal mucosa may be the one clear indication for emergency proctocolectomy. If possible, the rectum should be spared for later mucosal proctectomy with ileoanal anastomosis.

Acute Toxic Megacolon

- It can occur in both ulcerative colitis and Crohn's disease
- Its incidence is higher in ulcerative colitis
- Patients usually present clinically with the **onset of abdominal pain and severe diarrhea (greater than 10 stools per day), followed by abdominal distention and generalized tenderness**
- Once megacolon and toxicity develop, fever, leukocytosis, tachycardia, pallor, lethargy, and shock ensue. It is important to note that any of these manifestations **can be masked** by chronic steroid use and the generally poor nutritional condition of the patient
- An abdominal radiograph usually shows dilation of the transverse and occasionally the sigmoid colon that is greater than 5 cm and averages 9.2 cm. Thickening and nodularity of the bowel wall due to mucosal inflammation are also noted
- **Initial treatment for toxic megacolon includes intravenous fluid and electrolyte resuscitation, nasogastric suction, broad-spectrum antibiotics to include anaerobic and aerobic gram-negative coverage, and total parenteral nutrition to improve nutritional status.** Proctoscopy may be helpful in determining the etiology of the attack, as may culture of the stool.

Adipose Tissue Changes of Crohn's Disease

- Fat Hypertrophy
- **Fat Wrapping (Creeping fat)**
- More than **50%** of intestinal surface may be covered by fat, especially along the **antimesenteric border** and sometimes leading to the **obliteration of bowel mesentry angle**
- Creeping fat is well demonstrated by **CT scan**

Ulcers in GIT

- **Transverse ulcers: TB**
- **Longitudinal ulcer: Crohn's disease**
- **'Flask'-shaped ulcer: Amebic ulcer**

Tumors of Small Bowel

BENIGN:

- Adenoma
- Lipoma
- Angioma
- Hamartoma

MALIGNANT:
- Adenocarcinoma
- Carcinoid
- Lymphoma
- Sarcoma

Small Intestine

- **Blood Supply:** The small intestine receives its blood supply from the **superior mesenteric artery**, the second largest branch of the abdominal aorta
- **Peyer's patches** are lymph nodules aggregated in the submucosa of the small intestine. These lymphatic nodules are most abundant in the ileum, but the jejunum also contains them
- **Mucosa:** The mucosal surface of the small intestine contains numerous circular mucosal folds called the **plicae circulares (valvulae conniventes, or valves of Kerckring).** These folds are 3 to 10 mm in height; they are taller and more numerous in the distal duodenum and proximal jejunum, becoming shorter and fewer distally
- **Intestinal villi** barely visible to the naked eye resemble tiny finger-like processes projecting into the intestinal lumen.

Acute Mesenteric Ischemia and Infarction

- Classified as occlusive or nonocclusive
- ***Occlusion* accounts for about 75%** of acute intestinal ischemia
- Result from an arterial thrombus **(one-third of arterial occlusions)** or **embolus (two-thirds of arterial occlusions)** of the celiac or superior mesenteric arteries
- **Arterial embolus** occurs most commonly in patients with **chronic or recurrent atrial fibrillation, artificial heart valves, or valvular heart disease**
- **Arterial thrombosis** is usually associated with **extensive atherosclerosis or low cardiac output**
- **Venous occlusion is rare**; it is occasionally seen in women taking oral contraceptives
  - The major clinical feature of acute **mesenteric ischemia is severe abdominal pain, often colicky and periumbilical at the onset**, later becoming diffuse and constant
  - **Superior mesenteric arteries** are commonly involved
  - **Vomiting, anorexia, diarrhea, and constipation** are also frequent
  - Examination of the abdomen may reveal **tenderness and distention**
  - Bowel sounds are often normal even in the face of severe infarction. Some patients have a surprisingly normal abdominal examination in spite of severe pain
  - Mild gastrointestinal bleeding is often detected by examination of stool for occult blood; gross hemorrhage is unusual except in ischemic colitis. Leukocytosis is often present
  - Later in the course of the disease (24 to 72 h), **gangrene of the bowel occurs with diffuse peritonitis, sepsis, and shock**
  - Abdominal plain films in patients with **mesenteric ischemia** may reveal air-fluid levels and distention
  - Barium study of the small intestine reveals nonspecific dilation, poor motility, and evidence of thick mucosal folds **(thumb printing)**
  - Acute **mesenteric ischemia** is a grave condition with a high morbidity and mortality
  - **Arteriography** is diagnostic
  - **Embolectomy** is the treatment

Chronic Intestinal Ischemia

- It is called **abdominal angina**
- Occurs under conditions of **increased demand for splanchnic blood flow**
- The patient complains of **intermittent dull or cramping midabdominal pain 15 to 30 min after a meal,** lasting for several hours postprandially.

- Significant weight loss due to decreased food intake **(food fear)** may be present
- Arteriographic studies should be performed to confirm the diagnosis
- The only definitive treatment is **vascular surgery or balloon angioplasty** to remove the thrombus or the **construction of bypass arterial grafts to the ischemic bowel**

Appendix

- MC position is **retrocecal**
- Appendicular artery is an **end artery**
- **McBurney's point is in relation to appendicitis**

Acute Appendicitis

- The peak incidence of acute **appendicitis** is in the second and third decades of life
- It is relatively rare at the extremes of age
- The most commonly accepted theory of the pathogenesis of appendicitis is that it results from obstruction followed by infection. The lumen of the appendix becomes obstructed by hyperplasia of submucosal lymphoid follicles, a fecalith, tumor, or other pathologic condition. Once the lumen of the appendix is obstructed, the sequence of events leading to acute appendicitis
- Infection with **Yersinia** organisms cause the disease (PSEUDOAPPENDICITIS)
- Left sided appendicitis is diverticulosis
- Most commonly caused by a **fecalith**, which results from accumulation and inspissation of fecal matter around vegetable fibers
- **Enlarged lymphoid follicles** associated with viral infections (e.g. measles), inspissated barium, worms (e.g. Oxy uris)
- (Pinworms, *Ascaris*, and *Taenia*), and tumors (e.g. carcinoid or carcinoma) may also obstruct the lumen
- **Tenderness at Mcburney's point**
- Retrocecal appendicitis: Rigidity absent
- **Pelvic and postileal appendicitis: Diarrhea (MISSED FREQUENTLY)**
- Gangrene and perforation occur. If the process evolves slowly, adjacent organs such as the terminal ileum, cecum, and omentum may wall off the appendiceal area so that a localized abscess will develop, whereas rapid progression of vascular impairment may cause perforation with free access to the peritoneal cavity
- **Signs:**
  - **Hamburger sign (significant anorexia)**
  - **Pointing sign**
  - **Rovsing's sign**
  - **Psoas sign**
  - **Obturator test**
- Acute **appendicitis** may be the first manifestation of Crohn's disease
- Fever greater than 102 °F and leucocyte count greater than 18,000/mm^3 suggests **ruptured appendix**
- The history and sequence of symptoms are important diagnostic features of **appendicitis**
- The initial symptom is almost invariably *abdominal pain* usually poorly localized in the periumbilical or epigastric region with an accompanying urge to defecate or pass flatus, neither of which relieves the distress
- **Appendicitis** is the most common extrauterine condition requiring abdominal operation
- **USG is helpful in diagnosis**
- **USG and CT scan are confirmatory**
- The treatment is early operation and appendectomy as soon as the patient can be prepared
- The *only* circumstance in which operation is *not* indicated is the presence of a palpable mass 3 to 5 days after the onset of symptoms.

Mucocele of Appendix:

- **It is a benign tumor/retention cyst**
- **It can progress to malignancy.**

Appendicular Carcinoid:
- **Mc malignant tumor of appendix**
- **Adenocarcinoma of appendix is rare**
- **Treated by right hemicolectomy.**

Peritoneal cavity

- **It is the largest cavity in the body**
- Mc causative organism of **acute bacterial peritonitis** is ***E. coli*** followed by Klebsiella
- **Peritoneal mesotheliomas** are associated with asbestos exposure
- **Lymphoma and retroperitoneal sarcoma are the most common malignant lesions of retroperitoneum**
- **'Ormond's disease' is idiopathic retroperitoneal fibrosis**
- **'Peritoneal mice' is *Appendicis epiploicae***
- **Commonest site of intraperitoneal abscess is 'pelvic'.**

Pneumococcal Peritonitis

There are two forms of this disease: (1) primary, and (2) secondary to pneumonia
- **Primary** pneumococcal peritonitis is more common
- The patient is often an undernourished girl between 3 and 6 years of age, and it is probable that the infection sometimes occurs via the vagina and Fallopian tubes, for pneumococci have been cultured from patients' vaginas
- In males, the infection is blood-borne from the upper respiratory tract or the middle ear. After the age of 10, pneumococcal peritonitis is most unusual
- Associated with nephritic syndrome
- Children with nephritis are more liable to this condition than others.

Familial Mediterranean fever (periodic peritonitis)
- **Characterized by abdominal pain and tenderness, mild pyrexia, polymorphonuclear leucocytosis and occasionally pain in the thorax and joints**
- The duration of an attack is 24–72 hours, when it is followed by complete remission but exacerbations recur at regular intervals
- Most of the patients have undergone appendicectomy in childhood
- This disease, often **familial**, is limited principally to **Arabs, Armenians and Jews;** other races are occasionally affected
- The peritoneum—**particularly in the vicinity of the spleen and the Gallbladder is inflamed**
- There is no evidence that the interior of these organs is abnormal. Colchicine may prevent recurrent attacks.

Peritoneal bands and adhesions
- **Congenital bands and membranes**. Intestinal obstruction is rarely seen except by an obliterated vitellointestinal duct
- Peritoneal adhesions
- Peritoneal adhesions are abnormal deposits of fibrous tissue that form after peritoneal injury
- They follow operation or peritonitis and are the commonest cause of small bowel obstruction and secondary female infertility in developed countries.

Talc granuloma
- Talc (silicate of magnesium) should never be used as a **lubricant for rubber gloves** for it is a cause of peritoneal adhesions and granulomas in the Fallopian tubes.

Starch peritonitis
- Like talc, starch powder has found disfavor as a surgical glove lubricant
- In a few starch-sensitive patients, it causes a painful ascites, fortunately of limited duration.

Frequently asked

Subphrenic abscess

Anatomy

The complicated arrangement of the peritoneum results in the formation of four peritoneal and three extraperitoneal spaces in which pus may collect. Three of these spaces are on either side of the body, and one is approximately in the midline

Left superior (anterior) intraperitoneal (left subphrenic)

- It is bounded above by the diaphragm, and behind by the left triangular ligament and the left lobe of the liver, the gastrohepatic omentum and anterior surface of the stomach. To the right is the falciform ligament and to the left the spleen, gastrosplenic omentum and diaphragm
- Patient is toxic
- The common cause of an abscess here is an **operation on the stomach, the tail of the pancreas, the spleen or the splenic flexure of the colon.**

Left inferior (posterior) intraperitoneal (left subhepatic)

- It is another name for the 'lesser' sac
- The commonest cause of infection here is complicated **acute pancreatitis**. In practice, a perforated gastric ulcer rarely causes a collection here because the potential space is obliterated by adhesions.

Right superior (anterior) intraperitoneal (right subphrenic)

- Lies between the right lobe of the liver and the diaphragm. It is limited posteriorly by the anterior layer of the coronary and the right triangular ligaments, and to the left by the falciform ligament
- Common causes here are perforating cholecystitis, a perforated duodenal ulcer, a duodenal cap 'blow-out' following gastrectomy and appendicitis.

Right inferior (posterior) intraperitoneal (right subhepatic)

- It lies transversely beneath the right lobe of the liver in Rutherford Morison's pouch
- It is bounded on the right by the right lobe of the liver and the diaphragm. To the left is situated the foramen of Winslow and below this lies the duodenum. In front are the liver and the gallbladder, and behind, the upper part of the right kidney and diaphragm
- The space is bounded above by the liver and below by the transverse colon and hepatic flexure. It is the deepest space of the four and the commonest site of a subphrenic abscess which usually arises from appendicitis, cholecystitis, a perforated duodenal ulcer or following upper abdominal surgery.

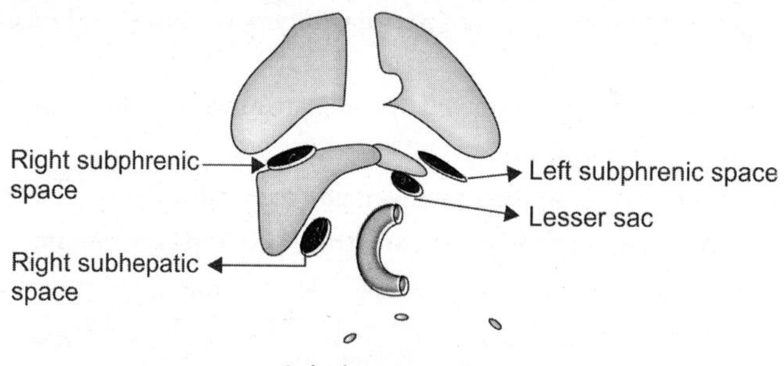

Subphrenic spaces

Syndromes Associated with Small Intestinal Neoplasms

- **Bessauds-Hillmand-Augier Syndrome**. Sexual infantilism associated with intestinal polyposis
- **Carter-Horsley-Hughes Syndrome**. Diffuse polyposis of the small and large intestine
- **Cowden's Disease or Multiple Hamartoma Syndrome**. Hamartomatous, juvenile, lipomatous, or inflammatory polyps are present mainly in the stomach and colon but are also present in the small intestine. Benign and malignant breast and thyroid disease are also found in these patients, as well as mucocutaneous lesions, trichilemmoma, acral keratoses, and oral papillomas
- **Cronkhite-Canada Syndrome**. This syndrome is characterized by generalized gastrointestinal polyposis and **ectodermal defects such as alopecia, excessive skin pigmentations, and nail atrophy**. In the intestinal polyps, dilated cystic glands are found in an edematous lamina propria. Loss of protein from the gut, along with calcium, magnesium, and potassium deficiencies, may occur
- **Familial Polyposis of the Colon**. This syndrome is customarily associated with polyps of the colon, but cases of generalized polyposis have been recorded, with associated malignancy.

- **Gardner's Syndrome**. This syndrome is generally characterized by **rectal and colonic polyposis,** but generalized polyposis has been recorded. These polyps are involved in the development of adenocarcinoma. The syndrome also includes **cysts of the skin, osteomas, fibrous and fatty tumors of the skin and mesentery, follicular odontomas, and dentigerous cysts and changes in the bony structures of the jaws**. This syndrome is familial and is transmitted as an autosomal dominant trait
- **Gordon's Disease**. This is a **protein-losing gastroenteropathy, usually manifested as Ménétrier's disease**, which involves mucosal hypertrophy, hyperplasia of the superficial epithelium, degeneration in the glandular layer, and hypoproteinemia due to leakage of proteins through the mucous membranes. A diffuse gastrointestinal polyposis associated with protein loss has also been reported
- **Juvenile Polyposis**. Juvenile polyposis is most commonly found in the colon and rectum, but isolated examples of generalized gastrointestinal polyposis have been reported with and without family history or other congenital abnormalities.

- **Muir-Torre Syndrome**. This syndrome was described to include **sebaceous adenomas, epidermoid cysts, fibromas, desmoids, lipomas, fibrosarcomas and leiomyomas with visceral cancers**
- **Peutz-Jeghers Syndrome.** This syndrome is characterized by **hamartomatous polyps** of the gastrointestinal tract (stomach, small bowel, colon) that are associated with mucocutaneous pigmentation (lips, oral mucosa, fingers, forearm, toes, umbilical area). The skin pigmentation may fade after puberty, but that of the mucous membrane is retained
- ***Pseudoxanthoma elasticum***. Benign **vascular lesions of the intestinal tract** have been reported in association with this disease
- **Rendu-Osler-Weber Disease.** This disease is described as **telangiectasia** of the nasopharynx or gastrointestinal tract
- **Turcot's Syndrome**. **Malignant brain tumors** are associated with inherited intestinal adenomatous polyposis
- **von Recklinghausen's Disease**. **Generalized neurofibromatosis** with café au lait skin pigmentation may also include **neurofibromas of the gastrointestinal tract.**

Non-neoplastic Polyps

- Hyperplastic polyps
- Hamartomatous polyp
- Inflammatory polyp
- Almost all other polyps are malignant
- Juvenile polyp is most common in children
- **Villous adenoma has the highest malignant potential than other histological types.**

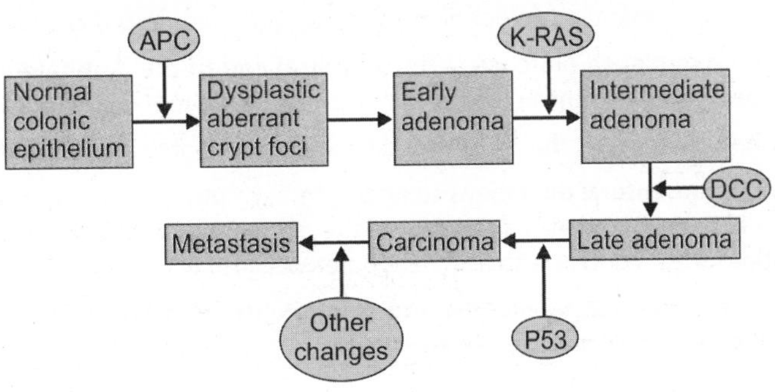

Malignant polyps

Meckel's Diverticulum

- **A true congenital diverticulum**
- It is a **vestigial remnant of the omphalomesenteric duct** (also called the **vitelline duct**), and is the most frequent malformation of the gastrointestinal tract
- Meckel's diverticulum is located in the **distal ileum**, usually within about 60-100 cm of the ileocecal valve
- It is typically **3–5 cm long**, runs **antimesenterically** and has its own blood supply
- It is a remnant of the connection from the umbilical cord to the small intestine present during embryonic development.

A Memory Aid is the Rule of 2s

- **2%** (of the population)
- **2** feet (from the ileocecal valve)
- **2** inches (in length)
- **2%** are symptomatic
- **2** types of common ectopic tissue (gastric and pancreatic)
- Most common age at clinical presentation is **2**
- Males are **2** times as likely to be affected.

- It can also be present as an indirect hernia, where it is known as a **'Hernia of Litter'**
- Furthermore, it can be attached to the umbilical region by the vitelline ligament, with the possibility of vitelline cysts, or even a patent vitelline canal forming a vitelline fistula when the umbilical cord is cut
- Torsions of intestine around the intestinal stalk may also occur, leading to **obstruction, ischemia, and necrosis**
- **Symptoms**
  - The majority of people afflicted with Meckel's diverticulum are **asymptomatic**. If symptoms do occur, they typically appear before the age of two
  - The most common presenting symptom is **painless rectal bleeding,** followed by intestinal obstruction, volvulus and intussusception. Occasionally, Meckel's diverticulitis may present with all the features of acute appendicitis
  - **A technetium-99m (99mTc) pertechnetate scan** is the investigation of choice to diagnose Meckel's diverticula
  - Other tests such as colonoscopy and screenings for bleeding disorders should be performed, and angiography can assist in determining the location and severity of bleeding. Meckel's diverticulitis occurs more often in males
  - Can be a leading point of intussusception.

Omphalomesenteric Duct Remnants

- Remnants of the omphalomesenteric (vitelline) duct may present as abnormalities related to the abdominal wall
- In the fetus, the omphalomesenteric duct connects the fetal midgut to the yolk sac. This normally obliterates and disappears completely. However, any or all of the fetal ducts may persist.

- **An umbilical polyp** is a small excrescence of **omphalomesenteric duct mucosa** that is retained in the umbilicus. Such polyps resemble umbilical granulomas except that they do not disappear after silver nitrate cauterization.
- **Umbilical sinuses** result from the continued presence of the **umbilical end of the omphalomesenteric duct**. These resemble umbilical polyps, but close inspection reveals the presence of a sinus tract deep to the umbilicus.
- Persistence of the **entire omphalomesenteric duct** is heralded by the passage of enteric contents from the umbilicus.
- **Cystic remnants of the omphalomesenteric duct** may persist and be asymptomatic for long periods of time. The **cysts** may be connected to the ileum with a fibrous band that is a remnant of the obliterated omphalomesenteric duct. Patients may present with acute volvulus and intestinal obstruction or with acute abdomen because of cyst infection.
- **Meckel's diverticulum** results when **the intestinal end of the omphalomesenteric duct persists.** This is a true diverticulum of the intestine with all layers of the intestinal wall represented.

Colonic Polyposis Syndromes

• **Gardner's Syndrome**	• Colonic cancer associated with soft tissue tumors (osteomas, lipomas, cysts, fibrosarcomas).
• **Turcot's Syndrome**	• Colonic cancer associated with central nervous system malignancies.
• **Cronkhite-Canada Syndrome**	• Intestinal polyps, hyperpigmentation with alopecia and absence of finger nails.
• **Hereditary Polyposis Coli Syndrome or** • **APC (Adenomatous Polyposis Coli)**	• Most important presenting with hundreds of polyps • 100% chances of malignant transformation • Autosomal dominant with involvement of chromosome 5.

• **Hereditary Non-Polyposis Coli Syndrome (Lynch Syndrome)**	• This consists of three family members having at leat two generations with colonic cancer • There is a high risk of associated ovarian and endometrial cancer in this syndrome.
• **Cowden's Syndrome**	• Hamartomas with increased risk of bleeding especially in a child presenting with rectal bleeding.

Colonic Diverticula

- Herniations or sac-like **protrusions of the mucosa** through the muscularis, at the point where a nutrient artery penetrates the muscularis
- Most commonly in the **sigmoid colon** and decrease in frequency in the proximal colon
- They **increase with age**
- Related to an **increase in intraluminal pressure**
- Diet, deficient in dietary fiber or roughage. Results in decreased fecal bulk, narrowing of the colon, and an increase in intraluminal pressure in order to move the smaller fecal mass
- Colonic diverticula are usually asymptomatic and are an incidental finding on barium enema or colonoscopy.

Diverticulitis

- Inflammation can occur in diverticular sac
- The cause is mechanical, related to retention in the diverticula of undigested food residue and bacteria, which may form a hard mass called a fecalith
- More often in the left as in the right colon
- Acute colonic diverticulitis is a disease of variable severity characterized by **fever, left lower quadrant abdominal pain, and signs of peritoneal irritation—muscle spasm, guarding, rebound tenderness**
- Rectal bleeding, usually microscopic, is noted in 25% of cases; it is rarely massive. Polymorphonuclear leukocytosis is common
- Massive hemorrhage from colonic diverticula is one of the most common causes of hematochezia in patients over age 60
- Complications include free perforation, which results in acute peritonitis, sepsis, and shock, particularly in the elderly
- Abscess formation or fistulas then occur as the inflammatory mass burrows into other organs. Severe pericolitis may cause a fibrous stricture around the bowel, which can be associated with colonic obstruction and may mimic a neoplasm
- **Diagnosis:** During the acute phase of diverticulitis, barium enema and sigmoidoscopy may be hazardous, since contrast material or air under pressure may lead to rupture of an inflamed diverticulum and convert a walled-off inflammatory lesion to a free perforation
- Colonoscopy or surgical excision may be required for accurate diagnosis. Abdominal computed tomography scan may demonstrate the presence of a pericolic abscess.

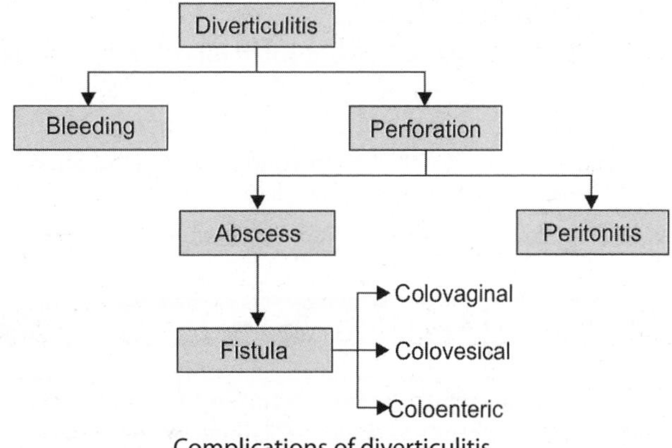

Complications of diverticulitis

Aganglionic Megacolon (Hirschsprung's Disease)

- Congenital disorder due to **absence of enteric neurons** (ganglions) in the distal colon and rectum
- Hirschsprung's disease or congenital aganglionic megacolon is caused by a congenital absence of the ganglion cells of both the Meissner and Auerbach plexuses
- It is the most common cause of lower intestinal obstruction in the neonatal period. In early childhood, it may present as chronic constipation with intermittent fecal soiling. It occurs predominantly in males and there is an increased family incidence
- The biopsy would reveal an absence of ganglion cells in the submucosal and myenteric plexuses
  - Some patients have an autosomal dominant form of the disease with mutations in the *RET* gene
  - The aganglionic and contracted segment of bowel is unable to relax to permit passage of stool, causing the **normal proximal colon to become greatly dilated**
  - Barium enema reveals a narrowed segment in the rectosigmoid, with **massive dilation above. (never forget)**
  - Diagnosis is made by **full-thickness surgical biopsy**
  - The treatment of choice is a **pull-through procedure** in which normally innervated colon is anastomosed to the distal rectum just above the internal sphincter, thus bypassing the contracted aganglionic segment and restoring normal defecation.

Acquired Megacolon

In **Central and South America,**

Infection with ***Trypanosoma cruzi* (Chagas disease)**

Result in **destruction of the ganglion cells of the colon**

Onset is in adult life

- Schizophrenia
- Depression
- Cerebral atrophy

Spinal cord injury and

- Parkinsonism also may cause megacolon
- Myxedema and primary systemic sclerosis also can reduce colonic motility and produce marked colonic distention.

Acute Intestinal Pseudo-obstruction

- Referred to as **Ogilvie's syndrome**
- Involving primarily the **colon** but occasionally also the small intestine

Examination reveals a:

- **Distended, tympanitic abdomen**
- **Reduced or absent bowel sounds**
- **Localized tenderness** over the distended colon is common
- Abdominal films reveal **massive dilation of the colon and small intestine, occasionally with the presence of air-fluid levels**

- **The cecum**, being the most capacious part of the colon, is often massively dilated and tender
- Management requires careful correction of fluid and electrolyte abnormalities, intubation of the stomach or small intestine for decompression, and avoidance of drugs that depress intestinal motility
- **Barium enema may be hazardous** because of the risk of perforating the already dilated bowel.

USMLE Case Scenario

A 79-year-old man with Pick's disease undergoes surgery for a fractured femoral neck. On the 6th postoperative day, his abdomen is grossly distended and tense, but not tender. He has occasional bowel sounds. The rectal vault is empty on digital

examination, and there is no evidence of occult blood. X-ray films show a few distended loops of small bowel and a much distended colon. The cecum measures 9.5 cm in diameter. The gas pattern of distention extends throughout the entire large bowel, including the sigmoid and rectum. No stool is seen in the films. Vital signs are normal for his age.
Most likely diagnosis is: Ogilvie Syndrome

Intussusception

- **Outer** tube: Intussuscipiens
- **Inner** Tube: Intussusceptum
- Stool **Red currant jelly**
- Lump Sausage-shaped
- Emptiness in Iliac Fossa **Sign de dance**
- Barium enema **Claw sign**

USMLE Case Scenario

A 6-month-old brought by his mother presents with episodes of distress and crying interspersed with quiet periods of normal behavior and playing. His mother says that he passes stool mixed with mucus and blood, the jelly stool. The abdomen is soft and nontender. A sausage-like mass may be palpable in the upper abdomen. Most likely diagnosis is: Intussusception

- **Volvulus of gut is** usually **clockwise**
- **Volvulus of sigmoid colon** is usually **anticlockwise**
- Intussusception is usually of type **ileocolic**

Ischemic Colitis

- Most often affects the **elderly**
- Ischemic colitis is almost always **nonocclusive**
- In **acute fulminant ischemic colitis**, the major manifestations are **severe lower abdominal pain, rectal bleeding, and hypotension**
- Dilation of the colon and physical signs of peritonitis are seen in severe cases
- Abdominal films may reveal **thumb printing from submucosal hemorrhage and edema**
- **Barium enema is hazardous** in the acute situation because of the risk of perforation. Sigmoidoscopy or colonoscopy may detect ulcerations, friability, and bulging folds from submucosal hemorrhage
- **Surgical resection may be required** in some patients with fulminant ischemic colitis to remove gangrenous bowel; others with lesser degrees of ischemia may respond to **conservative medical management**
- **Subacute ischemic colitis** is the most common clinical variant of ischemic colonic disease. It produces lesser degrees of pain and bleeding, often occurring over several days or weeks.

Angiodysplasia of the Colon

- **Vascular ectasias or arteriovenous malformations (AVMs)** that occur in the right colon of many older individuals and may cause bleeding
- Angiodysplasia is a degenerative lesion consisting of **dilated, distorted, thin-walled vessels lined by vascular endothelium**
- Lesions are **usually multiple and are found primarily in the cecum** and ascending colon, but in some patients, they may be distributed from the stomach to the rectum
- **Colonoscopy** is diagnostic which allows treatment by laser photocoagulation, electrocautery, or injection with sclerosant
- Some patients with massive uncontrolled bleeding or multiple sites of angiodysplasia may require **right hemicolectomy**
- Angiodysplasias may also respond to **chronic estrogen-progesterone therapy.**

Colorectal Cancer

- Most colorectal cancers, regardless of etiology, arise from **adenomatous polyps**
- Probability of an adenomatous polyp becoming a cancer depends on the gross appearance of the lesion, its histologic features, and its size
- *Adenomatous polyps may be* ***pedunculated (stalked) or sessile (flat-based)****. Cancers develop more frequently in sessile polyps*
- *Villous adenomas, most of which are sessile, become malignant more than three times as often as tubular adenomas*
- *The likelihood that any polypoid lesion in the large bowel contains invasive cancer is related to the size of the polyp, being negligible (< 2%) in lesions < 1.5 cm, intermediate (2 to 10%) in lesions 1.5 to 2.5 cm in size and substantial (10%) in lesions > 2.5 cm*
  - ***Mc site: Rectum***
  - ***Mc site in colon: Sigmoid colon***
  - ***Mc type: Adenocarcinoma***
  - ***Right-sided common in females***
  - ***Right-sided presents as anemia***
  - ***Left-sided presents as obstruction/pain.***

Etiology and Risk Factors

Risk factors for the development of colorectal cancer

- *Upper socioeconomic populations*
- *↑meat protein*
- *↑dietary fat and oil as well as elevations in the serum cholesterol*
- *↑alcohol*
- *Smoking*
- *Sedentary habits*
- *Obesity*
- *Deficiency of antioxidants*
- *Family history of the disease*
- ***Streptococcus bovis bacteremia***
- *Ureterosigmoidostomy*
- *UC*
- *Crohn's disease*
- *FAP*

Protective Factors

- **Aspirin and other nonsteroidal anti-inflammatory drugs**, which are thought to suppress cell proliferation by inhibiting prostaglandin synthesis
- **Oral folic acid supplements and oral calcium supplements** have been found to reduce the risk of adenomatous polyps and colorectal cancers in case-control studies
- **Ascorbic acid, tocopherols, and β-carotene**
- **Estrogen replacement therapy**

Clinical Features

- **Lesions of the right colon** commonly ulcerate, leading to chronic, insidious blood loss without a change in the appearance of the stool. Patients with tumors of the ascending colon often present with symptoms, such as **fatigue, palpitations, and even angina pectoris and are found to have a hypochromic, microcytic anemia indicative of iron deficiency**
- Radiographs of the abdomen often reveal characteristic annular, constricting lesions **('apple-core' or 'napkin-ring')**

- **Cancers arising in the rectosigmoid** are often associated with **hematochezia, tenesmus, and narrowing of the caliber of stool;** anemia is an infrequent finding
- Liver is the most common site of metastasis. 1/3rd patients show hepatic metastasis
- Surgery is treatment of choice
  - **Anterior resection:** for tumors of upper 2/3rd of rectum
  - **Combined abdominoperineal resection:** for extensive tumors of lower 1/3rd of rectum
  - **Immunotherapy:** for disseminated carcinoma colon

Anal Canal Above Dentate Line	Anal Canal Below Dentate Line
• Endodermal	• Ectodermal
• Cuboidal epithelium	• Stratified squamous
• Superior rectal artery • Superior rectal vein	• Inferior rectal artery • Inferior rectal vein
• Internal iliac group of lymph nodes	• Superficial inguinal group of lymph nodes
• Pain-insensitive	• Pain-sensitive

The Anal Valves of Ball

- These are a series of transversely placed semilunar folds linking the columns of Morgagni. They lie along and actually constitute the waviness of the dentate line.

The Crypts of Morgagni (syn. anal crypts)

- These are small pockets between the inferior extremities of the columns of Morgagni. Into several of these crypts, mostly those situated posteriorly, open one anal gland by a narrow duct
- Infection of an anal gland can give rise to an abscess, and infection of an anal gland is the most common cause of anorectal abscesses and fistulae.

The Anorectal Ring

- Marks the junction **between the rectum and the anal canal**
- It is formed by the joining of the **puborectalis muscle, the deep external sphincter, conjoined longitudinal muscle and the highest part of the internal sphincter**
- The anorectal ring can be **clearly felt digitally**, especially on its posterior and lateral aspects
- Division of the anorectal ring results in **permanent incontinence of feces**
- The position and length of the anal canal, as well as the angle of the anorectal junction, depend to a major extent on the **integrity and strength of the puborectalis muscle sling**.

Fistula-in-Ano

- A fistula-in-ano is a track, lined by granulation tissue, which connects deeply in the anal canal or rectum and superficially on the skin around the anus
- It usually results from an anorectal abscess which burst spontaneously or was opened inadequately
- The fistula continues to discharge and, because of constant reinfection from the anal canal or rectum, seldom, if ever, closes permanently without surgical aid
- An anorectal abscess may produce a track, the orifice of which has the appearance of a fistula, but it does not communicate with the anal canal or the rectum. By definition, this is not a fistula, but a sinus

Types of anal fistulae

- **Low-level fistulae** open into the anal canal below the anorectal ring
- **High-level fistulae** open into the anal canal at or above the anorectal ring.

Malignant Lesions of the Anus and Anal Canal

- Squamous cell carcinoma (most common)
- Basaloid carcinoma

- Mucoepidermal carcinoma
- Basal cell carcinoma
- Malignant melanoma
- Anal intraepithelial neoplasia (AIN)

Most Common Sites

- Typhoid ulcer: Terminal ileum
- Tuberculous ulcer: Terminal ileum
- Crohn's disease: Terminal ileum
- Gallstone ileus: Terminal ileum
- Ulcerative colitis: Rectum
- Amebic colitis: Sigmoid colon
- Volvolus: Sigmoid colon
- Diverticulae: Sigmoid colon

Referred Abdominal Pains

- Biliary colic to: Right shoulder
- Renal colic to: Groin
- Appendicitis to: Periumbilical to right iliac fossa
- Pancreatitis to: Back
- Ruptured aortic aneurysm to: Back
- Hip pain to: Knee

Important Signs in Patients with Abdominal Pain

Sign	Finding	Association
Cullen's sign	Bluish periumbilical discoloration	• ***Retroperitoneal hemorrhage (hemorrhagic pancreatitis, abdominal aortic aneurysm rupture)***
Kehr's sign	Severe left shoulder pain	• ***Splenic rupture ectopic pregnancy rupture***
McBurney's sign	Tenderness located 2/3rd distance from anterior iliac spine to umbilicus on the right side	• ***Appendicitis***
Murphy's sign	Abrupt interruption of inspiration on palpation of right upper quadrant	• ***Acute cholecystitis***
Iliopsoas sign	Hyperextension of right hip causing abdominal pain	• ***Appendicitis***
Obturator's sign	Internal rotation of flexed right hip causing abdominal pain	• ***Appendicitis***
Grey-Turner's sign	Discoloration of the flank	• ***Retroperitoneal hemorrhage (hemorrhagic pancreatitis, abdominal aortic aneurysm rupture)***
Chandelier's sign	Manipulation of cervix causes patient to lift buttocks off table	• ***Pelvic inflammatory disease***
Rovsing's sign	Right lower quadrant pain with palpation of the left lower quadrant	• ***Appendicitis***

Important Appearances

• Corkscrew esophagus	Diffuse esophageal spasm
• Rosary esophagus	Diffuse esophageal spasm
• 'Double Bubble sign in X-ray abdomen'	Annular pancreas, Duodenal atresia
• 'Scalloping of sigmoid colon'	Ulcerative colitis
• 'Microcolon on barium enema.'	Ileal atresia
• 'Bird of prey sign'	Sigmoid volvolus
• 'String sign'	Crohn's disease
• 'Pipestem colon'	Ulcerative colitis
• Saw tooth appearance of colon	Diverticular disease
• Apple core lesion/Napkin ring appearance	Lt Colonic Ca
• Coffee bean sign	Volvulus
• Claw sign/Signe de dance	Intussusception
• Thumb printing sign	Ischemic colitis

USMLE Case Scenario

Physical examination of the newborn reveals an infant with facial features suggestive of Down's Syndrome. The infant then has bilious vomiting. An X-ray film showing the kidneys, ureters, and bladder (KUB) is performed, which shows a distended and gas-filled stomach and proximal duodenum and the absence of gas in the distal bowel. Most likely diagnosis is: Duodenal Atresia.

USMLE Case Scenario

An 88-year-old male who was bedridden for past few months as a result of stroke presents with nausea, vomiting, colicky abdominal pain. X-rays show distended loops of bowel with large air shadow like parrot's beak. He would be assumed to be having volvilus

Burst Abdomen (syn. Abdominal Dehiscence)

- A **serosanguinous (pink) discharge** from the wound is a forerunner of disruption
- Most pathognomonic sign of impending wound disruption
- Signifies that intraperitoneal contents are lying extraperitoneally
- Patients often volunteer the information that they **'felt something give way'**
- If skin sutures have been removed, omentum or coils of intestine may be forced through the wound and will be found lying on the skin. Pain and shock are often absent
- There may be symptoms and signs of intestinal obstruction

Saphena varix

- A saccular **enlargement of the termination of the long saphenous vein,** usually accompanied by other signs of varicose veins
- The swelling **disappears completely when the patient lies flat**, while a femoral hernia sac is usually still palpable
- In both, there is an **impulse on coughing**
- A saphena varix will, however, **impart a fluid thrill to the examining fingers** when the patient coughs or when the saphenous vein below the varix is tapped with the fingers of the other hand. Sometimes a **venous hum** can be heard when a stethoscope is applied over a saphena varix.

- **Composition of a hernia**

As a rule, a hernia consists of three parts — the sac, the coverings of the sac and the contents of the sac.

- **The sac**

The sac is a diverticulum of peritoneum consisting of mouth, neck, body and fundus. The neck is usually well-defined, but in some direct inguinal hernias and in many incisional hernias, there is no actual neck. The diameter of the neck is important because strangulation of bowel is a likely complication where the neck is narrow, as in femoral and paraumbilical hernias.

- **The body of the sac**

The body of the sac varies greatly in size and is not necessarily occupied. In cases occurring in infancy and childhood, the sac is gossamer-thin. In long-standing cases, the wall of the sac may be comparatively thick.

- **The covering**

Coverings are derived from the layers of the abdominal wall through which the sac passes. In long-standing cases they become atrophied from stretching and so amalgamated that they are indistinguishable from each other.

- **Contents**

These can be:

  - ***Omentum = omentocele (syn. epiplocele)***
  - ***Intestine = enterocele. More commonly small bowel, but may be large intestine or appendix***
  - ***A portion of the circumference of the intestine Richter's hernia***
  - ***A portion of the bladder (or a diverticulum)***
  - ***Ovary with or without the corresponding Fallopian tube***
  - ***A Meckel's diverticulum = a Littre's hernia***
  - ***Fluid — as part of ascites or as a residuum thereof.***

Important Hernia to be remembered

• **Maydl's hernia**	Strangulated loops of bowel like W in abdomen
• **Pantaloon/Saddle bag hernia**	Occurrence of both direct and indirect inguinal hernia in the same patient
• **Sliding hernia**	Hernia with sigmoid colon on left and cecum on right side
• **Laugier's hernia**	Femoral hernia through lacunar ligament of Gimbernat
• **Narath's hernia**	Hernia with congenital dislocation of hip
• **Spigelian hernia**	An interparietal usually subumbilical hernia
• **Obturator hernia**	Hernia through obturator canal
• **Epigastric hernia**	Hernia through linea alba
• **Littre's hernia**	Hernia of Meckel's diverticulum
• **Richter's hernia**	Hernia of a portion of circumference of bowel
• **Morgagni's hernia**	Hernia between coastal and sterna parts of diaphragm

Hernia-en-Glissade

- Hernia-en-Glissade is also called **sliding hernia**
- The contents of hernia on **left side** are sigmoid colon and mesentery
- Most common content **is sigmoid colon**
- The contents of hernia on **right side** are the cecum
- Sliding hernia occurs mostly in **males**
- Five out of every six cases occur on **left side**
- The incidence of hernia increases with **increasing age**

Spigelian Hernia

- Spigelian hernia is an **interparietal** hernia
- It lies at the level of **arcuate line** mostly
- The arcuate line lies below umbilicus. Hence, it is a **subumbilical** hernia
- **Lies lateral to rectus abdominis**
- The **spigelian fascia** is present only below the umbilicus and most of the spigelian hernias are present subumbilically
- In addition to this, the fibrous bands of spigelian fascia **run transversely with small defects** in between which are the sites of spigelian hernia
- The spigelian hernia may contain **loops of bowel, colon, omentum** or a part of **circumference of bowel** only.

Other Hernias

- Beclard's hernia: Hernia through opening for saphenous vein
- Treitz's hernia: Duodenojujenal hernia
- Rokintansky hernia: Mucous membrane herniation through muscular layer of bowel

• Mc type of hernia in men:	• Indirect inguinal
• Mc type of hernia in women:	• Indirect inguinal
• Femoral herna is more common in:	• Women
• Femoral hernia is common on:	• Right side
• Inguinal hernia is common on:	• Right side
• **Femoral hernia strangulates:**	• **Commonly**

- **Reducible hernia: Contents can be replaced back**
- **Irreducible hernia: Contents cannot be replaced back**
- **Strangulated hernia: Compromised blood supply**
- **External hernia: Protrudes through all layers of abdominal wall**
- **Interparietal hernia: Hernia sac contained within musculoaponeurotic layer of abdominal wall**

Pancreas

- The pancreas occupies a **retroperitoneal position** in the abdomen, lying posterior to the stomach and lesser omentum
- It extends obliquely from the **duodenal C loop** to a more cephalad position in the **hilum of the spleen**
- The gland is divided into four portions: **the head (which includes the uncinate process), the neck, the body, and the tail**
- It includes the posteroinferior extension arising from the ventral primordium, designated the **uncinate process**

- **Pancreatic agenesis**

Very rarely, the pancreas may be totally absent, a condition usually (but not invariably) associated with additional severe malformations that are incompatible with life. IPF1 gene mutations on chromosome 13q12.1 have been associated with pancreatic agenesis

- **Pancreas divisum**

It is the most common clinically significant congenital pancreatic anomaly, with an incidence of 3% to 10%. It occurs when the fetal duct systems of the pancreatic primordia fail to fuse. As a result, the main pancreatic duct (Wirsung) is very short and drains only a small portion of the head of the gland, while the bulk of the pancreas (from the dorsal pancreatic primordium) drains through the minor sphincter. The relative stenosis caused by the bulk of the pancreatic secretions passing through the minor sphincter predisposes such individuals to chronic pancreatitis

- **Annular pancreas**

A ring of pancreatic tissue that completely encircles the duodenum. It can present with signs and symptoms of duodenal obstruction such as gastric distention and vomiting

- **Ectopic pancreas**

Aberrantly situated, or ectopic, pancreatic tissue occurs in about 2% of the population; favored sites are the stomach and duodenum, followed by the jejunum, Meckel's diverticulum, and ileum.

Causes of Pancreatic Injury

- During splenectomy
- During Billroth II gastrectomy
- During islet cell tumor surgeries
- During sphincterotomy

Heterotopic Pancreas

- The **development of pancreatic tissue outside the confines of the main gland** is a congenital abnormality referred to as heterotopic pancreas
- Most commonly, **heterotopic pancreatic tissue is found in the stomach (MC)**
- **Duodenum, small bowel, or Meckel's diverticulum**
- In most locations, heterotopic pancreatic tissue **resides in a submucosal location**, presenting as firm, yellow, irregular nodules that vary in size from millimeters to several centimeters
- The clinical significance of heterotopic pancreas is dependent on resultant complications. **Intestinal obstruction** may ensue, rarely as a result of the size of the mass, and more commonly following **intussusception**, with the ectopic pancreatic tissue serving as the intussusceptum. Other complications of heterotopic pancreas include **ulceration and hemorrhage.**

Pancreas Divisum

- Follows **failure of fusion of the two primordial ductal systems**
- **The major portion of the pancreas is drained via the duct of Santorini via the minor duodenal papilla**
- **The major duodenal papilla usually communicates with a small duct of Wirsung, which drains the ventral pancreas, consisting of the inferior head and uncinate process**
- The significance of pancreas divisum remains **controversial.** It is unknown whether the ductal anomaly has any causal relationship to the pancreatitis
- Normal pancreatic tissue completely or partially encircles the **second portion of the duodenum**
- Annular pancreas is thought to arise from failure of normal clockwise rotation of the **ventral pancreatic bud**
- Varying degrees of **duodenal obstructive symptoms** may be observed in this condition
- There is a common association with other serious congenital anomalies, such as **intracardiac defects, Down's syndrome, and intestinal malrotation**
- In adults, symptoms may appear to be those of **upper gastrointestinal obstruction, chronic pancreatitis, or peptic ulcer**
- **Obstructive symptoms** are an indication for operation
- Retrocolic **duodenojejunostomy** is treatment of choice

Acute pancreatitis: Causes: The vast majority of cases in the UK are caused by gallstones and alcohol. Popular mnemonic is **GET SMASHED**

- **G**allstones (Mc cause)
- **E**thanol
- **T**rauma
- **S**teroids
- **M**umps (other viruses include Coxsackie B)
- **A**utoimmune (e.g. polyarteritis nodosa), **A**scaris infection
- **S**corpion venom
- **H**ypertriglyceridemia, **H**yperchylomicronemia, **H**ypercalcemia, **H**ypothermia
- **E**RCP
- **D**rugs (azathioprine, sulfasalazine, didanosine, **bendroflumethiazide**, frusemide, pentamidine, steroids, sodium valproate)

Pain in a band form radiating to back with relief on sitting is a feature

A pancreatic pseudocyst may be palpable in the upper abdomen

- **Grey turner's sign (flanks)**
- **Cullen's sign (umbilicus)**

A faint blue discoloration around the umbilicus (Cullen's sign) may occur as the result of hemoperitoneum, and a blue-red-purple or green-brown discoloration of the flanks (Turner's sign) reflects tissue catabolism of hemoglobin

The diagnosis of acute pancreatitis

- ↑**level of serum amylase.** Values threefold or more above normal virtually clinch the diagnosis if overt salivary gland disease and gut perforation or infarction are excluded
- There is no definite correlation between the severity of pancreatitis and the degree of serum amylase elevation. After 48 to 72 h, even with continuing evidence of pancreatitis, total serum amylase values tend to return to normal
- However, **pancreatic isoamylase and lipase levels** may remain elevated for 7 to 14 days
- **Fetal fat estimation** diagnoses **insufficiency**
- Gallstone pancreatitis has best prognosis.

Plain abdominal X-ray shows:

- **Sentinel loop**
- **Colon cut-off sign**
- **Renal halo sign**

Purtscher's Retinopathy, a relatively unusual complication, is manifested by a sudden and severe loss of vision in a patient with **acute pancreatitis.** It is characterized by a peculiar funduscopic appearance with cotton-wool spots and hemorrhages confined to an area limited by the optic disk and macula; it is believed to be due to occlusion of the posterior retinal artery with aggregated granulocytes.

Pancreatitis in patients with AIDS The incidence of **acute** pancreatitis is increased in patients with AIDS for two reasons: (1) the high incidence of infections involving the pancreas, such as infections with **cytomegalovirus, cryptosporidium, and the mycobacterium *avium complex***; and (2) the frequent use by patients with AIDS of medications, such as **didanosine, pentamidine,** and **trimethoprim-sulfamethoxazole**

Chronic Pancreatitis

- The **classic triad of 'Pancreatic calcification, Steatorrhea, and Diabetes mellitus'** usually establishes the diagnosis of chronic pancreatitis and exocrine pancreatic insufficiency but is found in less than one-third of chronic pancreatitis patients
- The **secretin stimulation test**, which usually gives abnormal results when 60% or more of pancreatic exocrine function has been lost. The radiographic hallmark of chronic pancreatitis is the presence of scattered calcification throughout the pancreas

Hereditary Pancreatitis

Hereditary pancreatitis is a rare disease that is **similar to chronic pancreatitis** except for an early age of onset and **evidence of hereditary factors** (involving an autosomal dominant gene with incomplete penetrance). Genetic linkage analysis identified the hereditary pancreatitis gene on **chromosome 7.**

Macroamylasemia

- In macroamylasemia, amylase circulates in the blood in a polymer form too large to be easily excreted by the kidney
- Patients with this condition demonstrate an elevated serum amylase value, a low urinary amylase value, and a C_{am}/C_{cr} ratio of less than 1%
- Usually macroamylasemia is an incidental finding and is not related to disease of the pancreas or other organs
- Macrolipasemia has been documented in a few patients with cirrhosis or non-Hodgkin's lymphoma.

REURRENT PANCREATITIS OCCURS IN METHYL MALONIC ACADEMIA

Serum Amylase ↑ in:

- **Pancreatitis**
- **Renal failure**
- **Ca lung**
- **Ruptured ectopic**
- **Blocked salivary ducts**

Pancreatic Pseudocyst

- Pancreatic pseudocysts are localized collections of pancreatic secretions in a cystic structure that **lack an epithelial lining**
  - These are usually solitary
  - They are commonly attached to the surface of the gland and involve peripancreatic tissues such as the lesser omental sac or the retroperitoneum between the stomach and transverse colon or liver
  - They can range from 2 to 30 cm in diameter
  - **Since pseudocysts form by walling off areas of hemorrhagic fat necrosis, they are typically composed of necrotic debris encased by fibrous walls of granulation tissue lacking an epithelial lining**
- Mc site body or tail
- Mc cause: pancreatitis (adults)
- **Mc cause: trauma (children)**
- Pseudocysts contain high concentrations of pancreatic enzymes, including amylase, lipase, and trypsin
- Pancreatic pseudocysts develop in up to patients after an attack of acute alcoholic pancreatitis
- Pseudocysts are also associated with acute pancreatitis with other causes, as well as with **chronic pancreatitis, pancreatic trauma, and pancreatic neoplasm**
- Most often present with upper abdominal pain
- Physical examination reveals abdominal tenderness in the majority of patients
- A CT scan of the abdomen is the favored study in an initial assessment for determining the presence of a pancreatic pseudocyst

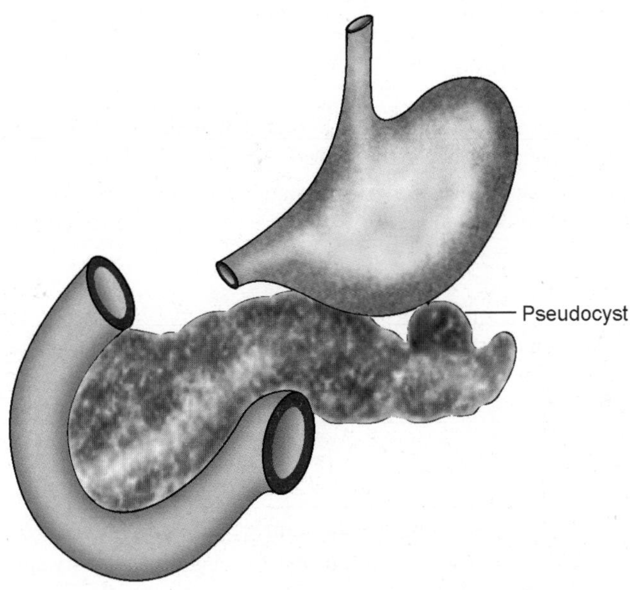

Pancreatic pseudocyst

Complications:
- Infection (MC)
- Rupture
- Hemorrhage
- < 5 cm managed conservatively
- **> 5 cm, cyst > 6 weeks, infection, complication:** Surgery
- Treatment of choice is **internal drainage (Cystojejunostomy)**.

Pancreatic Carcinoma

- *More common in males than in females and in blacks than in whites*
- *Cigarette smoking is the most consistent risk factor*
- *Chronic pancreatitis*
- *Diabetes mellitus*
- *Alcohol abuse or cholelithiasis are not risk factors for* ***pancreatic cancer***
- Hereditary pancreatitis, Peutz-Jeghers syndrome, VHL, Ataxia telangiectasia, Gardner's syndrome and Lynch syndrome II
- *Mutations in K-ras* genes

Clinical Features

- **Most common is:** Ductal adenocarcinomas
- **Most common in:** Pancreatic head (70% of cases)
- **Most common symptom is:** Pain and weight loss
- **Most common physical sign is:** Jaundice
  - Although the gallbladder is usually enlarged in patients with carcinoma of the head of the pancreas, it is palpable in 50% **(Courvoisier's sign)**
  - Other initial manifestations include **venous thrombosis and migratory thrombophlebitis (Trousseau's sign), gastrointestinal hemorrhage** from varices due to compression of the portal venous system by tumor, and **splenomegaly** caused by cancerous encasement of the splenic vein
  - **CECT** is the most effective technique for diagnosis
  - **Whipple's operation** is indicated for periampullary cancer or cancer head of pancreas
  - **'Gemcitabine', a deoxycytidine analogue**, produces improvement in the quality of life for patients with advanced **pancreatic cancer**.

Zollinger-Ellison Syndrome/Gastrinoma

- ***Mc site is duodenum followed by pancreas***
- ***Mc malignant pancreatic endocrine tumor***
- ***More common in males***
- ***Nonbeta cell tumor***
- ***Tumor of delta cells***

Zollinger-Ellison syndrome is a **NET (Neuroendocrine tumor) secreting gastrin**

- In ZES, characteristically **gastric acid hypersecretion** is present
- This gastric acid hypersecretion causes **peptic ulcer** disease often **refractory and severe**, associated with diarrhea
- The most common presenting symptom is **abdominal pain** (70–100%). Peptic ulcer can occur anywhere but the commonest location is the **duodenum** (50–70%) followed by **pancreas** (20–40%)
- ZES occurs in association with **MEN 1** (Hyperparathyroidism, Peptic ulcer disease and Pituitary tumors). About 20–25% patients have associated MEN1 and in most cases, Hyperparathyroidism is present before Hypergastrinemia
- Diagnosis is based on **fasting hypergastrinemia and increased basal acid output (BAO)**
- **Secretin injection test is used as most important investigation**
- **Proton pump inhibitors** are the **drugs of choice**
- Surgical cure is possible in only **30%** of patients
- SOMATOSTATIN and Omperazole used
- Hepatic metastasis occurs in **one-third** of patients.

Gastrinoma Triangle

90% of extrapancreatic gastrinomas lie here

Formed by:

- **3rd part of duodenum**

- **Cystic duct**
- **Pancreatic neck**

Ulcers in ZES

- *Unusual location*
- *Ulcers in absence of predisposing factors*
- *Ulcers in presence of hypercalcemia or family history of MEN 1*
- *Multiple ulcers*
- *Ulcers refractory to treatment*
- *Recurrence of ulcers*
- *Giant ulcers*
- *Ulcers with complications*

Insulinomas

- *Insulinomas are MC* ***endocrine tumors*** *of the pancreas thought to be derived* ***from beta cells*** *that autonomously secrete insulin, which results in hypoglycemia*
- *The most common clinical symptoms are due to the effect of the hypoglycemia on the central nervous system (neuroglycemic symptoms) and include confusion, headache, disorientation, visual difficulties, irrational behavior, or even coma*
- Also, most patients have symptoms due to excess catecholamine release secondary to the hypoglycemia, including sweating, tremor, and palpitations. Characteristically these attacks are associated with fasting
- Usually single
- **Whipple's triad is a feature**
- **Weight gain occurs**
- Insulinomas are **generally**, usually solitary (90%), and only 5 to 15% are malignant
- They almost invariably occur only in the pancreas, **distributed equally in the pancreatic head, body and tail**
- Insulinomas should be suspected in all patients with hypoglycemia, especially with a history suggesting attacks provoked by fasting or with a family history of MEN-1
- In insulinomas, in addition to **elevated plasma insulin levels, elevated plasma proinsulin levels are found and C-peptide levels can be elevated.**

Glucagonomas

- Glucagonomas are **endocrine tumors of the pancreas** that secrete **excessive amounts of glucagon that causes a distinct syndrome characterized by dermatitis, glucose intolerance or diabetes, and weight loss**
- Glucagonomas mainly occur in persons between 45 and 70 years old. They are heralded clinically by a characteristic dermatitis **(migratory necrolytic erythema**; accompanied by glucose intolerance weight loss, anemia, diarrhea and thromboembolism
- The characteristic rash usually starts as an **annular erythema at intertriginous and periorificial sites,** especially in the groin or buttock. It subsequently becomes raised and bullae form; when the bullae rupture, eroded areas form. The lesions can wax and wane
- A characteristic laboratory finding is **hypoaminoacidemia**
- Glucagonomas are generally large tumors at diagnosis, with an average size of 5 to 10 cm. Between 50 and 80% occur in the pancreatic tail and 50 to 82% have evidence of metastatic spread at presentation, usually to the liver. Glucagonomas are rarely extrapancreatic and usually occur singly.

Somatostatinoma Syndrome

Somatostatinomas are **endocrine tumors that secrete excessive amounts of somatostatin**, which causes a syndrome characterized by:

- **Diabetes mellitus**
- **Gallbladder disease**
- **Diarrhea**
- **Steatorrhea**

Somatostatinomas occur primarily in the pancreas and small intestine, and the frequency of the symptoms differs in each. Somatostatinomas occur in the pancreas in 56 to 74% of the cases, with the primary location being in the pancreatic head.

VIPomas

Are endocrine tumors that secrete excessive amounts of **VIP,** which causes a distinct syndrome characterized by **large-volume diarrhea, hypokalemia, and dehydration**. This syndrome is also called **Verner-Morrison syndrome, pancreatic cholera, or WDHA syndrome**

- **Watery diarrhea**
- **Hypokalemia**
- **Achlorhydria/hypochloridia**
- **Hypercalcemia**

Spleen

- **The gastrosplenic ligament** contains the short gastric arteries and veins
- **The splenorenal ligament** contains the splenic artery and vein, lymphatic structures, and often the tail of the pancreas
- **The arterial supply to the spleen** is derived from the celiac artery from both the splenic artery and the short gastric arteries, which usually arise as branches of the gastroepiploic or the splenic arteries
- **The splenic vein** is formed by a coalescence of polar veins in the splenic hilum and courses with the splenic artery along the dorsal surface of the pancreas to enter the portal system
- **The normal adult spleen** is a slightly concave, solid, dark red organ that measures approximately 3 × 8 × 14 cm
- **MC cyst of spleen is pseudocyst**

Wandering (Ectopic) Spleen/Splenosis

- Congenital deficiency or acquired laxity of the suspensory ligaments of the spleen may cause **extreme splenic mobility**
- Palpable in the **lower abdomen or in the pelvis**
- The majority of cases occur in **young and middle-aged women** in whom multiparity and laxity of the abdominal wall and splenic ligaments due to the hormonal effects
- **An elongated splenic pedicle** predisposes a wandering spleen to torsion, leading either to development of acute symptoms due to splenic volvulus and infarction or to chronic and intermittent abdominal discomfort due to spontaneous torsion and detorsion
- Splenic volvulus with infarction requires **emergency splenectomy**

Splenic Artery Aneurysm

- Occurs more frequently in **females**
- Medial dysplasia of the arterial wall. Atherosclerosis, pancreatitis, trauma or arteritis due to septic emboli, portal hypertension with splenomegaly
- Most splenic artery aneurysms are asymptomatic and characteristic **eggshell calcification** of an arteriosclerotic aneurysm may be an incidental finding on an abdominal radiograph.

- **Aneurysmal rupture** may occur and the rupture initially may be contained within the lesser sac
- Initial aneurysmal rupture into the **peritoneal cavity** or delayed rupture from the lesser sac are associated with findings of hemoperitoneum and exsanguinating hemorrhage. Rarely, a splenic artery aneurysm ruptures into the gastrointestinal tract, pancreatic duct, or splenic vein.

Splenic Abscess

Usually results from

- Bacteremia associated with a primary septic focus, such as bacterial endocarditis or lung abscess
- Secondary infection in an area of the spleen damaged by infarction (sickle cell anemia or leukemia), trauma, or parasitic infestation
- Clinical features of splenic abscess are those of **left subphrenic suppuration** and include fever, chills, left upper quadrant tenderness, and often splenomegaly
- Ultrasonography and radionuclide and CT scans are useful
- CT is the most direct way of evaluating the spleen.

Littoral Cell Angioma

- Littoral cell angioma is **a benign, vascular tumor** of spleen presenting as splenomegaly
- It may be associated with other malignancies and has malignant potential itself
- The tumor arises from the **littoral cells in the splenic red pulp sinuses**. Littoral cell angioma affects both men and women equally with no specific age predilection
- It is **usually asymptomatic** and is discovered incidentally
- Some of the patients with this entity may present with symptoms of **hypersplenism,** such as anemia, thrombocytopenia and splenomegaly, the latter seen in almost all patients with littoral cell angioma.

Splenunculi

These are single or multiple accessory spleens which are found

- **Near the hilum of the spleen**
- Splenic vessels
- Behind the tail of the pancreas in 30 percent
- In the splenic ligaments (gastrocolic, greater omentum, splenocolic)
- Mesocolon in the remainder
- Up to 20 percent of people have such splenunculi and most are no larger than 2 cm in diameter

Their importance lies in the fact that if not removed at the time of splenectomy, they will undergo hyperplasia and may well be the site of persistent disease.

Splenic Trauma

- Kehr's sign is occurrence of pain in the tip of shoulder due to presence of blood/irritant in peritoneal cavity
- Kehr's sign in left shoulder is considered a **characteristic sign of splenic rupture**
- Kehr's sign is a **classic example** of referred pain (phrenic nerve)

Other important conditions causing Kehr's sign are:

- **Diaphragmatic lesions**
- **Ectopic pregnancy**
- **Renal calculi**
- **Hemoperitonium**

The signs and symptoms of splenic trauma are those of hemoperitoneum. Generalized and nonspecific abdominal pain in the left upper quadrant occurs in approximately one-third of patients with splenic injury. Pain referred to the tip of the left shoulder (Kehr's sign) is inconstant, varying in incidence from 15 to 75%, and is unreliable for excluding splenic injury but is useful for enhancing the diagnostic probability if present. Kehr's sign is elicited by bimanual compression of the left upper quadrant after the patient has been in Trendelenburg's position for several minutes preceding the maneuver. On rare occasions, patients with splenic injury have a palpable tender mass in the left upper quadrant (Ballance's sign), caused by an extracapsular or subcapsular hematoma with omentum adherent to the injured spleen.

- Spleen is the most common organ injured in blunt abdominal injury
- Contrast-enhanced CT Scan is the investigation of choice for splenic injuries
- Features on X-ray suggestive of splenic injury are:

Obliteration of splenic shadow
Obliteration of psoas shadow
Fracture of lower left ribs
Elevation of left diaphragm
Indentation of stomach
Presence of fluid between coils of intestine

Spleen

- **Felty's Syndrome: Rheumatoid arthritis with Hypersplenism**
- **Banti's Syndrome: Congestive splenomegaly with Hypersplenism**
- **Egyptian Splenomegaly: Schistosomiasis**
- **Angiosarcoma: MC malignant tumor of spleen**
- **Splenosis: Rupture of spleen with dissemination into peritonium**
- **Spontaneous rupture is seen in Infectious mononucleosis typhoid, leukemia**

Splenectomy

- Mc indication for elective splenectomy: ITP
- HS
- G6PD
- Portal hypertension
- Hypersplenism
- Autosplenectomy is seen in sickle-cell anemia
- Pneumococcal vaccine and *N. meningitidis* vaccine given
- **Splenorrhaphy** is done in stable patient with lacerated spleen.

Not Done For

- Asymptomatic
- Splenomegaly with infection
- Splenomegaly with ↑ igm
- Hereditary hemolytic anemia
- Acute leukemia
- Agranulocytosis
- Porphyria

Complications

- Hemmorage
- Hematemesis
- Left basal atelectasis
- Pancreatitis, pancreatic abscess
- Risk of infections

Splenectomy Increases Risk for

- Pneumococcal infections
- *H. influenzae*
- Gram-negative enteric organisms
- Meningococcemia
- Babesia
- Malaria

An Overwhelming Postsplenectomy Infection (OPSI)

- **An overwhelming postsplenectomy infection (OPSI)** is a **rare but rapidly fatal infection** occurring in individuals following removal of the spleen. The infections are typically characterized by either meningitis or sepsis, and are caused by ***Streptococcus pneumoniae* mostly**
- The spleen contains many macrophages (part of the reticuloendothelial system), immune cells which phagocytose (eat) and destroy bacteria. In particular, these macrophages are activated when bacteria are bound by IgG antibodies (IgG1 or IgG3) or complement component C3b. These types of antibodies and complement are immune substances **called opsonizers,** molecules which bind to the surface of bacteria to make them easier for macrophages to phagocytose and destroy the bacteria
- When the spleen is gone, IgG and complement component C3b are still bound to bacteria, but they cannot be removed from the blood circulation because the spleen, which contained the macrophages, is gone. The bacteria, therefore, are free to cause infection
- Patients without spleens often need immunizations against pathogens that normally require opsonization and phagocytosis by macrophages in the spleen. These include common human pathogens with capsules
- ***Streptococcus pneumoniae***
- ***Salmonella typhi, Neisseria meningitidis, E. coli, Hemophilus influenzae, Streptococcus agalactiae, Klebsiella pneumoniae***
- **MC complication is left lower lobe atelectasis.**

Remember in Nutshell: About Overwhelming Postsplenectomy Infection

- *Infection due to* ***encapsulated bacteria***
- *Almost* ***50% due to Streptococcus. pneumoniae***
- Other organisms include: *hemophilus influenzae, Neisseria meningitidis*
- *Occurs postsplenectomy in* ***4% patients*** *without prophylaxis*
- *Mortality of OPSI is approximately* ***50%***
- *Greatest risk in* ***first 2 years postop.***

• Acute hematological effects of splenectomy	• Chronic hematological effects of splenectomy
– **Leukocytosis**	– Anisocytosis
– Thrombocytosis	– Poikilocytosis
– Heinz bodies	– Howell-Jolly bodies
– Basophilic stippling	– Nucleated erythrocytes

Liver

- 80% blood supply is from **portal vein. 20%** is from hepatic artery
- Liver is divided into surgical right and left lobes by a line between Gallbladder and middle hepatic vein. **Cantlie line**
- Portal venous system lacks valves

'Caterpillar Turn' or 'Moynihan's Hump'

- Normally the arterial supply of Gallbladder is from **cystic artery** which is a branch of **right hepatic artery**
- Sometimes an **accessory cystic artery** is also seen to arise from either **Gastroduodenal or right hepatic artery**
- The right hepatic artery takes a tortuous course called **'caterpillar turn'** or **'Moynihan's hump'**. This can be a source of profuse bleeding.

- **Orthoptic liver transplant** is replacement of patient liver with donor liver
- **Auxillary liver transplant** is transplanted alongside of part of patient's own liver.

Couinaud's segments of liver:

- Segment I: Caudate lobe. Rest of segments are clockwise
- Segment II: Lateral segment: left superior lobe
- Segment III: Lateral segment: left inferior lobe
- Segment IV: Quadrate lobe
- Segment V: Anterior segment: right inferior lobe
- Segment VI: Posterior segment: right superior lobe
- Segment VII: Posterior segment: right superior lobe
- Segment VIII: Anterior segment: right superior lobe
- Segment I has independent vascular supply

Portal Vein and Portal Hypertension

- Portal vein is an important vein formed behind the **neck of pancreas** by union of **splenic vein and superior mesentric vein. Have a look at the figure below**:
- Drains blood from **GIT AND SPLEEN**
- It is **8 cms in length**
- It is the major source of **blood supply to liver**
- It is **devoid of valves.**

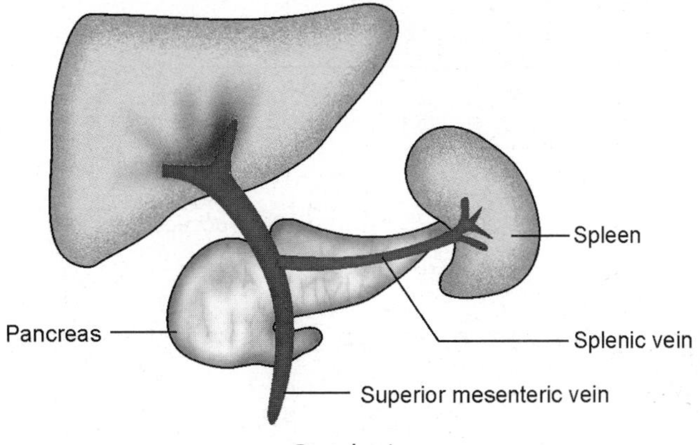

Portal vein

Portal Hypertension

- **(> 10 mm Hg)** most commonly results from increased resistance to portal blood flow
- Increased resistance can occur at three levels relative to the hepatic sinusoids:
  - ***Presinusoidal***
  - ***Sinusoidal***
  - ***Postsinusoidal***
- **'Cirrhosis' is the most common cause of portal hypertension** in the United States
- Portal venous pressure may be measured directly by percutaneous transhepatic **'skinny needle'** catheterization or indirectly through transjugular cannulation of the hepatic veins

Sites of portosystemic anastomosis involved in portal hypertension:

  - **Umbilicus: Caput medusae**
  - **Lower end of esophagus: Esophageal varices**
  - **Rectum and anal canal: Hemorrhoids**
  - **Bare area of liver**
  - **Posterior abdominal wall**
- **Bleeding varices: Propranolol is the drug of choice** for prophylaxis of bleeding
- **Octreotide** is the drug of choice for bleeding varices
- Barium swallow shows **string of beads** in esophagus.

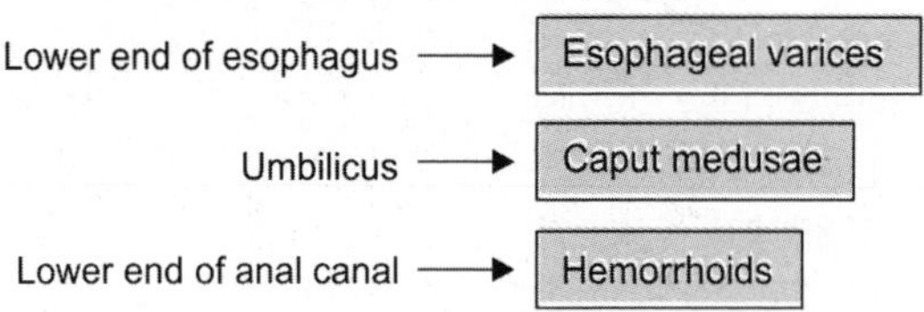

Sites of portosystemic anastomosis

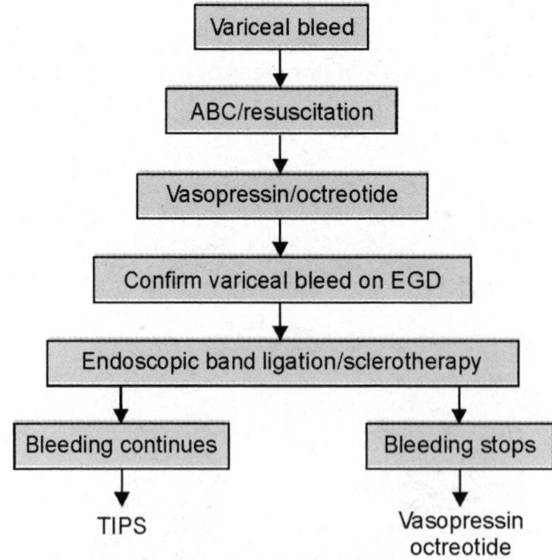

Management of variceal bleed

Amebic Liver Abscess

E. histolytica most often involves the **liver**

- Mc in **right lobe (posterosuperior surface)**
- Liquefaction necrosis is characteristic

- **Anchovy sauce pus: Chocolate-colored pus due to RBC Lysis**
- Scant inflammatory response at margins
- Some patients are febrile and have right upper-quadrant pain, which may be dull or pleuritic in nature and radiate to the shoulder
- Point tenderness over the liver and right-sided pleural effusion are common
- Jaundice is rare
- About one-third of patients with chronic presentations are febrile. Thus, the clinical diagnosis of an amebic **liver abscess** may be difficult to establish because the symptoms and signs are often nonspecific
- **Complications of Amebic Liver Abscess**
  - Pleuropulmonary involvement manifestations include sterile effusions, contiguous spread from the liver and rupture into the pleural space
  - Rupture into the pleural space
  - Rupture into the peritoneum
  - Rupture into the pericardium, usually from abscesses of the left lobe of the liver
- **DOC: Metronadizole**

Hydatid Disease

- **Echinococcosis** is also known as **hydatid disease**
- Hydatid cyst is a **parasitic infection** of humans by the tapeworm of genus *echinococcus*
- It is a **zoonosis**
  - **Echinococcus granulosus** causes ***Cystic Echinococcosis***
  - ***Echinococcus multilocularis*** causing ***Alveolar Echinococcosis***
  - ***Echinococcus vogeli*** causes ***Polycystic disease***

Echinococcus granulosus:

The **liver is the most common organ affected** followed by lungs, muscles, bones and kidneys

Passage of hydatid membrane in emesis is called **hydatid emesia**

Passage of hydatid membrane in stools is called **hydatid enterica**

Flushing and urticaria occur in rupture of hydatid cyst

1. **Abdominal tenderness** is the most common sign
2. Tender hepatomegaly signifies secondary infection of the cyst
3. Ascites is rare
4. Splenomegaly can be the result of portal hypertension or splenic echinococcosis

- **Brain involvement** depends on site of brain involved and may present as coma or herniation
- **Bone and muscle** involvement presents as visible masses
- Echinococcosis is caused by larval stages of parasite
- Man is an **accidental intermediate host**. Other intermediate hosts are sheep and cattle
- The **dog** is the **definitive host**
- **Serological assay (Weinberg reaction)** is a specific example of complement fixation test used in detection
- ELISA is also sensitive, blood culture not useful
- Eosinophilia is seen only in case of rupture of cysts
- Detachment of cysts and their collapse lead to characteristic **water Lily sign or floating membrane sign or camellotte sign**
- **Other X-ray signs of *echinococcus* are:**
  - **Serpent sign/Rising sun sign**
  - **Crumbled egg appearance**
  - **Anaphylaxis, intrapleural rupture, intraperitoneal rupture** are secondary complications
- **PAIR Technique** (Percutaneous aspiration, injection of scolicidal agents and reaspiration of cyst contents) has also been used for treatment
- **Albendazole** is the most effective drug most commonly used.

Hydatid Cyst of Lung

- Second most common site
- Less often seen in association with liver cyst
- Usually in lower lobes
- Calcification uncommon

Pyogenic Liver Abscess

- Has an increased incidence in **the elderly, diabetics and the immunosuppressed**, who usually present with anorexia, fevers and malaise accompanied by right upper quadrant discomfort
- The diagnosis is suggested by the finding of a **multiloculated cystic mass** on ultrasound or CT scan and is confirmed by aspiration for culture and sensitivity
- Usually single and large.
- The most common organisms are ***Escherichia coil*** and ***Streptococcus milleri*** but other enteric organisms such as *Streptococcus faecalis, Klebsiella* and *Proteus vulgaris* also occur and mixed growths are common. Opportunistic pathogens include Staphylococci. Treatment is with antibiotics and ultrasound-guided aspiration. Percutaneous drainage without ultrasound guidance should be avoided as an empyema may follow drainage through the pleural space
- Infection **through bile duct is the commonest route** followed by **hematogenous route**.

Hepatic Adenoma

- **Benign neoplasm**
- **Derived from hepatocytes**
- **Seen in women taking OCPS**
- **Usually asymptomatic but may bleed intraabdominally**
- **Seen as cold defects in hepatic scintigraphy**
- **Core biopsy contraindication**
- **Aspiration biopsy can be done**
- **> 6 cm tumor should be excised**

Focal nodular hyperplasia presents similarly but <u>without bleeding features</u>.

HEPATOCELLULAR CARCINOMA

Predisposing Factors

- Hepatitis B
- Hepatitis C
- Alcoholic liver disease
- Alpha 1 antitrypsin deficiency
- Hemachromatosis
- Tyrosinemia
- Aflatoxin B_1
- Vinyl chloride, Thorium and Androgenic hormones are also implicated

- AFP levels are raised. AFP is used as a **marker** for HCC
- Other markers are: Neurotensin, PIVKA 2
- Early stage tumors are successfully treated. If untreated, most patients die within 3–6 months of diagnosis. Early resection helps in survival for 1–2 years and, in selected cases, may even prolong life
- Surgical resection offers the only chance for cure

ULTRASOUND EXAMINATION IS FREQUENTLY USED TO SCREEN PATIENTS FOR HCC

Remember

- **Mc abdominal tumor. Mc solid tumor**
- **Mc in right lobe**
- **Mc symptom is abdominal pain**

Hepatocellular Carcinoma

Hepatocellular carcinoma: The principal reason for the high incidence of hepatocellular carcinoma in parts of Asia and Africa is the frequency of chronic infection with **hepatitis B virus (HBV) and hepatitis C virus (HCV).**

'Chronic liver disease' of any type is a risk factor and predisposes to the development of liver cell carcinoma. These conditions include **alcoholic liver disease, a1-antitrypsin deficiency, hemochromatosis** and **tyrosinemia.**

A small percentage of patients with hepatocellular carcinoma have a **paraneoplastic syndrome**

Erythrocytosis may result from erythropoietin-like activity produced by the tumor.

Hypercalcemia may result from secretion of a parathyroid-like hormone. Other manifestations may include **hypercholesterolemia, hypoglycemia, acquired porphyria, dysfibrinogenemia and cryofibrinogenemia**.

Imaging procedures to detect liver tumors **include ultrasound, CT, MRI, hepatic artery angiography and technetium scans**.

Ultrasound is frequently used to screen high-risk populations and should be the first test if hepatocellular carcinoma is suspected; it is less costly than scans, is relatively sensitive, and can detect most tumors > 3 cm.

Helical CT and MRI scans are being used with increasing frequency and have higher sensitivities.

AFP levels > 500 ug/L are found in about 70 to 80% of patients with hepatocellular carcinoma. Lower levels may be found in patients with large metastases from gastric or colonic tumors and in some patients with acute or chronic hepatitis.

High levels of serum AFP (> 500 to 1000 ug/L) in an adult with liver disease and without an obvious gastrointestinal tumor strongly suggest hepatocellular carcinoma.

Percutaneous liver biopsy can be diagnostic if the sample is taken from an area localized by ultrasound or CT. Because these tumors tend to be vascular, percutaneous biopsies should be done with caution.

Staging of hepatocellular carcinoma is based on **tumor size (< or > 50% of the liver), ascites (absent or present), bilirubin (< or > 3), and albumin (< or >3)** to establish **Okuda stages I, II, and III**. The natural history of each stage without treatment is: stage I, 8 months; stage II, 2 months; stage III, less than 1 month.

Fibrolamellar Carcinoma

Fibrolamellar carcinoma differs from the typical hepatocellular carcinoma in that it tends to occur in **young adults** without underlying cirrhosis

NOT associated with cirrhosis

This tumor **is nonencapsulated** but well circumscribed and contains fibrous lamellae

It **grows slowly** and is associated with a longer survival if treated

Surgical resection has resulted in 5-year survivals >50%; if the lesion is nonresectable, liver transplantation is an option, and the outcome far exceeds that observed in the nonfibrolamellar variety of liver cancer.

Hepatoblastoma is a **tumor of infancy** that typically is associated with very high-serum AFP levels

The lesions are **usually solitary**, may be resectable, and have a better 5-year survival than that of hepatocellular carcinoma.

Angiosarcoma consists of vascular spaces lined by malignant endothelial cells. Etiologic factors include prior exposure to **thorium dioxide (Thorotrast), polyvinyl chloride, arsenic, and androgenic anabolic steroids**.

Epithelioid hemangioendothelioma is of borderline malignancy

Most cases are benign, but bone and lung metastases occur.

This tumor occurs in early adulthood, presents with right upper quadrant pain, is heterogenous on sonography, hypodense on CT, and without neovascularity on angiography

Immunohistochemical staining reveals expression of factor VIII antigen. In the absence of extrahepatic metastases, these lesions can be treated by surgical resection or liver transplantation.

Indications for Liver Transplantation

Children	Adults
• **Biliary atresia**	• **Primary biliary cirrhosis**
• **Neonatal hepatitis**	• **Secondary biliary cirrhosis**
• **Congenital hepatic fibrosis**	• **Primary sclerosing cholangitis**
• **Alagille's disease**	• **Caroli's disease**
• **Byler's disease**	• **Cryptogenic cirrhosis**
• **α 1-Antitrypsin deficiency**	• **Chronic hepatitis with cirrhosis**
• **Inherited disorders of metabolism**	• **Hepatic vein thrombosis**
• **Wilson's disease**	• **Fulminant hepatitis**
• **Tyrosinemia**	• **Alcoholic cirrhosis**
• **Glycogen storage diseases**	• **Chronic viral hepatitis**
• **Lysosomal storage diseases**	• **Primary hepatocellular malignancies**
• **Protoporphyria**	• **Hepatic adenomas**
• **Crigler-Najjar disease type I**	
• **Familial hypercholesterolemia**	
• **Hereditary oxalosis**	
• **Hemophilia**	

Hepatic Dysfunction after Liver Transplantation

- Primary graft failure
- Vascular compromise
- Failure or obstruction of the biliary anastomoses, and rejection
- Postoperative jaundice may result from prehepatic, intrahepatic and posthepatic sources. *Prehepatic* sources represent the massive hemoglobin pigment load from transfusions, hemolysis, hematomas, ecchymoses and other collections of blood
- Vascular compromise associated with thrombosis or stenosis of the portal vein or hepatic artery anastomoses; vascular anastomotic leak; stenosis, obstruction, or leakage of the anastomosed common bile duct.

MELD

- The **'Model for End-Stage Liver Disease' (MELD) system** was implemented on February 27, 2002 to **prioritize patients waiting for a liver transplant**
- MELD is a numerical scale used for adult liver transplant candidates.
- **The range is from 6 (less ill) to 40 (gravely ill).** The individual score determines **how urgently a patient needs a liver transplant within the next three months.** The number is calculated using the most recent laboratory tests
- Within the MELD continuous disease severity scale, there are four levels. As the MELD score increases, and the patient moves up to a new level, a new waiting time clock starts
- Waiting time is carried backwards but not forward. If a patient moves to a lower MELD score, the waiting time accumulated at the higher score remains. When a patient moves to a higher MELD score, the waiting time at the lower level is not carried to the new level.

'Carcinoid Syndrome'

- Occurs in **less than 10% of patients with carcinoid tumors**
- The carcinoid syndrome is encountered **when venous drainage from the tumor gains access to the systemic circulation so that vasoactive secretory substances escape hepatic degradation**
- This situation obtains in three circumstances:
  - ***When hepatic metastases are present,***
  - ***When venous blood from extensive retroperitoneal metastases drains into paravertebral veins, and***
  - ***When the primary carcinoid tumor is outside the gastrointestinal tract, e.g. a bronchial, ovarian, or testicular tumor.***

- The principal features of carcinoid syndrome include **flushing, sweating, wheezing, diarrhea, abdominal pain, cardiac valvular fibrosis, and pellagra dermatosis**
- **Diarrhea is found in 83% of patients**, flushing in 49%, dyspnea in 20%, and bronchospasm in 6%
- Many patients develop **right-sided cardiac valvular disease** with congestive heart failure. **Serotonin** and possibly other neurohumors produced by the tumor cause fibrosis, as well as eventual incompetence of the tricuspid and pulmonic valves
- The lungs metabolize serotonin and the other mediators and protect the left heart from fibrosis. If one can establish that the tumor is slow-growing, patients with carcinoid-induced cardiac lesions are candidates for valve replacement
- Biochemical mediators
- The specific etiologic agents for each of the protean manifestations of carcinoid tumors are not known. **Serotonin, prostaglandins, 5-hydroxytryptophan, substance P, kallikrein, histamine, dopamine, and neuropeptide K are thought to be involved in the clinical manifestations of carcinoid tumors**
- **Serotonin is thought to be largely responsible for both the diarrhea and the fibrosis.** The cardiac lesions, and tricuspid and pulmonic insufficiency are components of this fibrosing phenomenon
- Other substances, such as histamine, VIP, and prostaglandins, may also **contribute to the systemic manifestations in the carcinoid syndrome**

Diagnosis

- **Urinary 5-HIAA or whole blood and platelet-poor plasma 5-HT is the most reliable test to confirm the diagnosis of carcinoid syndrome**
- Occasionally, measurement of plasma levels of **substance P and neurotensin** by radioimmunoassay may also be helpful
- Measurements of **neuron-specific enolase and chromogranins,** when available, provide nonspecific evidence of the presence of a neuroendocrine tumor
- **A useful diagnostic aid is the pentagastrin provocative test,** which induces facial flushing, gastrointestinal symptoms, elevation in circulating 5-HT

Appendicular Carcinoids

  - **Not** the commonest site
  - Mc site: tip
  - Presents as recurrent appendicitis
  - It has good prognosis
- **Carcinoid tumors occur in ileum and appendix**
- **Rectum is rarely involved**
- **5-year survival is more than 60%**
- **Females are affected less**

Congenital Abnormalities of the Gallbladder and Bile Ducts

Absence of the gallbladder

Occasionally the gallbladder is absent. Failure to visualize the gallbladder is not necessarily a pathological problem.

The Phrygian cap

The Phrygian cap is present in 2–6 percent of cholecystograms and may be mistaken for a pathological deformity of the organ. 'Phrygian cap' refers to hats worn by people of Phrygia, an ancient country of Asia Minor; it was rather like a Liberté cap of the French Revolution

Floating gallbladder

The organ may hang on a mesentery which makes it liable to undergo torsion.

Double gallbladder

Rarely, the gallbladder is twinned. One of the twins may be intrahepatic.

Absence of the cystic duct

This is usually pathological, as opposed to an anatomical anomaly and indicates the recent passage of a stone or the presence of a stone at the lower end of the cystic duct which is ulcerating into the common bile duct. The main danger at surgery is damage to the bile duct, and particular care to identify the correct anatomy is essential before division of any duct.

Low insertion of the cystic duct

The cystic duct opens into the common bile duct near the ampulla. All variations of this anomaly can occur. At operation, they are not important. Dissection of a cystic duct which is inserted low in the bile duct should be avoided as removal will damage the blood supply to the common bile duct and can lead to stricture formation.

An accessory cholecystohepatic duct

Ducts passing directly into the gallbladder from the liver do occur and are probably not uncommon. Nevertheless, larger ducts should be closed but before doing so, the precise anatomy should be carefully ascertained.

Extrahepatic biliary atresia

Etiology and pathology

Atresia is present in one per 14,000 live births, and affects males and females equally. The extrahepatic bile ducts are progressively destroyed by an inflammatory process which starts around the time of birth. Intrahepatic changes also occur and eventually result in biliary cirrhosis and portal hypertension. The untreated child dies before the age of 3 years of liver failure or hemorrhage.

The inflammatory destruction of the bile ducts has been classified into three main types:

- **Type I — atresia restricted to the common bile duct**
- **Type II — atresia of the common hepatic duct**
- **Type III — atresia of the right and left hepatic ducts**

Parasitic Infestation of the Biliary Tract

Biliary ascariasis

- The round worm, ***A. lumbricoides***, commonly infests the intestine of inhabitants of Asia, Africa and Central America
- It may enter the biliary tree through the ampulla of Vater and cause biliary pain
- Complications include **strictures, suppurative cholangitis, liver abscesses and empyema of the Gallbladder**. In the uncomplicated case, antispasmodics can be given to relax the sphincter of Oddi and the worm will return to the small intestine to be dealt with by antihelminthic drugs
- Operation may be necessary to remove the worm or deal with complications. Worms can be extracted via the ampulla of Vater by ERCP.

Clonorchiasis (Asiatic cholangiohepatis)

- The disease is **endemic in the Far East**
- Fluke, up to 25 mm long and 5 mm wide, inhabits the bile ducts, including the intrahepatic ducts
- **Fibrous thickening of the duct walls occur**. Many cases are asymptomatic. Complications include **biliary pain, stones, cholangitis, cirrhosis and bile-duct carcinoma**
- **Choledochotomy and T-tube drainage** and, in some cases, choledochoduodenostomy are required. Because a process of recurrent stone formation is set up, a choledochojejunostomy with Roux loop affixed to the abdominal parietes is performed in some centers to allow easy subsequent access to the duct system

Hydatid disease

- A large hydatid cyst may obstruct the hepatic ducts. Sometimes a cyst will rupture into the biliary tree and its contents cause obstructive jaundice or cholangitis, requiring appropriate surgery.

PREDISPOSING FACTORS

Cholelithiasis

Cholesterol and Mixed Stones

1. Familial disposition
2. Hereditary aspects
3. Obesity
4. Weight loss
5. Female sex hormones
6. Ileal disease or resection
7. Increasing age
8. Gallbladder hypomotility leading to stasis and formation of sludge:
   - Prolonged parenteral nutrition
   - Fasting
   - Pregnancy
   - Drugs such as octreotide
9. Clofibrate therapy
10. Decreased bile acid secretion
    - Primary biliary cirrhosis
    - Chronic intrahepatic cholestasis
    - Remember **fat, flatulent, female, fertile, forty/fifty**

Pigment Stones

1. Demographic/genetic factors: Asia, rural setting
2. Chronic hemolysis
3. Alcoholic cirrhosis
4. Chronic biliary tract infection, parasite infestation
5. Increasing age

Effects and Complications of Gallstones

In the gallbladder:

- Silent stones
- Chronic cholecystitis
- Acute cholecystitis
- Gangrene
- Perforation
- Empyema
- Mucocele
- Carcinoma

In the bile ducts:

- Obstructive jaundice
- Cholangitis
- Acute pancreatitis

In the intestine:

- Acute intestinal obstruction (gallstone ileus)

CBD Stone

- **Seen in 15% patients with gallstones**
- **Develop in gallbladder**
- **Obstructive pattern seen**
- **Mc cause of obstructive jaundice**
- **It can present with cholangitis**
- **Bile duct diameter > 6 mm on USG is suggestive**
- **ERCP, Sphincterotomy, with ballon clearance is standard treatment used**
- **In cholangiography appears as meniscus sign.**

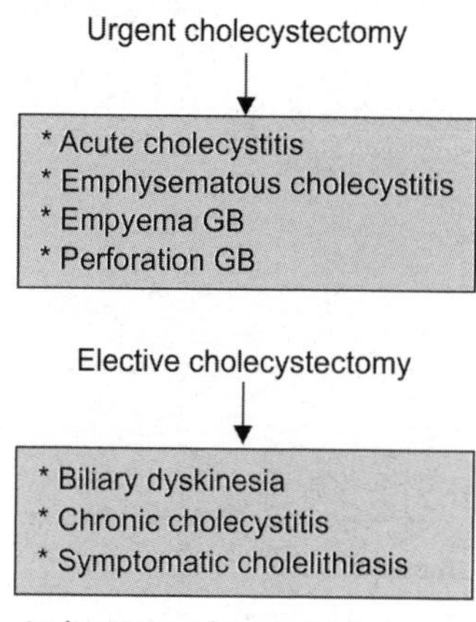

Urgent cholecystectomy
* Acute cholecystitis
* Emphysematous cholecystitis
* Empyema GB
* Perforation GB
Elective cholecystectomy
* Biliary dyskinesia
* Chronic cholecystitis
* Symptomatic cholelithiasis

Indications of cholecystectomy

Gallstone Ileus

- Gallstone ileus refers to **mechanical intestinal obstruction** resulting from passage of a large gallstone into bowel lumen
- This particular complication follows internal fistulas in which a **gallstone or common duct stone gains entrance into the intestinal tract** through an internal biliary fistula
- The usual potential complication is **ascending cholangitis**
- A typical presentation of gallstone ileus is a **history of frequent previous episodes of partial bowel obstruction** that exacerbate and abate as the stone negotiates its way into a narrower region of the intestinal tract. This phenomenon is called a **tumbling obstruction**
- Three-fourths of the spontaneous fistulas underlying gallstone ileus occur between the gallbladder and the duodenum
- Most gallstones that enter the gastrointestinal tract are either passed or vomited, but 10% to 15% may lead to gallstone ileus
- The common site of obstruction, found in two-thirds of patients, is the **ileum**
- The diagnosis is easily made if a **large mass lesion** is found at the site of bowel obstruction; this mass is readily identified if the gallstone is opaque. Sometimes, even if it is nonopaque, it can be observed because of the surrounding intestinal air
- In addition, the **finding of air in the biliary tree** makes the diagnosis almost certain
- The proper treatment of gallstone ileus is relief of the intestinal obstruction, usually by the performance of an **enterotomy and removal of the stone**
- Concomitant definitive correction of the internal fistula is advocated if the patient is in good condition and has sustained no prolonged desease.

ACUTE AND CHRONIC CHOLECYSTITIS

Acute Cholecystitis

- Usually follows obstruction of the cystic duct by a stone
- **Mc agent: *Escherichia coli, Klebsiella* spp**., group D *Streptococcus*, *Staphylococcus* spp., and *Clostridium* spp
- Deep inspiration or cough during subcostal palpation of the RUQ usually produces increased pain and inspiratory arrest (**Murphy's sign**)

- **The triad of sudden onset of RUQ tenderness, fever, and leukocytosis is highly suggestive.** Typically, leukocytosis in the range of 10,000 to 15,000 cells per microliter with a left shift on differential count is found
- The radionuclide **(e.g. HIDA) biliary scan is** IOC
- **Ultrasound** will demonstrate calculi in 90 to 95% of cases.

Acalculous Cholecystitis

Especially associated with:

- **Serious trauma or**
- **Burns**
- **Diabetes**
- TPN
- With the **postpartum period** following prolonged labor, and **orthopedic and other nonbiliary major surgical operations** in the postoperative period vasculitis, obstructing adenocarcinoma of the gallbladder, diabetes mellitus, torsion of the gallbladder, 'unusual' bacterial infections of the gallbladder (e.g. *Leptospira*, *Streptococcus*, *Salmonella*, or *Vibrio cholerae*), and parasitic infestation of the gallbladder
- Acalculous **cholecystitis** may also be seen with a variety of other systemic disease processes **(sarcoidosis, cardiovascular disease, tuberculosis, syphilis, actinomycosis, etc.)** and may possibly complicate periods of prolonged parenteral hyperalimentation
- USG is IOC.

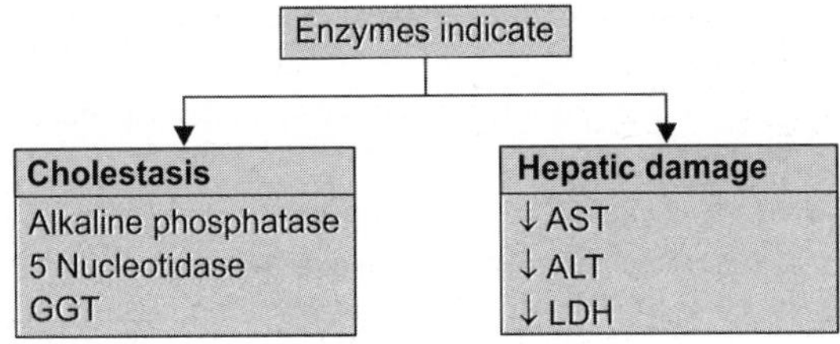

Enzyme elevation

Emphysematous Cholecystitis

- Begin with acute **cholecystitis** (calculous or acalculous) followed by ischemia or gangrene of the gallbladder wall and infection by gas-producing organisms
- Bacteria most frequently cultured in this setting include **anaerobes, such as *C. welchii* or *C. perfringens*, and aerobes, such as *E. coli***
- This condition occurs most frequently **in elderly men and in patients with diabetes mellitus**
- The diagnosis is usually made on plain abdominal film by the finding of gas within the gallbladder lumen, dissecting within the gallbladder wall to form a gaseous ring, or in the pericholecystic tissues. The morbidity and mortality rates with emphysematous **cholecystitis** are considerable. Prompt surgical intervention coupled with appropriate antibiotics is mandatory.

Chronic Cholecystitis

Chronic inflammation of the gallbladder wall is almost always associated with the presence of gallstones and is thought to result from repeated bouts of subacute or acute **cholecystitis** or from persistent mechanical irritation of the gallbladder wall. The presence of bacteria in the bile occurs in more than one-quarter of patients with chronic **cholecystitis**.

Cholangiocarcinoma

Adenocarcinoma of the extrahepatic ducts is more common. There is a slight male preponderance (60%), and the incidence peaks in the fifth to seventh decades.

Apparent predisposing factors include:

- **Some chronic hepatobiliary parasitic infestations**
- **Congenital anomalies with ectatic ducts**
- **Sclerosing cholangitis, chronic ulcerative colitis**
- **Occupational exposure to possible biliary tract carcinogens (employment in rubber or automotive plants)**
- **Perihilar mc location**

Nodular lesions often arise at the bifurcation of the **common bile duct (Klatskin tumors)** and are usually associated with a *collapsed gallbladder*

Patients with **cholangiocarcinoma** usually present with biliary obstruction, painless jaundice, pruritus, weight loss, and acholic stools

The diagnosis is most frequently made by cholangiography following ultrasound demonstration of dilated intrahepatic bile ducts.

Klatskin Tumor

Tumor of CBD between cystic duct and common hepatic duct

- ↓metastasis
- Slow growth
- Shows sclerosing features

Carcinoma of the Papilla of Vater

- The ampulla of Vater may be involved by extension of tumor arising elsewhere in the duodenum or may itself be the site of origin of a sarcoma, carcinoid tumor, or adenocarcinoma
- Papillary adenocarcinomas are associated with slow growth and a more favorable clinical prognosis than diffuse, infiltrative cancers of the ampulla, which are more frequently widely invasive
- **The presenting clinical manifestation** is usually **obstructive jaundice**
- **Endoscopic retrograde cannulation of the pancreatic duct is the preferred diagnostic technique** when ampullary carcinoma is suspected, because it allows for direct endoscopic inspection and biopsy of the ampulla and for pancreatography to exclude a pancreatic malignancy
- **Cancer** of the papilla is usually treated by **wide surgical excision**
- **Lymph node or other metastases are present** at the time of surgery in approximately 20% of the cases.

Cancer of the Gallbladder

- **Female/Male ratio** is 4:1
- The clinical presentation is most often one of **unremitting right upper quadrant pain associated with weight loss, jaundice, and a palpable right upper quadrant mass**
- Adenocarcinoma **most common type**
- Fundus is the **most common site**
- Biliary colic is the **most common presentation**
- Gallstones are the **most common predisposition.**

Risk Factors for GB Cancer

- The association between cancer of the **gallbladder** and **gallstones** is **well established.**
- A parallel exists between the epidemiology of cancer of the gallbladder and that of gallstones. There is no predilection for the development of carcinoma in a gallbladder containing single or multiple stones.
- It has been suggested that there may be some relationship between carcinoma and the **size of a stone.**
- A patient with a 3 cm gallstone is reportedly 10 times more likely to develop carcinoma than someone with a stone less than 1 cm.
- There are several other pathologic conditions of the gallbladder in addition to gallstones that are associated with the development of carcinoma.

- There is believed to be a 15% incidence of carcinoma of the gallbladder in patients who have or have had a **cholecystoenteric fistula** and the tumor may develop as much as 16 years later.
- There is believed to be a 15% incidence of carcinoma of the gallbladder in patients who have or have had a **cholecystoenteric fistula** and the tumor may develop as much as 16 years later.
- The incidence of carcinoma in a **calcified or porcelain gallbladder** is reported to range from 12.5 to 61%.
- It is now generally accepted that **adenoma of the gallbladder** is a precancerous lesion. Adenomas present as polypoid lesions which are best detected by ultrasonography.
- It has been suggested that **xanthogranulomatous cholecystitis,** a rare form of chronic cholecystitis that may grossly mimic cancer of the gallbladder, is also associated with a higher than expected incidence of carcinoma.
- Cancer of the gallbladder is more frequent in the presence of **congenital biliary dilatation** in which case there appears to be a lower incidence of associated gallstones.
- **Ulcerative colitis** has a well-known association with biliary tract malignancy.
- Although the majority of such malignancies involve the bile ducts, as many as 13% originate in the gallbladder.

- ***Rokitansky-Aschoff sinuses***: *Outpouching of Gallbladder Mucosa*
- *Mucosal Folds of Cystic Duct:* ***Valves of Heister***
- *Lymph node of GB* ***Cystic LN of Lund***
- ***Moynihans Hump*** *Tortuous course of Right Hepatic Artery in front of Cystic Duct. Also called* ***Caterpillar Turn***
- ***Callot's Triangle: Triangle bounded above by Liver, Medially by Common Hepatic Duct, Below by Cystic Duct***
- ***'Straw berry' Gallbladder*** *Cholesterosis*
- ***'Seagull or Mercedes Benz Sign'*** *Radiolucent gall shadow in cholelithiasis*
- ***Murphy's sign/Boas Sign*** Acute Cholecystitis

Acute Cholangitis

- **MC organisms:** ***E. coli***, *Klebsiella, Pseudomonas, Enterococcus*
- **Obstruction of CBD** leading to bacterial stasis, bacterial overgrowth, suppuration, biliary sepsis
- **Charcots triad:** Fever + RUQ pain + Jaundice
- **Reynolds pentad:** Fever + RUQ pain + Jaundice + Shock + Confusion
- **Suppurative cholangitis** has a high mortality rate

Sclerosing Cholangitis

- **Progressive, inflammatory, sclerosing, and obliterative process** affecting the **'extrahepatic <u>and/or</u> the intrahepatic bile ducts'**
- The disorder occurs in about 70% in association with **inflammatory bowel disease**, especially ulcerative colitis
- Also associated (albeit rarely) with **multifocal Fibrosclerosis Syndromes** such as:
  - ***Retroperitoneal, mediastinal, and/or periureteral fibrosis***
  - ***Riedel's struma***
  - ***Pseudotumor of the orbit***

Cholangiopancreatography may demonstrate a broad range of biliary tract changes as well as pancreatic duct obstruction and occasionally pancreatitis

- Often present with signs and symptoms of chronic or intermittent **biliary obstruction: jaundice, pruritus, RUQ abdominal pain, or acute cholangitis**
- Late in the course, complete biliary obstruction, secondary biliary cirrhosis, hepatic failure, or portal hypertension with bleeding varices may occur
- The diagnosis is established ***beaded appearance on cholangiography***

Complications

- **Adenocarcinoma colon**
- **Adenocarcinoma bile ducts**
- **Cirrhosis**

Hemobilia

- **Triad of:**
  - **Abdominal pain**
  - **Obstructive jaundice**
  - **Melana**
- **Occurs as a result of bleeding into biliary tract**
- **Causes:**
  - **Trauma**
  - **Gallstones**
  - **Cholangiohepatitis**
  - **Neoplasms of hepatobiliary system**
  - **Hepatic artery trauma**

Kidney

Renal tuberculosis

- Tuberculosis of the urinary tract arises from **hematogenous infection** from a distant focus which is often impossible to identify. The lesions are usually confined to one kidney
- A group of tuberculous granulomas in a renal pyramid coalesces and forms an ulcer. Mycobacteria and pus cells are discharged into the urine
- Sterile pyuria is a consistent feature
- Untreated, the lesions enlarge and **a tuberculous abscess** may form in the parenchyma
- The necks of the calyces and the renal pelvis stenosed by fibrosis confine the infection so that there is tuberculous pyonephrosis, which is sometimes localized to one pole of the kidney
- Extension of pyonephrosis or tuberculous renal abscess leads to perinephric abscess and the kidney is progressively replaced by caseous material **(putty kidney)** which may be calcified **(cement kidney)**
- At any stage, the plain radiograph may show areas of calcification **(pseudocalculi)**
- Less commonly the kidneys may be bilaterally affected as part of the generalized process of miliary tuberculosis
- Renal tuberculosis is often associated with tuberculosis of the bladder and typical tuberculous granulomas may be visible in the bladder wall. In the male, tuberculous epididymo-orchitis may occur without apparent infection of the bladder
- IVU is the most sensitive technique for detecting early renal TB.

Renal carbuncle

- An **abscess** in the **renal parenchyma** as the result of blood-borne spread of organisms, especially coliforms or *Staphylococcus aureus*, from a focus elsewhere in the body
- Occasionally the condition results from infection of a hematoma following a blow to the kidney
- Renal carbuncle is most commonly seen in **diabetic patients**, **intravenous drug abusers, those debilitated by chronic disease and patients with acquired immunodeficiency**.

Pathology: the renal parenchyma contains an encapsulated necrotic mass

Clinical features: There is an ill-defined tender swelling in the loin, persistent pyrexia and leucocytosis, signs that closely simulate those of perinephric abscess. In early cases, there is no pus or bacteria in the urine but they appear after a day or so. Urography shows a space-occupying lesion in the kidney which may be confused with a renal adenocarcinoma on ultrasonography and CT

Treatment: Resolution by antibiotic treatment alone is unusual. Formal open incision of the abscess may be necessary if the pus is too thick to be drained by percutaneous aspiration.

Idiopathic Retroperitoneal Fibrosis

- Rare condition in which one or both ureters become bound up in a **progressive fibrosis of the retroperitoneal tissues**
- The cause is unknown, although some cases may be drug-related
- The patient complains of backache, which is unremitting for several months
- The onset of anuria and renal failure prompts investigation of the renal tract which reveals hydronephrosis
- The excretion urogram typically shows displacement of the obstructed ureters ***towards the midline*** and the appearances on CT are diagnostic
- The sedimentation rate is markedly raised.

Randall's plaque and microliths

- Initial lesion in some cases of kidney stone was an **erosion at the tip of a renal papilla**
- **Deposition of calcium** on this erosion produced a lesion which has been called **Randall's plaque**
- Minute concretions **(microliths)** regularly occur in the renal parenchyma. These particles are carried by lymphatics to the subendothelial region where they may accumulate
- Ulceration of the epithelium exposes the potential calculus to the urine with the result that a stone forms. The importance of **Randall's plaques and Carr's microliths** is the pathogenesis for calculi
- Renal calculi overlie spine on lateral view
- **Renal colic + swelling in loin + disappearance of swelling with micturition = Dietl's crisis**
- **Pain in ureteric colic is due to ureteric peristalsis**
- **Noncontrast CT is the most sensitive diagnostic method for acute ureteric colic.**

'Renal Calculi'

- **Calcium stones:** Calcium oxalate and calcium phosphate stones make up **75 to 85% of the total renal calculi**
- **Most common**
- Calcium stones are **more common in men**; the average age of onset is the third decade. Approximately, 60% of people who form a single calcium stone eventually form another within the next 10 years
- In the urine, calcium oxalate monohydrate crystals **(whewellite)** usually grow as biconcave ovals that resemble red blood cells in shape and size but may occur in a larger, 'dumbbell' form.

- **Uric acid stones** are **radiolucent** and are also more common in men
- Half of patients with uric acid stones have gout; **uric acid lithiasis** is usually familial whether or not gout is present. In urine, uric acid crystals are **red-orange in color** because they absorb the pigment uricine
- Uric acid gravel appears like red dust, and the stones are also orange or red on some occasions.

- **Cystine stones** are uncommon, lemon yellow, and sparkle
- Radiopacity is due to the **sulfur content**
- Cystine crystals appear in the urine as flat, **hexagonal plates**.

- **Struvite stones** are common and **potentially dangerous**
- These stones occur mainly in **women** or patients who require chronic bladder catheterization and result from urinary tract infection with **urease-producing bacteria, usually *Proteus* species**
- **Grow in alkaline urine**
- **Grow in infected urine**
- The stones can grow to a large size and fill the renal pelvis and calyces to produce a **'staghorn' appearance**
- They are **radiopaque** and have a variable internal density. In urine, struvite crystals are **rectangular prisms** said to resemble **coffin lids**.

- On X-ray lateral view, renal stone is superimposed on shadow of vertebral column
- CT scan is the invstigation of choice for emergency.

- Most of ureteric calculi originate in kidney
- Sites of impaction of ureteric calculi:
  - **Pelviuretreric junction**
  - **At the crossing of iliac artery**
  - **Entering the bladder wall**
  - **Ureteric orifice**
- Small (< 2.5 cms) stone in proximal ureter: **ESWL**
- (> 2.5 cms) stone in proximal ureter: **Nephrolithotomy**
- Small stone in distal ureter: **Ureteroscopic removal**
- Large/long-standing stone in distal ureter: **Ureterolithotomy**
- **Stones hard to break in ESWL: Cysteine stones**

Stones (Calculi)

- **Whewellite:** (Calcium oxalate monohydrate crystals)
- **Weddilite:** (Calcium oxalate dihydrate crystals)
- **Staghorn/Coffin lid:** Struvite
- **Radiolucent:** Uric acid
- **Radio-opaque:** Calcium, Struvite, Cysteine

Acute Pyelonephritis

It is an infectious disease involving the kidney parenchyma and the renal pelvis. Gram-negative bacteria, such as *Escherichia coli, Proteus, Klebsiella*, and *Enterobacter*, are the most common causative organisms in acute pyelonephritis. Laboratory evaluation will often reveal leukocytosis with a left shift, and urinalysis typically shows pyuria, varying degrees of hematuria, and white cell casts. Since bacteremia is present, the patient should be hospitalized and empirically started on IV ampicillin and gentamicin.

Perinephric and Renal Abscesses

- The presentation of perinephric and renal abscesses is quite nonspecific
- Flank pain and abdominal pain are common
- At least 50% of patients are febrile
- Pain may be referred to the groin or leg, particularly with extension of infection.
- ***Perinephric or renal abscess should be most seriously considered when a patient presents with symptoms and signs of pyelonephritis and remains febrile after 4 or 5 days, by which time the fever should have resolved***
- **Renal ultrasonography and abdominal CT are the most useful diagnostic modalities**
- Treatment for perinephric or renal abscesses includes drainage of pus and antibiotic therapy directed at the organism(s) recovered
- For perinephric abscesses, percutaneous drainage is usually successful.

Renal Cell Carcinoma

SYNONYM: Hypernephroma, Grawitz tumor

- Accounts for 90 to 95% of malignant neoplasms arising from the kidney

Unusual features:

- **Refractoriness to cytotoxic agents**
- **Infrequent but reproducible responses to biologic response modifiers such as interferon and interleukin (IL) 2**
- **Spontaneous regression**

Epidemiology and Etiology

- **Cigarette smoking**
- **von Hippel-Lindau (VHL) syndrome. Tuberous sclerosis and polycystic kidney disease**
- **Abnormalities on chromosome 3 are most frequent**
- Most of the cancers arise from the **epithelial cells of the proximal tubules**
- Categories include:
  - Clear cell carcinoma (60% of cases)
  - Papillary (5 to 15%), chromophobic tumors (5 to 10%)
  - Oncocytomas (5 to 10%)
  - Collecting or Bellini duct tumors (RARER)

- The presenting signs and symptoms include **hematuria, abdominal pain, and a flank or abdominal mass.** This '**classic triad'** occurs in 10 to 20% of patients. Other symptoms are fever, weight loss, anemia, and a varicocele
- Causes expansile osteolytic lesions
- A spectrum of paraneoplastic syndromes has been associated with these malignancies, including:
  - **Erythrocytosis**
  - **Hypercalcemia**
  - **Nonmetastatic hepatic dysfunction (Stauffers' syndrome)**
  - **Acquired dysfibrinogenemia**

Erythrocytosis is present at presentation in only about 3% of patients

- **More frequently anemia, a sign of advanced disease**
- **Cushing's syndrome**
- **Galactorrhea**
- **Amyloidosis**
- **Hypertension**
- **PUO**

Staging by 'Robson' staging

- **Mc site of metastasis is lung,** soft tissue, bone, liver
- **Secondaries are 'expansile, osteolytic'**
  - The standard management for stage I or II tumors and selected cases of stage III disease is **radical nephrectomy**
  - There is no proven role for adjuvant chemotherapy, immunotherapy, or radiation therapy following successful surgical removal of the tumor, even in cases with a poor prognosis
  - **Surgery in the setting of metastases**: Nephrectomy may be indicated in highly selected cases for the alleviation of symptoms, including pain or recurrent urinary hemorrhage, and particularly if the latter is severe or associated with obstruction.

Pheochromocytoma

- Tumor of chromaffin cells
- (Headache) Hypertension is a common symptom but not a reliable symptom of pheochromocytoma
- Pheochromocytoma is a cause of '**Episodic/Paroxysmal' Hypertension** and not persistent hypertension
- Pheochromocytoma is also a cause of **'Orthostatic Hypotension.**'
- This rare tumor is most often found in the adrenal medulla, although it can also be found in other tissues derived from neural crest cells. The tumor cells secrete catecholamine hormones or their precursors, which can cause either paroxysmal or persistent hypertension. Urinary metabolites of epinephrine and norepinephrine are:
  - Vanillylmandelic acid (VMA) and homovanillic acid
  - So screening 24-hour urine collections for these substances can be helpful in establishing or excluding these diagnoses even in cases in which a physician does not observe one of the paroxysms and thus blood cannot be drawn for serum catecholamine levels at that time.

- NA production is ↑↑
  - **Bilateral in 10% cases**
  - **Extra-adrenal in 10% cases**
  - **Familial in 10% cases**
  - **Malignant in 10% cases**
  - **Multiple in 10% cases**
- **↑urinary VMA levels seen**
- **↑urinary metanephrine**
- MIBG scan is **most specific and sensitive for diagnosis**

Associated with:

- ***MEN 2 syndromes***
- ***von-Hippel-Lindau syndrome***
- ***Neurofibromatosis***
- ***Sturge-Weber syndrome***

Renal Artery Stenosis/Ischemic Renal Disease

- Accounts for 2 to 5% of hypertension
- Commonest cause in the **middle-aged and elderly** is an atheromatous plaque at the origin of the **renal artery**
- **In younger women**, *fibromuscular dysplasia* is the commonest cause

Renal artery stenosis should be suspected when hypertension develops in a previously normotensive individual over 50 years of age or in the young (under 30 years) with suggestive features: symptoms of vascular insufficiency to other organs, high-pitched epigastric bruit on physical examination, symptoms of hypokalemia secondary to hyperaldosteronism (muscle weakness, tetany, polyuria), and metabolic alkalosis

Understand the difference:

- The **'best initial screening test'** is a renal ultrasound
- A positive captopril test, which has a sensitivity and specificity of greater than 95%, constitutes an **'excellent follow-up procedure'** to assess the need for more invasive radiographic evaluation
- Magnetic resonance angiography (MRA) is the **'most sensitive (100%) and specific' (95%)** test for the diagnosis of renal arterial stenosis
- **The 'most definitive diagnostic procedure'** is **bilateral arteriography with repeated bilateral renal vein and systemic renin determinations**

Treatment

Interventional therapy (i.e. surgery or angioplasty) is superior to medical therapy, which, while controlling blood pressure, does little to salvage renal mass lost to ischemic injury.

Nutcracker phenomenon

- It is seen in varicocele
- It refers to **nut-inside-a-cracker**-like image
- The left renal vein is distended in varicocele on the left side
- As a result, **'Left renal vein gets compressed'** in between superior mesenteric artery and the aorta leading to renal vein hypertension
- The remedy is surgical transposition of left renal vein

The two diseases most commonly leading to renal failure and treatable by kidney transplantation are **glomerulonephritis and insulin-dependent diabetes mellitus**

Other important causes include:

- **Polycystic kidney disease**
- **Hypertensive nephrosclerosis**

- **Alport's disease**
- **IgA nephropathy**
- **Systemic lupus erythematosus**
- **Nephrosclerosis**
- **Interstitial nephritis**
- **Pyelonephritis**
- **Obstructive uropathy**
- **Hypertensive nephrosclerosis**

The left kidney is chosen, if possible, since its longer renal vein facilitates the recipient operation

However, if the arteriogram shows multiple renal arteries on one side, the **kidney with a single artery** is usually selected to facilitate the anastomosis

A flank incision is used. After Gerota's fascia is incised, the greater curvature of the kidney and the upper pole are mobilized, and the hilar structures are exposed

On the left side, the adrenal and gonadal veins are ligated so that the full length of the renal vein can be utilized

Traction on the renal artery should be avoided, since it causes spasm and decreased kidney perfusion, possibly compromising early function

The ureter should be mobilized, along with its blood supply and a generous amount of periureteric tissue. It is divided close to the bladder after ligating the distal end.

Carcinoma of the Bladder

Carcinoma arising within the bladder may be of three cell types: **transitional, squamous and adenocarcinoma [or mixed owing to metaplasia in a transitional cell carcinoma (TCC)]**

- Over 90 percent are **transitional cells in origin**
- Pure squamous carcinoma is uncommon **(Schistosomiasis, stones, irradiation, smoking)**
- Primary adenocarcinoma, which arises either from the **urachal remnant or from areas of glandular metaplasia,** accounts for 1–2 percent of cases
- Mc site: **Trigone and posterior wall**
- Mc symptom: **Painless hematuria.**

Transitional cell carcinoma

Following compounds may be carcinogenic:

- ***2-naphthylamine***
- ***4-aminobiphenyl***
- ***Benzidine***
- ***Chlornaphazine***
- ***4-chloro-o-toluidine***
- ***o-toluidine***
- ***4,4-methylenebis (2-choloraniline)***
- ***Methylene dianiline***
- ***Benzidine-derived azo dyes***

Occupations: Significantly excess risk of bladder cancer

- ***Textile workers***
- ***Dye workers***
- ***Tyre rubber and cable workers***
- ***Petrol workers***
- ***Leather workers***

- ***Shoe manufacturers and cleaners***
- ***Painters***
- ***Hairdressers***
- ***Lorry drivers***
- ***Drill press operators***
- ***Chemical workers***
- ***Rodent exterminators and sewage workers***

- **Cystoscopy** is the mainstay for evaluation
- Antigenic tests utilizing **NMP-22, MCM proteins** are used
- **Filling defect on IVU** is the most common sign
- Much said about **intravesical BCG** is advised for initial stage (Ta)
  - Kiss cancer is benign tumor of bladder
  - Tear drop bladder is pelvic hematoma
  - Secondary vesical calculus is stone in bladder after infection.

Schistosomiasis

- ***S. Haematobonium*** is causative agent
- Resides in **vesical venous plexus**
- Urticaria at the site of penetration occurs **(Swimmers' itch)**
- **Calcifications with small contracted bladder.**

Intermittent	**Painless**	**Terminal**	**Hematuria**

- **Praziquantel** is the DOC

Surgery is done in case of:

- Secondary bacterial cystitis
- Urinary calculi
- Ureteric stricture
- Seminal vesiculitis
- Fibrosis of bladder and bladder neck
- Cancer

Cystoscopic Features

- **'Pseudotubercles'** on cystoscopy are the earliest specific features. The pseudotubercles are larger, more prominent, more numerous, more yellow and more distinctly grouped.
- **'Nodules'** are due to fusion of tubercles.
- **'Sandy patches'** are a result of calcified dead ova.
- **'Ulceration'** is the result of sloughing of mucous membrane containing dead ova. Ulcers are shallow, bleed readily.
- **'Carcinoma'** is the end result of neglected bilharziasis.
- Carcinoma commences in ulcer and not papilloma.
- It is usually well advanced and requires radical cystectomy.

Special Forms of Lower Urinary Tract Infection

Acute abacterial cystitis (acute hemorrhagic cystitis)

- The patient presents with symptoms of severe UTI
- Pus is present in the urine, but no organism can be cultured.

- It is sometimes associated with abacterial urethritis and is commonly sexually acquired. Tuberculous infection and carcinoma *in situ* must be ruled out
- The underlying causative organism may be **mycoplasma or herpes**.

Frequency dysuria syndrome (urethral syndrome)

- This is common in women
- It consists of symptoms suggestive of urinary infection, but with negative urine cultures and absent pus cells
- Carcinoma *in situ*, tuberculosis and interstitial cystitis should be excluded
- Adopt general measures such as wearing cotton underwear, using simple soaps, general perineal hygiene and voiding after intercourse
- Other treatments include cystoscopy and urethral dilatation, although the benefits remain doubtful.

Tuberculous urinary infection

- Tuberculous urinary infection is **secondary to renal tuberculosis**
- Cystoscopy shows that early tuberculosis of the bladder **commences around the ureteric orifice or trigone,** the earliest evidence being **pallor of the mucosa** due to submucous edema
- Subsequently tubercles may be seen **cobble-stone appearance**
- Long-standing cases: There is much fibrosis and the capacity of the bladder is greatly reduced, scarred, fibrosed, small capacity **(thimble bladder)**
- Rigid wide-mouthed ureter **(golf hole ureter)**

Reiter's Syndrome

Patients typically present with the acute onset of arthritis (usually asymmetric and additive), with involvement of new joints occurring over a period of a few days to 2 weeks. Joints of the lower extremities are the most commonly involved, but wrists and fingers can also be affected. **Dactylitis (sausage digit),** a diffuse swelling of a solitary finger or toe, is a distinctive feature of Reiter's arthritis and psoriatic arthritis. **Tendonitis and fasciitis are common.** Spinal pain and low back pain are common. Conjunctivitis, urethritis, diarrhea, and skin lesions are also associated with Reiter's syndrome. Up to 75% of patients are **HLA-B27 positive**. Micro-organisms which can trigger Reiter's syndrome include ***Shigella spp., Salmonella spp., Yersinia spp., Campylobacter jejuni, and Chlamydia trachomatis.*** **Most patients are younger males.**

Incontinence

Genuine stress incontinence is defined as urinary leakage occurring during increased bladder pressure when this is solely due to increased abdominal pressure and not due to increased true detrusor pressure. It is caused by sphincter weakness. The commonest cause of leakage of urine in women is genuine stress incontinence (GSI), although in some parts of the world, vesicourethral fistulae owing to neglected labor are very common. GSI occurs secondary to weakness of the distal sphincter mechanism associated with laxity of the pelvic floor. It is usually found in multiparous women with a history of difficult labor often accompanied by the use of forceps.

Chronic urinary retention with overflow incontinence. This is recognized by a large residual volume of urine and is usually associated with high pressures during bladder filling.

Neurogenic incontinence. The common causes include:

- **Myelodysplasia**
- **Multiple sclerosis**
- **Spinal cord injuries**
- **Cerebral dysfunction [cerebrovascular accident (CVA), dementia]**
- **Parkinson's disease (paralysis agitans)**

These conditions lead to a combination of neurogenic vesical dysfunction often associated with loss of mobility. Careful investigation of the whole urinary tract is always required, and the treatment needs to strike a fine balance between preventing hydronephrosis from abnormally high bladder pressures, yet at the same time maintaining continence.

The mainstay of management is accurate urodynamic assessment to assess bladder emptying, incontinence and the risks to the upper tract. The upper tracts should be assessed with regular ultrasound scanning, and assessment of the patient's mobility, intelligence and motivation is vital. The important factors to assess urodynamically are:

- Bladder emptying
- Bladder capacity and bladder pressure during filling
- Continence

Small bladder capacity. The capacity of the bladder may be considerably diminished in several conditions. This can cause crippling urinary frequency and incontinence. It may follow tuberculosis, radiotherapy or interstitial cystitis. Radiotherapy for pelvic cancer can also cause this problem.

Drug-induced incontinence. The detrusor muscle is basically under postganglionic parasympathetic control and the main neurotransmitter system is cholinergic. A number of drugs can induce urinary retention **(anticholinergic agents, tricyclic antidepressants, lithium and some antihypertensives)**.

Constant dribbling of urine coupled with normal micturition. This occurs when there is a ureteric fistula or an ectopic ureter associated with a duplex system opening into the urethra beyond the urethral sphincter in females, or into the vagina. The history is diagnostic, and intravenous pyelography or ultrasound scanning may reveal the upper pole segment which is often poorly functioning. These segments are very liable to infection. Treatment is by excision of the aberrant ureter and portion of kidney which needs it. A ureteric fistula can be difficult to diagnose and may require retrograde ureterography and a high degree of suspicion to demonstrate.

Rupture of the Bladder

This may be **intraperitoneal (20 percent)** or **extraperitoneal (80 percent)**

Intraperitoneal rupture may be secondary to a blow, kick or fall on a fully distended bladder and it is more common in the male than in the female, and usually follows a bout of beer drinking. More rarely, it is due to surgical damage. Extraperitoneal rupture is usually caused by a fractured pelvis or is secondary to major trauma or surgical damage.

- **Sudden, agonizing pain in the hypogastrium, often accompanied by syncope**
- **The shock later subsides and the abdomen commences to distend**
- **No desire to micturate**
- **Varying degrees of abdominal rigidity and abdominal distension are present on examination**
- **No suprapubic dullness, but there is tenderness**
- **There may be shifting dullness**
- **If the urine is sterile, symptoms and signs of peritonitis are delayed**

Extraperitoneal rupture

In many cases of pelvic trauma, this is difficult to distinguish from rupture of the membranous urethra.

Confirming a suspected diagnosis of intraperitoneal rupture

- Plain X-ray in the erect position may show the ground-glass appearance of fluid in the lower abdomen
- Intravenous urography (IVU) may confirm a leak from the bladder
- A peritoneal 'tap' may be of value if facilities for radiological examination are not available
- If doubt still exists and if there is no sign of fracture, then retrograde cystography can be performed safely. With careful asepsis, a small [14 French gauge (FG)] catheter is passed. Usually some blood-stained urine will drain. A solution made from 60 ml of 35 percent Hypaque® or Conray® with 120 ml of sterile isotonic saline is injected into the bladder and radiographs are taken.

Ectopia vesicae (syn. exstrophy of the bladder)

Caused by the incomplete development of the infraumbilical part of the anterior abdominal wall, associated with incomplete development of the anterior wall of the bladder owing to delayed rupture of the cloacal membrane.

Clinical features of ectopia vesicae:

- One in 50,000 births (four male: one female)
- **Characteristic appearance because of the pressure of the viscera behind it**
- **Edges of abdominal wall can be felt**
- **Umbilicus is absent**

Urethral Stricture

The causes of urethral stricture are:

- Congenital
- Traumatic; MC Cause
- Inflammatory:
  - **Postgonorrheal**
  - **Posturethral chancre**
  - **Tuberculous**
- Instrumental:
  - **Indwelling catheter**
  - **Urethral endoscopy**
- Postoperative:
  - **Open prostatectomy**
  - **Amputation of penis**

Extravasation of Urine

Superficial extravasation is likely with **complete rupture of the bulbar urethra** and in ruptured urethral abscess.

- The extravasated urine is **confined in front of the midperineal point** by the attachment of Colles fascia to the triangular ligament, and by the attachment of Scarpa's fascia just below the inguinal ligament. The external spermatic fascia stops it getting into the inguinal canals
- Extravasated urine **collects in the scrotum and penis and beneath the deep layer of superficial fascia in the abdominal wall.**

Treatment is by **urgent operation** to drain the bladder by suprapubic cystostomy. This prevents further extravasation.

Deep extravasation occurs with **extraperitoneal rupture of the bladder or intrapelvic rupture of the urethra**

- It can also occur if the ureter is damaged or if there is perforation of the prostatic capsule or bladder during transurethral resection
- Urine extravasates in the layers of the **pelvic fascia and the retroperitoneal tissues.**

Treatment is by **suprapubic cytostomy** and drainage of the retropubic space.

- Urethral injury associated with pelvis: Membranous urethral injury
- Urethral injury associated with high-flying prostate: Membranous urethral injury
- Bladder injury associated with pelvis: Extraperitoneal rupture.

Injuries to the Male Urethra

Rupture of the bulbar urethra

Rupture of the bulbar urethra is the **most common urethral injury**

There is a **history of a blow to the perineum** usually due to a fall astride a projecting object. Cycling accidents, loose manhole covers and gymnasium accidents astride the beam account for a number of cases

Clinical features:

The triad of signs of a ruptured bulbar urethra is:

- **Retention of urine**
- **Perineal hematoma**
- **Bleeding from the external urinary meatus**

Rupture of the membranous urethra

Extraperitoneal rupture of the urethra

Intrapelvic rupture of the membranous urethra occurs near the apex of the prostate. Like extraperitoneal rupture of the bladder, it may be due to penetrating wounds but in civilian life, it is usually a result of **pelvic fracture**.

Fracture of the pubic and ischial rami is most likely to result when sudden force is applied to one lower limb in a car accident or in landing on one leg after falling from a height. There is an associated disruption of the sacroiliac joint so that one half of the pelvis and ischiopubic ramus is pushed up above the other. This applies a traction force on the prostate which is firmly bound by ligaments to the back of the symphysis pubis. The torn ends of the urethra may be widely displaced by this type of injury

Catheterization is best avoided.

Congenital Valves of the Posterior Urethra

- These are symmetrical folds of urothelium which can cause obstruction to the urethra of boys
- They are **usually found just distal to the verumontanum** but they may be within the prostatic urethra. They behave as flap valves. So, although urine does not flow normally, a urethral catheter can be passed without difficulty.
- In some instances, the valves are incomplete and the patient remains without symptoms until adolescence or adulthood
- In such cases, the prostatic urethra is grossly dilated and saccules and diverticula are present within it.

Other Important Points about Posterior Urethral Valves

- Symmetrical folds of **urothelium**
- Common **distal to verumontanum**
- Occur **in males** only
- MC cause of urinary obstruction in male infant
- Cause **obstruction to passage of urine and catheter**
- Diagnosis is by **VCUG** and endoscopy
- Associated with **VURD syndrome** (urethral valves, unilateral reflux, renal dysplasia)

Hypospadias

- Hypospadias occurs in one in 350 male births
- It is the most common congenital malformation of the urethra
- The external meatus opens on the underside of the penis or the perineum and the inferior aspect of the prepuce is poorly developed **('hooded prepuce')**
- **Meatal stenosis** also occurs
- **Bifid scrotum.**

Hypospadias is classified according to position of the meatus.

Glandular hypospadias — this is the **most common type** and does not usually require treatment. The normal site of the external meatus is marked by a blind pit, although it occasionally connects by a channel to the ectopic opening on the underside of the glans.

Coronal hypospadias — the meatus is placed at the junction of the underside of the glans and the body of the penis.

Penile and penoscrotal hypospadias — the opening is on the **underside of the penile shaft.**

Perineal hypospadias — this is the **most severe abnormality**. The scrotum is split and the urethra opens between its two halves. There may be testicular maldescent which may make it difficult to determine the sex of the child.

The more severe varieties of hypospadias represent an absence of the urethra and corpus spongiosum distal to the ectopic opening. The absent structures are represented by a fibrous cord which deforms the penis in a downward direction **(chordee).** The more distant the opening from its normal position, the more pronounced the bowing

6-10 months of age is the best time for surgery.

Cryptorchidism

The term 'cryptorchidism' (Greek cryptos = hidden, orchis = testis) should be reserved for impalpable, usually abdominal, testes

- There is a higher incidence of undescended testes in **premature** than in full-term babies.

- Two-thirds of undescended testes in newborn infants will descend, usually by 6 weeks in term and 3 months in preterm babies
- There is an increased incidence of cryptorchidism in **anencephalics** and other cerebral anomalies

Ectopic testes

These have descended as far as the external inguinal ring and then become deviated into the:

- **Superficial inguinal pouch**
- **Perineal**
- **Suprapubic or**
- **Femoral ectopic sites**
- The commonest by far is the superficial inguinal pouch, above and lateral to the external inguinal ring.

Retractile testes

The cremasteric reflex in young children will draw the testes into the region of the superficial inguinal pouch very readily but they can be manipulated back down to the bottom of the scrotum. The testis would normally reside in the scrotum if such a child is in a warm bath or is relaxed in bed.

Ascending testis

Some boys with recorded testicular descent at routine clinic checks in infancy may be found later at preschool or school medicals to have an undescended testis. This phenomenon of the 'ascending testis' was noted first by Atwell. It has been suggested that this is caused by failure of elongation of the spermatic cord during differential body growth, so that the testis is drawn up by absorption of the processus vaginalis.

Anorchia

Anorchia may be on one or both sides. If on one side alone, there may be ipsilateral renal agenesis. If the baby is fully masculinized but both testes are absent, it must be assumed that they have atrophied subsequent to torsion or infarction during development. **Absence of testicular tissue** and, therefore, lack of Müllerian inhibitory hormone during early gestation can lead to Müllerian development along the female lines. The lack of androgenic stimulation (testosterone) from the testes leads to failure of Wolffian duct development.

Predisposing Factors for Torsion of Testis are

- Inversion of testis
- Long mesorchium
- Undescended/ectopic testis
- High investment of tunica vaginalis
- Initiating factors: Spasm of cremaster
- **Torsion of spinal cord involves twisting of spermatic cord along its long axis. Left testis rotates anticlockwise and right testis rotates clockwise i.e. away from midline**
- **'De torsion' is the initial treatment.**

- Torsion of the testicle should be corrected as soon as possible after the diagnosis is entertained
- Incomplete torsion can cause partial strangulation, the effects of which may be overcome if surgical intervention is accomplished within 12 hours, whereas severe torsion with complete compromise of the blood supply results in loss of the testis unless surgical intervention occurs within approximately 4 hours
- The contralateral scrotum should also be explored at the time of the operation, since the primary anatomic defect—insufficient attachment of the testicle to the scrotal sidewall—most often is a bilateral phenomenon
- If the contralateral scrotum is not explored, the patient runs a very high risk of undergoing torsion on the other side and the possible complication of loss of both testes.

Hazards of Incomplete Descent are

- Sterility in bilateral cases
- Pain due to trauma
- An associated indirect inguinal hernia that is often present and, in older patients, it is frequently the hernia which causes symptoms
- Torsion
- Epididymo-orchitis that, in an incompletely descended testis, is extremely rare but of interest because, on the right side, it mimics appendicitis
- Atrophy of an inguinal testis that can occur even before puberty, possibly due to recurrent minor trauma
- Increased liability to malignant disease. All types of malignant testicular tumor are more common in incompletely descended testes even if they have been brought down surgically
- **Operate at between 9 and15 months of age.**

Testicular torsion	Epididymitis
• Usually < 30 yrs of age	• Usually > 30 yrs of age
• Pain stays same/worsens with testicular elevation (Prehn's test)	• Pain ↓ with testicular elevation
• Immediate exploration needed	• Immediate exploration NOT needed

Remember

- **Aspermia:** No ejaculate
- **Oligospermia:** Sperm count less than 20 million/ml
- **Polyzoospermia:** Count >350 million/ml
- **Azoospermia:** No spermatozoa in semen
- **Asthenozoospermia:** Reduced sperm motility
- **Necrozoospermia:** Spermatozoa are dead
- **Teratozoospermia:** >70% Spermatozoa with abnormal morphology

Oligospermia, by definition, indicates a sperm count of less than 20 million per ml. and under such circumstances, fertility is difficult

The principal causes of defective spermatogenesis include:

- Congenital inadequacy of the seminiferous tubules;
- Testicular damage as a consequence of infection, trauma, or infarction;
- Klinefelter's syndrome;
- Hypopituitarism;
- Varicocele; and
- Cryptorchidism
- Other causes of oligospermia may relate to the transport of spermatozoa. Chronic prostatitis and seminal vesiculitis may result in fibrosis and impede transport and delivery of sperm. Infection spreading into the vas deferens may induce fibrosis and stricture even to the point of total occlusion.

Azoospermia, complete absence of spermatozoa in the ejaculate, may be caused by:

- Total occlusion of the sperm transport system, vasa, seminal vesicles, or ejaculatory ducts. Congenital absence of the vasa and seminal vesicles may occur as an isolated anatomic defect, and congenital absence of the vasa is the rule in males with cystic fibrosis
- Gonococcal epididymitis and vasitis may cause complete stenosis and azoospermia
- Complete nonresponsiveness of the germinal epithelium as in primary gonadal failure may also produce a picture of azoospermia despite elevated follicle-stimulating hormone levels
- Trauma to the vasa in the course of an inguinal hernia operation or orchidopexy

Testicular Cancer

- **Primary germ cell tumors (GCTs) of the testis** constitute 95% of all testicular neoplasms. Infrequently, GCTs arise from an extragonadal site, including the mediastinum, retroperitoneum and, very rarely, the pineal gland
- **Bilateral in 10% cases**
- **Cryptorchidism** is associated with a several fold higher risk of GCT
- **Abdominal cryptorchid testes are at a higher risk** than inguinal cryptorchid testes
- Orchiopexy should be performed before puberty, if possible
- **Testicular feminization syndromes** increase the risk of testicular GCT
- **Klinefelter's syndrome** is associated with mediastinal GCT
- An isochromosome of the short arm of chromosome 12 is pathognomonic for GCT
- **A painless testicular mass** is pathognomonic for a testicular malignancy

Mc tumor of testis: Seminoma

Mc histological subtype: Mixed

Mc tumor in infants: Yolk sac tumor

Mc tumor in aged elderly: Lymphoma

Commonest testicular malignancy is: Seminoma

Most malignant testicular cancer is: Choriocarcinoma

Seminoma

- It has a median age in the fourth decade
- Generally follows a more indolent clinical course
- Seminomas are radiosensitive
- **But surgery is the TOC**
- Seminomas metastasize by lymphatics
- Seminomas correspond to dysgerminomas of ovary.

Spermatocele

- Spermatocele is a **unilocular retention cyst**
- It **almost always** lies in relation to the head of the epididymis
- The fluid **contains spermatozoa and resembles 'barley fluid'**
- Treatment for small spermatoceles is conservative follow-up while larger ones should be aspirated or excised
- A spermatocele is a diverticulum of the epididymis that contains cloudy fluid with spermatozoa. It is unilocular or multilocular and often confused with hydrocele because both a spermatocele and a hydrocele can be transilluminated. Differential diagnosis of spermatocele and hydrocele is aided by the localization of the mass: hydrocele generally surrounds the testis, while the spermatocele is more eccentric, can often be palpated in direct conjunction with the epididymis, and is often tender.

Cysts Connected with the Epididymis

Epididymal cysts

These are filled with a **crystal-clear fluid** (as opposed to the barley-water fluid of a spermatocele or the amber fluid of a hydrocele). They are very common, usually multiple and vary greatly in size at presentation. They represent cystic degeneration of the epididymis

Cyst of a testicular appendage

Cyst of a testicular appendage is usually unilateral and is felt as a small globular swelling at the superior pole. Such cysts are liable to torsion and should be removed if they cause symptoms.

Spermatocele

- This is a unilocular retention cyst derived from some portion of the sperm-conducting mechanism of the epididymis. A spermatocele **nearly always lies in the head of the epididymis** above and behind the upper pole of the testis
- It is usually softer and laxer than other cystic lesions in the scrotum but like them it transilluminates
- The fluid contains spermatozoa and resembles barley water in appearance
- Spermatoceles are usually small and unobtrusive. Less frequently they are large enough to make the patient think that he has three testicles.

Infantile hydrocele

Infantile hydrocele does not necessarily appear in infants. The tunica and processus vaginalis are distended to the inguinal ring but there is no connection with the peritoneal cavity.

Congenital hydrocele

The processus vaginalis is patent and connects with the general peritoneal cavity. The communication is usually too small to allow herniation of intra-abdominal contents. Digital pressure on the hydrocele does not usually empty it but the hydrocele fluid may drain into the peritoneal cavity when the child is lying down. Ascites or even ascitic tuberculous peritonitis should be considered if the swellings are bilateral.

Encysted hydrocele of the cord

There is a smooth oval swelling near the spermatic cord which is liable to be mistaken for an inguinal hernia. The swelling moves downwards and becomes less mobile if the testis is pulled gently downwards

Hydrocele of the canal of Nuck is a similar condition. It occurs in females and the cyst lies in relation to the round ligament. Unlike a hydrocele of the cord, a hydrocele of the canal of Nuck is always at least partially within the inguinal canal.

Postherniorrhaphy hydrocele

Postherniorrhaphy hydrocele is a relatively rare complication of inguinal hernia repair. It is possibly due to interruption to the lymphatics draining the scrotal contents.

Hydrocele of a hernial sac

Hydrocele of a hernial sac occurs when the neck is plugged with omentum or occluded by adhesions.

Filarial hydroceles and chyloceles

Filarial hydroceles and chyloceles account for up to 80 percent of hydroceles in some tropical countries where the parasite is endemic. Filarial hydroceles follow repeated attacks of filarial epididymo-orchitis. They vary in size and may develop slowly or very rapidly.

Occasionally the fluid contains liquid fat which is rich in cholesterol. This is due to rupture of a lymphatic varix with discharge of chyle into the hydrocele. Adult worms of the Wuchereria bancrofti have been found in the epididymis removed at operation or at necropsy. In long-standing chyloceles, there are dense adhesions between the scrotum and its contents. Filarial elephantiasis supervenes in a small number of cases.

Acute tuberculous epididymitis should come to mind when the **vas is thickened** and there is little response to the usual antibiotics

Acute epididymo-orchitis of mumps

- Develops in about 18 percent of males suffering from mumps, usually as the parotid swelling is waning
- The main complication is **testicular atrophy** which may cause infertility if the condition is bilateral (which is not usual). Partial atrophy is associated with persistent testicular pain. The epididymitis of mumps sometimes occurs in the absence of parotitis, especially in infants. The epididymis and testis may be involved by infection with other enteroviruses and in brucellosis and lymphogranuloma venereum.

USMLE Case Scenario

A 35-year-old man comes to the clinic with a 3-day history of severe left-sided scrotal pain and swelling. He is sexually active and has multiple sexual partners. He has no history of sexually transmitted diseases. His temperature is 38.7°C, blood pressure is 126/70 mm Hg, and pulse is 84/min. Examination shows unilateral intrascrotal tenderness and swelling. Testicular support makes the pain less intense. Most likely diagnosis would be: Epididymitis.

Idiopathic Scrotal Gangrene

Idiopathic scrotal gangrene **(syn. Fournier's gangrene)** is an uncommon and nasty condition. It is a vascular disaster of infective origin which is characterized by:

- Sudden appearance of scrotal inflammation;
- Rapid onset of gangrene leading to exposure of the scrotal contents;
- Absence of any obvious cause in over half the cases.

It has been known to follow minor injuries or procedures in the perineal area, such as a bruise, scratch, urethral dilatation, injection of hemorrhoids or opening of a periurethral abscess.

The **hemolytic streptococcus** (sometimes microaerophilic) is associated with other organisms (staphylococcus, E. coli, Clostridium welchii) in a fulminating inflammation of the subcutaneous tissues which results in an obliterative arteritis of the arterioles to the scrotal skin

Varicocele

- Dilatation and tortuosity of the veins of the **pampiniform plexus**
- Most commonly observed on the **left**
- Development of a varicocele may be an **indicator of left renal tumor** because the left spermatic vein system drains into the renal vein and obstruction at that point could produce dilatation of the veins of the left cord
- There may be a **heavy, dragging, aching sensation** in the scrotal compartment
- **Bag of Worms**
- May be a feature of renal cancer
- Negative transillumination test
- Reducible
- Cough impulse +
- MC cause of surgically treated male infertility.

Hydrocele

The tunica vaginalis, derived from the peritoneum as the processus vaginalis at the time of testicular descent, is a secretory membrane. Fluid is generated by the serous surface of the tunica vaginalis

- Congenital hydrocele may follow **failure of obliteration of the processus vaginalis**, and fluid formed within the peritoneal cavity may gravitate into the tunica vaginalis
- There may sometimes be an **associated palpable inguinal hernia**
- In older persons, hydrocele is frequently the result of **epididymo-orchitis or trauma**
- **Lord's plication is used for hydrocele.**

Prostate Gland

- Shape: Chest-nut-shaped
- Type: Fibromusculoglangular organ
- Corresponding female organ: Paraurethral glands of Skene
- Volume: 8-12 ml
- Carcinoma arises from: Peripheral zone
- BHP arises from: Periurethral zone
- Fracture of the bony pelvis may often result in laceration and transection of the membranous urethra just distal to the prostate and urinary extravasation as well as bleeding may displace the prostate and bladder superiorly
- MC site of urethral cancer is also membranous urethra.

Benign Prostatic Hypertrophy (BPH, BHP)

Fibromusculoglandular hyperplasia (All 3 elements involved in varying proportion)

It is the **most common cause of bladder outlet obstruction** in men older than 50 years of age

Mechanical pressure phenomena cause:

- *Upward displacement of the base of the bladder*
- *Fish-hooking of the lower ureters due to trigonal displacement*
- *Hypertrophy of the bladder wall with trabeculation*
- *Cellule formation*
- *Diverticula* of the bladder
- *Complete bladder outlet obstruction may result in decompensation of the detrusor muscle and total urinary retention*
  - In the early stages, the patient complains of **diminished size and force of the urinary stream**
  - **Hematuria** may be caused by prostatic enlargement with engorgement of the small mucosal vessels covering the adenomatous gland, ruptured as a consequence of straining to urinate
  - Rectal examination shows most often **symmetric enlarged prostate and rubbery**
  - As enlargement progresses, the gland protrudes posteriorly, compressing the anterior rectal wall and sometimes producing symptoms of **constipation**
  - The size of the gland **bears little relationship** to the degree of symptomatic difficulty
  - **Anticholinergic drugs and antihistamines should be avoided** because they may precipitate urinary retention

Indications for a surgical procedure include:

- **Residual urine of more than 100 ml**, particularly when there is associated azotemia of any degree
- **Persistent or recurrent urinary infection** refractory to usual therapeutic methods; gross hematuria on more than one occasion
- **Acute urinary retention**
- **Chronic urinary retention** with overflow dribbling
- **Conservative therapy** is by drugs

Surgical procedures are:

- TURP
- Transvesical prostatectomy
- Retropubic prostatectomy
- Perineal prostatectomy

Ho: YAG laser is used

- **MC complication of TURP: Retrograde ejaculation**
- **Irrigation fluid used now in TURP: 1.5% Glycine**
- **Altered sensorium with drowsiness after TURP might indicate: Hyponatremia**

Complications of Prostatectomy

- Hemorrhage
- Bladder perforation
- Retrograde ejaculation/Impotence
- Incontinence
- Urethral stricture
- Hyponatremia
- Sepsis
- Osteitis pubis

Minimally Invasive Procedures

- Transurethral needle ablation of prostate (TUNA)
- Transurethral microwave therapy (TUMT)

- Transurethral US-guided laser-induced prostatectomy (TULIP)
- Transurethral vapourization of prostate (TUVP)
- Transurethral incision of prostate (TUIP)

Carcinoma of the Prostate

- **Adenocarcinoma** of the prostate is the most common
- Most often has its origin in **glandular acini of the peripheral group of glands located in the posterior and posterolateral regions of the prostate**
- Mc Neals Zone is referred to as **cancer zone**
- Peripheral zone is the commonest site
- PSA is the initial **screening test/marker**
- Unique qualities of prostatic carcinoma are that many tumors produce an enzyme, **acid phosphatase**, which can be detected in the serum of patients **with metastatic disease** or at least a very large local lesion
- **Prostate-specific antigen density (PSAD)** is calculated by dividing the serum PSA level by the estimated prostate weight calculated from transrectal ultrasonography (TRUS). **Values > 0.15 suggest** the presence of cancer. PSAD levels also increase with age
- **PSA velocity** is derived from calculations of the rate of change in **PSA before** the diagnosis of cancer was established. Increases of > 0.75 ng/mL per year are suggestive of cancer
- The noninvasive proliferation of epithelial cells within ducts is termed **'Prostatic intraepithelial neoplasia' (PIN)**. It is considered the precursor of cancer, but not all PIN lesions develop into invasive cancers
- Histologic grade is based most commonly on the **'Gleason system'**
- **Direct spread** is most common to seminal vesicles
- **Blood-borne** metastasis is most common to bones
- **Lymphatic spread** is most common to obturator nodes
- Secondaries are **osteoblastic**
- Metastasis to vertebrae is through **Batson's vertebral venous plexus**
- Carcinoma characteristically is **hard, nodular and irregular**
- **Digital rectal examination plus PSA levels are used for screening**
- **Gleason's staging is used for Ca prostate.**

Phimosis

Adhesions between the foreskin and the glans penis may persist until the boy is 6 years of age or more, giving the false impression that the prepuce will not retract. Rolling back the prepuce causes its inner lining to pout and the meatus comes into view. This condition should not be confused with true phimosis in small boys where there is scarring of the prepuce which will not retract without fissuring. In these cases, the aperture in the prepuce may be so tight as to cause urinary obstruction.

Paraphimosis

- When the tight foreskin is retracted, it may sometimes be difficult to return and a paraphimosis results
- In this condition, the venous and lymphatic return from the glans and distal foreskin is obstructed and these structures swell alarmingly causing even more pressure within the obstructing ring of prepuce. Gangrene may occur
- Ice bags, gentle manual compression and injection of a solution of hyaluronidase in normal saline may help to reduce the swelling
- Such patients can be treated by **circumcision** if careful manipulation fails
- A dorsal slit of the prepuce under local anesthetic may be enough in an emergency.

Balanoposthitis: Inflammation of the prepuce is known as posthitis; inflammation of the glans is balanitis. The opposing surfaces of the two structures are often involved — hence the term **balanoposthitis.**

Chordee. Chordee (French = corded) is a fixed bowing of the penis due to hypospadias or, more rarely, chronic urethritis. Erection is deformed and sexual intercourse may be impossible. Treatment is usually surgical.

Peyronie's Disease

- Peyronie's disease is a relatively common cause of deformity of the erect penis
- On examination, hard plaques of fibrosis can be palpated in the tunica of one or both corpora cavernosa. The plaques may be calcified. The presence of the unyielding plaque tissue within the normally elastic wall of the corpus cavernosum causes the erect penis to bend, often dramatically, towards the side of the plaque
- The etiology is uncertain, but it may be a result of past trauma — there is an association with Dupuytren's contracture
- Usually self-limiting.

Paget's disease of the penis (syn. erythroplasia of Quérat) is 'a persistent rawness of the glans like a long-standing balanitis followed by cancer of the substance of the penis' (Sir James Pager). Treatment is by circumcision, observation and excision if the lesion does not resolve.

Buschke–Lowenstein tumor is uncommon. It has the histological pattern of a verrucous carcinoma. It is locally destructive and invasive, but appears not to spread to lymph nodes or to metastasize. Treatment is by surgical excision.

Cancer of the Penis

- It is a rare tumor
- It has a much higher proportion in populations where **circumcision and personal hygiene are not well established**
- The most common form of cancer of the penis is **squamous cell carcinoma**
- It is seen associated with **chronic balanoposthitis** from lack of circumcision
- Lymphadenopathy is common

Premalignant lesions

- **Buschke-Lowenstein tumor**
- **Erythroplasia of Quérat/ Paget's disease of penis**
- **Bowen's disease**
- **Leukoplakia**
- **Balanitis xerotica obliterans**
  - Diagnosis is established by **biopsy**
  - Treatment consists of **partial or total penectomy**; a proximal margin-free tumor of at least 1.5 cm is desirable
  - Inguinal node dissection with excision of both superficial and deep inguinal nodes is advocated when clinically palpable nodes persist after amputation
  - Lymphadenopathy may occur from secondary infection seen in most cases of advanced penile carcinoma.

Peyronie's Disease

- A **localized induration of the fibrous investments of the penile shaft**, first described by the French surgeon Peyronie
- After age of 40 years usually
- **Penile fibromatosis**
- A **firm fibrotic thickening of the 'Fascia of the Corpora Cavernosa'** is observed, usually involving the dorsolateral aspects of the penile shaft or the intracavernous septum between the corpora cavernosa
- Histologically similar to **Keloid or Dupuytren's contracture**
- The fibrous plaques themselves **may be painless**
- Often **compromise of erectile capacity of the penis** with **'deviation of the penis on erection'** and **pain as a consequence** of this derangement
- Deviation of the penis that **interferes with intromission and coitus**
- Progression is slow, and spontaneous remissions are observed
- **Nesbitt's operation** is done

Priapism

- **P**rolonged
- **P**athologic
- **P**ainful erection of the **p**enis
- In recognition of the Greek god of sexual excess, **P**riapus
- **P**elvic venous thrombosis predisposes to priapism, **metastatic malignant diseases, leukemia, pelvic trauma, sickle-cell disease or trait, trauma to the corpora, or spinal cord injury**
- **P**rompt recognition and therapy are essential because prolonged unrelieved priapism almost inevitably leads to subsequent Permanent impotence from fibrosis of the corpora cavernosa.

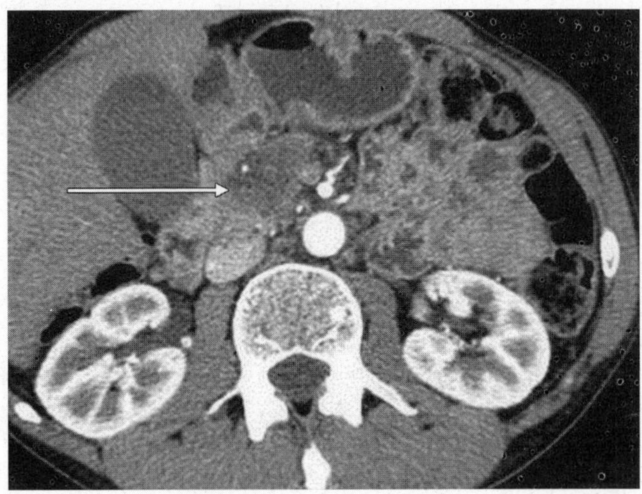

CTs scan of cancer pancreas

Neurosurgery

Glioblastoma
- Most common primary bone tumor
- Prognosis : grave
- Pseudopalisading pattern of tumor cells

Meningioma
- Psammoma bodies
- Arises from arachnoid cells
- Second most common brain tumor in adults

Oligodendroglioma
- Most common in frontal lobes
- Fried egg appearance of tumor cells

Schwannomas
- Origin from Schwann cells
- Bilateral schwannomas found in NF2
- Two patterns: Antoni A and Antoni B

Pituitary tumors
- Secrete prolactin
- Derived from Rathke's Pouch

CNS Tumors

- MC site of CNS Lipoma Corpus Callosum
- MC site of Germinoma Pineal Gland
- MC site of Chordoma Clivus
- MC source of Metastasis to Brain (females) Breast
- MC source of Metastasis to Brain (males) Lung
- Imaging of choice is: Contrast-enhanced MRI
- Most specific test: Stereotactic needle biopsy
- Bleeding brain tumors: Glioblastoma multiforme

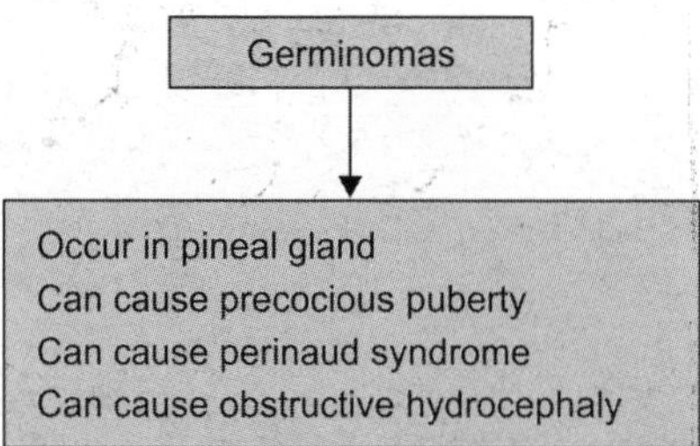
Germinomas
Occur in pineal gland
Can cause precocious puberty
Can cause perinaud syndrome
Can cause obstructive hydrocephaly

• **Calcification of cerebral cortex (Railroad calcification)**	• Sturge-weber syndrome
• **Diffuse nodular calcification**	• Toxoplasmosis
• **Amorphous supracellular calcification**	• Craniopharyngioma
• **Basal ganglia calcification**	• Hypoparathyroidism (commonest)
• **Rice grain calcification**	• Cysticercosis
• **Periventricular calcification**	• CMV infection
• **Sunray calcification with spicules of brain**	• Meningioma
• **Bone thickening at the site of brain tumor**	• Meningioma
• **Punched out rarefication**	• Multiple myeloma, sarcoidosis, Gout
• **Pepper pot or Salt and pepper app**	• Hyperparathyroidism
• **Beaten silver app**	• Raised intracranial pressure
• **Postclenoid erosion**	• Raised intracranial pressure
• **Candle grease dripping or trouser leg appearance**	• Intramedullary tumors in myelography

Waterhouse-Friderichsen Syndrome

- **Massive bilateral adrenal cortical hemorrhage** occurs in cases of fulminating **meningococcal septicemia** and in some cases of streptococcal, staphylococcal or pneumococcal septicemia
- Most cases occur in infants and young children, but it can happen in adults with severe hemorrhage or burns. The onset is catastrophic, with rigors, hyperpyrexia, cyanosis and vomiting
- Petechial hemorrhages into the skin which coalesce rapidly into purpuric blotches are a constant feature. Profound shock follows, and before long the patient passes into coma
- The condition is one of overwhelming sepsis that pursues a galloping course, death occurring in most cases within 48 hours of the onset of symptoms unless correct treatment is given without delay.

Conditions Involving Pituitary Gland

Craniopharyngioma

Craniopharyngiomas represent 3 to 5% of intracranial neoplasms and arise from either sellar or extrasellar remnants of **Rathke's pouch**

These tumors **usually affect children** and produce symptoms of increased **intracranial pressure** (headache, vomiting, somnolence) as well as visual disturbances

Calcification within the tumor is readily seen on CT

Transfrontal resection is the treatment of choice for craniopharyngioma

Craniopharyngiomas are **generally resistant to radiation therapy**.

Pituitary Apoplexy

Pituitary apoplexy follows **sudden hemorrhage into or infarction of** a pituitary tumor. Symptoms occur suddenly due to **expansion of blood within the sella** and include severe headache, **stiff neck, loss of vision, and extraocular nerve palsies**

Secondary adrenal insufficiency may lead to hypotension and shock

Pituitary apoplexy most often occurs in an undiagnosed pituitary tumor but can appear during radiation therapy for pituitary tumors, during anticoagulation, or after closed-head trauma

Acute pituitary apoplexy is a neurosurgical emergency that requires acute transsphenoidal decompression of the sella.

Sheehan's Syndrome

Pituitary necrosis may occur rarely after **postpartum hemorrhage and hypovolemia**. The degree of subsequent hypopituitarism reflects the extent of pituitary necrosis and may include adrenal insufficiency, hypothyroidism and amenorrhea. An inability to breastfeed postpartum due to destruction of oxytocin containing neurons of the posterior pituitary is an early clue to this diagnosis.

Empty Sella Syndrome

Results from **arachnoid herniation through an incomplete diaphragma sellae.** This syndrome may occur in the absence of a recognized pituitary tumor and is either primary due to a congenital diaphragmatic defect or secondary due to an injury to the diaphragm by pituitary surgery, radiation, or infarction.

Primary empty sella syndrome occurs in **obese, multiparous, hypertensive women who experience headaches but have no underlying neurologic disorders**. Pituitary function is usually normal, but occasionally PRL is increased and GH reserve is reduced. Secondary empty sella syndrome is observed in patients with otherwise benign CSF hypertension and in patients with a loss of pituitary function due to apoplexy or surgical therapy.

ICU Management: A to J

A	:	**Asepsis/Airway**
B	:	**Bed sore/encourage Breathing/Blood pressure**
C	:	**Circulation/encourage Coughing/Consciousness**
D	:	**Drains**
E	:	**ECG**
F	:	**Fluid status**
G	:	**GI losses/Gag reflex**
H	:	**Head positioning/Height**
I	:	**Insensible losses**
J	:	**Jugular venous pulse**

Postoperative Respiratory Complications

Several factors militate against normal respiratory function in the early postoperative period:

- **Effects of general anesthesia, mechanical ventilation and postoperative analgesia, which depress the respiratory system and suppress reflexes such as coughing, which clears secretions and periodic deep breathing and yawning, which expand collapsed alveoli**
- **Depression of the immune system by trauma or sepsis**
- **Progressive reduction in vital capacity by 50 to 70% during the initial 12 to 18 hours after thoracotomy and laparotomy.**

Atelectasis and Pneumonia

1. Atelectasis is the most common complication of operations performed under general anesthesia, with radiologic evidence in up to 70% of patients after thoracotomy and laparotomy
2. If air passages are occluded by secretions, perhaps in association with bronchospasm, alveolar air is absorbed and the alveoli collapse. This is the most likely explanation for collapse that involves the entire segment or lobe of a lung, especially if the patient has thick, tenacious secretions. However, atelectasis is often patchy and diffuse, appearing as plates of collapsed tissue on chest films
3. First clinical signs of atelectasis are rales, diminished breath sounds, and bronchial breathing, often accompanied by fever, tachycardia, and radiologic evidence of consolidation due to the associated pneumonia.

Pulmonary Aspiration

Aspiration of material from the alimentary tract into the airway can lead to two distinct complications: aspiration pneumonitis, which is due to the chemical composition of the aspirate; and aspiration pneumonia, which is due to its bacterial content. The two can coexist, with aspiration pneumonia as a complication of aspiration pneumonitis.

Aspiration Pneumonitis

Aspiration pneumonitis is caused by the aspiration of gastric contents, which are normally sterile. The consequences depend on the nature of the aspirated material. If the pH of the aspirate is less than 2.5, it can cause a chemical burn to the airways. The syndrome was first described by Mendelson.

The clinical features of dyspnea, cyanosis, and tachycardia usually appear within half-an-hour of aspiration, with rales and expiratory wheezes on auscultation. Chest films reveal interstitial pulmonary edema. Arterial blood gases demonstrate hypoxia and hypercapnia. The condition may rapidly deteriorate into respiratory failure and is associated with high mortality.

Aspiration Pneumonia

Aspiration pneumonia is usually due to inhalation of contents from the oropharynx that are normally at physiologic pH but contain bacteria, particularly anaerobes. It is a common cause of postoperative pneumonia and is particularly associated with poor oral hygiene and the prolonged use of nasogastric and endotracheal tubes.

Pulmonary Edema

Pulmonary edema in a postoperative patient may be due to left ventricular failure following cardiac complications or to injury to the alveolar membrane as a result of sepsis, oxygen toxicity, and so forth, but it is generally the result of circulatory overload following excessive administration of intravenous fluids. Circulatory overload may also follow absorption of fluids used for irrigation of the peritoneum or hollow viscera, such as the bladder, or it may occur during mechanical bowel preparation, especially in those with a history of cardiac disease.

Immediate Postoperative Respiratory Depression

Respiratory depression immediately following operation is usually due to the persistent effects of narcotic analgesia used during anesthesia, or to the sustained action of muscle relaxants. Narcotics depress the respiratory center in the brainstem and can usually be reversed by antagonists such as naloxone.

Acute Respiratory Failure

Acute respiratory failure is defined as a direct, life-threatening inability to maintain adequate gas exchange in the lungs. Although criteria for instituting mechanical ventilation require an assessment of arterial blood gases, ventilation, dead space, and muscle strength, in practice, respiratory failure is considered to be imminent if arterial partial pressure of oxygen (PaO_2) is less than 60 mm Hg when one is breathing room air, or the arterial partial pressure of carbon dioxide ($PaCO_2$) is greater than 60 mm Hg in the absence of metabolic alkalosis.
Postoperative respiratory failure can be caused by one or a combination of pulmonary defects: hypoventilation, imbalance between ventilation and perfusion and diminished alveolar oxygen diffusion.

Important Surgical Points in Diabetes

The most common site of infection in diabetics is the urinary tract

- **Pyelonephritis**
- **Papillary necrosis**
- **Emphysematous pyelonephritis**
- **Perinephric abscesses** are all more common in diabetics

Unusual infections are also seen, including:

- **Rhinocerebral mucormycosis**, an invasive fungal infection of the nose and sinuses
- **Malignant external otitis**, an invasive bacterial infection of the auditory canal usually caused by *Pseudomonas aeruginosa*
- **Necrotizing cellulitis** and especially in the perineal region of male diabetics who have recently had urethral catheterization known as **Fournier's gangrene**
- Impaired Wound Healing
- Cholelithiasis
- **Gangrene of the gallbladder**
  - **A peripheral, symmetric sensorimotor neuropathy** with the most common manifestation is **peripheral neuropathy of the feet** and distal lower extremity, with loss of protective sensation in the foot
  - Minor trauma may develop into a serious necrotizing infection with tissue loss
  - Normal adjustments of the foot in weight bearing do not occur, and **heavy calluses** form over pressure points, adding to the pressure and causing necrosis under the callus
  - **Foot problems are the most common indication for hospital admission in diabetics. Necrobiosis lipoidica diabeticorum.**

Gas Gangrene

Results from the following clostridial species:

- Clostridium welchii
- Clostridium oedematiens
- Clostridium septicum
- Microscopy of wound **exudate shows gram-positive bacilli**
- Anaerobic culture on blood agar shows **hemolytic colonies** *(Clostridium welchii)*
- **'Stormy' clot reaction** with litmus milk
- *Clostridium welchii* also shows **positive Nagler's reaction**, due to lecithinase reaction of alpha exotoxin

Clinical features

- Patients are generally toxic and unwell
- Often have features of shock, jaundice, haemolysis or acute renal failure

Local signs of gas gangrene include:

- **Myositis or myonecrosis**
- Gas formation with **palpable crepitus**
- Mottled discoloration of the overlying skin
- Plain X-ray often shows **gas in the subcutaneous tissue and fascial plains**

Interesting Facts in Relation to Fruits and Vegetables, etc.

• ***Potato nodes***	• *Sarcoidosis*
• ***Potato tumor***	• *Chemodectoma*
• ***Potato/oyster ovary***	• *PCOD*
• ***Strawberry Gallbladder***	• *Cholesterosis*

• ***Strawberry tongue***	• *Scarlet fever*
• ***Strawberry cervix***	• *Trichomonas vaginalis*
• ***Strawberry hemangioma***	• *Nevus vasculosus*
• ***Barley colored fluid cyst***	• *Spermatocele*
• ***Apple jelly nodules***	• *Lupus vulgaris*
• ***Apple core lesion***	• *Ca colon*
• ***Raspberry tumor***	• *Umbilical adenoma*
• ***Raspberry thorn sign***	• *Crohn's disease*

SURGICAL ONCOLOGY

Latest Tumor Markers

• **Alphafetoprotein**	• Hepatocellular carcinoma
• **CEA**	• Adenocarcinoma colon, pancreas, lung, ovary
• **PSA**	• Prostate cancer
• **Neuron-specific enolase**	• Small cell lung cancer, Neuroblastoma
• **LDH**	• Lymphoma
• **Catoecolamines**	• Pheochromocytoma
• **Beta 2 microglobulin**	• Multiple myeloma • Lymphoma
• **Bladder tumor antigen**	• Bladder tumor, UTI, Renal calculi
• **CA 27.29**	• Breast cancer
• **CA 72.4**	• Ovarian and pancreatic cancer
• **LASA–P (Lipid Associated Sialic Acid)**	• Ovarian cancer
• **NMP 2**	• Bladder cancer
• **HCG**	• Gestational trophoblastic disorders
• **CA 125**	• Ovarian cancer
• **Placental Alkaline Phosphatase**	• Seminoma
• **S100**	• Melanoma, neural tumors

Also Remember

• **Intermediate filament**	• Tumor
• **Keratin**	• Carcinoma
• **Vimentin**	• Sarcoma
• **Desmin**	• Muscle
• **Neurofilaments**	• Phechromocytoma, Neuroblastoma
• **Glial Fibrillary Acidic Protein (GFAP)**	• Astrocytomas, Ependymomas

Types of Secondaries

Osteolytic Secondaries	Osteoblastic Secondaries
• **Kidney**	• Prostate, Seminoma
• **Lung**	• Breast, Uterus, Ovary
• **Thyroid**	• Carcinoid
• **GIT**	• Osteosarcoma

Spontaneous Regression is seen in

- Renal cell carcinoma
- Retinoblastoma
- Choriocarcinoma
- Neuroblastoma
- Malignant melanoma

Pulsating Tumors

- RCC secondaries
- Osteosarcoma
- Osteoclastoma
- Sec from follicular Ca thyroid

Screening and Tumors

- **Breast cancer: Self-examination + mammography**
- **Cervical cancer: Pap smear examination**
- **Colorectal cancer: Fecal occult blood test, digital rectal examination, sigmoidoscopy and colonoscopy in high-risk group particularly**
- **Prostate: Digital rectal examination and PSA level**

'Important Surgeries' (Frequently asked)

Nissen's Fundoplication Hiatus Hernia

Ramstedt's Pyloromyotomy Hypertrophic Pyloric Stenosis

Whipple's Pancreaticoduodenectomy

Heller's Operation Achalasia Cardia

Prolapse Rectum

- Thiersch's Surgery
- Ripstein's Surgery
- Delorme's Surgery
- Wells Surgery
- Lauhats Surgery

Hydronephrosis

- Anderson-Hynes Pyeloplasty

Inguinal Hernia Repair

- Bassini Repair
- Shouldice Repair
- Lytle Plication

Femoral Hernia

- Mc Eveddy
- Losenthein
- Lockwood

Varicose veins

- Trendelenburg
- Cockett and Dodd

Hirschsprung's Disease
- Modified Duhamel
- Swenson's
- Soave's

USMLE and ENT

Congenital Disorders of Ear

- **Bat ear/Lop ear:** Abnormally long protruding ear
- **Microtia:** Small pinna
- **Macrotia:** Abnormally large pinna
- **Anotia:** Absent pinna
- **Preauricular sinus:** Incomplete fusion of tubercles
- **Preauricular appendages:** Skin-covered tags containing cartilage.

Subperichondrial Hematoma

Blunt trauma to the pinna causes a **subperichondrial hematoma**

When bleeding occurs between the cartilage and the perichondrium, the pinna becomes a **reddish purple** shapeless mass

Because the perichondrium carries the blood supply to the cartilage, the cartilage undergoes **avascular necrosis** if the hematoma is present on both sides of the cartilage, and with time, the pinna becomes shriveled.

Hematoma may become organized and calcify, which produces the **cauliflower ear characteristic of wrestlers and boxers**

Cauliflower ear is Perichondritis in wrestlers.

INFECTIOUS DISEASES

External Otitis

External Otitis. Infection of the ear canal occurs in a:
- **Diffuse form** involving the entire canal, termed **otitis externa diffusa**
- A **localized form due to furunculosis**, termed **otitis externa circumscripta.**

Malignant External Otitis
- An unusually virulent form of external otitis due to **infection with *P. aeruginosa*** occurs in **immunosuppressed diabetics,** particularly elderly diabetics with poor metabolic control
- It produces pain, **purulent otorrhea, and hearing loss**
- **Facial nerve is most common cranial nerve involved**
- **Granulation tissue found**

Acute Suppurative Otitis Media (ASOM)

Mc organism in **children: *Strepae pneumonia***

Mc organism in **neonates: Group B streptococci**

A myringotomy is indicated when bulging of the tympanic membrane persists despite antibiotic therapy or when the pain and systemic symptoms and signs, such as fever, vomiting and diarrhea are severe

Complications of acute otitis media are:
- **Acute mastoiditis**

- **Petrositis**
- **Labyrinthitis**
- **Facial paralysis**
- **Conductive and sensorineural hearing loss**
- **Epidural abscess**
- **Meningitis**
- **Brain abscess**
- **Lateral sinus thrombosis**
- **Subdural empyema, and**
- **Otitic hydrocephalus**
- **Mastoid reservoir phenomenon seen**

Serous/Secretory Otitis Media/Glue Ear

Manifested as **effusions in the middle ear**

↓Mobility of tympanic membrane

- **Air bubbles** behind TM
- **Marginal perforation seen:**
  - **Straw/amber**-colored TM
  - **Blue tympanic membrane**
  - **B-shaped tympanogram**
  - **Medical treatment not effective much here**
  - **Myringotomy with ventilation tube insertion is used as treatment.**

Cholesteatoma/Epidermosis/Keratoma

- **A cholesteatoma** occurs when the middle ear is lined with **stratified squamous epithelium (white, amorphous debris in the middle ear)**
- The stratified squamous epithelium **desquamates** in this closed space
- **Basically a bone erosion.**
- The desquamated epithelial debris cannot be cleared and accumulates in ever-enlarging concentric layers. This debris serves as a culture medium for microorganisms.
- Cholesteatomas have the ability to destroy bone, including the tympanic ossicles, probably because of the elaboration of collagenase
- **Usually found in apex of petrous temporal bone**
- **Attic/posterior superior marginal region is usually involved.**
- Pars flaccida and marginal perforations are frequently associated with cholesteatomas
- **Lateral semicircular canal** is the commonest to perforate.
- The presence of a cholesteatoma greatly **increases the probability of the development of a serious complication,** such as purulent labyrinthitis, facial paralysis, or intracranial suppurations. Intracranial infections include meningitis, brain abscess, lateral sinus thrombosis, subdural empyema, and epidural abscess
- **Modified radical mastoidectomy is used for treatment**

Complications of CSOM

- Commonest complication is **Mastoiditis**
- **Commonest cause of brain abscess is CSOM**
  - **Luc's abscess (Root of Zygomatic Process)**

- **Bezold's abscess (Sternomastoid)**
- **Citelli's abscess (Digastric triangle)**
- **Labrynthitis**
- **Petrositis**
- **Gradenigo's syndrome (Photophobia, Lacrimation, V and VI Cranial Nerve Involvement)**
- **Osteomyelitis**
- **Septicemia**
- **Lateral sinus thrombosis**

Lateral sinus thrombosis (LST)

(Griesinger's sign) Tenderness and edema over mastoid are path gnomonic of lateral sinus thrombosis (LST)

Classic symptoms of LST include a **'picket fence' fever** pattern; chills; progressive anemia (especially with beta-hemolytic strep); and, symptoms of septic emboli, headache and papilledema may indicate extension to involve the cavernous sinus

The Tobey-Ayer test is measured by monitoring the CSF pressure during a lumbar puncture. No increase in CSF pressure during external compression of the internal jugular vein on the affected side, and an exaggerated response on the patent side, is suggestive of LST.

- **Radical mastoidectomy:** Here the **middle ear, including the attic and the antrum, and the mastoid air cell area are converted into one cavity** that communicates with the exterior through the ear canal
- **Modified radical mastoidectomy:** If the cholesteatoma lies superficial to the remnants of the tympanic membrane and ossicles, a **modified radical mastoidectomy** can be performed. The modified radical mastoidectomy **spares the tympanic membrane remnants and ossicles and preserves the remaining hearing**
- **It is the commonest operation done for CSOM.**

- **Schwartz operation is simple or cortical mastoidectomy**
- **Radical mastoidectomy** is done for: **Atticoantral cholesteatoma.**

Most Common Organisms

• **Otomycosis**	Aspergillus niger > candida
• **Furuncle**	*Staph. aureus*
• **Ramsay Hunt Syndrome**	Herpes Zoster virus
• **Malignant otitis externa**	*Pseudomonas aureginosa*
• **Bullous myringitis**	Viral (Influenza virus)
• **Hemorrhagic otitis externa**	Influenza
• **Perichondritis**	*Pseudomonas aeruginosa*

Ramsay Hunt Syndrome

It is also called herpes zoster oticus: It is an infection of facial nerve that is accompanied by a painful rash and facial muscle weakness, among other signs and symptoms. The cause of Ramsay Hunt syndrome is *varicella-zoster* virus. Signs and symptoms of Ramsay Hunt syndrome include:

- A painful red rash with fluid-filled blisters on your eardrum, external ear canal, the outside of your ear, the roof of your mouth (palate) or your tongue
- Facial weakness (palsy) on the same side as the affected ear
- Difficulty closing one eye
- Ear pain
- Hearing loss
- Ringing in ears (tinnitus)
- A sensation of spinning or moving (vertigo)
- A change in taste perception or loss of taste

- *H. influenzae* **used to be** the most common cause of bacterial meningitis under 5 years
- Since the introduction of vaccine, its occurrence has **greatly decreased**
- Risk factors for *H. influenzae* include **Otitis media**, Sinusitis, Pharyngitis and other URTI
- As such, its occurrence also is **associated with significant sensorineural hearing loss in up to 20 percent of cases**
- It is recommended to give steroids immediately along with antibacterials to **decrease hearing loss.**

Otosclerosis

- Autosomal dominant
- Begins in 'fissula ante fenestram.'
- Common in females
- Family history positive
  - The most common cause of a progressive conductive hearing loss usually bilateral in an adult with a normal eardrum
  - **Reversible conductive deafness seen**
  - Otosclerosis is a disease of the bone of the otic capsule, with a predilection for the anterior part of the oval window
  - **Flamingo pink tympanic membrane seen**
  - **But in majority, TM is normal (kindly remember)**
  - **Paracusis willisii** (ability to hear better in noisy environment)
  - Positive Schwartz test
  - **Carhart's notch** at **2000 Hz** present
  - **Gelle's test is done for otosclerosis**
  - **Stapedectomy** is surgery of choice
  - **Sodium fluoride is of benefit**
  - **Used in pinkish tympanic membrane**
  - **Other operations done are: Fenestration and stapedectomy.**

- **Commonest site of Otosclerosis: Oval window**
- **Commonest bone affected in otosclerosis: Stapes**

Meniere's Disease/Endolymphatic Hydrops/Ear Glaucoma

Meniere's disease is characterized by **triad of:**

- **Hearing loss**
- **Tinnitus**
- **Recurrent prostrating vertigo**

Tinnitus is nonpulsatile

Low-frequency sensorineural hearing loss is seen

The pathologic change in the inner ear is **generalized dilation of the membranous labyrinth,** or **endolymphatic hydrops**.

Only one ear is involved in **85%** of patients with Meniere's disease

- **Females** are more commonly affected
- **Diplacusis** (Same sound perceived as two different pitch has in two ears)
- **Hennebert's sign:** Vertigo and Nystagmus induced by pressure to stapedial footplate
- **Tulio's phenomenon:** Vertigo and Nystagmus induced by loud noise

Benign Paroxysmal Positional Vertigo and Nystagmus

- Vertigo that occurs with **changes in position** may follow lesions in the inner ear, eighth nerve, brainstem, or cerebellum
- Positional vertigo and nystagmus arising from **the inner ear** are termed benign paroxysmal positional vertigo and nystagmus.

- The patient experiences vertigo **when lying on or rolling over onto the affected ear or when tilting the head back to look up.** There is a **latency of a few seconds** after assuming the provocative position before the vertigo and nystagmus begin
- The vertigo is characterized by an intense sensation of spinning, and the **nystagmus is rotary and counterclockwise when the affected right ear is placed under and clockwise when the affected left ear is placed under**
- **The quick component of the nystagmus is always toward the affected ear**
- The finding of basophilic calcium-containing concretions in the ampulla of the posterior semicircular canal has led some to refer to this condition as **cupulolithiasis.**

Bell's Palsy

Bell's palsy is a **unilateral facial paralysis** that develops suddenly and is accompanied by pain in the postauricular area **(LMNL).**

It is thought to be of **viral etiology**.

All divisions of the nerve are paralyzed; this distinguishes the disease from a supranuclear lesion. The lesion is in the internal auditory meatus or the intratemporal course of the nerve. The initial pathologic changes are **hyperemia and edema**

- **Acute onset**
- **Spontaneous remission**
- **Increased predisposition in diabetes mellitus**

The **edema compresses the blood supply to the nerve** because of the bony confines of the fallopian canal. A conduction block develops without death or degeneration of the axons. Release of the pressure on the nerve produces rapid recovery of function. This type of paralysis is termed **neurapraxia**.

Corticosteroid therapy is initiated as soon as possible after the onset of the paralysis and is continued for 10 days to minimize the inflammatory reaction.

It is an indication for decompression of the facial nerve by removing the bone of the fallopian canal. **Approximately 85% of all patients with idiopathic facial nerve paralysis recover spontaneously**.

Chemodectomas

These nonchromaffin paragangliomas are termed **glomus jugulare or glomus tympanicus** tumors, depending on their site of origin.

The glomus tympanicus tumor arises from the **area of Jacobson's nerve in the tympanic plexus on the promontory of the middle ear.**

The glomus jugulare tumor arises from the glomus jugulare body in the jugular bulb. Both tumors consist of rich networks of vascular spaces surrounded by epithelioid cells

Usually the neoplasms grow slowly, and symptoms may not be evident until the neoplasm is quite large

- **Pulsatile tinnitus**
- **Facial nerve paralysis**
- **Otorrhea**
- **Hemorrhage**
- **Vertigo**
- **Paralysis of cranial nerves IX, X, XI, and XII are often the presenting symptoms and signs.**

Characteristically, a **'red mass'** that **pulsates and blanches with compression with a pneumatic otoscope** can be seen in the ear canal or middle ear **(Brown sign).**

The pulsation can also be demonstrated with tympanometry. There may be evidence of bone erosion in the mastoid process, middle ear, or petrous pyramid on CT. The extent of the lesion is best demonstrated with MRI with enhancement with gadolinium. Angiography is a necessary part of the preoperative evaluation.

Glomus Tumor (Continued)

- One of the **most common benign tumors** of middle ear
- **Squamous cell carcinoma is the commonest.**

- Arises from **glomus bodies** in the jugular bulb of internal jugular vein
  - **Red reflex**
  - **Rising sun appearance**
  - **Bluish reflex through tympanic membrane** is a feature
- **Earliest symptom** is **deafness and tinnitus**
- Deafness is of **conductive type**
- **Vertigo** and **cranial nerves IX and XII** may get involved
- **Multicentric with lymphatic metastasis**
- **Modified radical mastoidectomy and excision of petrous temporal bone are standard procedures.**

Acoustic Neurinomas/Vestibular Schwannoma

They arise more often from the **vestibular division** of the eighth nerve.

Superior vestibular nerve is most commonly involved.

These neoplasms are derived from **Schwann cells**.

Compromise most of **CP angle tumors**

- **Cranial nerve V** is **involved first**
- **Loss of corneal reflex**
- **Deafness** is the earliest symptom
- **Deafness is retrocochlear type.**

The **NF2 gene** (Schwannomerlin, Schwannomin, MERL_HUMAN, MERLIN—Moesin-Ezrin-Radixin-Like Protein) is located on the long (q) arm of chromosome **22**.

Upon microscopic examination, the acoustic neurinoma presents two distinctive architectural patterns, designated **Antoni A and Antoni B**. Both are created by spindle cells with elongated nuclei and fibrillated cytoplasm, predominantly those of Schwann cells. The two tissue patterns differ in cellular weave and density.

- **Antoni A** tissue is compact, with a prominence of interwoven fascicles
- **Antoni B** tissue is porous and less structured.

In Neurofibromatosis type II, bilateral acoustic neuromas are the hallmark

There is public concern that **use of mobile phones** could increase the risk of brain tumors. If such an effect exists, acoustic neuroma would be of particular concern because of the proximity of the acoustic nerve to the handset.

Hitselberger's Sign: In acoustic neuroma, loss of sensation in the ear canal supplied by Arnold's nerve (branch of vagus nerve to ear)

The most useful (i.e. sensitive and specific) test to identify acoustic neuromas is a **Gadolinium-enhanced MRI of the head**

Surgical removal is the treatment of choice

However, stereotactic radiotherapy by using gamma knife or X knife may be used.

Memorize

• AC > BC	Normal
• AC < BC (**Negative Rinne**) • Sound lateralized to deaf ear (**Weber**) • Absolute bone conduction (ABC) normal	Conductive deafness
• AC > BC • Sound lateralized to better ear • Absolute bone conduction • (ABC) Shortened	Sensorineural deafness

FOR FEIGNED HEARING LOSS, STENGER'S TEST IS DONE

Ototoxic Drugs

- **Salicylates**
- **Quinine and its synthetic analogues**
- **Aminoglycoside antibiotics (Gentamycin, kanamycin)**
- **Loop diuretics such as furosemide and ethacrynic acid**
- **Cancer chemotherapeutic agents such as cisplatin**

Hereditary Prenatal Causes of Deafness

There are a large number of syndromes in which deafness is a recognized factor:

- Leopard syndrome
- Lentigines
- ECG abnormalities
- Ocular hypertelorism
- Pulmonary stenosis
- **Abnormal genitalia**
- **Growth retardation**
- **Sensorineural deafness**
- **Pendred syndrome: Deafness + goiter**
- **Usher's syndrome:** Deafness + mental retardation + seizures + retinitis pigmentosa + cataracts
- **Waardenburg's Syndrome: White Forelock** + hyperpigmented patches + deafness + displacement of inner canthi
- **Klippel-Feil syndrome:** A **short neck** limits head movements, the **hairline is low** at the back, there may be paralysis of the external rectus muscle in one or both eyes and there is sensorineural hearing loss which may be severe
- **Alport's syndrome:** It is **X-linked dominant** and affects boys more severely than girls. There is severe progressive glomerulonephritis and a progressive sensorineural loss which does not show itself until the boy is about 10 years old
- **Refsum's syndrome** consists of **ichthyosis, ataxia, retinitis pigmentosa, night blindness, mental retardation and a sensorineural deafness**
- **Jervell and Lange-Nielsen syndrome** is autosomal recessive with a cardiac arrhythmia and a profound sensorineural deafness. These children may present with syncopal attacks and, if untreated, these attacks can be fatal.

Other Syndromes

- Crouzon
- Apert
- Klippel-Feil
- Down
- Goldenhar
- Pierre Robinson
- van der Hoeve
- Stickler
- Wilder Ranch Syndrome

Presbycusis

- **Presbycusis** (age-associated hearing loss) is the **most common cause of sensorineural hearing loss in adults**
- In the early stages, it is characterized by **symmetric, gentle to sharply sloping high-frequency hearing loss**
- With progression, the hearing loss involves all frequencies.

- More importantly, the hearing impairment is associated with **significant loss in clarity**
- There is a **loss of discrimination for phonemes, recruitment (abnormal growth of loudness), and particular difficulty in understanding speech in noisy environments**
- Hearing aids may provide limited rehabilitation once the word recognition score deteriorates below 50
- Significant advancements and improvements in cochlear implants have made them the treatment of choice.

Important Questions Asked

Ramsay Hunt's syndrome is caused by **herpes zoster virus**

- It is characterized by a **facial palsy** and is often associated with facial pain and the appearance of vesicles on the eardrum, ear canal and pinna
- Vertigo and sensorineural hearing loss (**VIII nerve**) accompany it
- Treatment with aciclovir is effective if given early.

Ear Signs

- **Brown Sign**—blanching of redness on increasing pressure more than systemic pressure seen in **Glomus jugulare**
- **Hitselberger's sign:** In **Acoustic neuroma**—loss of sensation in the ear canal supplied by Arnold's nerve (branch of vagus nerve to ear)
- **Light house Sign**—seeping out of secretions in **acute otitis media**
- **Lyre's Sign**—splaying of carotid vessels in **carotid body tumor**
- **Milian's Ear Sign—Erysipelas** can spread to pinna (cuticular affection), whereas cellulitis cannot
- **Tragus Sign—External otitis**, Pain on pressing tragus
- **Waquino's Sign** is the blanching of the tympanic mass with gentle pressure on the carotid artery. Seen in **Glomus tumors**.
- **Bezold's Sign:** Inflammatory edema at the tip of the mastoid process in **Mastoiditis**.

Anatomy of the Nose and Paranasal Sinuses

- The skeleton of the nose consists of the **nasal bones, the ascending processes of the maxilla, the upper lateral cartilages, the lower lateral cartilages, and the septal cartilage**. The nasal septum is the medial wall of each nasal cavity
- **The lateral wall** of each nasal cavity provides the attachment for the **three turbinates.**
- Nasal mucosa is largely supplied by branches of external carotid artery
- Pale, edematous nasal mucosa indicates nasal allergy
- Warming, moistening and filtration are functions of nasal cavity
- Deviated dorsum and septum are crooked nose
- Depressed nasal bridge is seen in trauma, abscess and syphilis
  - The **nasolacrimal duct** opens into the **inferior meatus.** The middle meatus lies between the middle turbinate and the inferior turbinate
  - The **ostia of the maxillary and anterior ethmoid cells** and the **nasofrontal duct** are in the **middle meatus**. The superior meatus lies between the superior turbinate and the middle turbinate
  - The **ostia of the posterior ethmoid** cells are in the **superior meatus**
  - **The ostium of the sphenoid sinus** is in the posterior part of the superior meatus, the **sphenoethmoid recess.**
- Terms relating to disorders of smell include:
  - **Anosmia**, an absence of the ability to smell
  - **Hyposmia**, a decreased ability to smell; hyperosmia (an increased sensitivity to an odorant); dysosmia (distortion in the perception of an odor); phantosmia, perception of an odorant where none is present; and **agnosia**, inability to classify, contrast, or identify odor sensations verbally, even though the ability to distinguish between odorants or to recognize them may be normal
  - **Parosmia is the perception of bad smell.**

Ozena, or atrophic rhinitis
- It is characterized by **atrophied mucosa overlaid by foul-smelling dry crusts** (Greek ozein, 'stench')
- **Klebsiella ozaenae** is often isolated from nasal cultures
- **Young's operation done in atrophic rhinitis.**

Rhinoscleroma: Klebsiella rhinoscleromatis
- It is a **chronic granulomatous disease** of the upper respiratory tract mucosa
- **Mikulicz cells (foamy histiocytes)** are seen in the submucosa of biopsy specimens
- **Russell bodies are also a feature**
- Rhinoscleroma can be treated with streptomycin, trimethoprim-sulfamethoxazole, a quinolone, or tetracycline for 2 months.

Glanders: Pseudomonas mallei
- A respiratory disease of horses. Infection is rare in humans; nasal inoculation may produce a purulent nasal discharge followed by granulomatous intranasal lesions that ulcerate
- Treatment is with sulfadiazine.

Neonatal congenital syphilis
- It may present as **rhinitis (snuffles)**, and the generalized osteochondritis that follows may result in a **'saddle-nose' deformity**.

Rhinosporidiosis
- **Rhinosporidium seeberi** is a fungus-like organism, not yet cultured, that causes **Rhinosporidiosis**
- **'Pedunculated nasal masses'** that grow over months or years cause obstruction and a foul odor and must be surgically excised.

Blastomyces dermatitidis
- A fungus prevalent in the Mississippi and Ohio River valleys, usually causes **pulmonary disease** but may cause **chronic ulcerative lesions of the skin and nasal mucosa**.

Mucormycosis
- A life-threatening fungal illness that occurs **primarily in diabetic patients**, may present as **black eschars** in the nasal cavity

Important Points Related to Nose

Oblique # of nasal septum: **Jarjavay #**

Horizontal # of nasal septum: **Chaevellet #**

Rhinophyma: Sebaceous gland hypertrophy.

CSF Rhinorrhea
- # Cribriform plate of ethmoid, Nasoethmoid #
- Beta 2 transferrin levels high
- Contains glucose
- Less proteins.

Apple jelly nodules on nasal septum. Lupus vulgaris

Mucormycosis

- ***Rhizopus*** and ***Rhizomucor*** species are ubiquitous, appearing on decaying vegetation, dung, and foods of high sugar content
- **Mucormycosis** is uncommon and is largely confined to patients with serious pre-existing diseases
- **Mucormycosis** originating in the paranasal sinuses and nose predominantly affects **patients with poorly controlled diabetes mellitus, organ transplantation, who have a hematologic malignancy, or who are receiving long-term deferoxamine therapy**
- **Vascular invasion by hyphae** is a prominent feature
- Ischemic or hemorrhagic necrosis is the foremost histologic finding.

- **Mucormycosis** originating in the nose and paranasal sinuses produces a characteristic clinical picture. **Low-grade fever, dull sinus pain, and sometimes nasal congestion or a thin, bloody nasal discharge are followed in a few days by double vision, increasing fever and obtundation**
- Examination reveals a unilateral generalized reduction of ocular motion, chemosis, and proptosis. The nasal turbinates on the involved side may be dusky red or necrotic
- A sharply delineated **area of necrosis**, strictly respecting the midline, may appear in the hard palate. The skin of the cheek may become inflamed. Fungal invasion of the globe or ophthalmic artery leads to blindness
- Opacification of one or more sinuses is detected by computed tomography (CT) or by magnetic resonance imaging (MRI)
- Carotid arteriography may show invasion or obstruction of the carotid siphon. Coma is due to direct invasion of the frontal lobe.

Trauma and Foreign Bodies

Nasal Fracture. The nose is a vulnerable leading part. **Fractures of the nasal bones are the most common fractures of the facial bones.** Fractures of the nose may involve the ascending processes of the maxillae and the nasal processes of the frontal bones as well as the nasal bones. A fracture of the nose is **usually an open fracture**

The **most common deformity** is a **deviation of the nasal bones to the right,** with depression of the nasal bones on the left, characteristically occurring with a right hook. Fractures of the nose may be associated with **septal fractures and hematomas**

Trauma to the facial bones is often associated with a cerebrospinal fluid rhinorrhea.

Septal hematomas lie between the quadrangular cartilage and the perichondrium. When the perichondrium has been elevated from both sides of the septal cartilage, the cartilage undergoes avascular necrosis. Septal hematomas **frequently become infected and abscess formation produces avascular and septic necrosis of the septal cartilage**, which causes a **saddle deformity of the nose**. Septal hematomas are **incised and drained as soon as the diagnosis is made**

Septal abscesses are located between the cartilage and the perichondrium. They may involve both sides of the cartilage. Septal abscesses are incised and drained under general anesthesia as soon as the diagnosis is established. Incisions are made bilaterally if there is pus on both sides of the septum.

ACUTE BACTERIAL SINUSITIS

Pains of Sinusitis

Symptoms of acute sinusitis include purulent nasal or postnasal drainage, nasal congestion, and sinus pain or pressure whose location depends on the sinus involved.

- **Maxillary sinus pain** is often perceived as being located in the cheek or upper teeth;
- **Ethmoid sinus pain**, between the eyes or retro-orbital;
- **Frontal sinus pain,** above the eyebrow;
- **Sphenoid sinus pain,** in the upper half of the face or retro-orbital with radiation to the occiput. Sinus pain is frequently worse when the patient bends over or is supine.

Important Points About Sinusitis

- **Maxillary sinus is the commonest sinus involved followed by frontal, ethmoid and sphenoid**
- **Mucopus in middle meatus is a feature of maxillary sinusitis**
- **Periodicity is seen in frontal sinusitis**
- **Frontal sinusitis doesn't occur at birth**
- **Definitive diagnosis of sinusitis is done by Sinoscopy.**

In children and adults, ***Streptococcus pneumoniae*** and ***Haemophilus influenzae*** (not type b), the most common pathogens respectively.

Chronic sinusitis is characterized by symptoms of **sinus inflammation lasting 3 months.**

Orbital complications of sinusitis, such as **orbital cellulitis and orbital abscess**, usually arise from ethmoid sinusitis, since the ethmoid is separated from the orbit by only a very thin bone (the lamina papyracea). Patients present with fever, unilateral periorbital edema and erythema, conjunctival injection and chemosis, and proptosis.

Another extracranial complication of sinusitis is **frontal subperiosteal abscess (Pott's puffy tumor) from frontal sinusitis.**

Intracranial complications such as:

- **Epidural abscess**
- **Subdural empyema**
- **Meningitis**
- **Cerebral abscess**
- **Dural-vein thrombophlebitis may result from sinusitis**, particularly from frontal or sphenoid infections. Because the sphenoid sinus sits between the two cavernous sinuses, **sphenoid sinusitis is a major cause of cavernous sinus thrombophlebitis**.

Epistaxis

Ninety percent of the time, epistaxis occurs from a plexus of vessels **(Kiesselbach's plexus)** in the **anteroinferior part of the septum (Little's area)**

Which is an area of anastomosis between ICA and ECA

Arteries contributing to Little's area:

- **Sphenopalatine**
- **Anterior ethmoidal**
- **Superior labial**
- **Greater palatine artery**

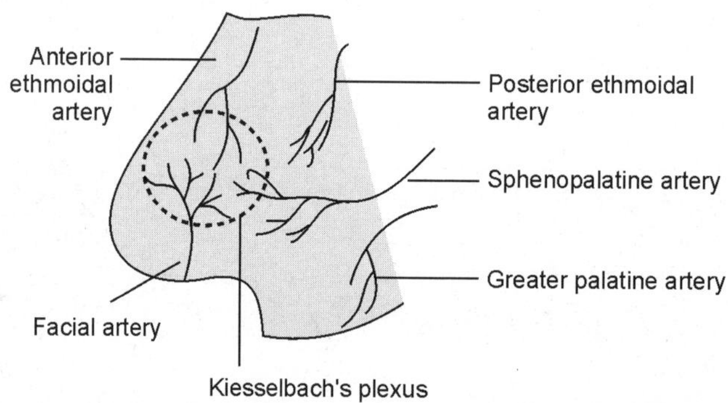

Recurrent epistaxis is seen in:

- **DNS**
- **Atrophic rhinitis**
- **Maxillary carcinoma**

- In the other 10% of cases, nasal bleeding occurs from the **posterior part of the nose,** particularly from far posterior in the inferior meatus at the junction of the inferior meatus and the nasopharynx
- **Woodruff's area under the posterior end of inferior turbinate where sphenopalatine artery anastomoses with posterior pharyngeal artery may be the source of posterior epistaxis**
- It is from this area that individuals with **arteriosclerosis and hypertension** are likely to bleed
- This type of bleeding may be difficult to control

Silver nitrate is preferred as the cauterizing agent, since it produces satisfactory intravascular coagulation without a severe burn of the mucous membrane.
Nose pricking is the **commonest cause of epistaxis in children**
Hypertension is the **commonest cause of epistaxis in adults** Mc cause of epistaxis in pubescent male: Angiofibroma Mc cause of epistaxis in pubescent female: Bleeding disorder Mc cause of epistaxis in children: Trauma
A particularly debilitating form of epistaxis occurs in **hereditary hemorrhagic telangiectasia (Rendu-Osler-Weber disease).** Patients with this disease have frequent bleeding from the nose and gastrointestinal tract.

Congenital Malformations

Choanal Atresia. Choanal atresia is a malformation in which the **opening of the nasal cavity into the nasopharynx is obstructed by a partition of mucous membrane and bone**
The malformation may occur unilaterally or bilaterally
If it occurs bilaterally, it produces respiratory distress in the neonate
Newborn infants are obligatory nasal breathers. If there is obstruction to the nasal airway, asphyxia occurs
The newborn presses his tongue against the roof of his mouth during the inspiratory effort. Fortunately, crying, with its attendant mouth breathing, often allows some ventilatory exchange
This diagnosis should be made in the **delivery room**
Choanal atresia should be considered in an infant who makes respiratory effort but fails to accomplish ventilatory exchange
The immediate solution to the problem is the insertion of an oral airway

ORAL CAVITY

Ludwig's Angina

- **Edema of floor of mouth**
- Involves **submandibular, sublingual spaces**
- Bilateral usually is a rapidly spreading, life-threatening cellulitis of the sublingual and submandibular spaces that usually starts in an infected lower molar. **Patients are febrile and may drool the secretions they cannot swallow**
- **A brawny, board-like edema in the sublingual area pushes the tongue up and back**
- **Airway obstruction may result as the infection spreads to the supraglottic tissues**

Vincent's Angina

- **Vincent**'s angina, also called **acute necrotizing ulcerative gingivitis or trench mouth**
- These have **halitosis and ulcerations of the interdental papillae**
- **Oral anaerobes are the cause**
- Therapy with oral penicillin plus metronidazole or with clindamycin alone is effective in both this condition and gingivitis.

Ranula

- Sublingual
- Thin-walled, **retention cyst**
- Due to **obstruction of mucous glands**

- Lined by columnar epithelium
- Complete excision is the ideal treatment

Cancrum oris

- **Rapidly developing gangrene in oral cavity**
- Postmeasles usually
- Does not involve jaw
- ***Noma***, or *cancrum oris*, is a fulminant gangrenous infection of the oral and facial tissues that occurs in severely malnourished and debilitated patients and is especially common among children. **Beginning as a necrotic ulcer in the gingiva of the mandible**, noma is caused by oral anaerobes, especially fusospirochetal organisms **(e.g. *Fusobacterium nucleatum*)**
- It is treated with high-dose penicillin, debridement, and correction of the underlying malnutrition.

Oral Cancer Predispositions for Oral Cancer

MC malignant tumor of adult males

- **Smoking**
- **Spirits (alcohol)**
- **Sharp jagged tooth**
- **Sepsis**
- **Syndrome (Plummer-Vinson)**
- **Syphilis**
- **Betel nut**

Premalignant Conditions

- Leukoplakia
- Erythroplakia
- Chronic candidiasis
- Papillomas tongue/cheek
- OSMF (oral submucous fibrosis)
- Surgery treatment of choice
- Radiosensitive.

Anatomy of the Pharynx

For descriptive purposes, the pharynx can be divided into the:

- **Nasopharynx**
  - Oval-shaped
  - Eustachian tube opens into it
- **Oropharynx**
- **Hypopharynx**

However, from a functional point of view, the pharynx remains united by the constrictors of the pharynx. They have a common insertion in the median pharyngeal raphe and form a musculomembranous tubular passage from the base of the skull to the opening of the esophagus.

Waldeyer's ring: The lymphoid structures of the pharynx include the pharyngeal tonsil or adenoid the palatine tonsils, the Tubal bands and the lingual tonsils.

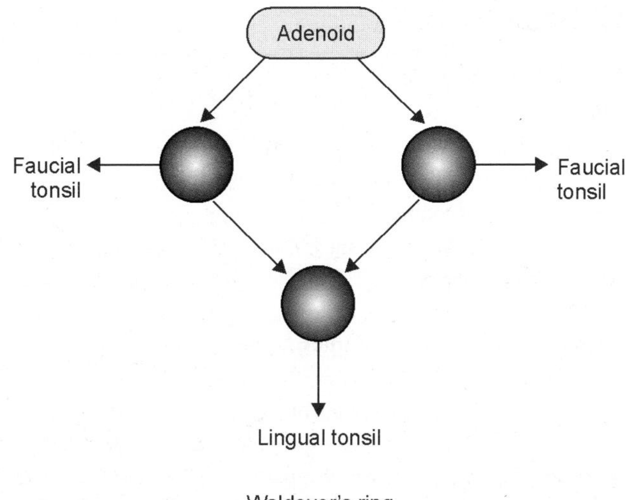

Waldeyer's ring

Foreign Bodies

Foreign bodies of the pharynx are likely to be found in four locations: the palatine tonsils, the lingual tonsils, the valleculae, and the pyriform sinuses

- Foreign bodies in the palatine tonsil are removed by grasping the foreign body with a hemostat
- Foreign bodies in the nasopharynx require general anesthesia for their removal
- Foreign bodies of the hypopharynx are removed during direct laryngoscopy under local anesthesia.

Nasopharynx

Adenoids

- Nasopharyngeal tonsil
- No crypts and no capsule
- Adenoid hypertrophy in childhood often leads to obstruction of the eustachian tubes and the choanae. Nasal obstruction, nasal discharge, sinusitis, epistaxis and voice change
- **Adenoid facies:**
  - Elongated face with dull expression
  - Open mouth
  - Prominent crowded upper teeth
  - Hitched up upper lip
- This lymphoid hyperplasia may be physiologic or secondary to infectious and allergic manifestations
- Obstruction of the eustachian tubes leads to serous or secretory otitis media, recurrent acute otitis media, and exacerbations of chronic otitis media

Tornwaldt's Cyst

- Cysts occasionally form in the region of the **medial recess of the nasopharynx**. These cysts become symptomatic when they become infected
- There may be persistent purulent drainage that has a foul taste and odor
- **Symptoms of eustachian tube obstruction and sore throat may be prominent**
- Excision or marsupialization of the cyst with an adenotome is the treatment of choice.

BENIGN NEOPLASMS OF THE NASOPHARYNX

Juvenile Nasopharyngeal Angiofibroma

Juvenile angiofibromas are **benign**, **vascular** neoplasms

They are commonin **pubescent males**

They cause **recurrent epistaxis**

Mc site is the posterior part of nasal cavity close to sphenopalatine foramen

Biopsy is contraindicated in nasopharyngeal angiofibroma

They may encroach upon the paranasal sinuses, the orbit, and the intracranial cavity. Histologically, these neoplasms are composed of fibrous tissue and numerous thin-walled vessels without contractile elements

Miller's sign seen

The extent of the neoplasm can be determined with **CT and angiography**

Contrast-enhanced CT is DOC

The pterygomaxillary fissure is often widened on the sagittal plane of the CT of the lateral part of the nasopharynx by the extension of the neoplasm into the infratemporal fossa. These neoplasms have a characteristic vascular pattern on angiography

Treatment with estrogens and embolization of the internal maxillary artery at angiography have been used to reduce the operative blood loss

These neoplasms are **responsive to radiation therapy**

Surgery is the TOC.

Nasopharyngeal Carcinoma

Lymphoepithelioma or squamous cell carcinoma is the most common type.

Carcinoma of the nasopharynx occurs at relatively young ages, and there is an unusually high incidence among the **Chinese**

Bimodal age distribution seen

Mc site is lateral wall of nasopharynx (Fossa of Rosenmuller)

Mc cranial nerve involved is VII CN.

Epstein-Barr virus is implicated.

Cervical lympadenopathy is the **commonest presentation**

Others present with **nasal or eustachian tube obstruction**

Obstruction of the eustachian tube may cause a middle-ear effusion

Serous otitis media seen.

The nasal obstruction may be associated with **purulent, bloody rhinorrhea and frank epistaxis.** The more dramatic symptoms caused by cranial nerve paralysis and cervical lymph node metastasis are, unfortunately, common presenting complaints.

The diagnosis is made by **biopsy of the primary tumor**

Trotter's Triad

- Conductive deafness
- Palatal paralysis
- Temporoparietal neuralgia is seen.

The **treatment of choice** for carcinoma of the nasopharynx is **irradiation with a supervoltage source**. The radiation should be delivered to the primary tumor-bearing area of the nasopharynx and to both sides of the neck, whether or not there is clinically demonstrated metastasis. Operations have no role in the initial therapy of carcinoma of the nasopharynx. Those cervical metastases that remain clinically palpable following radiation therapy or that subsequently become apparent should be eradicated by radical neck dissection.

Peritonsillar Abscess/Quinsy

Peritonsillar abscess called Quinsy

MC organism: *Streptococcus*.

Peritonsillar cellulitis and abscess are complications of acute tonsillitis in which the infection has spread deep to the tonsillar capsule

Pus forms between the tonsillar capsule and the superior constrictor of the pharynx

The tonsil is displaced medially

The **uvula** becomes tremendously edematous and is **displaced to the opposite side**

The soft palate is very red and **displaced forward**

- There is marked **trismus** due to irritation of the **pterygoid muscles**, and the head is held tilted toward the side of the abscess. It is painful for the patient to talk and to swallow
- **Odynophagia**
- **Hot potato voice**
- **Referred otalgia via IX cranial nerve are a feature**

Swallowing is so painful that the patient drools. The breath is foul-smelling

Peritonsillar cellulitis or abscess is rare in children under the age of 10 to 12 years and is usually caused by a group A beta-hemolytic streptococcus or anaerobe

Tonsillectomy done usually 6 weeks after appearance.

Parapharyngeal Abscess

Parapharyngeal abscess may occur in infants and young children as well as in adults

- The abscess is usually secondary to streptococcal pharyngitis or tonsillitis
- Pus forms in the parapharyngeal space secondarily from the breakdown of lymphadenitis
- The pus is **located lateral to the superior constrictor of the pharynx and adjacent to the carotid sheath**
- The tonsil and soft palate may be displaced medially but there may be no inflammatory reaction in the pharynx
- There is marked swelling in the anterior cervical triangle.

Retropharyngeal Abscess

Retropharyngeal abscess occurs in infants and young children and is rare after the age of 10 years

These infections are **located between the constrictors of the pharynx and the prevertebral fascia**

Dysphagia fever torticollis bulge in posterior pharyngeal wall are a feature.

Anatomy of the Larynx

The skeleton of the larynx consists of the **thyroid cartilage, the cricoid cartilage, the arytenoid cartilages with corniculate and cuneiform cartilages, and the epiglottis.**

The primary function of the larynx is protection of lower respiratory tract that of a sphincter

During deglutition, both the true vocal cord sphincter and the false vocal cord sphincter are closed, and the epiglottis is drawn posteriorly over the closed sphincter and serves as a watershed, deflecting food and fluid into the pyriform sinuses.

The larynx serves as the **sounding source for speech**. A fundamental tone is produced by the movement of the vocal cords, which is brought about by the flow of exhaled air past lightly approximated vocal cords

Abductor of vocal cord is **posterior cricoarytenoid**

Adductors of vocal cord: Lateral crocoarytenoid, transverse arytenoid

Vocal cords in larynx are lined by stratified squamous epithelium.

- **The internal laryngeal nerve is sensory to larynx above vocal cords.**
- **The recurrent laryngeal nerve is sensory to larynx below vocal cords.**
- **All muscles of larynx except cricothyroid are supplied by recurrent laryngeal nerve.**
- **Cricothyroid is supplied by external laryngeal nerve.**

Laryngomalacia

- **Mc cause of stridor in a newborn**
- **Inspiratory stridor seen**
- **Omega-shaped epiglottis**
- **Reassurance is the treatment modality**

Vocal Nodules. Vocal nodules are caused by **using a fundamental frequency that is unnaturally low and using the voice too loudly and too long**

Vocal nodules are condensations of hyaline connective tissue in the lamina propria at the **junction of the anterior one-third and the posterior two-thirds of the true vocal cord.** These nodules produce hoarseness and give the voice a breathy quality. In adults, these lesions are removed during direct laryngoscopy to restore the voice. However, it is necessary to begin voice therapy prior to surgical therapy, because if the underlying misuse of the voice is not corrected, the nodules recur. In children, surgical removal is not usually necessary, because the vocal nodules regress with voice therapy, which consists of voice rest, reduction in intensity and duration of voice production, and elevation of the pitch.

Vocal Cord Paralysis

Vocal cord paralysis follows traumatic, infectious, and neoplastic involvement of the vagus and recurrent laryngeal nerves and degenerative neurologic disorders.

Unilateral vocal cord paralysis produces hoarseness and aspiration

Bilateral vocal cord paralysis causes upper airway obstruction with little adverse effect on the voice

- Bilateral **INCOMPLETE** vocal cord paralysis causes maximum stridor
- **Most dangeous is bilateral abductor paralysis**
- **Total thyroidectomy is the mc cause of vocal cord palsy**
- **Bilateral recurrent laryngeal nerve palsy occurs in thyroid malignancy.**

Heimlich maneuver (abdominal thrust). In this maneuver, the operator places his arms around the choking individual from behind, grasps the fist of one hand in the other hand, and brings both hands up in the subxiphoid area briskly to apply pressure to the diaphragm. The pressure increases the intrathoracic pressure and may expel the foreign body. This should maneuver fail, an alternative airway must be established by the prompt performance of a tracheostomy.

Laryngotracheobronchitis

Laryngotracheobronchitis is **Croup**

MC causative agent: ***Parainfluenza***

Haemophilus influenzae is the most frequently isolated agent in bacterial croup, but *Staphylococcus* and *Streptococcus* may also cause croup.

Painful croupy cough, hoarseness and stridor.

Narrowing of subglottic region on X-ray **(Steeple sign)**

Epiglottitis

***H. influenzae* type b** is the predominant microorganism in epiglottitis

Epiglottitis or supraglottic laryngitis is more likely to cause abrupt and complete airway obstruction

MC cause of death is also complete airway obstruction

- Child prefers sitting position (Tripod sign)
- Lateral X-ray shows swollen epiglottis (Thumb sign)
- Hospitalization with IV antibiotics, steroids, humidification and intubation are a sequence.

- **Hot potato voice: Quinsy**
- **Median rhomboid glossitis: Candidiasis**
- **Thumb sign: Epiglottitis**
- **Hour glass sign: Subglottic edema**
- **Seals bark cough: Croup**
- **Steeple sign: Croup**
- **Trench mouth: Vincent's angina**

Laryngoceles

Laryngoceles are epithelium-lined diverticula of the laryngeal ventricle and may be located internal or external to the laryngeal skeleton

An internal laryngocele may displace and enlarge the false vocal cord and may cause hoarseness and airway obstruction

External laryngoceles pass through the **thyrohyoid membrane** and present as a mass in the neck over the thyrohyoid membrane

The mass rises with the larynx on swallowing. Internal and external laryngoceles may co-exist

Laryngoceles are more common in glassblowers, wind instrument musicians, and others who develop high intraluminal pressures. Initially, laryngoceles are filled with air and expand and collapse with changes in the intraluminal pressure

They are expanded during the Valsalva maneuver. They appear as smooth, ovoid, air-filled masses on CT scans of the neck.

Papilomas of Larynx

- HPV-implicated
- Common in children and infants
- **Multiple**
- **Recurrent**
- Treated by removal/Surgical excision

Premalignant Lesions

- **Leukoplakia**
- **Keratosis**
- **Smoking**
- **Papilloma**
- **Chronic laryngitis**

Malignant Neoplasms of the Larynx

The majority of malignant neoplasms of the larynx are **squamous cell carcinomas**

Carcinoma may arise from the mucous membrane of any part of the larynx; however, there is a predilection for the true vocal cords, particularly the anterior portions of the true vocal cords. For purposes of clinical staging and end-result reporting, carcinomas of the larynx can be divided into:

- **Supraglottic lesions** involve the epiglottis, aryepiglottic fold, and false vocal cords
- **Glottic lesions** are limited to the area of the true vocal cords
- **Subglottic lesions** include the glottic area as well as the subglottic area
- **Hypopharyngeal lesions** may be divided into lesions of the pyriform sinus, area, and posterior pharyngeal wall.

Supraglottic carcinomas

Smoking is a common factor

Pain is the mc manifestation.

Second mc laryngeal tumor

Early lymphatic spread seen

They may produce hoarseness by secondary involvement of the vocal cords, or they may produce pain on swallowing as the first symptom. Often the pain radiates to the ears

Not infrequently, a patient with a supraglottic carcinoma presents with the chief complaint of a swelling in the neck that represents a metastasis

Early supraglottic carcinoma is successfully treated with radiation therapy to the primary lesion and both sides of the neck, but in advanced lesions, better survival rates are obtained with a combination of radiation therapy and surgical therapy.

Glottic cancers

Mc cancers

Hoarseness is the mc manifestation

Hoarseness is the earliest manifestation

Best prognosis

No lymphadenopathy usually

Subglottic lesions

- Represent more advanced glottic carcinomas in which the neoplasm has secondarily invaded the subglottic area as well as the supraglottic area
- Metastasis to the same side is present in 50% of patients
- Subglottic extension of the carcinoma requires a total laryngectomy and radical neck dissection
- With thyroid lobectomy on the same side.

Pyriform sinus carcinomas

- Tend to remain asymptomatic for long periods of time
- Often the patient presents with dysphagia and pain on swallowing that may radiate to the ear on the same side
- A combination of preoperative or postoperative radiation therapy and operation yields better survival rates than operation alone

Postcricoid carcinoma

- The presenting complaint is usually pain on swallowing and dysphagia
- Metastasis to both sides of the neck is common
- A combination of preoperative or postoperative radiation and surgical therapy is usually employed, and the operation required is pharyngectomy, total laryngectomy, and, if there are palpable metastases, radical neck dissection on one side followed by radical neck dissection on the other side in approximately 6 weeks
- Verrucous carcinoma larynx is treated by endoscopic surgery.

Some Important Signs

- **BOCCA'S SIGN** — Absence of postcricoid crackle (MUIR's crackle) in **carcinoma postcricoid**
- **BOYCE SIGN—Laryngocele**—Gurgling sound on compression of external laryngocele with reduction of swelling
- **DODD'S SIGN/CRESCENT SIGN—**X-ray finding—Crescent of air between the mass and posterior pharyngeal wall
- **Positive in AC polyp.** Negative in angiofibroma
- **FURSTENBERGER'S SIGN—**This is seen when nasopharyngeal cyst is communicating intracranially, there is enlargement of the cyst on crying and upon compression of jugular vein
- **HITSELBERGER'S SIGN—**In **acoustic neuroma**—Loss of sensation in the ear canal suppllied by Arnold's nerve (branch of Vagus nerve to ear)
- **HONDOUSA SIGN—**X-ray finding in **angiofibroma** indicating infratemporal fossa involvement characterized by widening of gap between ramus of mandible and maxillary body
- **HENNEBERT SIGN—**False fistula sign (**cong. Syphilis, Meniere's**)
- **IRWIN MOORE'S SIGN—**Positive sueeze test in **chronic tonsillitis**
- **RACCOON SIGN—**Indicates **subgaleal hemorrhage** and not necessarily base of skull #

- **STEEPLE SIGN**—X-ray finding in **Acute laryngotracheobronchitis**
- **STANKIEWICZ'S SIGN**—Indicates **orbital injury during FESS**. Fat protrudes into nasal cavity on compression of eyeball from ouside
- **THUMB SIGN**—X-ray finding A/c **epiglottitis**
- **TRAGUS SIGN—EXTERNAL OTITIS**, Pain on pressing tragus
- **TEAPOT SIGN** is seen in **CSF rhinorrhoea**
- **BATTLE SIGN**—Bruising behind ear at mastoid region, due to petrous temporal bone fracture (middle fossa #)
- **OODS SIGN**—Palpable jugulodigastric lymph nodes

Orthopedics and USMLE

Biochemical Markers in Bone Metabolism (USMLE Favorite)

Markers in 'Bone mineralization'

Role in **'Bone mineralization'**

- **Bone-specific Alkaline Phosphatase**
- **Osteocalcin (bone-GLA protein)**
- **Propeptide of Type I Collagen**
- **Osteonectin**
- **Osteopontin**

Urinary Markers for 'Bone resorption'

- Urinary and serum cross-linked N telopeptide
- Urinary and serum cross-linked C telopeptide
- Urine hydroxyproline
- **Serum bone sialoprotein**
- **Serum Tartrate Acid Phosphatase (TRAP)**

Classification of Fractures (USMLE Favorite)

- *A single fracture line is referred to as a **'simple' fracture.***
- *When multiple fracture lines and bone fragments exist, the fracture is said to be **'comminuted' fracture***
- *Penetrating injury producing a fracture, or fracture fragments protruding through the skin, constitutes an **'open' fracture**.*
- *When no such wound is present, the fracture is classified as **'closed' fracture.***
- *More subtle trauma such as the activities of daily living may also produce fractures in elderly patients with osteoporosis, in patients with metabolic bone-wasting disease, or in patients with tumor of the bone. Such injuries are referred to as **pathologic fractures**. The most common causes of pathologic fracture are **osteoporosis** and **metastatic carcinoma.***
- *Healthy bone may fracture with the repetitive application of minor trauma, as in **'Fatigue' or 'Stress' fractures**. These fractures are seen in the metatarsals after a long hike or in the tibia, fibula, femur, or other skeletal locations in individuals involved in regular athletic activities.*

Fractures in Children

The **periosteum is extremely strong** in children.

Children's **bones are much more resilient** and less brittle than those of adults.

Bending moments applied to the bone of a child may cause a **Greenstick fracture**, in which there is distraction of the cortex on the convex side and compression of bone on the concave side. (**Cortex intact**)

Commonly Asked Terminology

- **Dislocation** means that the articular surfaces are not opposed or congruous and that the restraining ligaments and probably the capsule have been partially or completely torn.
- **Subluxation** means a partial displacement of one side of the joint on the other, but with less severe distortion than a dislocation. Soft tissue interposition may prevent complete reduction in either instance.
- **Reduction** refers to the action required to obtain anatomic alignment.
- **Arthoplasty:** Joint is excised and bones are so kept to avoid fusion.

Commonly Asked Fractures (USMLE Favorite)

• **Aviators #**	• **Neck of talus**
• **BOXERS #**	• **Neck of fifth metacarpal**
• **Bennett's #**	• **(Intra-articular) Base of 1st metacarpal**
• **Rolando's #**	• **(Extra-articular) Base of 1st metacarpal**
• **Chauffer's #**	• **Radius above styloid process**
• **Chance #**	• **Horizontal # through vertebrae due to sudden deceleration**
• **Clay shoveler's #**	• **Spinous process of T1**
• **Cotton's #**	• **Trimalleolar #**
• **Galeazi #**	• **Distal radius with dislocation of distal radioulnar joint**
• **Jefferson's #**	• **Burst fracture of Atlas (C1)**
• **Jones #**	• **Base of 5th metatarsal**
• **Hangman's #**	• **Axis**
• **Monteggia's #**	• **Proximal ulna with dislocation head of radius**
• **March #**	• **Stress # shaft of second or third metatarsal**
• **Maisonneuver #**	• **Neck of fibula**
• **Pott's #**	• **Bimalleolar ankle**
• **Smith's#**	• **Reverse of colles**
• **Pond #**	• **Depressed skull # in infants**
• **Toddler's #**	• **Spiral # of tibia**
• **Crescent #**	• **Iliac bone with sacroiliac disruption**

Factors effecting Fracture Healing

1. **Degree of immobilization is the 'most important factor'**. Repeated disruptions of repaired tissue significantly impairs healing
2. **Age**: Young patients heal rapidly
3. **Nutrition**: Good nutrition plays a vital role
4. **Diseases** like Diabetes mellitus, Osteoporosis, Immunocompromised states, Marfan's syndrome, Ehler-Danlos syndrome cause delayed healing
5. **Hormones**: Growth hormone, Calcitonin promote growth healing. Corticosteroids delay healing of fractures
6. **Type of bone**: Cancellous bones heal quickly due to increased vascularity
7. **Severe degree of trauma** and secondary infection cause delayed fracture healing
8. **Inadequate blood supply** near talus, NOF cause delayed fracture healing
9. **Intra-articular fractures** communicate with synovial fluid which contains collagenases and retards fracture healing
10. **Separation of bone ends**: Normal apposition is also important, inadequate reduction, excessive traction or interposition of soft tissue prevents healing
11. **Infection**: Infections cause necrosis and edema, impair healing and increase mobility of fracture site.

Important Bursitis (USMLE Favorite)

1. **Prepatellar Bursitis**	• **Housemaid's Knee**
2. **Infrapatellar Bursitis**	• **Clergyman's Knee/Vicar's Knee**
3. **Olecranon Bursitis**	• **Student's elbow**
4. **Ischial Bursitis**	• **Weaver's bottom**
5. **Lateral Malleolus Bursitis**	• **Tailor's ankle**
6. **Great Toe Bursitis**	• **Bunion**

Important Casts used in Orthopedics

1. **Minerva cast**	• **Cervical spine disease**
2. **Turnbuckle cast**	• **Scoliosis**
3. **Risser's cast**	• **Scoliosis**
4. **Milwaukee's brace**	• **Scoliosis**
5. **Boston brace**	• **Scoliosis**
6. **Frog leg cast**	• **CDH**
7. **Cylinder cast**	• **# Patella**
8. **Hip spica**	• **# Femur**
9. **Hanging cast**	• **# Humerus**
10. **Tube cast**	• **Knee**

Nerve Injuries of Upper Limb (USMLE Favorite)

Ulnar Nerve 'Musicians Nerve'

- **Injured especially at the level of medial** condyle of Humerus (Lower end)
- Ulnar nerve supplies medial 1/3 of palm **(Hypothenar area)**
- Ulnar nerve in hand supplies:
  - **(3, 4 Lumbricals)**
  - **Palmar and dorsal interossei**
  - **Adductor pollicis**
  - **Hypothenar muscles**
- Ulnar nerve in hand supplies
  - **Flexor carpi ulnaris**
  - **Medial half of flexor digitorum profundus**
- **Lesion of ulnar nerve causes:**
  - **Weakness of ulnar deviation**
  - **Weakness of wrist flexion**
  - **Adductor pollicis paralysis with loss of thumb adduction**

In Ulnar Nerve Palsy, there is

1. **Positive card test**
2. **Positive book test/Froment sign**
3. **Positive Egawa's test**
4. **Ulnar claw hand**

Median Nerve: 'Laborers Nerve'

- Does not supply arm
- Supplies all flexors except flexor carpi ulnaris and medial half of flexor digitorum profundus in forearm
- **Supplies:**
  - **L**umbrical 1 and 2,
  - **O**pponens pollicis,
  - **A**bductor pollicis brevis,
  - **F**lexor pollicis brevis in hand **(LOAF)**.

Implicated in:
- **Ape thumb deformity**
- **Carpal tunnel syndrome**
- **Pointing index**
- **Loss of opposition and abduction of thumb**
- **Pen test is positive in median nerve injury**

Radial Nerve

- Supplies **Extensor** Compartment of Arm and Forearm
- Commonly involved in **'Spiral groove/Radial groove'**
- **Accompanied by Profunda Brachii vessels**
- **Supplies:**
  - **BEAST** Muscles (**B**rachioradialis, **E**xtensors of wrist and fingers, **A**nconeus, **S**upinator, **T**riceps)

- Implicated in **'Crutch Palsy'**
- Implicated in **'Saturday Night Palsy'**
- Implicated in **'Wrist Drop'**

Important 'Sites' of Injury

1. Injury to Upper End of Humerus	• **Axillary nerve damage**
2. Injury (Anterior Dislocation of Shoulder)	• **Axillary nerve damage**
3. Injury to Mid Humerus	• **Radial nerve**
4. Injury to Lower end (Medial) of Humerus	• **Ulnar nerve**
5. Injury to Supracondylar area of Humerus	• **Median nerve**
6. Injury to Upper Trunk of Brachial Plexus	• **Erb palsy**
7. Injury to Lower Trunk of Brachial Plexus	• **Klumpke's palsy**

IMPORTANT CONDITIONS AFFECTING UPPER LIMB

Ganglion cysts

- These cystic swellings occur on the hands, particularly on the dorsal aspect of the wrists, and are usually near or attached to tendon sheaths and joint capsules
- Most common sites:
  - **Scapholunate joint on the back of the wrist**
  - **Distal volar aspect of the radius**
  - **Flexor tendon sheaths.**

- The lesions appear to be degenerative and the gelatinous material found in the center has a high hyaluronic acid content
- Many ganglion cysts regres spontaneously or after needle aspiration of the contents. Recurrent ganglia or ganglia that are cosmetically unacceptable to the patient can be surgically excised, but may recur after excision.

1. **Infections from thumb and index finger spread to thenar spaces**
2. **Infections from middle and ring fingers spread to mid palmar spaces**
3. **Infections from little finger spread to ulnar bursa and forearm space of Parona**

Carpal Tunnel Syndrome

- Entrapment of **Median Nerve** in Carpal Tunnel leading to tingling, parasthesias, weakness in hand
- Painful
- Associated with:
  - **Trauma**
  - **Pregnancy**
  - **Acromegaly**
  - **Rheumatoid arthritis**
  - **Amyloidosis**
  - **Multiple myeloma**
  - **Hypothyroidism**
- **Tinnel's sign** +
- **Phalen's sign** +
- **Electrodiagnostic tests**, USG imaging and MRI are useful adjuncts

Dupuytren's Contracture

- **Progressive**
- **Painless**
- **Puckering of skin of Palmar Fascia**
- **Flexion of MCP joints of ring and little fingers**

Colles' Fracture

- **Fall on outstretched hands**
- **Common in elderly women**
- **Distal fragment displaced dorsally, angulated dorsally, supinated**
- **'Dinner Fork' Deformity**
- **Commonest complication is 'Stiffness of fingers'**

Scaphoid Fracture

- **Scaphoid is one of the carpal bones which undergo fracture commonly as well as avascular necrosis**
- **Avascular necrosis of 'proximal' fragment is seen**
- **Injury occurs by fall on outstretched hands**
- **MC site of injury is 'waist'**
- **Tenderness in 'Anatomical snuff box' may be seen**
- **Best radiological view is Oblique view**
- **In absence of radiological findings, suspect scaphoid fracture**
- **Most common site is between proximal 1/3 and distal 2/3**

Nerve Injuries

- **Neurapraxia: Complete recovery possible**
- **Axonotmesis: Rupture of nerve fiber with intact sheath**
- **Neurotmesis: Rupture of nerve fiber and sheath**
  - Best recovery is seen in **pure motor nerve (radial nerve)**
  - In mixed nerve, recovery is poor because sensory and motor fibers may unite with each other.

Volkmann's Ischemic Contracture (Features) (P)

- **Pallor**
- **Pain (most important sign)**
- **Paralysis**
- **Paresthesias**
- **Pulselessness**
  - **Median nerve mostly involved**
  - **Deformity:** Flexion of wrist, extension of fingers at MCP, flexion at IP, pronation of forearm
  - **Seddons area of Affection** is infarct of muscles in the form of an ellipsoid where the axis is in the line of anterior interosseous artery and central line in middle of forearm called Seddons area
  - **Flexor digitorum profundus and flexor pollicis longus** are muscles damaged.

Important Nerves Involved in

Wrist drop	**Radial nerve palsy**
Foot drop	**Common peroneal nerve palsy**
Meralgia paresthetica	**Lateral cutaneous nerve of thigh**
Winging of scapula	**Long thoracic nerve of Bell**
Erb's Palsy	**Upper trunk of brachial plexus**
Klumpke's palsy	**Lower trunk of brachial plexus**

Dislocation of Shoulder Joint

- **Shoulder is the 'most common' joint to dislocate in human body**
- **'Subcoracoid' dislocation/inferior dislocation is the commonest type**
- **Posterior dislocation of shoulder is rare and associated with epileptic convulsions**
- **Bankart's (Glenoid Labrum) and Hill-Sachs lesion (Humeral Head) are seen.**
  - **Hamilton Ruler Test**
  - **Dugas' Test**
  - **Callaway's Test are used**
- **Reduction is by Kocher's maneuver**
- **Recurrent dislocation is treated by Putti-Platt and Bankart's Operation**

Congenital Dislocation of Hip

- **It is a developmental anomaly**
- **Associated with 'oligohydramnios'**
- **Females are more prone**
- **Most common in western race.**

- Shallow acetabulum is predisposing factor
- Common in first born baby
- Incidence is common in Frank breech

Tests used:

- *Ortolani's Test (Click of entrance)*
- *Von Rosen's sign*
- *Barlow's sign are useful in Diagnosis*

Remember:

- Lurching gait (Unilateral CDH)
- Waddling gait (Bilateral CDH)
- Ultrasonography is used for Diagnosis
- Shenton's line is broken
- von Rosen Splint is used in Treatment

USMLE Case Scenario

A physician delivers a healthy-looking baby girl, who had a breech presentation. He is taken to an orthopedician because his father notices that the baby cannot abduct the thighs when the hips and knees are flexed, but a click cannot be elicited when the physician tries to manually dislocate or reduce the femoral heads. Both the legs are of same length and gluteal folds are symmetrical.

Remember

- Commonest type of hip dislocation: posterior
- Flexion, adduction and internal rotation are a feature
- Posterior dislocation can be seen on per rectal examination

LOWER LIMB ORTHOPEDICS

Tarsal Tunnel Syndrome

- It is entrapment of 'Posterior Tibial Nerve' in the Tarsal tunnel
- Occurs in association with:
  - 'Rheumatoid arthritis'
  - Ankylosing spondylitis
  - Neural tumors or perineural fibrosis
- Pain and sensory disturbances over plantar aspect of foot is seen

Congenital Talipes Equinovarus (CTEV)

- Also called Clubfoot
- IE deformity:
  - *Inversion deformity*
  - *Equinus deformity*
- Associated with:
  - *Idiopathic causes*
  - *Neurological disorders*
  - *Spina bifida*
  - *Arthrogyrophosis multiplex*

- **Foot in <u>Equines, Varus and Adduction</u>**
- **Usually bilateral**
- **Manipulation should begin 'immediately after birth by mother'**
- **At 2 years' treatment is 'posteromedial soft tissue release'**
- **Treatment of chronic cases is 'Triple Arthodesis'**

Options for Treatment of CTEV

- **< 3 years: Soft tissue release**
- **4–8 years: Evans surgery**
- **8–11 years: Wedge tarsectomy**
- **> 12 years: Triple arthrodesis**
- **Already operated: Ilizarov technique.**

Important Terms

- **Tennis Elbow is Medial Epicondylitis (Affects Common Flexor Origin)**
- **Golfer's Elbow is Lateral Epincondylitis (Affects Common Extensor Origin)**
- **Student's elbow is Olecranon bursitis**
- **Painful arc syndrome is Supraspinatus Tendinitis in which patient can't abduct his arm beyond 30° without pain**
- **Frozen shoulder: Active movement at shoulder is not possible at all.**

Remember 'new'Important points in Orthopedics

- **Guyon's Canal**: Fibro-osseous canal bound by hamate and pisiform bone through which **ulnar artery and nerve pass.**
- **Bowler's Thumb**: Traumatic neuropathy of **ulnar digital nerve to thumb.**
- **Pronator Syndrome**: **High carpal tunnel syndrome**: Entrapment of **Median nervenerve at elbow**.
- **Anterior interosseous syndrome**: Compression of AIN (**Anterior Interosseous Nerve)** 4-6 cms below elbow causing weakness of FPL, FDP and pronator quadrates
- **Cubital Tunnel Syndrome**: Compression of**ulnar nerve** during its passage around medial aspect of elbow.
- **Radial Tunnel Syndrome**: Resistant Tennis Elbow due to entrapment **of Posterior Interosseous nerve** in the lateral aspect of Proximal forearm.
- **Wartenberg's Syndrome**: Entrapment of **Sensory branch of Radial nerve** as it emerges beneath Brachioradialisproximal to Radial Styloid process.
- **Meralgia Paresthetica: Lateral cutaneous nerve of thigh**
- **Anterior Tarsal Tunnel Syndrome**: **Deep peroneal nerve**
- **Tarsal Tunnel Syndrome**: **Posterior tibial nerve**
- **Jogger's Foot**: **Medial plantar nerve**
- **Hip Pointer**: **Iliac crest**
- **Tennis Leg**: **Gastrocnemius Soleus strain**

Prolapse of Intervertebral Disk

- Most common site **L4-L5**
- Burst # occurs due to **compression**
- Most common cause is **trauma**
- Extrusion of nucleus pulposus into body of vertebrae is **Schmorl's node**

Spondylosis

- It is **degeneration** of Intervertebral disk
- Spondylolysis is a **bony defect in the pars interarticularis** (a segment near the junction of the pedicle with the lamina) of the vertebra

Spondylolisthesis

- It is the **anterior slippage of the vertebral body, pedicles, and superior articular facets,** leaving the posterior elements behind
- Spondylolisthesis is **associated with spondylolysis** and degenerative spine disease and occurs more frequently in women
- The slippage may be asymptomatic but may also cause low back pain, nerve root injury (the L5 root most frequently), or symptomatic spinal stenosis
- A **'step'** may be present on deep palpation of the posterior elements of the segment above the spondylolisthetic joint
- The trunk may be shortened and the abdomen protuberant as a result of extreme forward displacement of L4 on L5 in severe degrees of spondylolisthesis
- **Spondylolisthesis** is **slipping** of one vertebrae over other
- **Beheaded Scottish Terrier sign is seen**
- **Beheaded Scottish Terrier sign is seen in oblique view.**

Tests Suggesting Disk Prolapse

- **Naffezier's test**
- **Milgram's test**
- **Sitting root test**

Vertebrae and Corresponding Spinal Level

• Cervical Region	**C1-C7 Add 1**
• Upper Thoracic Lesion	**T1 –T6 Add 2**
• Lower Thoracic Lesion	**T7-T9 Add 3**
• T10	**Corresponds to L1-L2**
• T12-L1	**Corresponds to L5-S1**

Remember Eponyms

• **Marble bone disease**	• **Osteopetrosis**
• **Spotted bone disease**	• **Osteopoikilosis**
• **Stripped bone disease**	• **Osteopathia striata**
• **Candle bone disease**	• **Melorheostosis**

- **Normal carrying angle: males: 10-15 degrees, Females: 15-18 degrees**
- **Cubitus varus:** Reduction in normal carrying angle
- **Cubitus valgus:** Increase in carrying angle
- **Cubitus rectus:** No valgus or varus angulation

Slipped FEMORAL EPIPHYSIS (SCFE)

- **It is displacement of 'Proximal Femoral Epiphysis'**
- **Common in children (obese) in 2nd decade**
- **Pain is the initial and most common complaint**
- **'Epiphysis' slips 'downwards and posteriorly'**

- Limping is the associated feature
- Flexion, Abduction and Medial Rotation are limited
- Diagnosis is by:
  - Trethowan's sign
  - Capener's sign
  - Trendelenburg's sign may be positive

Perthes Disease

- Is chronic disease with ischemia of upper end of femur causing 'avascular necrosis'
- Osteochondritis of femoral head
- Boys are affected more
- Adduction of limb is unaffected
- Not obese
- Pain is the initial and most common complaint
- Limping is the associated feature
- MRI is the investigation of choice

Coxa vara

Term used to describe a hip in which angle between neck and shaft of femur is less than 125°

Osteochondritis

1. Perthes disease	• Osteochondritis of Femoral head
2. Panner's disease	• Osteochondritis of Capitulum
3. Kienbock's disease	• Osteochondritis of Lunate
4. Osgood-Schlatter disease	• Osteochondritis of Tibial tubercle
5. Sever's disease	• Osteochondritis of Calcaneum
6. Kohler's disease	• Osteochondritis of Navicular
7. Frieberg's disease	• Osteochondritis of Metatarsal head
8. Scheuermann's disease	• Osteochondritis of vertebrae

Different Vertebral Types in Different Diseases

1. Picture frame vertebrae	• Paget's disease (P-P)
2. Square-shaped vertebrae	• Ankylosing spondylitis
3. Hamburger vertebrae	• Osteopetrosis
4. Beak-shaped vertebrae	• Mucopolysaccharidosis
5. Wedge-shaped vertebrae	• Osteoporosis
6. Fish head vertebrae	• Osteoporosis
7. Fish mouth vertebrae	• Osteogenesis imperfecta • Ehler-Danlos syndrome • Homocystinuria • Marfan's syndrome
8. Vertebrae plana	• Eosinophilic granuloma

Commonly asked Limb Deformities in USMLE

• **Limb abducted and externally rotated in**	• **Anterior dislocation Hip**
• **Limbflexed, adducted and internally rotated in**	• **Posterior dislocation Hip**
• **Cubitus varus (Gunstock deformity)**	• **Supracondylar # of humerus**
• **Cubitus valgus**	• **# Lateral condyle humerus**

Differentiae Limb Deformities

- **Flexion, adduction, internal rotation: Posterior dislocation of hip (FADIR)**
- **Flexion, abduction, external rotation: Anterior dislocation of hip (FABER)**
- **Flexion, adduction, external rotation: #NOF (FADER)**

USMLE Case scenario

A 44-year-old passenger in a lorry accident hits the dashboard with his knees and complains of severe pain in his right knee. He has right lower extremity shortened, adducted, and internally rotated. The likely diagnosis is:
Posterior dislocation of the knee

BONE TUMORS (HIGH YIELD FACTS COMMONLY ASKED)

Benign Tumors

The common benign bone tumors include:

- **Enchondroma, osteochondroma, chondroblastoma, and Chondromyxoid fibroma, of <u>cartilage origin</u>**
- **Osteoid osteoma and osteoblastoma of <u>bone origin</u>**
- **Fibroma and desmoplastic fibroma of <u>fibrous tissue origin</u>**
- **Hemangioma of <u>vascular origin</u>**
- **Giant cell tumor of <u>unknown origin</u>**
- **Malignant Tumors**: The most common malignant tumors of bone are **plasma cell tumors**. The four most common malignant nonhematopoietic bone tumors are:
  a. **Osteosarcoma**
  b. **Chondrosarcoma**
  c. **Ewing's sarcoma**
  d. **Malignant fibrous histiocytoma**

Rare malignant tumors include:

- **Chordoma** (of notochordal origin)
- **Malignant giant cell tumor**
- **Adamantinoma (of unknown origin)**
- **Hemangioendothelioma (of vascular origin)**

Tumors According to Location

Epiphyseal	Metaphyseal	Diaphyseal
• Chondroblastoma	• Chondrosarcoma	• Round cell tumors
• Osteoclastoma	• Enchondroma	• Ewing's sarcoma
	• Osteochondroma	• Multiple myeloma
	• Osteoblastoma	• Adamantinoma
	• Osteosarcoma	• Osteoid osteoma
	• Bone cyst	
	• Osteomyelitis	

Diaphyseal Metaphyseal

- **Fibrous dysplasia and other fibrous tumors of Bone**
- **Fibrosarcoma**
- **Fibroxanthoma**
- **Chondromyxoid fibroma**
- **Fibrous cortical defect**
- **Nonossifying fibroma**

Different Appearances of Bony Tumors

Onion skin appearance	Ewing's sarcoma
Honey comb appearance	Adamantinoma
Breech of Cortex	Osteoclastoma, Aneurysmal bone cyst
Soap bubble appearance	**Osteo<u>clastoma</u>**
Codman's triangle	**Osteo<u>sarcoma</u>**
Sun ray appearance	**Osteo<u>sarcoma</u>**
Chicken wire pattern	Chondroblastoma
Linear Striations	**Vertebral Hemangioma**
Physaliphorous cells	**Chordoma**
Cotton wool/Ground Glass Appearance	**Fibrous Dysplasia**

Ewing's Sarcoma

- **Affects children < 15 years usually**
- **Diaphysial Tumor**
- **Common in second decade**
- **Onion skin lesions on X-ray**
- **Translocation (t; 11:22)**
- **Mimics Osteomyelitis**
- **PAS Positive material (Glycogen) found**
- **Most radiosensitive bone tumor**

Osteosarcoma

- **Second most common primary malignant bone marrow**
- **Metaphyseal tumor**
- **Affects knee joint**
- **MC site <u>lower</u> end of femur**
- **Sunburst appearance**
- **Codman's triangle**
- **Presents with secondaries in lungs with pneumothorax**
- **Pulsating bone tumor**
- **Chemotherapy + limb salvage surgery used for treatment**

USMLE Case Scenario

A 15-year-old has a lesion in the metaphyseal end of his distal femur. Areas of lytic bone destruction mixed with areas of reactive and tumor bone formations are seen. This tumor rapidly permeates through the overlying cortex into the subperiosteal space and produces a characteristic appearance of trabecular bone oriented at right angles to the underlying cortical surface. Likely diagnosis is: Sarcoma

Osteoclastoma

- **Epiphyseal tumor**
- **Soap bubble appearance**
- **Breech of cortex**
- **Lower end of Femur is most common site**

Chondrosarcoma

- **Metaphyseal Tumor**
- **Dense Punctate Calcifications**
- **Associated with endosteal scalloping**

Multiple Myeloma

- This malignant neoplasm of marrow cell origin is **the 'most common primary malignant neoplasm' of bone.**
- Myeloma is often encountered in the **late decades of life** and is seen more frequently in **males** than in females.
- The symptoms vary from local pain and discomfort to systemic symptoms of
  - **Anemia**
  - **Fever**
  - **Hypercalcemia**
  - **Renal failure** related to extensive skeletal involvement
  - **Abnormal production of immunoglobulins**
- Myeloma characteristically produces **lytic destruction of bone** with little if any reactive bone formation
- These lesions are described as **'geographic or punched out'** in appearance.
- **The absence of reactive bone formation** is borne out by the observation that myeloma lesions are often **silent on radionuclide scanning**
- Pathologic fracture is often the presenting symptom.
- The diagnosis of myeloma is made by **marrow aspiration or the demonstration of abnormal plasma cells at the site of bony destruction.**
- Fifty percent of patients with disseminated disease have **Bence Jones protein in their urine**
- Serum **electrophoresis demonstrates an abnormal amount of immunoglobulins.**
- Urine electrophoresis is also helpful when the diagnosis is in doubt and may demonstrate abnormal proteins in patients with a normal serum electrophoretic pattern.
- Microscopically, myeloma produces **sheets of plasma cells**. Usually these are well-differentiated cells in which the characteristic arrangements of nuclear chromatin can be recognized with '**Russel Bodies'.**

Aneurysmal Bone Cyst

- Aneurysmal bone cyst is **metaphyseal lesion**
- **It has blood filled spaces**
- **Pulsatile in elderly**
- Aneurysmal bone cyst is **expansile radiolucent** lesion
- Aneurysmal bone cyst may show **'focal cortical destruction, cortical breech'**.
- Aneurysmal bone cyst most commonly occurs in Lower end of **HUMERUS**

Unicameral Bone Cyst

- **Usually a single cavity with connective tissue lining**
- **Gaint cells seen**
- **Lytic lesion usually in children**

Chondroblastoma

- Chondroblastoma is a **benign** cartilaginous tumor
- Chondroblastoma is **epiphyseal** tumor

Chondroblastoma is characterized by

- **Multi nucleate giant cells**
- **PAS positive reaction**
- 'Dense punctuate/stippled or mottled calcification with sclerotic rim'

Most common site is **proximal humerus**

Adamantinoma

- Epithelial tumor from **dental epithelium**
- Mc sites: **Mandible, Tibia**
- **Diaphyseal tumor**
- **Slowly growing, locally invasive benign, cystic lesion**
- **Occurs in late adolescence/middle age**
- **'Bubble defect' in anterior tibial cortex** is a feature

Osteoid Osteoma

- One of the **commonest benign bone tumor**
- Severe **Pain at night responding to NSAIDS**
- Mc site: **Femur and tibia**

USMLE Case Scenario

A 12-year-old has a solitary lesion in his left femur which is exquisitely painful. Pain is described as a persistent discomfort unrelated to activity or rest and is often worse at night. Curiously, pain is relieved for several hours by the use of Nonsteroidal anti-inflammatory drugs. The lesion is composed of a central nidus of closely packed trabeculae of woven bone. Most likely lesion is: Osteoid Osteoma

Most Common Sites

1. Bone secondaries	**Vertebrae**
2. Multiple myeloma	**Vertebrae**
3. Adamantinoma	**Mandible**
4. Paget's disease	**Pelvis**
5. Ivory osteoma	**Frontal sinus**
6. Simple bone cyst	**Upper end of Humerus**
7. Aneurysmal bone cyst	**Lower end of Humerus**
8. Osteoclastoma	**Lower end of Femur**
9. Rhabdomyosarcoma	**Head and neck region**

Paget's Disease

Paget's disease is a focal disorder of bone remodeling that results in increased bone turnover and abnormal bone architecture. Patients are often asymptomatic but may present with gross skeletal abnormalities (bowing, long-bone fractures, increased skull circumference), deafness, nerve compression syndromes, or simply an abnormally elevated alkaline phosphatase. Serum calcium and phosphorus levels are usually normal

- Paget's Disease is also called **Osteitis Deformans.**

- It is because of **extensive osteoclastic activity and disorganized new bone formation.**
- **Commonly** involved bones are**: Pelvis, tibia, skull, spine**
- **Pelvis being the commonest site**
- **Serum calcium and phosphate levels are normal**
- **Alkaline phosphatase and Osteocalcin levels are increased**

Pain is the most common presenting feature

Complications include:

- High output cardiac failure
- Fractures
- Hypercalcemia
- Cranial nerve palsies and spinal stenosis
- Deafness due to otosclerosis
- Steal Syndrome
- Osteosarcoma (dangerous)

Bisphosphonates are the 'drug of choice'.

USMLE Case Scenario

A bony disease is characterized increased generation and overactivity of osteoclasts and the calcification rate is characteristically increased with increased urinary excretion of small peptides containing hydroxyproline reflects: Paget's Disease

Differentiate

- **Paget's disease of nipple:** Which is associated with underlying ductal malignancy of breast
- **Paget's disease of vulva**: Which is not associated with underlying malignancy but can cause vulval cancer
- **Paget's recurrent fibroid**: A **spindle cell sarcoma** of low potential **occurring in abdominal wall or thighs**
- **Paget's cells**: Upward spread of breast cancer cells into epidermis which are mucin positive.

Fibrous Dysplasia

- Fibrous dysplasia is a **tumor like lesion**
- It is **benign**
- It is **developmental in origin** and **hormone dependent**
- Pathology is replacement of bone by fibrous tissue
- X-ray shows '**Ground glass' appearance and 'Chinese lettering of bone'**
- Rarely **osteosarcoma** can occur in fibrous dysplasia
- Sexual precocity in girls with polyostotic fibrous dysplasia and cutaneous pigmentation constitutes '**McCune Albright Syndrome'**
- Fibrous dysplasia and McCune-Albright syndrome represent a phenotypic spectrum of disorders caused by **activating mutations in the GNAS1 gene**

Radiologic Changes

The roentgenographic appearance of the lesions is that of a radiolucent area with a well-delineated, smooth or scalloped border, typically associated with focal thinning of the cortex of the bone

Fibrous dysplasia can cause **bones to become larger** than normal, a feature characteristic of Paget's disease as well.

The **'ground-glass' appearance** is due to the thin spicules of calcified woven bone.

Deformities can include:

- **Coxa vara**
- **Shepherd's-crook deformity of the femur**
- **Bowing of the tibia**
- **Harrison's grooves**
- **Protrusio acetabuli**
- **Involvement of facial bones, may create a leonine appearance (leontiasis ossea).**
- **Fibrous dysplasia of the temporal bones can cause progressive loss of hearing and obliteration of the external ear canal**
- Advanced skeletal age in girls is correlated with **sexual precocity** but can occur in boys without sexual precocity
- Occasionally, a focus of fibrous dysplasia may undergo cystic degeneration, with an enormous distortion of the shape of the **bone**, and mimic the so-called **aneurysmal bone cyst.**

Acute Pyogenic Arthritis (SEPTIC)

- Joint infection with pyogenic organisms occurs as a result of **hematogenous seeding of the joint,** extension of adjacent osteomyelitis, or penetrating wounds of the joint
- Hematogenous pyarthrosis is most commonly observed in children under the age of 5 years
- **S. aureus is the most common etiologic agent**, followed by Hemophilus influenzae, Streptococcus, Gonococcus, and Pneumococcus
- Acute pyarthrosis is **almost always monoarticular**
- Patients with immune deficiency may present with multiple joint involvement
- **The hip joint** is the most frequently involved.

Clinical Considerations

- The onset of pyogenic arthritis is **acute, with fever, irritability and pain**
- In the early stages of infection, a **limp** may develop, which rapidly progresses to severe pain, preventing ambulation
- On examination, one observes swelling, overlying erythema, and exquisite tenderness to direct palpation. Any attempt at joint motion produces paroxysms of pain.

Laboratory studies demonstrate:

- **Elevated** white blood cell count and an
- **Elevated** erythrocyte sedimentation rate
- Aspiration of the involved joint under sterile conditions reveals a **cloudy, turbid synovial fluid, with a cell count ranging from 50,000 to 200,000 polymorphonuclear neutrophils per cu cm**
- A Gram's stain of the involved joint fluid shows organisms in 50% of cases. The joint fluid is sent for aerobic and anaerobic culture
- **Blood cultures** are frequently positive.

Radiographs in the early stages of septic arthritis reveal no bony change

- There is distention in the joint capsule secondary to increased pressure within the joint, and the joint may appear abnormally widened
- In severe cases, there may be pathologic dislocation of the joint or pathologic separation of the epiphysis. In untreated or inadequately treated cases, destruction of articular cartilage eventually produces joint narrowing.

Treatment

Pyogenic arthritis is an emergency

When the diagnosis has been established, intravenous antibiotics are administered without awaiting the results of culture.

Septic Arthritis

It is microbial invasion of the synovial space. Pathogens enter the synovial space by either hematogenous spread, local spread from contiguous infection, or a traumatic or surgical infection of the joint space. Accumulating fluid and pus rapidly raise the intra-articular

Pressure and permanently injure vessels and articular cartilage. More than 90% of cases of septic arthritis affect the joints of the lower extremity, with the knee most commonly involved. Acute septic arthritis is bacterial, with Staphylococcus.

Septic Arthritis	Transient Synovitis
• **Less** common	• **Mc cause** of hip pain and limpin children
• Patient is **sick**	• Patient is not sick
• High grade fever usual	• High grade feverun usual
• Pain is **severe**	• Pain is not severe
• **ESR, CRP, WBC↑**	• ESR, CRP, WBC usually normal

Osteomyelitis

- **Osteomyelitis is the term used to denote infection of bone**
- **Earliest site of bone involvement is in Metaphysis**
- The majority of bone infections are the result of **Staphylococcus aureus**
- The **isolated necrotic bone** within the abscess cavity is called a **sequestrum**
- New bone formation occurring about the periphery of the abscess represents the body's attempt to wall off the infection. This new bone is called **involucrum**
- In some instances, a static abscess cavity remains without further enlargement. This equilibrium between host and organism is known as a **Brodie's abscess in long bones**
- Young children may demonstrate the phenomenon known as **pseudoparalysis.** These children refuse to move the involved limb, mimicking a neurologic deficit
- **Radiographs:** It takes some time for osteomyelitic lesions to appear on radiographs
- The lesion of osteomyelitis appears on radiograph in not less than two weeks
- As a result alternative diagnostic modalities are used to pick-up osteomyelitis in the form of **MRI and Bone scans**
- Most cases of acute osteomyelitis are due to Staph Aureus and MRSA strains are common nowadays
- It is not advisible to wait for radiological changes to appear in case of acute osteomyelitis and then to start treatment.

Diagnosis

1. ESR Increased
2. CRP Increased
3. TLC Increased
4. MRI (90% sensitive 95% specific)
5. Bone scans 60% sensitive and 33% specific)
6. Blood cultures positive in 65% cases (Confirmatory)

Radiographic Changes in Osteomyelitis

1. Hazziness
2. Loss of density of effected bones
3. Subperiosteal reaction
4. Bone death and appearance of **(sequestrum)**
5. Periosteal new bone formation **(involucrum)**

Time Related Changes in Acute Osteomyelitis

- **Soft tissue swelling**: Less than a week
- **Periosteal reaction**: After ten days
- **Lytic changes**: After two weeks

- Early diagnosis of acute **osteomyelitis** is critical because prompt antibiotic therapy may prevent the necrosis of bone
- The evaluation usually begins with plain radiographs because of their ready availability, although they frequently show no abnormalities during early infection
- In 95% of cases, the technetium radionuclide scan using **^{99m}Tc diphosphonate is positive within 24 h of the onset of symptoms.** Falsely negative scans usually indicate obstruction of blood flow to the bone. Because the uptake of technetium reflects osteoblastic activity and skeletal vascularity, the bone scan cannot differentiate **osteomyelitis** from fractures, tumors, infarction, or neuropathic osteopathy
- **Ga citrate- and ^{111}In-labeled leukocyte** or immunoglobulin scans, which have greater specificity for inflammation, may help distinguish infectious from noninfectious processes and indicate inflammatory changes within bones that for other reasons are already abnormal on radiography and technetium scanning
- **Ultrasound can be used to diagnose osteomyelitis** by the detection of subperiosteal fluid collections, soft tissue abscesses adjacent to bone, and periosteal thickening and elevation
- **MRI is as sensitive as the bone scan for the diagnosis of acute osteomyelitis** because it is able to detect changes in the water content of marrow. MRI yields better anatomic resolution of epidural abscesses and other soft tissue processes than CT and is currently the imaging technique of choice for vertebral **osteomyelitis.**

Remember Most Commons of USMLE

- Most common organism of acute osteomyelitis: **Staph aureus**
- Most common organism of acute osteomyelitis in **drug addicts**: **Pseudomonas**
- Most common mode of infection: **Hematogeneous**
- Most common site in bone: **Metaphysis**
- Most common site of acute osteomyelitis in **Infants**: **Hip**
- Most common site of acute osteomyelitis in **children**: **Femur**
- Most common site in **adults**: **Thoracolumbar spine**

- Osteomyelitis in **sickle cell disease:** Salmonella
- Osteomyelitis after **foot wound:** Pseudomonas aeruginosa
- Osteomyelitis involving **prosthetic joints:** S. aureus
- Osteomyelitis involving **IV drug abusers:** S. aureus

Types of Sequestrum

Ring Sequestrum	Amputation stumps
Tubular Sequestrum	Osteomyelitis (Hematogeneous)
Rice grain Sequestrum	Tuberculosis

Skeletal Tuberculosis

- In bone and joint disease, pathogenesis is related to **reactivation of hematogenous foci** or to spread from adjacent paravertebral lymph nodes
- **Weight-bearing joints** (spine, hips, and knees ¾ in that order) are affected most commonly
- Spinal tuberculosis **(Pott's disease or tuberculous spondylitis)** often involves two or more adjacent vertebral bodies
- Upper thoracic spine is the most common site of spinal tuberculosis in children
- The lower thoracic and upper lumbar vertebrae are usually affected in adults. From the anterior superior or inferior angle of the vertebral body, the lesion reaches the adjacent body, also destroying the intervertebral disk
- With advanced disease, collapse of vertebral bodies results in **kyphosis (gibbus)**
- A **paravertebral 'cold' abscess** may also form

- In the upper spine, this abscess may track to the chest wall as a mass; in the lower spine, it may reach the inguinal ligaments or present as a psoas abscess
- **Pathologic Considerations**
- The histologic appearance of the tuberculous lesion in bone resembles that observed in visceral tuberculosis. Histiocytes, Langhans giant cells, and fibroblastic proliferation are all present
- Caseous necrosis is **less frequently** seen in joint lesions than in pulmonary lesions
- The destruction produced by granulomatous inflammation is **characteristically slow**
- Within the joint, invasion of bone tends to occur at the margins where synovium is attached to bone, producing a characteristic marginal defect
- As destruction proceeds, the joint becomes filled with necrotic products and fragments of articular cartilage, material called **rice bodies** because of its resemblance to grains of rice
- **Computed tomography (CT) or magnetic resonance imaging (MRI)** reveals the characteristic lesion and suggests its etiology, although the differential diagnosis includes other infections and tumors
- **Aspiration of the abscess or bone biopsy confirms the tuberculous etiology**, as cultures are usually positive and histologic findings highly typical
- **Skeletal tuberculosis responds to chemotherapy**, but severe cases may require surgery

Skeletal Actinomycosis

- **Actinomyces Israelii is the MC organism**
- **Orocervicofacial form is the MC type of skeletal actinomycosis**
- **'Lower jaw' (Mandible) is the commonest site**
- **Induration and Sinus Formation are a feature**
- **Pencillin G is the DOC**

Rickets

- Rickets is characterized by **defective mineralization** of bones and cartilage
- Osteomalacia is **defective mineralization** of bones
- Rickets is **seen before** closure of growth plates

Causes

- Nutritional rickets: vit D deficiency, Malabsorption
- Accelerated loss of vit D: Phenytoin, Rifampicin, Barbiturates
- Impaired hydroxylation in liver and Kidney
- Liver disease, Hypoparathyroidism, Renal failure, Renal Tubular Acidosis
- Vit D Resistant rickets, Fanconi's syndrome, Wilson's disease.

Clinical Features

Failure of calcification of cartilage and osteoid.

Epiphyseal enlargement occurs (thickening of knees, ankles, wrists)

- **Craniotabes**
- **Genu valgum**
- **Coxa vara**
- **Short stature**
- **Protrubent abdomen**

- **Wide open fontanelle**
- Enlargement of costochondral junction. **(Ricketic rosary)**
- Lateral indentation of chest due to pull of diaphragm on ribs. **(Harrison's groove)**
- **Triradiate pelvis**
- Forward projection of sternum. **(Pectus Carinatum)**
- **Kyphoscoliosis**

Radiographic Features

- **Thickening and widening of epiphysis**
- **Cupping and fraying of metaphysis**
- **Irregular metaphyseal margins**
- **Flaring of anterior ends of ribs**
- **Bowing of diaphysis**

Biochemical

- **Serum calcium: normal or low**
- **Serum phosphate: low**
- **Alkaline phosphatase: high**
- **PTH: high**

Fracture NOF (Neck of Femur)

- Fracture NOF is the **most common** site of fracture in elderly
- Velocity of trauma in most cases is **trivial**. (low velocity trauma)
- Most common patients are **elderly females** with predisposing causes like
  - **Osteoporosis**
  - **Osteomalacia**
  - **Diabetes**
  - **Stroke patients**
  - **Alcoholics**
  - **Caisson's disease**
  - **Steroid therapy**
- Limb is shortened, adducted and externally rotated
- Pain around hip with **flexion, adduction and external rotation** is suggestive of Intracapsular Fracture NOF
- **(Telescopic Test is done)**
- Tenderness of hip on palpation with painful movements at hip joint is a feature.

Classification of Fracture Neck of Femur (# NOF)

- **Intracapsular**: Subcapital, Transcervical
- **Extracapsular:** Basal, Pertrochanteric

Avascular necrosis is seen in

- Head of femur
- Scaphoid
- Talus

Disease Association of Avascular Necrosis

- **Gaucher's disease**
- **Sickle cell disease**
- **Chronic steroid use**
- **HIV Infection**

[99mTc] pertechnetate or [99mTc] diphosphonate scintigraphy may be useful in avascular necrosis

SICKLE CELL DISEASE

Sickle cell disease is associated with several musculoskeletal abnormalities

- Children under the age of 5 may develop diffuse swelling, tenderness, and warmth of the hands and feet lasting from 1 to 3 weeks. The condition, referred to as **sickle cell dactylitis or hand-foot syndrome** has also been observed in sickle cell disease and sickle cell thalassemia. Dactylitis is believed to result from infarction of the bone marrow and cortical bone leading to periostitis and soft tissue swelling. Radiographs show **periosteal elevation, subperiosteal new bone formation, and areas of radiolucency and increased density involving the metacarpals, metatarsals, and proximal phalanges**
- Sickle cell crisis is often associated with **periarticular pain and joint effusions**
- Patients with sickle cell disease may also develop **osteomyelitis**, which commonly involves the **long tubular bones.** These patients are particularly susceptible to bacterial infections, especially **Salmonella infections**, which are found in more than half of cases. Radiographs of the involved site show **periosteal elevation initially**, followed by disruption of the cortex
- Sickle cell disease is also associated with **bone infarction resulting from thrombosis** secondary to the sickling of red cells
- **Avascular necrosis of the head of the femur** is seen
- It also occurs in the humeral head and less commonly in the distal femur, tibial condyles, distal radius, vertebral bodies, and other juxta articular sites
- **Septic arthritis is occasionally encountered in sickle cell disease**. Multiple joints may be infected. Joint infection may result from hematogenous spread or from spread of contiguous osteomyelitis
- Microorganisms identified include **Staphylococcus, Streptococcus, Escherichia coli, and Salmonella**
- **The latter is not seen as frequently in septic arthritis as it is in osteomyelitis**
- **The bone marrow hyperplasia in sickle cell disease results in widening of the medullary cavities, thinning of the cortices and coarse trabeculations and central cupping of the vertebral bodies.**

Osteogenesis Imperfecta (OI)

OI is also called **Brittle bone disease** or **'Lobstein syndrome'**

- Basic defect is in **Collagen Type 1**
- It is transmitted either as AD or AR Inheritance
- **Type 1 OI** is THE **MOST COMMON TYPE**
- OI is inherited as **autosomal dominant trait mostly**
- **'Blue sclera'** is present in several types of OI But not all
- **Grey sclera** is a feature as well**.** Other ocular features of OI are**:**
  - **Saturn ring, Arcus juvenilis, Hypermetropia and Retinal Detachment are seen**
  - The sclera is **normal** in some types of OI
  - Feature of OI is **generalized osteopenia** with recurrent fractures and skeletal deformity. Fracture healing however is normal. Fracture in utero may be seen. Laxity of joint ligaments leads to **hypermobility**
- Some people have associated **'dentogenesis imperfecta'**: small fragile and discolored teeth
- **Dermis** may be abnormally thin and skin is susceptible to easy bruising
- **Hearing loss** due to involvement of inner and middle ear bones may produce deafness
- **Wormian bones** are a feature
- **'Popcorn calcification'and 'whorls of radiodensities'** are a radiographic feature
- Treatment is largely **supportive**

Osteopetrosis

Osteopetrosis is also called:
- **Albers Schonberg disease** or
- **Marble bone disease**
- It is characterized by
  - **Anemia**
  - **Hepatoslpenomegaly**
  - **Infections**
  - **Pathological fractures**
- There is **osteoclast dysfunction**
- Radiographically there is **increased opacity** of bones
- **Endobones (bone within a bone)** is seen

Osteoporosis

Osteoporosis is defined as a **reduction of bone mass (or density)** or the presence of a fragility fracture. This reduction in bone tissue is accompanied by deterioration in the architecture of the skeleton, leading to a markedly increased risk of fracture

Several noninvasive techniques are now available for estimating skeletal mass or density

These include:
- **Dual-energy X-ray absorptiometry (DXA)**
- **Single-energy X-ray absorptiometry (SXA)**
- **Quantitative computed tomography (CT)**
- **Ultrasound**

The diagnosis of Osteoporosis is made when a patient has characteristic osteoporotic fracture. In absence of such a fracture, evaluation of osteoporosis is done by T score measurement based on bone mass.

- T score > – 1 Normal
- T score Between – 1 and – 2.5 Osteopenia
- T Score < – 2.5 Osteoporosis

Major factors for osteoporosis

- **Low cacium intake**
- **Sedentary lifestyle**
- **Cigarette smoking**
- **Excessive alcohol**
- **Excessive caffeine**
- **Medications (corticosteroids, thyroxine)**
- **Female gender**
- **Early menopause**
- **Slender build**
- **Positive family history**

Glucocorticoid-Induced Osteoporosis is by

- **Inhibition of osteoblast function** and potential increase in osteoblast apoptosis, resulting in impaired synthesis of new bone
- **Stimulation of bone resorption**, probably as a secondary effect
- **Impairment of the absorption of calcium** across the intestine, probably by a vitamin D-independent effect

- **Increase of urinary calcium loss** and induction of some degree of secondary hyperparathyroidism
- **Reduction of adrenal androgens** and suppression of ovarian and testicular secretion of estrogens and androgens
- **Potential induction of glucocorticoid myopathy**, which may exacerbate effects on skeletal and calcium homeostasis, as well as Increase the risk of falls.

Remember Electrolyte Disturbances in Related Disorders

• **Pr. Hyperparathyroidism**	↑Ca	↓PO_4	↑PTH
• **Sec Hyperparathyroidism**	↓Ca	↓PO_4	↑PTH
• **Malabsorption**	↓Ca	↓PO_4	↑PTH
• **Renal Failure**	↓Ca	↑PO_4	↑PTH
• **Paget's Disease**	Ca (N)	PO_4 (N)	

Rheumatoid arthritis (RA)

I provide this topic in detail as lots of questions are asked from here.

- **Rheumatoid arthritis (RA)** is a **chronic multisystem disease** of unknown cause
- Disease of synovium (synovial membrane)
- **Disease starts in synovium**
- **Synoviumis the part affected most**
  - The characteristic feature of RA is **persistent inflammatory synovitis**, usually involving peripheral joints in a **symmetric distribution**
  - **Familial, immunological and infective causes are implicated.**
  - **Women** are affected approximately three times more often than men.
  - The **class II major histocompatibility complex** allele **HLA-DR4** and related alleles are known to be major genetic risk factors for RA.
  - Microvascular injury and an increase in the number of synovial lining cells appear to be the **earliest lesions in rheumatoid synovitis.**
  - RA most often causes symmetric arthritis with characteristic involvement of certain specific joints such as the **proximal interphalangeal and metacarpophalangeal joints**
  - The distal interphalangeal joints are rarely involved. Synovitis of the wrist joints is a nearly uniform feature of RA and may lead to limitation of motion, deformity, and **median nerve entrapment (carpal tunnel syndrome).**
  - Synovitis of the elbow joint often leads to flexion contractures that may develop early in the disease. The knee joint is commonly involved with synovial hypertrophy, chronic effusion, and frequently ligamentous laxity. Pain and swelling behind the knee may be caused by extension of inflamed synovium into the popliteal space **(Baker's cyst).**
  - On occasion, inflammation from the synovial joints and bursae of the upper cervical spine leads to **atlantoaxial subluxation.** This usually presents as pain in the occiput but on rare occasions may lead to compression of the spinal cord.

Characteristic changes of the hand include:

- **Radial deviation at the wrist with ulnar deviation of the digits**, often with palmar subluxation of the proximal phalanges **('Z' deformity)**
- Hyperextension of the proximal interphalangeal joints, with compensatory flexion of the distal interphalangeal joints (**swan-neck deformity)**
- Flexion contracture of the proximal interphalangeal joints and extension of the distal interphalangeal joints (**boutonniere deformity)**
- Hyperextension of the first interphalangeal joint and flexion of the first metacarpophalangeal joint with a consequent loss of thumb mobility and pinch
- **Trigger finger** also occurs.

Criteria for Classification of Rheumatoid Arthritis

Any 4 criteria must be present to diagnose rheumatoid arthritis; criteria 1 through 4 must have been present for > = 6 wk.

- **Morning stiffness for > = 1 h**
- **Arthritis of > = 3 joint areas**
- **Arthritis of hand joints (wrist, metacarpophalangeal or proximal interphalangeal joints)**
- **Symmetric arthritis**
- **Rheumatoid nodules (PATHOGONOMIC)**
- **Serum rheumatoid factor, by a method positive in < 5% of normal control subjects**
- **Radiographic changes (hand X-ray changes typical of rheumatoid arthritis that must include erosions or unequivocal bony decalcification)**

- **Extra-articular Manifestations** As a rule, these manifestations occur in individuals with **high titers of autoantibodies to the Fc component of immunoglobulin G (rheumatoid factors).**
- **Rheumatoid nodules** develop in 20 to 30% of persons with RA.
- Clinical weakness and atrophy of skeletal muscle are common. **Muscle atrophy** may be evident within weeks of the onset of RA.
- **Rheumatoid vasculitis** Neurovascular disease presenting either as a mild **distal sensory neuropathy or as mononeuritis multiplex** may be the only sign of vasculitis. **Cutaneous vasculitis** usually presents as crops of small brown spots in the nail beds, nail folds, and digital pulp. Larger ischemic ulcers, especially in the lower extremity, may also develop. Myocardial infarction secondary to rheumatoid vasculitis has been reported, as has vasculitic involvement of lungs, bowel, liver, spleen, pancreas, lymph nodes testes. Renal vasculitis is rare.
- Pleuropulmonary manifestations, which are more commonly observed in men, include **pleural disease, interstitial fibrosis, pleuropulmonary nodules, pneumonitis, and arteritis**
- Clinically apparent heart disease attributed to the rheumatoid process is rare, but evidence of **asymptomatic pericarditis** is found at **autopsy in 50% of cases.**
- RA tends to spare the central nervous system directly, although vasculitis can cause peripheral neuropathy. Neurologic manifestations may also result from **atlantoaxial or midcervical spine subluxations**. Nerve entrapment secondary to proliferative synovitis or joint deformities may produce **neuropathies of median, ulnar, radial (interosseous branch), or anterior tibial nerves.**
- The rheumatoid process involves the eye in fewer than 1% of patients. Affected individuals usually have long-standing disease and nodules. The two principal manifestations are **episcleritis**, which is usually mild and transient, and **scleritis**, which involves the deeper layers of the eye and is a more serious inflammatory condition. Histologically, the lesion is similar to a **rheumatoid nodule** and may result in thinning and **perforation of the globe (scleromalacia perforans).**

- **Felty's syndrome** consists of chronic RA, splenomegaly, neutropenia, and on occasion, anemia and thrombocytopenia.
- **Osteoporosis** secondary to rheumatoid involvement is common and may be aggravated by glucocorticoid therapy.
- RA in the Elderly **Aggressive disease** is largely restricted to those patients with **high titers of rheumatoid factor**. By contrast, elderly patients who develop RA without elevated titers of rheumatoid factor (seronegative disease) generally have less severe, often self-limited disease
- The **presence of rheumatoid factor does not establish the diagnosis of RA** as the predictive value of the presence of rheumatoid factor in determining a diagnosis of RA is poor. **Thus fewer than one-third of unselected patients with a positive test for rheumatoid factor will be found to have RA.** Therefore, the rheumatoid factor test is **not useful as a screening procedure**

A number of additional autoantibodies may be found in patients with RA, including:

- Antibodies to filaggrin
- Antibodies to citrulline
- Antibodies to calpastatin
- Antibodies to components of the spliceosome (RA-33), and an unknown antigen, Sa.

Goals of therapy of RA

- Relief of pain
- Reduction of inflammation
- Protection of articular surfaces
- Maintenance of function
- Control of systemic involvement

- **First Aspirin and NSAIDS are used**
- **Second line involves use of low dose glucocorticoids**
- **Third line involves use of DMARDS (Disease modifying anti rheumatic drugs) Methotrexate, Gold Compounds, Pencillamine, Hydroxychloroquine and Sulfasalazine**
- **Fourth line is use of TNF alpha blockers (Infliximab and Etanercept)**
- **Fifth line is use of Immunosupressants and Cytotoxic drugs**

CPPD Deposition Disease

Clinical manifestations of CPPD deposition include:

- The **knee is the joint most frequently affected** in CPPD arthropathy. Other sites include the wrist, shoulder, ankle, elbow, and hands. Rarely, the temporomandibular joint and ligamentum flavum of the spinal canal are involved
- Clinical and radiographic evidence indicates that CPPD deposition is **polyarticular in at least two-thirds of patients**
- If radiographs reveal punctate and/or linear radiodense deposits in fibrocartilaginous joint menisci or articular hyaline cartilage **(chondrocalcinosis)**, the diagnostic certainty of CPPD is further enhanced
- Definitive diagnosis requires **demonstration of typical crystals** in synovial fluid or articular tissue
- Acute attacks of CPPD arthritis may be precipitated by **trauma, arthroscopy, or hyaluronate injections.** Rapid diminution of serum calcium concentration, as may occur in severe medical illness or after surgery (especially parathyroidectomy), can also lead to **pseudogout** attacks
- Polarization microscopy usually reveals **rhomboid crystals with weak positive birefringence**

TREATMENT

Treatment by **joint aspiration and NSAIDs, or colchicine**, or intra-articular glucocorticoid injection may result in return to prior status in 10 days or less

Uncontrolled studies suggest that **radioactive synovectomy (with yttrium 90)**

Patients with progressive destructive large-joint arthropathy usually require **joint replacement**

- **Deposition of Calcium Pyrophosphate crystals**
- **Crystals are Rhomboid in shape**
- **Thery are positively Birefringent**
- **Usually Large joints affected**

Gout

- **Metatarsopharyngeal joints involved**
- **Usually great Toe. (Podagra)**
- **Assymetric joint involvement usually**
- **Negatively birefringent crystals seen**
- **NSAIDS, colchicines, Allopurinol used in treatment**

Psoriatic Arthritis

- **Distal Interphalangeal Joints usually involved**
- **Rheumatoid-like polyarthritis**
- **Asymmetrical oligoarthritis: typically affects hands and feet**

- **Sacroilitis**
- **DIP joint disease**
- **Arthritis mutilans (severe deformity fingers/hand, 'telescoping fingers')**

Joint Involvement

• **PIP joint involvement**	• **RA, OA, Psoriatic arthritis**
• **PIP and DIP**	• **OA, Psoriatic arthritis**
• **PIP and DIP and MCP and wrist**	• **Psoriatic arthritis**

Ankylosing spondylitis

- **Typically a young man who presents with lower back pain and stiffness**
- **HLA 27 association**
  - Stiffness is usually worse in the morning and improves with activity
  - **Enthesopathy** is characteristic
  - **Bamboo spine**
  - **Squaring of vertebrae**
  - **Pain improves with exercise**
  - Peripheral arthritis (25%, more common if female)

Other features – **the 'A's**

- **Apical fibrosis**
- **Anterior uveitis**
- **Aortic regurgitation**
- **Achilles tendonitis**
- **AV node block**
- **Amyloidosis and cauda equina syndrome**

X-rays are often normal early in disease, later changes include:

- **Sacroilitis: Subchondral erosions, sclerosis**
- **Squaring of lumbar vertebrae**
- **'Bamboo spine' (late and uncommon)**

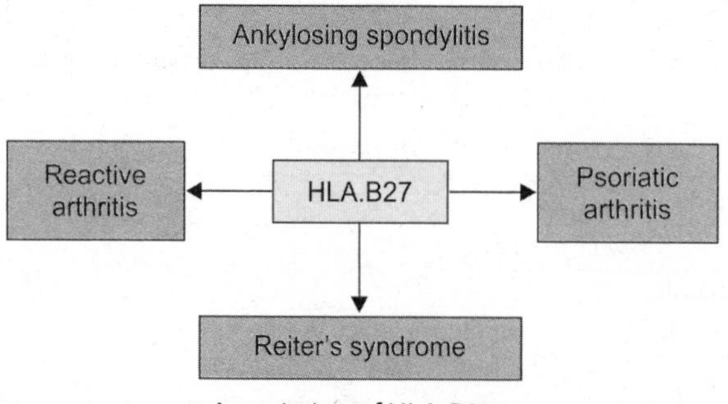

Association of HLA-B27

Osteoarthritis/OA

- Involves hip, knee usually
- Disease of elderly and obese usually

- Does not affect MCP joints
- The earliest structural changes in osteoarthritis include enlargement, proliferation, and disorganization of the chondrocytes in the superficial part of the articular cartilage. This process is accompanied by increasing water content of the matrix with decreasing concentration of the proteoglycans
- Gross examination at this stage reveals a soft granular articular cartilage surface. Eventually, full-thickness portions of the cartilage are lost, and the subchondral bone plate is exposed. Friction smoothens and burnishes the exposed bone, giving it the appearance of polished ivory **(bone eburnation).** The underlying cancellous bone becomes sclerotic and thickened. Small fractures can dislodge pieces of cartilage and subchondral bone into the joint, forming loose bodies **(joint mice)**
- The fracture gaps allow synovial fluid to be forced into the subchondral regions to form fibrous walled cysts. Mushroom-shaped **osteophytes (bony outgrowths)** develop at the margins of the articular surface
- Herberden's nodes **(DIP)** involved
- Bouchard's nodes seen **(PIP)** involved
- Ankylosis occurs
- **Radiological features:**
  - **Osteophyte formation**
  - **Subchondral sclerosis**
  - **Cyst formation occurs**

Remember

- **Epiphyseal widening** is a feature of Rickets
- **Epiphyseal dysgenesis** is a feature of Hypothyroidism
- **Epiphyseal enlargement** is a feature of Juvenile Rheumatoid Arthritis

Hemophilic Arthropathy

- Hemophilia is a **sex-linked recessive genetic disorder** characterized by the **absence or deficiency of factor VIII (hemophilia A, or classic hemophilia)** or **factor IX (hemophilia B, or Christmas disease)**
- **Hemophilia A is more common type**
- **Spontaneous hemarthrosis is a common problem** with both types of hemophilia and can lead to a chronic deforming arthritis
- The frequency and severity of hemarthrosis are **related to the degree of clotting factor deficiency**
- Hemarthrosis becomes evident after 1 year of age, when the child begins to walk and run
- In order of frequency, the joints most commonly affected are the **knees**, ankles, elbows, shoulders, and hips. Small joints of the hands and feet are occasionally involved.
- **Squaring of patella** is a feature
- In the initial stage of arthropathy, hemarthrosis produces a **warm, tensely swollen, and painful joint.** Widening of the femoral intercondylar notch, enlargement of the proximal radius, and squaring of the distal end of the patella are seen
- The patient holds the affected joint in flexion and guards against any movement
- Blood in the joint remains liquid because of the absence of intrinsic clotting factors and the absence of tissue thromboplastin in the synovium
- The blood in the joint space is resorbed over a period of a week or longer, depending on the size of the hemarthrosis
- **Recurrent hemarthrosis leads to the development of a chronic arthritis**
- **Bleeding into muscle and soft tissue** also causes musculoskeletal disorders
- When bleeding involves periosteum or bone, a pseudotumor forms. These occur distal to the elbows or knees in children and improve with treatment of the hemophilia.

Orthopedic Importance of Knee Joint

- **Most common site of Septic arthritis**
- **Most common site of Syphilitic arthritis**

- **Most common site of Gonococcal arthritis**
- **Most common site of Pseudogout**
- **Most common site of Hemophilic arthritis**
- **Most common site of Osteochondritis dessicans**

X-ray Examinations of Different Types of Arthritis

1.	**Osteophytes**	• **Osteoarthritis**
2.	**Syndesmophytes**	• **Ankylosing spondylitis**
3.	**Bamboo spine**	• **Ankylosing spondylitis**
4.	**Pencil-in-cup deformity**	• **Psoriatic arthritis**
5.	**Calcification of Articular cartilage**	• **Pseudogout**
6.	**Erosions with ↓Joint space**	• **Rheumatoid Arthritis**
7.	**Arthritis mutilans**	• **Psoriatic arthritis**
8.	**Piano key sign**	• **Rhematoid arthritis**
9.	**Sausage digits**	• **Psoriasis**

The Reflex Sympathetic Dystrophy Syndrome (RSDS)

- The reflex sympathetic dystrophy syndrome (RSDS) is now referred to as **complex regional pain syndrome, type 1**, by the new Classification of the International Association for the Study of Pain
- It is characterized by:
  - Pain and swelling
  - Usually of a distal extremity, accompanied by vasomotor instability
  - Trophic skin changes
  - The rapid development of bony demineralization
- **A precipitating event** can be identified in at least two-thirds of cases. These events include:
  - **Trauma, such as fractures and crush injuries**
  - **Myocardial infarction**
  - **Strokes**
  - **Peripheral nerve injury**
  - **Use of certain drugs, including barbiturates, anti-tuberculous drugs and, more recently, cyclosporine** administered to patients undergoing renal transplantation
  - The pathogenesis of RSDS is thought to involve **abnormal activity of the sympathetic nervous system** following a precipitating event.

Remember

- **Iliotibial tract syndrome**: Synovium deep to iliotibial tract is inflamed where it rubs on lateral femoral condyle. Common in marathon runners
- **Medial shelf syndrome**: Synovial fold above medial meniscus is inflamed
- **Fat pad syndrome**: Tenderness deep to patellar tendon may be caused by fat caught in tibiofemoral joint.

Scoliosis

Associations

- **Hemivertebrae**
- **Wedge vertebrae**
- **Block vertebrae**

- **Unsegmented bar**
  - **Turnbuckle cast scoliosis**
  - **Risser's cast scoliosis**
  - **Milwaukee's brace scoliosis**
  - **Boston brace scoliosis**
- **Cobb's angle** is measured in **scoliosis**

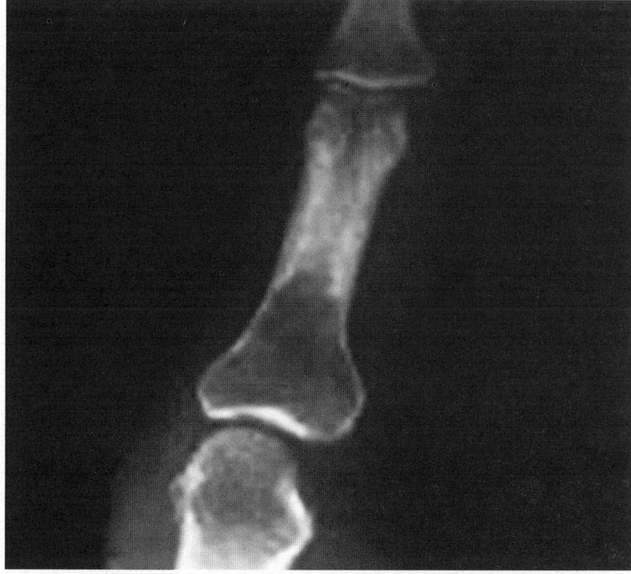

X-ray enchondroma

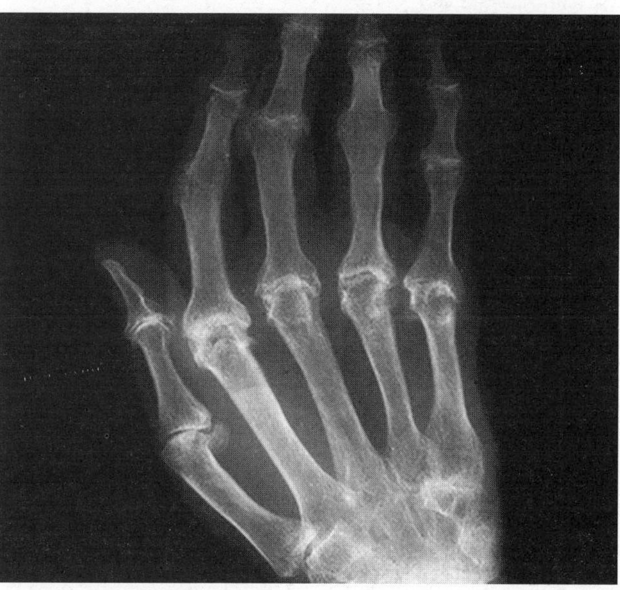

X-ray demonstrating rheumatoid hand

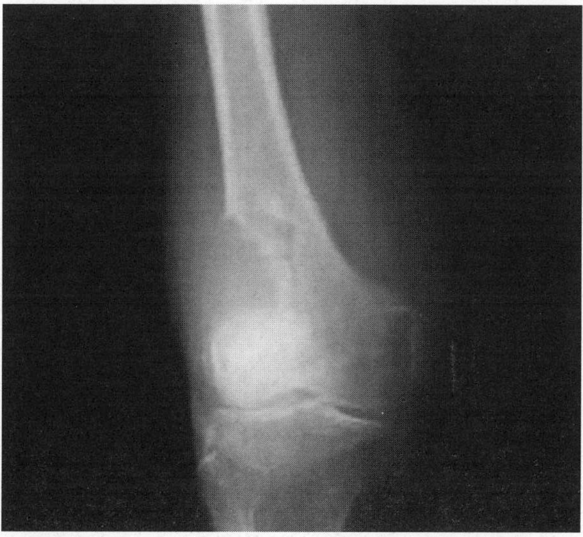

X-ray demonstrating osteolytic metastasis of femur from a primary cancer in breast

Identify bone tumors by

1. Clues by appearance of lesion
2. Clues by location of lesion

3. Clues by type of periosteal reaction
4. Clues by matrix of lesion
5. Clues by density of lesion
6. Clues by number of lesion

Sclerotic cortical lesions
- Osteoid osteoma
- Brodie's abscess
- Stress fracture

Lytic lesions in children
- Eosinophilic granuloma
- Neuroblastoma
- Leukemia

Lytic lesions in adult
- Metastatic lesions (lung, kidney, thyroid)
- Multiple myeloma
- Primary bone tumor

Blastic lesion in children
- Medulloblastoma
- Lymphoma

Blastic lesion in adult
- Metastatic disease (breast, prostate)
- Lymphoma
- Paget's disease

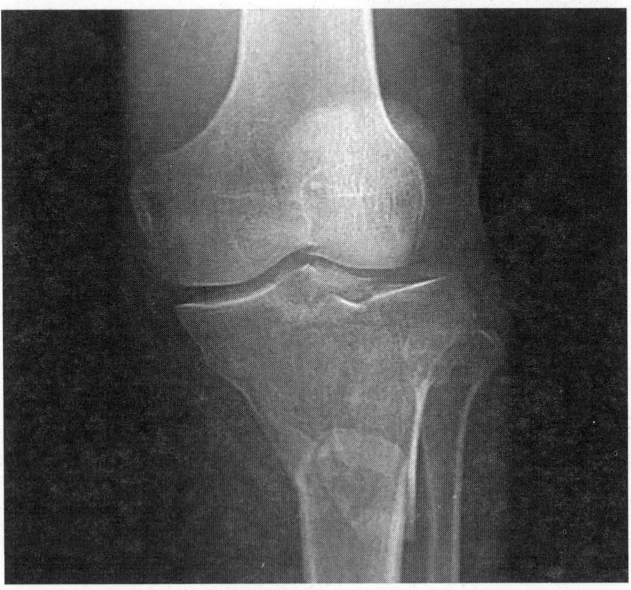

Fracture proximal tibia

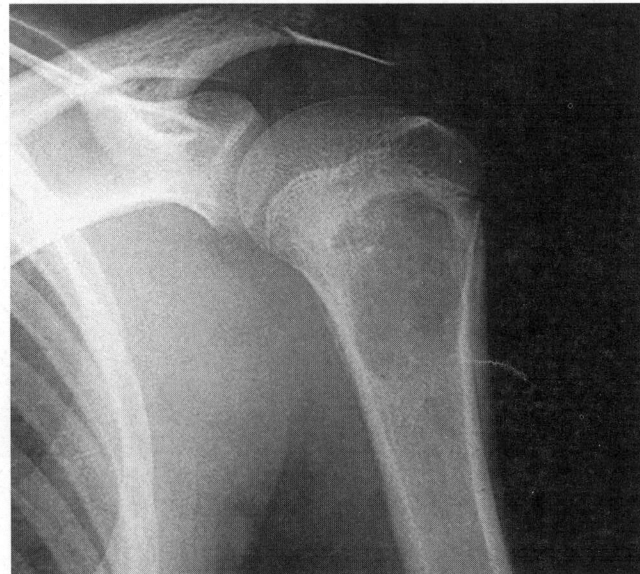

X-ray demonstrating osteosarcoma
osteochondroma femur

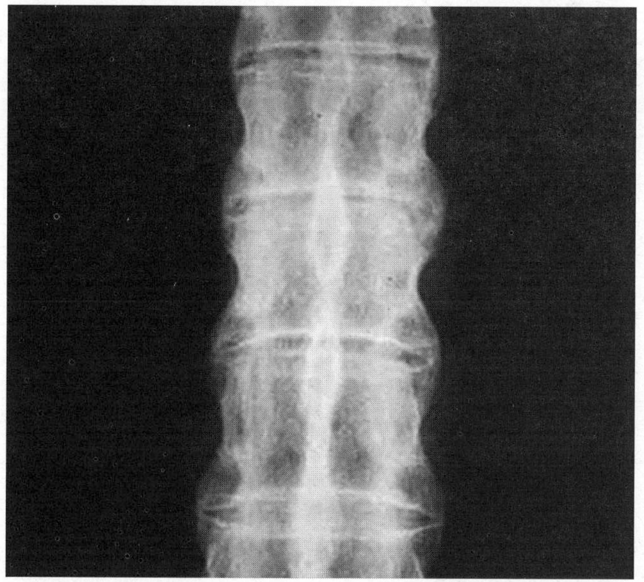

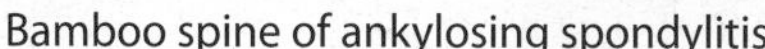

Bamboo spine of ankylosing spondylitis

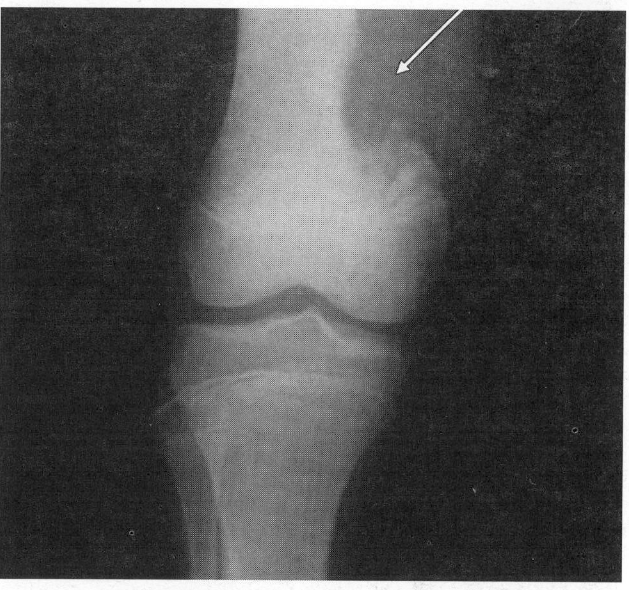

X-ray demonstrating osteosarcoma

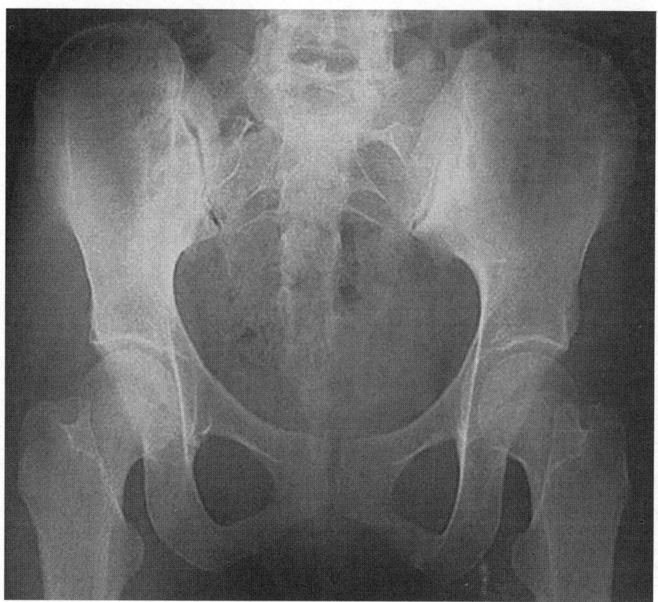

Sacroilitis of left side

Important Diseases

• **Burton's Disease**	Combination of scurvy and rickets
• **Engelmann Disease**	Progressive diaphyseal dysplasia
• **Trevor's Disease**	Dysplasia epiphysis hemimelica
• **Caffey's Disease**	Osteomyelitis of Jaw
• **De Quervain's Disease**	Tenovaginitis of APL and EPB (tendon)
• **Blount's Disease**	Tibia vara

Important Tests Frequently Asked

- Barlow's test CDH
- Ortolani's test CDH
- Galeazzi test CDH
- Alli's test CDH
- Hart's test CDH

- ***Thomas test fixed flexion deformity***
- ***Allen's test palmar arch integrity***
- ***Gaenslen's test sciatica***
- ***McMurray's test menisci***
- ***Anterior drawer test–Anterior cruciate ligament***
- ***Lachman's test–Anterior cruciate ligament***
- ***Pivot shift test–Anterior cruciate ligament***

Posterior drawer test–post cruciate ligament

Apprehension test/sign	Anterior shoulder joint dislocation
Gaenslen's test	Sacroiliac joint pain
Phalen's test	Carpal tunnel syndrome
Finkelstein's test	De Quervain's disease
Adson's test	Thoracic outlet syndrome
Wringing test	Lateral epicondylitis
Cozen's test	Lateral epicondylitis
Lift-off test	Subscapularis

NEWER TOPICS

Pycnodysostosis

- Pycnodysostosis is an **autosomal recessive form of osteosclerosis** that superficially resembles osteopetrosis
- It is a **form of short-limbed dwarfism associated with bone fragility** and a tendency to fracture with minimal trauma
- Life span is usually **normal**
- In addition to a generalized **increase in bone density**, features include:
  - **Short stature**
  - **Separated cranial sutures**
  - **Hypoplasia of the mandible**
  - **Kyphoscoliosis and deformities of the trunk**
  - **Persistence of deciduous teeth**
  - **Progressive acro-osteolysis of the terminal phalanges**
  - **High, arched palate**
  - **Proptosis**
  - **Blue sclerae**
  - **A pointed, beaked nose**
- Patients usually present because of frequent fractures
- **(*Remember the clinical presentation*)**

Osteomyelosclerosis

- In osteomyelosclerosis, **the marrow cells are replaced by diffuse fibroplasia**, occasionally accompanied by **osseous metaplasia and increased skeletal density on roentgenograms**

- It is a **myeloproliferative disorder** and is characteristically accompanied by **extramedullary hematopoiesis**
- **Hyperostosis corticalis generalisata (van Buchem's disease)** is characterized by **osteosclerosis of the skull (base and calvaria), lower jaw, clavicles and ribs and thickening of the diaphyseal cortices of the long and short bones**. Alkaline phosphatase levels in the serum are elevated, and the disorder may be due to increased formation of bone of normal structure. The major manifestations are due to neural compression and consist of optic atrophy, facial paralysis, and perception deafness
- **In hyperostosis generalisata with pachydermia,** the sclerosis is due to increased formation of subperiosteal spongy bone and involves the epiphyses, metaphyses and diaphyses. Pain, swelling of joints, and thickening of the skin of the lower arms are common.

Progressive Diaphyseal Dysplasia

- **CAMURATI-ENGELMANN DISEASE**
- This is an **autosomal dominant** disorder:
- **Symmetric thickening and increased diameter of the diaphyses of long bones** occur, particularly in the femur, tibia, fibula, radius, and ulna
- **Pain over affected areas,** fatigue, abnormal gait, and muscle wasting are the major manifestations
- **Serum alkaline phosphatase levels may be elevated**, and, on occasions, hypocalcemia and hyperphosphatemia may be found
- Other abnormalities include **anemia, leukopenia, and an elevated erythrocyte sedimentation rate.**

Melorheostosis

- This rare, sporadic condition usually begins in childhood and is characterized by a slowly **progressive linear hyperostosis in one** or more bones of one limb
- Usually in a lower extremity
- All segments of the bone may be involved, with sclerotic areas that have a **'Candle Dripping Wax'** or **'flowing' distribution**
- The involved limb is often extremely painful.

Osteopoikilosis

Osteopoikilosis is characterized by **dense spots of trabecular bone <1 cm in diameter**, usually of uniform density, located in the epiphyses and adjacent parts of the metaphyses

All bones may be involved **except the skull, ribs, and vertebrae.**

Stress Fractures

- Stress fractures are undisplaced fatigue fractures, which develop as a result of **repeated loading**. The lower limbs are most frequently affected
- **The metatarsals (march fractures) and the tibia being the most frequently involved** bones
- **March fracture involves 2, 3 metatarsals most commonly**
- Younger children and even toddlers can present with stress fractures but they are more common in adolescents where the proximal third of the tibia is the most frequent site
- Symptoms of localized pain develop insidiously and are usually relieved by rest
- Treatment involves **protection from further trauma, which sometimes involves immobilization and always involves abstinence from the causative stress,** usually running. Once symptoms have resolved, a gradual return to activity can be begun.

Adolescent Hallus Valgus

- Hallux valgus or 'bunions' in adolescents is **usually familial** rather than the result of **poor footwear**
- There is often an associated bunionette of the fifth toe and patients often have a characteristically broad forefoot with varus of the first metatarsal (metatarsus primus varus)

- Surgery is best deferred until skeletal maturity is reached
- Surgical treatment gives good results for symptomatic feet with a painful bunion but caution should be exercised in the pain-free patient who may be disappointed if surgery leaves a better looking but painful foot.

Enthesitis-related Arthritis

Enthesitis is defined as **inflammation of the insertion of tendons into bones**. This new diagnostic group is intended to define those with disease related to the HLA antigen B27, and avoids the term 'juvenile spondyloarthropathy'; inaccurate because of the rarity of spinal involvement in children

Enthesitis-related arthritis is defined as arthritis and enthesitis; or arthritis; or enthesitis with at least two of the following features:

1. **Sacroiliac joint tenderness and/or inflammatory spinal pain**
2. **Presence of HLA B27**
3. **Family history in at least one first- or second-degree relative of medically confirmed HLA B27-associated disease**
4. **Anterior uveitis that is usually associated with pain, redness, or photophobia**
5. **Onset of arthritis in a boy after 8 years of age**

Ehlers–Danlos syndrome

- Ehlers-Danlos syndrome (EDS) consists of a **group of disorders of connective tissue** characterized by:
- **Joint hypermobility plus fragility and laxity of the skin**
- These conditions are characterized by abnormalities in collagen genes resulting in the **production of abnormal collagen and consequent tissue fragility**
- EDS has **soft, hyperextensible skin, 'cigarette paper' scars, easy bruising and marked hypermobility**. EDS type II is similar to type I but less severe
- Also seen is serious involvement with a **high incidence of rupture of the arteries, the colon or the pregnant uterus.** Management of EDS consists of patient education and support, with genetic counseling for the more severe forms.

Synovial chondromatosis

- It is a disorder characterized by **multiple focal metaplastic growths of normal-appearing cartilage in the synovium or tendon sheath.** Segments of cartilage break loose and continue to grow as **loose bodies**
- When calcification and ossification of loose bodies occur, the disorder is referred to as **synovial osteochondromatosis**
- The disorder is **usually monoarticular** and affects **young to middle-aged individuals**. The knee is most often involved, followed by hip, elbow and shoulder
- Symptoms are pain, swelling, and decreased motion of the joint
- Radiographs may show several rounded calcifications within the joint cavity.
- **Treatment is synovectomy**; however, the tumor may recur.

Causes of 'Loose' Bodies

- **Trauma**
- **Osteochondritis dissecans**
- **Synovial chondromatosis**
- **Osteoarthritis**

• An infant presents with failure to thrive, Pancytopenia. Bones are brittle and fracture easily. Defect is found in osteoclasts	• **Infantile osteopetrosis**
• A two-year-old presents with multiple fractures in different stages of healing brought by overconcerned parents	• **Battered baby syndrome**

• A six-year-old with b/l symmetrical fractures and blue sclera. Bones are osteopenic and brittle	• **Osteogenesis imperfecta**
• An athelete after trauma and hematoma formation at elbowcomes to you with hard calcific mass found in the muscle Belly	• **Myositis ossificans**
• A patient with multiple injuries on day 2 develops Tachycardia, Tachypnea, ↓Po2 and rash.	• **Fat embolism**
• A patient after hip replacementdevelops chest pain and cvs collapse	• **Pulmonary thromboembolism**

Clinical Scenarios

• An itching, squeezing pain sensation after amputation that an amputated limb is still attached and functioning with intensly painful sensations	• **Phantom limb pain**
• Complex and progressive disease with pain swelling and changes in skin **without** demonstrable nerve lesions after injury	• **Reflex sympathetic dystrophy/ Sudeck's atrophy**
• Complex and progressive disease with pain swelling and changes in **skin with** demonstrable nerve lesions after injury	• **Causalgia**
• A 13-year-old boy with a hot, tender swelling arising from diaphysis of bone with characteristic feature of onion skinning	• **Ewing's sarcoma**
• An obese boy in 2nd decade presents with pain and with limited flexion, abduction and femoral head seen downwards and posteriorly	• **Slippped femoral epiphysis**
• A 10-year-old boy with pain and limp. X-ray shows distorted femoral neck and head	• **Perthes' disease**
• An elderly boy after trauma presents with expansile osteolytic and cystic bony lesion with thin wall	• **Aneurysmal bone cyst**
• An elderly man presents to orthopedic clinic with pain in bones. On X-ray, **cortical widening of** bones. **'Molten wax'** or **'Candle Dripping Wax' appearance** of bones is noted	• **Melorheostosis**
• A male presents with triad of lytic bony lesions on skull, diabetes Insipidus and exomphalos	• **Hand-schuller-christian disease**

USMLE Case Scenario

A 6-month-old brought by his mother presents with episodes of distress and crying interspersed with quiet periods of normal behavior and playing. His mother says that he passes stool mixed with mucus and blood, the jelly stool. The abdomen is soft and nontender. A sausage-like mass may be palpable in the upper abdomen. Most likely diagnosis is:

1. Sigmoid volvulus
2. Cecal volvulus
3. Colonic atresia
4. Hirschsprung's disease
5. Ladd's bands
6. Annular pancreas
7. Intussusception
8. Tracheoesophageal fistula
9. Congenital hypertrophic pyloric stenosis

Ans. 7. Intussusception

USMLE Case Scenario

A 35-year-old patient has tumor in the adrenal medulla, who has paroxysmal hypertension. Urinary metabolites of:

1. 17-ketosteroids in 24-hour urine collections can be helpful in establishing diagnoses
2. 5 HIAA in 24-hour urine collections can be helpful in establishing diagnoses
3. DHEA in 24-hour urine collections can be helpful in establishing diagnoses
4. VMA in 24-hour urine collections can be helpful in establishing diagnoses

Ans. 4. VMA in 24-hour urine collections can be helpful in establishing diagnoses

USMLE Case Scenario

Hirschsprung's disease is one of the most common causes of lower intestinal obstruction in the neonatal period. In early childhood, it may present as chronic constipation with intermittent fecal soiling. It occurs predominantly in males and there is an increased family incidence. It is due to:

1. Congenital absence of the aganglionic cells of Auerbach's plexus
2. Acquired absence of the ganglion cells of Auerbach's plexus
3. Acquired absence of the ganglion cells of Meissner's plexus
4. Congenital absence of the aganglionic cells of both the Meissner's and Auerbach's plexuses
5. Congenital absence of the ganglion cells of both the Meissner's and Auerbach's plexuses

Ans. 5. Congenital absence of the ganglion cells of both the Meissner's and Auerbach's plexuses

USMLE Case Scenario

A patient (44 years old) from New York presents with fatigue, weight loss, and muscle aches. Laboratory abnormalities present as hypoglycemia, hyponatremia and hyperkalemia are seen. This patient has:

1. Cushing's disease
2. SIADH
3. Hypothyroidism
4. Adrenal hyperfunction
5. Adrenal insufficiency

Ans. 5. Adrenal insufficiency

USMLE Case Scenario

A syndrome is associated with the rare occurrence of malignant infiltration of the colonic sympathetic nerve supply in the region of the celiac plexus in which sometimes massive cecal and colonic dilation is seen in the absence of mechanical obstruction. Such an entity is described as:

1. Maffucci syndrome

2. Ortner's syndrome
3. Ollier's syndrome
4. Holt-Oram syndrome
5. Ogilvie's syndrome

Ans. 5. Ogilvie's syndrome

USMLE Case Scenario

Whipple's triad summarizes the clinical findings in patients with insulinomas: (1) attacks precipitated by fasting or exertion; (2) fasting blood glucose concentrations below 50 mg/dL; (3) symptoms relieved by oral or intravenous glucose administration. These tumors are treated surgically and simple excision of an adenoma is curative in the majority of cases. The cell of origin of such tumors is:

1. Alpha cells
2. Beta cells
3. Delta cells
4. Argentaffin cells

Ans. 2. Beta cells

USMLE Case Scenario

A nonsuppurative inflammatory process of the retroperitoneum that causes problems by extrinsic compression of retroperitoneal structures, such as the ureters, aorta, and inferior vena with ureteral obstruction as one of the most common presentations of this disease process is:

1. Retroperitoneal hematoma
2. Retroperitoneal sarcoma
3. Idiopathic retroperitoneal fibrosis
4. Ogilvie's syndrome

Ans. 3. Idiopathic retroperitoneal fibrosis

USMLE Case Scenario

A 55-year-old female after receiving trauma from a vehicular accident notices pain of sudden onset, sharp in nature with a swelling in the right lower quadrant of abdomen. Later, she also has fever, leukocytosis, anorexia, and nausea. CT scan shows a mass within the rectus sheath.

Most likely diagnosis is:

1. Pancreatic pseudocyst
2. Epigastric hernia
3. Divarication of recti
4. Rectus sheath hematoma
5. Umbilical adenoma

Ans. 4. Rectus sheath hematoma

USMLE Case Scenario

In children, usually surgical intervention is not needed in:

1. Omphalocele
2. Gastroschisis
3. Patent urachal duct
4. Patent omphalomesenteric duct
5. Umbilical hernias

Ans. 5. Umbilical hernias

- Omphalocele and gastroschisis result in evisceration of bowel and require emergency surgical treatment to effect immediate or staged reduction and abdominal wall closure.
- Patent urachal or omphalomesenteric ducts result from incomplete enclosure of embryonic connections from the bladder and ileum, respectively, to the abdominal wall. They are appropriately treated by excision of the tracts and closure of the bladder or ileum. In most children, umbilical hernias close spontaneously by the age of 4 and need not be repaired.

USMLE Case Scenario

A 42-year-old nonalcoholic presents to a gastroenterologist with multiple episodes of chest pain, regurgitation of saliva and undigested food. The characteristic appearance of the esophagram shows a tapered 'bird's beak' deformity at the level of the esophagogastric junction. Further manometry yields high resting pressures of the lower esophageal sphincter, which fails to relax. Most likely the disease is:

1. Carcinoma esophagus
2. GE junction growth
3. Diffuse esophageal spasm
4. Nutcracker esophagus
5. Achalasia

Ans. 5. Achalasia

USMLE Case Scenario

True about somatostatin are all except:

1. Somatostatin is produced by D cells in the pancreatic islets
2. It is an inhibitor of secretion of growth hormone
3. It inhibits the secretion of insulin
4. It stimulates the secretion of glucagon
5. It inhibits the secretion of gastrin
6. It inhibits the secretion of secretin
7. It inhibits the secretion of VIP
8. It inhibits intestinal, biliary, and gastric motility

Ans. 4. It stimulates the secretion of glucagon

USMLE Case Scenario

A 46-year-old woman presents with chronic widespread musculoskeletal pain, fatigue, and frequent headaches. She states that her musculoskeletal pain improves slightly with exercise. On examination, painful trigger points are produced by palpitation of the trapezius and lateral epicondyle of the elbow. Signs of inflammation are absent and laboratory studies are within normal. Most likely diagnosis is:

1. CFS
2. Fibromyalgia
3. Encephalitis
4. Osteoarthritis

Ans. 2. Fibromyalgia

The patient is presenting with signs and symptoms of fibrositis (fibromyalgia). Examination typically reveals painful trigger points produced by palpation of the trapezius and the lateral epicondyle of the elbow.

USMLE Case Scenario

An 80-year-old woman complains of a 4-month history of worsening gait and low back pain that is worse on walking. She denies any trauma and is not incontinent. She has been fairly healthy and only takes iron supplements. On examination, she has hypoactive muscle stretch reflexes in the legs. The plain X-rays of the lumbosacral region show degenerative changes that seem age-appropriate. Which of the following is the most likely diagnosis?

1. Acute lumbar disc herniation
2. Cervical stenosis

3. Lumbar stenosis
4. Myopathy
5. Normal pressure hydrocephalus (NPH)

Ans. 3. Lumbar stenosis

It is caused by degenerative changes in the lumbosacral spine. The history is that of vague low back pain with subtle physical examination findings referable to impingement on motor and sensory roots.

USMLE Case Scenario

The most common malignancy found in Marjolin's ulcer is:

1. Basal cell carcinoma
2. Squamous cell carcinoma
3. Malignant fibrous histiocytoma
4. Neurotrophic malignant melanoma

Ans. 2. Squamous cell carcinoma

USMLE Case Scenario

A 45-year-old from New Jersey on his sixth postoperative day has salmon-colored fluid on dressing. Most appropriate diagnosis would be:

1. Wound dehiscence
2. Wound infection only
3. Wound healing
4. Granulation

Ans. 2. Wound dehiscence

USMLE Case Scenario

A 35-year-old man presenting in GI clinic with dysphagia for liquids more than solids and regurgitating undigested food would most likely be having:

1. Achalasia cardia
2. Mallory-Weiss syndrome
3. GI malignancy
4. Gastritis
5. Hirschsprung's disease

Ans. 1. Achalasia cardia

USMLE Case Scenario

A 60-year-old elderly man, who is a smoker and drinks as well, has progressive dysphagia and loses weight. He would most likely be having:

1. Achalasia cardia
2. Mallory-Weiss syndrome
3. GI malignancy
4. Gastritis
5. Hirschsprung's disease

Ans. 3. GI malignancy

USMLE Case Scenario

A 34-year-old male engineer complains of burning retrosternal pain aggravated by bending, lying flat. He has no dysphagia, weight loss. He most likely is having:

1. Achalasia cardia
2. Mallory-Weiss syndrome

3. GI malignancy
4. Gastritis
5. Hirschsprung's disease
6. GERD

Ans. 6. GERD

USMLE Case Scenario

There is metaplasia of the normal squamous mucosa of the esophagus to a columnar (glandular) type of epithelium, and it is usually seen as a response to repeated acid exposure to the distal esophagus. This leads to:

1. Adenocarcinoma
2. Squamous cell carcinoma
3. Papilloma
4. Transitional cell carcinoma

Ans. 1. Adenocarcinoma

Barrett's esophagus may occur in a small number of patients who have gastroesophageal reflux disease (GERD). This condition is a metaplasia of the normal squamous mucosa of the esophagus to a columnar (glandular) type of epithelium and is usually seen as a response to repeated acid exposure to the distal esophagus. Tobacco and alcohol use are also thought to contribute to the process. The significance of Barrett's esophagus is that it may lead to the development of low-grade dysplasia, high-grade dysplasia, or esophageal adenocarcinoma.

USMLE Case Scenario

A 45-year-old marine worker, after a heavy drink and violent episode of vomiting, feels severe epigastric pain and is diaphoretic. Among the below given options, most likely diagnosis would suggest:

1. Achalasia cardia
2. Boerhaave's rupture
3. Mallory-Weiss syndrome
4. GI malignancy
5. Gastritis
6. Hirschsprung's disease
7. GERD

Ans. 2. Boerhaave's rupture

USMLE Case Scenario

A 42-year-old nonalcoholic presents to a gastroenterologist with multiple episodes of chest pain, regurgitation of saliva and undigested food. The characteristic appearance of the esophagram shows a tapered 'bird's beak' deformity at the level of the esophagogastric junction. Further manometry yields high-resting pressures of the lower esophageal sphincter, which fails to relax. Most likely the disease is:

1. Achalasia cardia
2. Boerhaave's rupture
3. Mallory-Weiss syndrome
4. GI malignancy
5. Gastritis
6. Hirschsprung's disease
7. GERD

Ans. 1. Achalasia cardia

USMLE Case Scenario

An elderly man, who is a heavy drinker, faints during his job. His examination shows occult blood in stools. He has altered bowel habbits, is pale and fatigues easily. He should be investigated for:

1. Achalasia cardia
2. Boerhaave's rupture

3. Mallory-Weiss syndrome
4. GI malignancy
5. Gastritis
6. Hirschsprung's disease
7. GERD

Ans. 4. GI malignancy

USMLE Case Scenario

A 55-year-old patient of ulcerative colitis presents to a gatro clinic in New Orleans with severe abdominal pain, leukocytosis and high temperature with massively distended colon on X-ray. Most likely diagnosis would be:

1. Toxic megacolon
2. Pseudomembranous colitis
3. Boerhaave's rupture
4. Mallory-Weiss syndrome
5. GI malignancy
6. Gastritis
7. Hirschsprung's disease

Ans. 1. Toxic megacolon

USMLE Case Scenario

A patient postoperatively on clindamycin complains of watery diarrhea and, crampy abdominal pain. This clinical scenario would be suggestive of:

1. Toxic megacolon
2. Ischemic colitis
3. Pseudomembranous colitis
4. Boerhaave's rupture
5. Mallory-Weiss syndrome
6. GI malignancy
7. Gastritis
8. Hirschsprung's disease

Ans. 3. Pseudomembranous colitis

USMLE Case Scenario

A 77-year-old woman reports that she had an operation 35 years earlier for intractable ulcer symptoms. She recalls of gastrectomy surgery of some kind.
Review of her prior medical records indicates that she underwent an antrectomy and a gastrojejunostomy.
Which of the following is she most at risk for developing?

1. Bacterial overgrowth
2. Bleeding from the lower gastrointestinal tract
3. Chronic pancreatitis
4. Constipation
5. Pancreatic insufficiency

Ans. 1. Bacterial overgrowth

USMLE Case Scenario

A 48-year-old patient with perianal pain cannot sit down with fever and chills with tender, fluctuant mass between anus and ischial tuberosity. This would be suggestive of:

1. Psoas abscess
2. Subphrenic abscess

3. Ischiorectal abscess
4. Pelvic abscess
5. Ischemic colitis
6. Pseudomembranous colitis

Ans. 3. Ischiorectal abscess

USMLE Case Scenario

A six-year-old boy passes a bloody bowel movement. This would most likely suggest:

1. Psoas abscess
2. Subphrenic abscess
3. Ischiorectal abscess
4. Pelvic abscess
5. Ischemic colitis
6. Meckel's diverticulitis
7. Pseudomembranous colitis

Ans. 6. Meckel's diverticulitis

USMLE Case Scenario

A young boy complains of right flank colicky pain radiating to inner thigh or scrotum. Microscopy of urine shows hematuria. This suggests most likely:

1. Psoas abscess
2. Ureteric colic
3. Renal cancer
4. BHP
5. Prostate cancer
6. Subphrenic abscess
7. Ischiorectal abscess
8. Pelvic abscess
9. Ischemic colitis
10. Meckel's diverticulitis
11. Pseudomembranous colitis

Ans. 2. Ureteric colic

USMLE Case Scenario

A 25-year-old medical student has enlarged hair follicles in otherwise normal skin in the anal region. The follicle holds a single hair shaft surrounded by rings of keratin. The cavity contains pus under pressure and a wall of edematous fat; polymorphonuclear cells predominate. The cavity has a wall of fibrous tissue lined by granulation tissue of lymphocytes, and giant cells. The cavity is laden with *Staphylococcus aureus* and other organisms, including anaerobes. Most likely diagnosis is:

1. Subphrenic abscess
2. Ischiorectal abscess
3. Pelvic abscess
4. Ischemic colitis
5. Pilonidal sinus
6. Anal abscess

Ans. 5. Pilonidal sinus

USMLE Case Scenario

A 33-year-old young man presents to ask for advice regarding the future management of his ulcerative colitis. He has had pancolitis for the past 15 years and has been told by his physician that he is at an increased risk for developing colorectal cancer. He asks for the physician's recommendation regarding appropriate surveillance. Which of the following is the most appropriate response?

1. Annual stool guaiac testing
2. Barium meal
3. Barium enema
4. Colonoscopy
5. Colonoscopy with multiple biopsies
6. Flexible sigmoidoscopy
7. Flexible sigmoidoscopy with multiple biopsies
8. Laparoscopy

Ans. 5. Colonoscopy with multiple biopsies

Patients with longstanding extensive ulcerative colitis for a long duration are at an increased colon cancer risk. Appropriate surveillance involves annual or biannual colonoscopy with multiple biopsies at regular intervals, even of normal-appearing mucosa, to check for dysplasia.

USMLE Case Scenario

A prematurely born infant fails to tolerate attempted feeding. Bilious vomiting is observed and initiates a diagnostic evaluation. Plain X-ray of the abdomen demonstrates one air bubble in the stomach and the second in the duodenum proximal to the obstruction. Most likely diagnosis is:

1. Esophageal atresia
2. Duodenal atresia
3. Annular pancreas
4. Pyloric stenosis

Ans. 2. Duodenal atresia

USMLE Case Scenario

An 85-year-old man with Pick's disease undergoes surgery for a fractured femoral neck. On the 6th postoperative day, his abdomen is grossly distended and tense, but not tender. He has occasional bowel sounds. The rectal vault is empty on digital examination, and there is no evidence of occult blood. X-ray films show a few distended loops of small bowel and a much distended colon. The cecum measures 9.5 cm in diameter. The gas pattern of distention extends throughout the entire large bowel, including the sigmoid and rectum. No stool is seen in the films. Vital signs are normal for his age. Which of the following is the most likely diagnosis?

1. Fecal impaction
2. Mechanical intestinal obstruction
3. Ogilvie syndrome
4. Paralytic ileus
5. Volvulus of the sigmoid colon

Ans. 3. Ogilvie syndrome

USMLE Case Scenario

A 6-month-old brought by his mother presents with episodes of distress and crying interspersed with quiet periods of normal behavior and playing. His mother says that he passes stool mixed with mucus and blood, the jelly stool. The abdomen is soft and nontender. A sausage-like mass may be palpable in the upper abdomen.

Most likely diagnosis is:

1. Diverticulitis
2. Appendicitis
3. Mesenteric adenitis
4. Volvulus
5. Duodenal atresia
6. Annular pancreas
7. Intussusception

Ans. 7. Intussusception

USMLE Case Scenario

A 27-year-old baseball player goes to the team physician 2 hours before game time, complaining of abdominal pain. The symptoms began approximately 7 hours earlier in a diffuse fashion. Two hours later, he began feeling nauseated and vomited twice. Over the past 4 hours, the abdominal pain has become more severe and well localized in the right lower quadrant. His examination now reveals well-localized pain in the right lower quadrant inferolateral to the umbilicus. Which of the following is the most likely diagnosis?

1. Acute obstruction of the appendiceal lumen by a fecalith
2. Acute onset of ileocolitis
3. Acute onset of ischemic colitis
4. Acute *Yersinia* infection
5. Obstruction of the ileocecal valve by a mass

Ans. 1. Acute obstruction of the appendiceal lumen by a fecalith

USMLE Case Scenario

A 77-year-old presents with acute abdominal pain in the left lower quadrant. Examination reveals fever, leukocytosis, physical findings of peritoneal irritation in the left lower quadrant and sometimes a palpable mass. Among the options given below, most likekly diagnosis would be:

1. Renal colic
2. Cholecystitis
3. Pancreatitis
4. Diverticulitis
5. Hepatitis
6. Cholangitis
7. Pseudo-obstruction

Ans. 4. Diverticulitis

USMLE Case Scenario

A 45-year-old female complains of colicky right hypochondriac pain with radiation to right scapula. She is obese and has GERD as well. LFT and KFT are within normal limits. Urine examination is normal. The scenario should be suggesting:

1. Acute cholecystitis
2. Acute nephritis
3. Acute pyelonephritis
4. Acute hepatitis

Ans. 1. Acute cholecystitis

USMLE Case Scenario

A patient is brought to the hospital with history of RTA 8 hours back. A few drops of blood were noted at the external urethral meatus. He has not passed urine and his bladder is palpable per abdomen. What is the probable diagnosis?

1. Ureteral injury with extravasations of urine in the retroperitoneum
2. Urethral injury
3. Rupture bladder
4. Anuria due to hypovolemia

Ans. 2. Urethral injury

USMLE Case Scenario

An 88-year-old male, who was bedridden for the past few months as a result of stroke, presents with nausea, vomiting, colicky abdominal pain. X-rays show distended loops of bowel with large air shadow like parrot's beak. He would be assumed to be having:

1. Ischemic colitis
2. Meckel's diverticulitis

3. Pseudomembranous colitis
4. Volvulus
5. Intussusception
6. Colonic atresia
7. Annular pancreas

Ans. 4. Volvulus

USMLE Case Scenario

Which of the following polyps is not premalignant:

1. Juvenile polyposis syndrome
2. Familial polyposis syndrome
3. Juvenile polyp
4. HNPCC

Ans. 3. Juvenile polyp

USMLE Case Scenario

A cirrhotic develops malaise, right hypochondriac pain with weight loss and AFP levels which are elevated. This suggests a diagnostic work-up for:

1. Endodermal sinus tumor
2. Yolk sac tumor
3. Renal cell carcinoma
4. Metastatis from GIT
5. Wilms' tumor
6. Hepatoma

Ans. 6. Hepatoma

USMLE Case Scenario

A person with colonic cancer shows nodularities in liver with CEA levels elevated. Most likely cause would be:

1. Endodermal sinus tumor
2. Yolk sac tumor
3. Renal cell carcinoma
4. Metastatis
5. Wilms' tumor
6. Hepatoma

Ans. 4. Metastatis

USMLE Case Scenario

A 30-year-old female on OCPS develops sudden onset abdominal pain with tachycardia and hypotension. No history of trauma. Blood coagulation profile is within normal limits. Most likely cause would be:

1. Lower GI bleed
2. Portal hypertension
3. Variceal bleed
4. Hemophilia
5. Antiphospholipid antibody syndrome
6. Bleeding from ruptured hepatic adenoma

Ans. 6. Bleeding from ruptured hepatic adenoma

USMLE Case Scenario

A 55-year-old has progressive jaundice with weight loss, increased alkaline phosphatase, nagging epigastric and back pain USG reveals dilated intra- and extrahepatic ducts with thin-walled GB. Most likely cause is:

1. Pancreatitis
2. Cholecystitis
3. Hepatitis
4. Pancreatic cancer
5. Hepatic cancer
6. Bladder cancer

Ans. 4. Pancreatic cancer

USMLE Case Scenario

After treatment of acute pancreatitis, the patient comes after 7 weeks with ill-defined epigastric mass. This would suggest:

1. Solitary renal cyst
2. Pancreatic cyst
3. Hepatic cyst
4. Splenic cyst
5. Polycystic kidney

Ans. 2. Pancreatic cyst

USMLE Case Scenario

After an automobile accident, the patient comes after 7 weeks with ill-defined epigastric mass. This would suggest:

1. GI perforation
2. Splenic trauma
3. Solitary renal cyst
4. Pancreatic pseudocyst
5. Hepatic cyst
6. Splenic cyst
7. Polycystic kidney

Ans. 4. Pancreatic pseudocyst

USMLE Case Scenario

A 34-year-old female presents with abdominal mass accompanied by pain, nausea, and vomiting. The mass is diagnosed on physical examination. It displays a characteristic lateral mobility and is associated with the bowel mesentery. The most likely diagnosis is:

1. Pancreatic pseudocyst
2. Mesenteric cyst
3. Hepatic cyst
4. Splenic cyst
5. Polycystic kidney

Ans. 2. Mesenteric cyst

USMLE Case Scenario

A 35-year-old patient presents with intermittent pain and moves around a lot because he cannot get comfortable. He has costovertebral angle tenderness, urinary frequency and urgency. Most likely diagnosis would be:

1. Renal colic
2. Cholecystitis
3. Pancreatitis

4. Diverticulitis
5. Hepatitis
6. Cholangitis
7. Pseudoobstruction

Ans. 1. Renal colic

USMLE Case Scenario

A patient with recurrent peptic ulcer disease *H. pylori* was not detected. There are multiple ulcers on first and second portions of duodenum. This would make a medical student think about:

1. Glucagonoma
2. Carcinoid
3. Gastrinoma
4. Insulinoma
5. Pheochromocytoma

Ans. 3. Gastrinoma

USMLE Case Scenario

A 26-year-old woman comes to the emergency room complaining of severe abdominal pain. She has had burning, midepigastric pain for the past 2 years. The pain has been relieved by antacids, but it seems to have become progressively worse. Today, she vomited from the pain and noticed dark, 'coffee-ground' material. She has no past medical history of any significance. When asked specifically, she denies any use of nonsteroidal anti-inflammatory drugs (NSAIDs) or alcohol. In emergency department, her blood pressure was recorded as 110/70 mm Hg and pulse was 104/min. Upon gastric lavage, brown particulate matter is aspirated. She is admitted to the hospital for further work up. The next morning, she undergoes upper endoscopy, which reveals multiple small ulcers in the antrum, duodenum, and proximal jejunum.

Biopsies for the presence of *Helicobacter pylori* are negative. A lesion in which of the following locations would most likely explain these findings?

1. Liver
2. Endocrine pancreas
3. Exocrine pancreas
4. Pituitary
5. Small intestine

Ans. 3. Endocrine pancreas

This patient has a gastrinoma, a classic cause of multiple severe ulcers in odd locations.

USMLE Case Scenario

A 40-year-old woman from Alaska comes to a physician after four months of intermittent abdominal cramps and diarrhea accompanied by skin flushing that is most pronounced in the head and neck area. Physical examination reveals a murmur heard over the tricuspid valve. Urine-special studies for 5-hydroxyindoleacetic acid show excretion of 99 mg/day, which indicates a great increase in levels. CT scan of the liver demonstrates a 2 cm small lesion. Most likely diagnosis is:

1. Carcinoid tumor, metastatic
2. Cholangiocarcinoma, primary
3. Hepatocellular carcinoma, primary
4. Mucinous adenocarcinoma of the colon, metastatic
5. Squamous cell carcinoma of the esophagus, metastatic

Ans. 1. Carcinoid syndrome is the term used for the cluster of cutaneous flushing, abdominal cramps, and diarrhea that is seen in patients who have excess amounts of circulating vasoactive substances, including serotonin.

USMLE Case Scenario

A 44-year-old female has migratory necrolytic dermatitis. She is diabetic and thin. She might be having an underlying:

1. Glucagonoma
2. Carcinoid

3. Gastrinoma
4. Insulionma
5. Pheochromocytoma

Ans. 1. Glucagonoma

USMLE Case Scenario

A 33-year-old male with pounding headache, palpitations, perspirations and increased VMA levels is suffering from:

1. Glucagonoma
2. Carcinoid
3. Gastrinoma
4. Insulinoma
5. Pheochromocytoma

Ans. 5. Pheochromocytoma

USMLE Case Scenario

A 55-year-old female with flushing, non healing diahorreas and bronchospasm with increased 5HIAA levels:

1. Glucagonoma
2. Carcinoid
3. Gastrinoma
4. Insulinoma
5. Pheochromocytoma

Ans. 2. Carcinoid

USMLE Case Scenario

A 40-year-old woman comes to a physician after 4 months of intermittent abdominal cramps and diarrhea accompanied by skin flushing that is most pronounced in the head and neck area. Physical examination reveals a murmur heard over the tricuspid valve. Urine-special studies for 5-hydroxyindoleacetic acid show excretion of 99 mg/day [reference range 0.5–9.0 mg/day]. CT scan of the liver demonstrates a 2 cm lesion. Most likely diagnosis is:

1. Glucagonoma
2. Carcinoid
3. Gastrinoma
4. Insulinoma
5. Pheochromocytoma

Ans. 2. Carcinoid

USMLE Case Scenario

A 20-year-old female with hypertension not responding to antihypertensives with bruit over renal area suggests:

1. Renal artery duplication
2. Fibromuscular dysplasia
3. Benign hypertension
4. Malignant hypertension

Ans. 2. Fibromuscular dysplasia

USMLE Case Scenario

A 75-year-old with hypertension not responding to antihypertensives with bruit over renal area is suffering from:

1. Renal artery stenosis
2. Fibromuscular aplasia
3. Benign hypertension
4. Malignant hypertension

Ans. 1. Renal artery stenosis

USMLE Case Scenario

A nonsuppurative inflammatory process of the retroperitoneum that causes problems by extrinsic compression of retroperitoneal structures such as the ureters, aorta and inferior vena with ureteral obstruction as one of the most common presentations of this disease process is:

1. Pseudomyxoma
2. Renal artery stenosis
3. Retroperitoneal tumor
4. Retroperitoneal fibrosis

Ans. 4. Retroperitoneal fibrosis

USMLE Case Scenario

True statement is:

1. BPH is a risk factor for prostatic cancer and after simple prostatectomy, patients are still at risk of developing prostate cancer
2. BPH is a risk factor for prostatic cancer and after simple prostatectomy, patients are not at risk of developing prostate cancer
3. BPH is not a risk factor for prostatic cancer and after simple prostatectomy, patients are still at risk of developing prostate cancer
4. BPH is not a risk factor for prostatic cancer and after simple prostatectomy, patients are not at risk of developing prostate cancer

Ans. 3. BPH is not a risk factor for prostatic cancer and after simple prostatectomy, patients are still at risk of developing prostate cancer. Simple prostatectomy involves shelling out the prostate adenoma and leaving the pseudocapsule (true prostate) behind. Therefore, these patients are still at risk of developing prostate cancer, although BPH in and of itself is not a risk factor for prostatic cancer.

USMLE Case Scenario

The most common source of arterial emboli is/are:

1. Superficial veins of lower limb
2. Deep veins of lower limb
3. Veins of pelvis
4. Heart
5. Lungs

Ans. 4. Heart

The heart is the most common source of arterial emboli and accounts for 90% of cases. Within the heart, sources include diseased valves, endocarditis, the left atrium in patients with unstable atrial arrhythmias, and mural thrombus on the wall of the left ventricle in patients with a myocardial infarction.

USMLE Case Scenario

A patient is evaluated for subclavian steal syndrome. On being subjected to exercise, left arm of a carpenter develops relative ischemia. Atherosclerotic occlusion of the subclavian artery proximal to the vertebral artery is seen. The dynamics of blood flow suggest that in this syndrome:

1. Reversal of blood occurs through carotid artery with decreased flow to brain
2. Reversal of blood occurs through carotid artery with increased flow to brain
3. Reversal of blood occurs through vertebral artery with decreased flow to brain
4. Reversal of blood occurs through vertebral artery with increased flow to brain

Ans. 3. Reversal of blood occurs through vertebral artery with decreased flow to brain

USMLE Case Scenario

The presence of air in the mediastinum after an episode of vomiting and retching is virtually pathognomonic of:

1. Spontaneous rupture of lung bullae
2. Spontaneous rupture of trachea

3. Spontaneous rupture of the esophagus (Boerhaave's syndrome)
4. Spontaneous rupture of the esophagus (Mallory-Weis Tear)

Ans. 3. Spontaneous rupture of the esophagus (Boerhaave's syndrome)

Patients with Mallory-Weiss syndrome typically present with a massive, painless hematemesis after severe vomiting or retching. The majority of tears occur just below the gastroesophageal junction.

USMLE Case Scenario

An elderly 88-year-old man from Kansas presents with nausea, vomiting, abdominal distention, colicky abdominal pain, and obstipation. A lesion radiographically on plain film of the abdomen appears as an upside-down U or 'bent inner tube'. Most likely diagnosis is:

1. Intussusception
2. Sigmoid volvulus
3. Acute mesenteric ischemia
4. Chronic mesenteric ischemia
5. Annular pancreas
6. Strangulated intestinal hernia

Ans. 2. Sigmoid volvulus

USMLE Case Scenario

Pancreatectomy is a highly skilled procedure. The metabolic consequences of total pancreatectomy are manifold. They include all except:

1. Weight loss
2. Malabsorption
3. Hypocalcemia
4. Hypophosphatemia
5. Diabetes mellitus
6. Diarrhea
7. Iron deficiency
8. Pernicious anemia
9. Megaloblastic anemia

Ans. 9. Megaloblastic anemia

USMLE Case Scenario

A lesion has been identified as a source of gastrointestinal bleeding. It is characteristically located within 6 cm distal to the gastroesophageal junction. It typically consists of an abnormally large submucosal artery that protrudes through a small, solitary mucosal defect. Most likely the lesion is:

1. Marginal artery lesion
2. Sudeck artery lesion
3. Arc of Rion
4. Brodel's line
5. Prepyloric vein of Myo
6. Moynihan's hump
7. Dieulafoy's lesion

Ans. 7. Dieulafoy's lesion

USMLE Case Scenario

Most specific statement about carcinoid tumor is that is:

1. Carcinoid tumors arise from the ectoderm, are a type of apudoma and the most common site is the small bowel.
2. Carcinoid tumors arise from the neuroectoderm, are a type of apudoma and the most common site is the small bowel.
3. Carcinoid tumors arise from the neuroectoderm, are a type of apudoma and the most common site is the appendix.

4. Carcinoid tumors arise from the ectoderm, are a type of apudoma and the most common site is the large bowel.
5. Carcinoid tumors arise from the neuroectoderm, are a type of apudoma and the most common site is the large bowel.

Ans. 2. Carcinoid tumors arise from the neuroectoderm, are a type of apudoma and the most common site is the small bowel.

USMLE Case Scenario

In a 44-year-old man, it is found that the entire colon, from cecum to rectum, is involved with a grossly continuous inflammatory process microscopically confined to the mucosa and submucosa of the colon. With crypt abscesses and superficial ulcerations, disease is suggestive of:

1. Ischemic bowel disease
2. Irritable bowel disease
3. Pseudomembranous colitis
4. Ulcerative colitis
5. Crohn's disease

Ans. 4. Ulcerative colitis

USMLE Case Scenario

The classic Quincke triad of abdominal pain in the right upper quadrant, jaundice and gastrointestinal bleeding is present in patients with:

1. Peutz-jeghers syndrome
2. Gardner's syndrome
3. Turcot's syndrome
4. Hemobilia
5. Angiodysplasia

Ans. 4. Hemobilia

USMLE Case Scenario

A 44-year-old has findings of bilateral hydronephrosis and hydroureter proximal to the site of extrinsic compression of the ureters. The ureters are seen to be fibrosed over a substantial distance, starting inferiorly and progressing superiorly. The ureters are deviated medially toward the midline. Most likely diagnosis is:

1. Ormond's disease
2. Caffey's disease
3. Ollier's disease
4. Trevor's disease

Ans. 1. Ormond's Disease

USMLE Case Scenario

An 81-year-old man with Alzheimer disease, who lives in a nursing home, undergoes surgery for a fractured femoral neck. On the 5th postoperative day, it is noted that his abdomen is grossly distended and tense, but not tender. He has occasional bowel sounds. The rectal vault is empty on digital examination and there is no evidence of occult blood. X-ray films show a few distended loops of small bowel and a very distended colon. The cecum measures 9 cm in diameter and the gas pattern of distention extends throughout the entire large bowel, including the sigmoid and rectum. No stool is seen in the films. Other than the abdominal distention and the ravages of his mental disease, he does not appear to be ill. Vital signs are normal for his age. The most likely diagnosis is:

1. Ogilvie's syndrome
2. Ormond's disease
3. Turcot's syndrome
4. Gardner's syndrome
5. FAP
6. HNPCC
7. Muir-Torre syndrome

Ans. 1. Ogilvie's syndrome

USMLE Case Scenario

An 85-year-old male presents with adenomatous polyposis; osteomas of the mandible, skull, and long bones; and a sebaceous cyst. Most likely diagnosis is:

1. Turcot's syndrome
2. Gardner's syndrome
3. FAP
4. HNPCC
5. Muire-Torre syndrome

Ans. 2. Gardner's syndrome

USMLE Case Scenario

A 16-year-old female has firm, rubbery mass in right breast moving with palpation. It suggests of:

1. Fibroadenoma
2. Giant fibroadenoma
3. Fibrocystic disease
4. Intraductal papilloma
5. Breast abscess

Ans. 1. Fibroadenoma

USMLE Case Scenario

A 16-year-old female has firm, rubbery mass in right breast, which is 8 cms in diameter. It suggests of:

1. Fibroadenoma
2. Giant fibroadenoma
3. Fibrocystic disease
4. Intraductal papilloma
5. Breast abscess

Ans. 2. Giant fibroadenoma

USMLE Case Scenario

A bloodstained discharge from the nipple indicates one of the following:

1. Breast abscess
2. Fibroadenoma
3. Duct papilloma
4. Fat necrosis of breast

Ans. 3. Duct papilloma

USMLE Case Scenario

A 42-year-old woman hit her breast with a broom handle while doing housework. She noticed a lump in that area at the time, and 1 week later, the lump was still present. She then sought medical advice. On physical examination, she had a 3 cm hard mass deep inside the affected breast, and some superficial ecchymosis over the area.
Which of the following is the most appropriate next step, or steps, in management?

1. Reassess in about 2 months, with no specific therapy
2. Hot packs, analgesics, and surgical evacuation of the hematoma
3. Mammogram, and no further therapy if the report does not identify cancer
4. Mammogram and biopsy of the mass
5. Mastectomy

Ans. 4. Mammogram and biopsy of the mass

USMLE Case Scenario

A 30-year-old female has bloody discharge from nipple. No other palpable masses are seen.
1. Fibroadenoma
2. Giant fibroadenoma
3. Fibrocystic disease
4. Intraductal papilloma
5. Breast abscess

Ans. 4. Intraductal papilloma

USMLE Case Scenario

A 55-year-old woman has 3.5 cm hard mass in her left breast with ill-defined borders and not mobile. The skin overlying has orange peel appearance:
1. Fibroadenoma
2. Giant fibroadenoma
3. Fibrocystic disease
4. Intraductal papilloma
5. Breast abscess
6. Breast Ca

Ans. 6. Breast Ca

USMLE Case Scenario

A 65-year-old male from Australia has an indolent, pale, raised, waxy, 1.0 cm skin mass over the bridge of the nose. The mass has been slowly growing over the past 4 years. There are no enlarged lymph nodes in the neck. Which of the following is the most likely diagnosis?
1. Lipoma
2. Sebaceous cyst
3. Basal cell carcinoma
4. Invasive melanoma
5. Keratoacanthoma
6. Pyogenic granuloma
7. Squamous cell carcinoma

Ans. 3. Basal cell carcinoma

It affects sun-exposed areas, particularly the mid and upper face, in patients lacking protective pigmentation. One of its morphologic forms is that of a raised, waxy, pale lesion that grows very slowly and doesn't metastasize to lymph nodes.

USMLE Case Scenario

A 65-year-old has sudden onset, tearing chest pain radiating to back with BP 220/120 with unequal arm pressures and normal cardiac enzymes:
1. Subclavian steal syndrome
2. AAA (Abdominal Aortic Aneurysm)
3. Dissecting aneurysm of thoracic aorta
4. Coarctation of aorta

Ans. 3. Dissecting aneurysm of thoracic aorta

USMLE Case Scenario

A 20-year-old with BP 195/120 in upper limb with normal BP in lower limbs and rib-notching might be considred to be having:
1. Subclavian steal syndrome
2. AAA (Abdominal Aortic Aneurysm)
3. Dissecting aneurysm of thoracic aorta
4. Coarctation of aorta

Ans. 4. Coarctation of aorta

USMLE Case Scenario

The Sistrunk procedure is done for:
1. Thyroglossal cyst
2. Branchial cyst
3. Sublingual cyst
4. Ectopic thyroid

Ans. 1. Thyroglossal cyst

Most common congenital, cystic, midline neck mass. Thyroglossal duct cysts are benign cysts that can arise anywhere along the embryonic path of descent of the thyroid gland (from the foramen cecum to the level of the thyroid).
- **Thyroglossal duct cysts can become infected, demonstrating rapid enlargement and tenderness, but are otherwise generally nontender and asymptomatic.**
- **Treatment is with surgical excision.**
- **The Sistrunk procedure, in which the cyst, the middle third of the hyoid bone, and the thyroglossal duct tract are all excised, is associated with the lowest rate of recurrence.**

USMLE Case Scenario

An 11-year-old girl is brought by her parents to Washington with round 1 cm mass in midline of neck moving with movement of tongue. There is no history suggesting night sweats, weight loss, and pruritus. Most likely diagnosis is:
1. Thyroglossal duct cyst
2. Branchial cyst
3. Cystic hygroma
4. Lymphoma

Ans. 1. Thyroglossal duct cyst

USMLE Case Scenario

A 15-year-old girl from Ohio has a round 1 cm mass on side of neck beneath and in front of sternocleidomastoid. It is said to be a remnant of 2nd cleft. The diagnosis would be:
1. Thyroglossal duct cyst
2. Branchial cyst
3. Cystic hygroma
4. Lymphoma

Ans. 2. Branchial cyst

USMLE Case Scenario

A 6-year-old presents with a swelling which seems to be fluid-filled translucent mass in supraclavicular area. It most likely represents:
1. Thyroglossal duct cyst
2. Branchial cyst
3. Cystic hygroma
4. Lymphoma

Ans. 3. Cystic hygroma

USMLE Case Scenario

A 35-year-old present with enlarged lymph nodes in cervical region with night sweats and pruritus plus axillary lymphadenopathy. The swelling seen by a surgeon is non translucent, solid. Most likely the diagnosis suggests:
1. Thyroglossal duct cyst
2. Branchial cyst
3. Cystic hygroma
4. Lymphoma

Ans. 4. Lymphoma

USMLE Case Scenario

A well-differentiated follicular carcinoma of thyroid can be best differentiated from a follicular adenoma by:

1. Hurthle cell change
2. Lining of tall columnar and cuboidal cells
3. Vascular invasion
4. Nuclear features

Ans. 3. Vascular invasion

USMLE Case Scenario

A pathologist is observing a slide. He Treports seeing perineural invasion. In which one of the following is perineural invasion most commonly seen?

1. Adenocarcinoma
2. Adenoid cystic carcinoma
3. Basal cell adenoma
4. Squamous cell carcinoma

Ans. 2. Adenoid cystic carcinoma

USMLE Case Scenario

Three days after catheterization, a young patient presents with skin findings in the distal extremities of livedo reticularis, ischemic ulcerations, cyanosis, gangrene. This would suggest a likely diagnosis of:

1. Cholesterol emboli syndrome
2. Pseudoaneurysm
3. Inguinal hernia
4. Pneumothorax

Ans. 1. Cholesterol emboli syndrome

USMLE Case Scenario

A 67-year-old man comes to the clinic complaining of steady, dull back pain over the past 3 weeks. He states that he has recently moved after retiring from a career in banking and is searching for a new primary care physician. He denies trauma to his back and otherwise feels well. On physical examination, his blood pressure is 170/93 mm Hg with a pulse of 88/min. He has no tenderness over the spinal processes or paraspinal areas. His abdomen is obese but there is a suggestion of a nontender, pulsatile mass in the epigastric region. The remainder of the physical examination is normal. Which of the following diagnoses should be considered at this time?

1. Abdominal aortic aneurysm (AAA)
2. Acute aortic dissection
3. Cauda equina syndrome
4. Lumbosacral disk herniation
5. Pancreatitis

Ans. 1. Abdominal aortic aneurysm (AAA)

It is imperative to recognize the potential presence of an abdominal aortic aneurysm (AAA). The combination of the history of hypertension and smoking, the new back pain, and a pulsatile mass on examination is highly suggestive of abdominal aneurysm. The back pain occurs as the expanding mass compresses structures in the retroperitoneum. It is particularly important to make the diagnosis because large aneurysms (greater than 5 cm in diameter) are associated with a very high risk of rupture and subsequent mortality.

USMLE Case Scenario

A 55-year-old obese female presents with fatty deposits on limbs/trunk with facial sparing and multiple painful lipomas. This would suggest a likely diagnosis of:

1. Gardner's disease
2. Turcot's disease

3. Dercum's disease
4. De Quervain's disease

Ans. 3. Dercum's disease

USMLE Case Scenario

A 58-year-old woman had a mitral valve replacement, and was placed on anticoagulants and prophylactic antibiotics following her surgery. Five days after her surgery, she developed a sharply demarcated, erythematous rash on her left thigh. Two days after the rash appeared, large hemorrhagic bullae began to form in the area of the rash. Which of the following medications most likely caused the patient's rash?

1. Aspirin
2. Cefazolin
3. Heparin
4. Vancomycin
5. Warfarin

Ans. 5. Warfarin

USMLE Case Scenario

A 33-year-old man comes to the clinic with a 2-day history of severe left-sided scrotal pain and swelling. He is sexually active and has multiple sexual partners. He has no history of sexually transmitted diseases. His temperature is 38.7 °C, blood pressure is 126/70 mm Hg, and pulse is 84/min. Examination shows unilateral intrascrotal tenderness and swelling. Testicular support makes the pain less intense. Which of the following is the most likely diagnosis?

1. Epididymitis
2. Prostatitis
3. Testicular torsion
4. Urethritis
5. Varicocele

Ans. 1. Epididymitis

This patient has epididymitis, most likely due to Chlamydia trachomatis. Epididymitis refers to inflammation of the epididymitis, which leads to unilateral intrascrotal pain, swelling, and fever. Testicular support usually relieves the pain to some extent.

USMLE Case Scenario

A 35-year-old drug addict from Downtown Mexico, who is homosexual, presents complaining of pain with defecation. He denies any symptoms of diarrhea, abdominal pain, or fevers. On physical examination, he is afebrile and has an unremarkable abdominal examination. On examination of the perianal area, there is a group of clustered ulcers adjacent to the anal orifice and extending into the anal canal. A sigmoidoscopy reveals normal rectosigmoid mucosa. Which of the following is the most likely diagnosis?

1. Crohn's disease
2. Cytomegalovirus infection
3. Herpes infection
4. Neisseria gonorrhea
5. Shigella dysenteriae
6. Ulcerative colitis

Ans. 5. Herpes infection

The grouped ulcers are characteristic of a herpetic infection. The ulcers begin as vesicular lesions and then painfully ulcerate.

USMLE Case Scenario

The midcervical region from 2 cm above the clavicle to the angle of the mandible is:

1. Zone I
2. Zone II

3. Zone III
4. Zone IV

Ans. 2. Zone II

Zone I is the base of the neck from 2 cm above the clavicles to the level of the clavicles.
Zone II is the midcervical region from 2 cm above the clavicle to the angle of the mandible.
Zone III is the top of the neck from the angle of the mandible to the base of the skull.

USMLE Case Scenario

A widened mediastinum on chest radiograph with hypotension after history of trauma is most likely to be diagnostic of:
1. Syphilis
2. Esophageal rupture
3. Bronchial injury
4. Thoracic aortic aneurysm
5. Thoracic aortic rupture

Ans. 4. Thoracic aortic aneurysm

USMLE Case Scenario

A 45-year-old consults a surgeon as he has been having periods of Headache. He also has frequent episodes of rapid heartbeat accompanied by sweating, flushing, and a sense of impending doom. Physical examination is unrevealing, with no evidence of arrhythmia at the time of the exam. Urinary measurement of which of the following would most likely be diagnostic in this case?
1. 5 HIAA
2. Acetylcholine
3. Dehydroepiandrosterone (DHEA)
4. Human chorionic gonadotropin (hCG)
5. 17-ketosteroids
6. Vanillylmandelic acid (VMA)

Ans. 6. Vanillylmandelic acid (VMA)

Pheochromocytoma↑Urinary metabolites of epinephrine and norepinephrine are seen. Vanillylmandelic acid (VMA) and homovanillic acid.

USMLE Case Scenario

Truth about Indirect hernias is:
1. Indirect hernias are the most common type in males only
2. Indirect hernias are the most common type in females only
3. Indirect hernias are the most common type in both sexes and all age groups
4. Direct hernias are the most common type in both sexes and all age groups

Ans. 3. Indirect hernias are the most common type in both sexes and all age groups

USMLE Case Scenario

A 25-year-old alcoholic male presents to emergency OPD half-an-hour after onset of pain around umbilicus which radiates to the back. His USG done one year back had demonstrated gallstones. Serum amylase is not elevated. He has nausea, vomiting and anorexia. Most likely cause is:
1. Acute gastritis
2. Acute pancreatitis
3. Acute mesenteric adenitis
4. Acute cholecystitis
5. Acute appendicitis

Ans. 2. Acute pancreatitis

USMLE Case Scenario

It is said that a patient, who is hungry and asking for food, does not have appendicitis. This is called:

1. Coffee-bean sign
2. Hamburger sign
3. Psoas sign
4. Obturator sign
5. Rovsing sign

Ans. 2. Hamburger sign

USMLE Case Scenario

A biliary fistula is an established and abnormal connection between any portion of the biliary tree and some other area. If this abnormal connection is between the biliary tree and the exterior, it is termed as external fistula; a connection between the biliary tree and an internal structure constitutes an internal fistula. There are four important complications of biliary fistula. They are:

1. Hyponatremia, Weight loss, Infection, Gallstone Ileus
2. Hyponatremia, Weight gain, Infection, Gallstone Ileus
3. Hypernatremia, Weight loss, Infection, Gallstone Ileus
4. Hypernatremia, Weight gain, Infection, Gallstone Ileus

Ans. 1. Hyponatremia, Weight loss, Infection, Gallstone Ileus

USMLE Case Scenario

Seminomas are characterized by features of:

1. Most common testicular malignant lesions, are nonuniform in gross and histologic appearance, characterized by slow growth and late invasion
2. Most common testicular malignant lesions, are nonuniform in gross and histologic appearance, characterized by rapid growth and early invasion
3. Most common testicular malignant lesions, are uniform in gross and histologic appearance, characterized by slow growth and late invasion
4. Most common testicular malignant lesions, are uniform in gross and histologic appearance, characterized by rapid growth and early invasion

Ans. 3. Most common testicular malignant lesions, are uniform in gross and histologic appearance, characterized by slow growth and late invasion.

USMLE Case Scenario

Fluid within the tunica is resorbed at a constant rate through the extensive venous and lymphatic systems of the spermatic cord. Hydrocele, the excessive accumulation of this serous fluid, results when there is increased production or decreased resorption. The fluid accumulates in:

1. The tunica albuginea derived from the testis
2. The tunica vasculosa derived from the testis
3. The tunica albuginea derived from the peritoneum
4. The tunica vasculosa derived from the peritoneum
5. The tunica vaginalis derived from the peritoneum
6. The tunica vaginalis derived from the testis

Ans. 5. The tunica vaginalis derived from the peritoneum

USMLE Case Scenario

Congenital hydrocele may follow:

1. Success of obliteration of the tunica vaginalis
2. Failure of obliteration of the tunica vaginalis

3. Success of obliteration of the processus vaginalis
4. Failure of obliteration of the processus vaginalis

Ans. 4. Failure of obliteration of the processus vaginalis

Congenital hydrocele may follow failure of obliteration of the processus vaginalis, and fluid formed within the peritoneal cavity may gravitate into the tunica vaginalis.

USMLE Case Scenario

In a 55-year-old, a painless firm fibrotic thickening of the fascia of the corpora cavernosa is observed involving the dorsolateral aspects of the penile shaft or the intracavernous septum between the corpora cavernosa. These lesions are histologically similar to:

1. Rodent ulcer
2. Papilloma
3. Melanoma
4. Keloid
5. Ear
6. Thyroid cartilage
7. Tendon
8. Ligament

Ans. 4. Keloid

Peyronie's disease. A firm fibrotic thickening of the fascia of the corpora cavernosa is observed, usually involving the dorsolateral aspects of the penile shaft or the intracavernous septum between the corpora cavernosa, histologically similar to keloid or Dupuytren's contracture.

USMLE Case Scenario

Impotence may be one of the earliest signs of Leriche's syndrome, which is thrombotic obstruction of the:

1. Varicose veins
2. Iliac veins
3. Iliac arteries
4. Femoral arteries
5. Femoral veins
6. Testicular arteries
7. Testicular veins

Ans. 3. Iliac arteries

USMLE Case Scenario

A 54-year-old after a trauma has hypoxia, confusion. Petechiae are found over the chest, conjunctivae, and uvula. Neurological examination shows confusion, agitation, stupor. Respiratory abnormalities include tachypnea, profound hypoxia. Blood examination shows thrombocytopenia, hypofibrinogenemia, and prolongation of the partial thromboplastin time.

Electrocardiogram shows prominent S waves in lead 1, prominent Q waves in lead 3, ST segment depression and right axis strain.

Arterial PO_2 is 50 mm Hg on room air.

Most likely diagnosis is:

1. Pulmonary embolism
2. Air embolism
3. Fat embolism
4. Pulmonary infarct
5. ARDS
6. DIC

Ans. 3. Fat embolism

USMLE Case Scenario

The type of lymphedema most commonly involving the dorsum of the foot and lower extremity up to the level of the knee with a familial history is:

1. Lymphedema congenita
2. Lymphedema praecox
3. Lymphedema tarda
4. Milroy's disease

Ans. 4. Milroy's disease

USMLE Case Scenario

The type of lymphedema most commonly involving the dorsum of the foot and lower extremity up to the level of the knee with a familial history is:

1. Anterior commissure in the midline
2. Posterior commissure in the midline
3. Anterior commissure away from the midline
4. Posterior commissure away from the midline

Ans. 2. Posterior commissure in the midline

USMLE Case Scenario

A 34-year-old has frontal osteomyelitis with marked overlying soft tissue swelling that is secondary to frontal sinusitis. It is referred to as:

1. Sebaceous cyst
2. Cylindroma
3. Keratoacanthoma
4. Pott's puffy tumor

Ans. 4. Pott's puffy tumor

USMLE Case Scenario

A 56-year-old man from Australia has a skin cancer. Diagnosis of melanoma is made. These are seen to most melanomas occurring in patients with:

1. Fair, nonfreckled skin that does not burn easily, blond hair, blue eyes
2. Fair, freckled skin that burns easily, blond hair, nonblue eyes
3. Fair, nonfreckled skin that burns easily, blond hair, blue eyes
4. Fair, freckled skin that burns easily, blond hair, blue eyes

Ans. 4. Fair, freckled skin that burns easily, blond hair, blue eyes

USMLE Case Scenario

The ligament which attaches the liver to the anterior abdominal wall from the diaphragm to umbilicus and incorporates the ligamentum teres hepaticus in its dorsal border is:

1. Falciform ligament
2. Coronary ligament
3. Gastrohepatic ligament
4. Hepatoduodenal ligament

Ans. 1. Falciform ligament

1. **The falciform ligament, which attaches the liver to the anterior abdominal wall from the diaphragm to umbilicus and incorporates the ligamentum teres hepaticus in its dorsal border. In persons with portal hypertension, the umbilical vein recanalizes and connects the periumbilical superficial venous system with the portal system.**
2. **The anterior and posterior right and left coronary ligaments, which in continuity with the falciform ligament connect the diaphragm to the liver.**

3. The gastrohepatic and hepatoduodenal ligaments, which consist of the anterior layer of lesser omentum and are continuous with the left triangular ligament. The hepatoduodenal ligament contains the hepatic arteries, portal vein, and extrahepatic bile ducts. It forms the anterior boundary of the epiploic foramen of Winslow and the communication between the greater and lesser peritoneal cavities.

USMLE Case Scenario

After a dissection by an anatomist, a tongue-like projection of liver tissue is seen extending inferiorly from the right lobe. The condition is more frequently encountered in the female and in living, this condition usually causes no symptoms. The projection is:

1. Caudate lobe
2. Quadrate lobe
3. Riedel's lobe
4. Azygos lobe
5. Uncinate process
6. Omental tuberosity

Ans. 3. Riedel's lobe

USMLE Case Scenario

A pathologist reports that a disease is confined to the mucosal and submucosal layers of the colonic wall, with superficial ulcers, increased cellular infiltration of the lamina propria, and cyst abscesses beginning in the rectum and advancing proximally to involve the entire colon. On gross inspection, the colonic mucosa demonstrates healed granular superficial ulcers superimposed on a friable and thickened mucosa with increased vascularity. The most likely cause is:

1. Crohn's disese
2. Ulcerative colitis
3. Diverticulosis
4. Colonic cancer

Ans. 2. Ulcerative colitis

USMLE Case Scenario

A 55-year-old presents with profound nausea and vomiting, abdominal distention, postprandial epigastric pain, and weight loss. Vascular compression of the duodenum is believed to produce this constellation of symptoms. It is commonly known as Wilkie's syndrome. The artery involved is:

1. Celiac trunk
2. Superior mesenteric artery
3. Inferior mesenteric artery
4. Short gastric artery
5. Gastroepiploic artery

Ans. 2. Superior mesenteric artery

USMLE Case Scenario

An elderly patient who usually takes high-fiber diet presents with acute onset of severe colicky pain, nausea, vomiting, and obstipation. On abdominal examination, a compressible mass extending from the right lower quadrant to the midabdominal region is felt. Plain abdominal roentgenogram reveals marked distention of the cecum as well as small bowel dilatation. Barium enema classically reveals the narrowing accompanying the twisting of the colon (so-called bird's neck deformity). Most likely cause is:

1. Meckel's diverticulitis
2. Pseudo-obstruction
3. Intussusception

4. Cecal volvulus
5. Sigmoid cancer
6. Right colonic cancer

Ans. 4. Cecal volvulus

USMLE Case Scenario

A 65-year-old male presents with pulsatile tinnitus, hemorrhage, vertigo, and paralysis of cranial nerves IX, X, XI as presenting symptoms and signs. A red mass that pulsates and blanches with compression with a pneumatic otoscope can be seen in the ear canal. These were found to be nonchromaffin paragangliomas. Most likely tumor is:

1. Cholesteatoma
2. Angiofibroma
3. Glomus jugulare
4. Glomus tympanicum

Ans. 4. Glomus tympanicum

USMLE Case Scenario

A 25-year-old medical student from New York has enlarged hair follicles in an otherwise normal skin. The follicle holds a single hair shaft surrounded by rings of keratin. The cavity contains pus under pressure and a wall of edematous fat; polymorphonuclear cells predominate. The cavity has a wall of fibrous tissue lined by granulation tissue of capillaries, lymphocytes and giant cells. The cavity is laden with *Staphylococcus aureus* and other organisms, including anerobes. Most likely diagnosis is:

1. Posterior midline crypt
2. Hidradenitis suppurativa
3. Carbuncle
4. Pilonidal abscess

Ans. 4. Pilonidal abscess

USMLE Case Scenario

A prematurely born infant fails to tolerate attempted feeding. Bilious vomiting is observed and initiates a diagnostic evaluation. Plain X-ray of the abdomen demonstrates one air bubble in the stomach and the second in the duodenum proximal to the obstruction. Most likely diagnosis is:

1. Tracheoesophageal atresia
2. Meckel's diverticulitis
3. Cecal volvulus
4. Sigmoid volvulus
5. Duodenal atresia

Ans. 4. Sigmoid volvulus

USMLE Case Scenario

Neuhauser's sign is seen in:

1. Paralytic ileus
2. Meconium ileus
3. Pyloric stenosis
4. Annular pancreas
5. Duodenal atresia
6. Jejunal atresia
7. Ileal atresia
8. Imperforate anus

Ans. 2. Meconium ileus
A ground-glass appearance in the right lower quadrant (Neuhauser's sign or the soap-bubble sign) may be observed and represents viscid meconium mixed with air.

USMLE Case Scenario

An infant presents with abdominal distention and failure to pass meconium in the first 24 hours of life. Plain abdominal radiographs demonstrate loops of distended bowel with air-fluid levels. Barium enema shows a microcolon extending up to the descending at which point the colon becomes dilated and copious intraluminal material (thick meconium plug) is observed. Following instillation of the contrast material, large pieces of inspissated meconium is passed and the obstruction is completely relieved. Most likely cause is:

1. Cystic fibrosis
2. Aganglionic megacolon
3. Meconium plug syndrome
4. Colonic atresia
5. Rectal atresia

Ans. 3. Meconium plug syndrome

USMLE Case Scenario

A combination of omphalocele, anterior diaphragmatic hernia, sternal cleft, ectopia cordis and intracardiac defects is called pentalogy named as:

1. Pentalogy of Fallot
2. Pentalogy of Cantrell
3. Pentalogy of Charcot
4. Pentalogy of Alport
5. Pentalogy of St. Mary Joseph

Ans. 2. Pentalogy of Cantrell

USMLE Case Scenario

An infant appears dyspneic, tachypneic, and cyanotic and has severe retractions with an increased chest diameter. Bowel sounds are heard on auscultation of the affected chest. An anteroposterior chest X-ray demonstrates air-filled viscera in the chest. Compression of ipsilateral lung, which is hypoplastic, is also noted. Most likely diagnosis is:

1. Choanal atresia
2. Tracheoesophageal fistula
3. Congenital diaphragmatic hernia
4. Acquired diaphragmatic hernia
5. Congenital cystic lung

Ans. 3. Congenital diaphragmatic hernia

USMLE Case Scenario

A severe force is exerted laterally on the ring of C1, and the arches fracture at the thinnest and weakest points with sparing of the spinal cord. The fracture fragments spread outward. The fracture is diagnosed on lateral cervical spine roentgenograms. It is a description of:

1. Jefferson's fracture
2. Hangman's fracture
3. Boxer's fracture
4. Bennett fracture
5. Monteggia fracture

Ans. 1. Jefferson's fracture

USMLE Case Scenario

An 86-year-old woman from a nursing care center presents complaining of very severe abdominal pain, which began abruptly 7 hours ago. She describes the pain as severe. She has had episodes of atrial fibrillation in the past. On physical examination, she appears extremely uncomfortable. Her temperature is 102.9 °F, blood pressure is 180/110 mm Hg, and pulse is 100/min and irregular. An abdominal examination reveals mild distention and no hepatosplenomegaly. The abdomen is soft but very tender to palpation. A rectal examination reveals brown, guaiac positive stool. She has no audible bowel sounds. Which of the following is the most likely diagnosis?

1. Diverticulitis
2. Crohn's disease
3. Ulcerative colitis
4. Ischemic colitis
5. Mesenteric ischemia
6. Pancreatitis
7. Small bowel obstruction

Ans. 5. Mesenteric ischemia

Embolic occlusion of the superior mesenteric artery. These patients will present with severe pain out of proportion to their objective physical findings. The diagnosis should be suspected clinically and immediate superior mesenteric arteriogram should be performed.

USMLE Case Scenario

Polyploidy conditions can affect the alimentary tract of children. Not a Polypoid condition is:

1. Peutz-Jeghers syndrome
2. Cronkhite-Canada syndrome
3. Familial polyposis
4. Fanconi's syndrome
5. Gardner's syndrome
6. Turcot's syndrome
7. Juvenile polyposis coli

Ans. 4. Fanconi's syndrome

USMLE Case Scenario

A 34-year-old male is suspected to have torsion of testis. It is confirmed that torsion of testis is the final diagnosis. Management:

1. Can be delayed and limited to the affected side
2. Can be delayed but should include the asymptomatic side
3. Should be immediate and limited to the affected side
4. Should be immediate and include the asymptomatic side

Ans. 4. Should be immediate and include the asymptomatic side

Torsion of the testicle should be corrected as soon as possible after the diagnosis is entertained. The opposite scrotum should also be explored at the time of the operation, since the primary anatomic defect is most often a bilateral phenomenon.

USMLE Case Scenario

Congenital berry aneurysms are especially common at a few specific locations. Most of these aneurysms are located at:

1. The junction of the posterior communicating artery and the internal carotid artery
2. Vertebral arteries
3. The first major branches of the middle cerebral artery
4. Bifurcation of the basilar artery

Ans. 1. The junction of the posterior communicating artery and the internal carotid artery

USMLE Case Scenario

Congenital anomalies of the female genital system consist of those derived from remnants of the mesonephric duct or the Wolffian duct. The most common of these is the parovarian cyst which represents:

1. The lower Wolffian duct and may grow to be as large as 20 cm
2. The upper Wolffian duct and may grow to be as large as 20 cm
3. The upper mesonephric duct and may grow to be as large as 20 cm
4. The lower mesonephric duct and may grow to be as large as 20 cm

Ans. 2. The upper Wolffian duct and may grow to be as large as 20 cm

USMLE Case Scenario

An 18-year-old man shot once in the left chest has a blood pressure of 80/50 mm Hg, a heart rate of 130 beats per minute and distended neck veins. Immediate treatment might include:

1. Administration of one liter of Ringer's lactate solution
2. Subxiphoid pericardiotomy
3. Needle decompression of the left chest in the second intercostal space
4. Emergency thoracotomy to cross-clamp the aorta

Ans. 3. Needle decompression of the left chest in the second intercostal space

USMLE Case Scenario

Of the visceral aneurysms, which is the most common?

1. Celiac
2. Superior mesenteric
3. Hepatic
4. Splenic

Ans. 4. Splenic aneurysms are the most common visceral type

USMLE Case Scenario

Features of tumor lysis syndrome are:

1. Hyperuricemia, hyperphosphatemia, hypercalcemia
2. Hyperuricemia, hypophosphatemia, hypocalcemia
3. Hypouricemia, hyperphosphatemia, hypercalcemia
4. Hyperuricemia, hyperphosphatemia, hypocalcemia

Ans. 4. Hyperuricemia, hyperphosphatemia, hypocalcemia

USMLE Case Scenario

Whenever antibiotics are used, they exert a selective pressure on the endogenous flora of the patient and on exogenous bacteria that colonize sites at risk. Bacteria that remain are resistant to the antibiotics being used and become the pathogens. It is seen that a new infection develops during antibiotic treatment for the original infection. Such infections are called:

1. Super infections
2. Restricted infections
3. Anti-infections
4. Neoinfections

Ans. 1. Super infections

USMLE Case Scenario

The most life-threatening conditions, requiring instantaneous intervention as in laryngeal fracture with complete upper airway obstruction, is referred to as:

1. Exigent
2. Emergency

3. Urgent
4. Deferrable

Ans. 1. Exigent

1. **Exigent—the most life-threatening conditions, requiring instantaneous intervention (e.g. laryngeal fracture with complete upper airway obstruction and tension pneumothorax).**
2. **Emergency—those conditions requiring immediate intervention, certainly within the first hour (e.g. ongoing hemorrhage and intracranial mass lesions).**
3. **Urgent—those conditions requiring intervention within the first few hours (e.g. open contaminated fractures, ischemic extremity and hollow viscous injuries).**
4. **Deferrable—those conditions that may or may not be immediately apparent but will subsequently require treatment (e.g. urethral disruption and facial fractures).**

USMLE Case Scenario

A 34-year-old female presents with abdominal mass accompanied by pain, nausea, and vomiting. The mass is diagnosed on physical examination. It displays a characteristic lateral mobility and is associated with the bowel mesentery. The most likely diagnosis is:

1. Ovarian cyst
2. Umbilical cyst
3. Liver cyst
4. Splenic cyst
5. Mesenteric cyst

Ans. 5. Mesenteric cyst

USMLE Case Scenario

A 44-year-old has findings of bilateral hydronephrosis and hydroureter proximal to the site of extrinsic compression of the ureters. The ureters are seen to be fibrosed over a substantial distance, starting inferiorly and progressing superiorly. The ureters are deviated medially toward the midline. Most likely diagnosis is:

1. Ortner's disease
2. Ollier's disease
3. Ogilvie's disease
4. Ormond's disease

Ans. 4. Ormond's disease

USMLE Case Scenario

During an abdominal examination, a 45-year-old patient from New Jersey is seen to lie quietly in the medical emergency. He appears acutely ill with tachypnea and tachycardia. Hypotension is present, respirations are shallow, and deep breathing or coughing produces severe abdominal pain. The patient is febrile. Percussion reveals the abdomen to be extremely tender, especially in the epigastric region. Palpation of the abdomen reveals a firm board-like appearance, with rigidity of the rectus muscles.

Rebound tenderness is seen, present in all four quadrants, and is worse in the epigastric region. Auscultation of the abdomen reveals hypoactive bowel sounds that progress to absent bowel sounds.

These findings confirm:

1. Acute cholecystitis
2. Acute hepatitis
3. Acute cholangitis
4. Acute mesenteric adenitis
5. Generalized peritonitis
6. Small bowel obstruction
7. Large bowel obstruction

Ans. 5. Generalized peritonitis

USMLE Case Scenario

A 45-year-old female presents with peritoneal infection, cirrhosis and poor hepatic function. A diagnosis of spontaneous bacterial peritonitis is made. The clinical features include ascites, fever, abdominal pain, and encephalopathy. Rebound tenderness is also seen. The diagnosis was established by peritoneal fluid aspiration with Gram stain and assessment of polymorphonuclear leukocytes. Most likely causative agent is:

1. *Streptococcus*
2. *Pneumococcus*
3. *Meningococcus*
4. *Listeria*
5. *Escherichia coli*
6. *Proteus*
7. *Pseudomonas*
8. *Klebsiella*

Ans. 5. *Escherichia coli*

USMLE Case Scenario

Kasabach-Merritt syndrome consists of triad of:

1. Giant fibroadenoma, Thrombocytosis, Coagulopathy
2. Giant fibroadenoma, Thrombocytopenia, Coagulopathy
3. Giant hemangioma, Thrombocytopenia, Coagulopathy
4. Giant hemangioma, Thrombophilia, Coagulopathy

Ans. 3. Giant hemangioma, Thrombocytopenia, Coagulopathy

USMLE Case Scenario

An infant presents with macrocephaly and hydrocephalus. Further cerebral ischemia but high-output cardiac failure due to the tremendous arteriovenous shunting is seen on evaluation. Most likely cause is:

1. Sigmoid sinus thrombosis
2. Vein of Galen aneurysm
3. Arnold-Chiari malformation
4. Cavernous sinus thrombosis
5. Subclavian steal syndrome

Ans. 2. Vein of Galen aneurysm

It is a vascular malformations of the brain are common causes of intracerebral hemorrhage in the pediatric age group. The classic arteriovenous malformation (AVM) is the most common, with cavernous angiomas and venous angiomas less commonly associated with hemorrhage.

USMLE Case Scenario

A bacterium is the cause of nonclostridial necrotizing soft tissue infections. The most common pathogen recovered when no prior injury or operation is the cause of the infection is:

1. *Clostridium perfringens*
2. *Staphylococcus aureus*
3. *Shigella*
4. *Yersinia*
5. *Pseudomonas*
6. *Beta-hemolytic Streptococcal pyogenes*

Ans. 6. *Beta-hemolytic Streptococcal pyogenes*

- The only bacterium commonly reported as the sole cause of nonclostridial necrotizing soft tissue infections is *beta-hemolytic S. pyogenes.*
- This happens to be the most common pathogen recovered when no prior injury or operation is the cause of the infection.

- Postoperative and postinjury cases of necrotizing soft tissue infection are most often caused by mixed bacterial species, including aerobic and anaerobic pathogens, both gram-positive and gram-negative, a very similar spectrum to that seen in intra-abdominal infections.

USMLE Case Scenario

Palpating left iliac fossa and then quickly releasing your hand, the patient feels pain at a point two-thirds of the way from the umbilicus to the anterior superior iliac spine. This is diagnostic of:

1. Cholecystitis and called Boas' sign
2. Mesenteric adenitis and called McBurney's sign
3. Pancreatitis and called Cullen's sign
4. Appendicitis and called McBurney's sign
5. Appendicitis and called Rovsing's sign

Ans. 5. Appendicitis and called Rovsing's sign

USMLE Case Scenario

In a 66-year-old female in Wales, subtotal thyroidectomy is performed, but following the surgery, the woman is extremely hoarse and can barely speak above a whisper. This hoarseness is most probably related to damage to a branch of which of the following cranial nerves?

1. Facial
2. Glossopharyngeal
3. Hypoglossal
4. Trigeminal
5. Vagus

Ans. 5. Vagus

USMLE Case Scenario

A 43-year-old man from Toledo develops a mass on the back of his left hand. He is reluctant to get it checked but on persistent pressure from his wife, he consults a dermatologist. On consulting a dermatologist after a few days it is seen that the lesion on his left hand consists of a round, firm, flesh-colored, 1.2 cm nodule with sharply rising edges and a central crater. Keratotic debris can be expressed from the central crater. The lesion has developed very rapidly over about a two-month period. Which of the following is the most likely diagnosis?

1. Wart
2. Solar keratosis
3. Sebaceous cyst
4. Keratoacanthoma
5. Lipoma
6. Malignant melanoma
7. Pyogenic granuloma
8. Seborrheic keratosis

Ans. 4. Keratoacanthoma

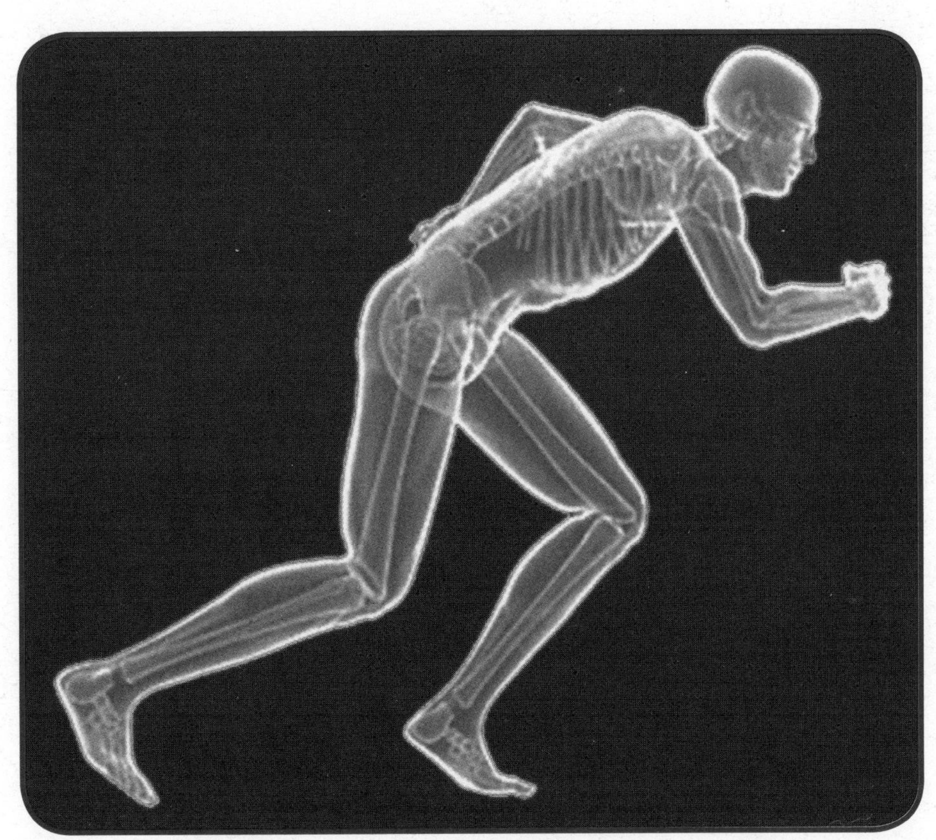

ORTHOPEDICS

Orthopedics | 6

USMLE Case Scenario

The Neural structure most commonly injured as a result of an anterior dislocation of the shoulder is the:

1. Musculocutaneous nerve
2. Axillary nerve
3. Axillary artery
4. Median nerve

Ans. 2. Axillary Nerve

The axillary nerve is at greatest risk for injury. Occasionally a more severe neurologic deficit can occur as a result of injury to the brachial plexus.

USMLE Case Scenario

A 45-year-old carpenter describes a fall on the outstretched hand during routine activities. Multiple radiographic views show no distinct fracture. He is tender to palpation in the anatomic snuffbox. The most suitable method of management is:

1. Diagnose sprained wrist and apply an elastic bandage
2. Diagnose suspected scaphoid fracture and apply a short-arm cast to include the thumb
3. Immobilize the wrist
4. Prescribe NSAIDS/Salicylates and permit continued activity
5. Do an open reduction
6. Wait and watch till any complication occurs

Ans. 2. Diagnose suspected scaphoid fracture and apply a short-arm cast to include the thumb

A short-arm cast to include the thumb is the most appropriate treatment. Salicylates and continued activity would not treat scaphoid fracture. Fracture scaphoid is a tricky thing to diagnose.

If no fracture is noted initially, the cast is applied and films are taken at 10 days to 2 weeks since nondisplaced scaphoid fractures are often more easily visualized at that time.

USMLE Case Scenario

Dislocation of the Radial head with a fracture of the Proximal Third of the ulna is known as:

1. Monteggia's deformity
2. Galezzi deformity
3. Colles deformity
4. Subluxation
5. Nursemaids elbow

Ans. 1. Monteggia's deformity

USMLE Case Scenario

Compartment Syndrome results from increasing pressures in the fascial compartments of the arm or leg. Pulselessness, Extreme, pallor of the extremity, motor paralysis and paresthesias are all components of the syndrome. Pain is usually seen as:

1. Pain on active flexion of the fingers or toes
2. Pain on passive flexion of the fingers or toes

3. Pain on lateral movements of the fingers or toes
4. Pain on passive extension of the fingers or toes

Ans. 4. Pain on passive extension of the fingers or toes

The patient will usually hold the injured part in a position of flexion to maximally relax the fascia and reduce the pain; passive extension will usually produce severe pain.

USMLE Case Scenario

Osteitis fibrosa cystic or Recklinghausen disease of the bone:

1. Is bone mineralization due to rapid mobilization of mineral salts
2. Is bone mineralization due to nonmobilization of mineral salts
3. Is bone demineralization due to rapid mobilization of mineral salts
4. Is bone demineralization due to nonmobilization of mineral salts

Ans. 3. Is bone demineralization due to rapid mobilization of mineral salts

USMLE Case Scenario

In Erb (Erb-Duchenne) palsy, the upper roots of the brachial plexus are injured (C5–6). A deformity resulting in paralysis of the shoulder and arm muscles; the arm hangs limply to the side and is extended and internally rotated is usually due to:

1. C5 –C6 injury
2. C7 –C8 injury
3. C2 –C3 injury
4. C8 –T1 injury

Ans. 1. C5–C6 injury

In Erb (or Erb-Duchenne) palsy, the upper roots of the brachial plexus are injured (C5–6). Lower trunk is involved in Klumpkes Palsy

USMLE Case Scenario

Podagra is usually seen as:

1. Pain in the thoracic vertebrae
2. Pain in the lumbar vertebrae
3. Pain in the metacarpal phalangeal joint
4. Pain in the metatarsal phalangeal joint
5. Pain in the Hip joint
6. Pain in the knee joint

Ans. 4. Pain in the metatarsal phalangeal joint

USMLE Case Scenario

A 32-year-old construction worker working in a high rise building arrives in the emergency department of New York after an accident on the job. The tendon of the biceps brachi in the arm at the elbow has been severed by a laceration due to a sharp instrument that extends 2.1 cm medially from the tendon. Which of the following structures is likely to have been injured by medial extension of the laceration?

1. Brachial artery
2. Ulnar nerve
3. Musculocutaneous nerve
4. Profunda brachii artery
5. Radial nerve
6. Axillary nerve

Ans. 1. Brachial artery

The brachial artery is immediately medial to the tendon of the biceps brachii at the elbow. As the artery enters the forearm, it is covered by the bicipit alaponeurosis, a broadening of the biceps tendon.

USMLE Case Scenario

An 80-year-old woman residing in South Texas complains of nearly 4 month history of worsening gait and low back pain that is worse on walking. She has been fairly healthy and only takes iron supplements. On examination, she has hypoactive muscle stretch reflexes in the legs. The plain X-rays of the lumbosacral region show degenerative changes that seem age-appropriate. Which of the following is the most likely diagnosis?

1. Acute lumbar disk herniation
2. Cervical stenosis
3. Lumbar stenosis
4. Myeloma
5. Myopathy
6. Normal pressure hydrocephalus (NPH)

Ans. 3. Lumbar stenosis

It is caused by degenerative changes in the lumbosacral spine. The points in favor are of history of low back pain with subtle physical examination findings referable to impingement on motor and sensory roots in the lumbar canal.

USMLE Case Scenario

A 15-year-old boy was treated for retinoblastoma at the age of 1 year presented with pain and swelling around the knee, X-ray showed some typical appearance. Most likely diagnosis is:

1. Osteosarcoma
2. Osteoclastoma
3. Osteoid osteoma
4. Bone cyst
5. Chondroma
6. Chondrosarcoma

Ans. 1. Osteosarcoma

Association of Retinoblastoma and Osteosarcoma is well established.

USMLE Case Scenario

A 46-year-old woman presents with chronic widespread musculoskeletal pain, fatigue, and frequent headaches. She states that her musculoskeletal pain improves slightly with exercise. On examination, painful trigger points are produced by palpitation of the trapezius and lateral epicondyle of the elbow. Signs of inflammation are absent and laboratory studies are within normal. Most likely diagnosis is:

1. Chronic Fatigue
2. Malignancy
3. Myositis
4. Neuropathy
5. Fibromyalgia

Ans. 5. Fibromyalgia

USMLE Case Scenario

A 30-year-old woman consults a physician because of a small but painless, pea-like lesion on the extensor aspect of her right wrist. She finds the lesion causing cosmetic disfigurement. Grossly the lesion is white and translucent and oozes gelatinous material when cut. Most likely diagnosis is:

1. Osteosarcoma
2. Osteoclastoma
3. Osteoid Osteoma
4. Bone cyst
5. Chondroma
6. Chondrosarcoma
7. Ganglion cyst

Ans. 7. Ganglion cyst

USMLE Case Scenario

A 72-year-old man, a farmer by occupation from comes for a follow-up visit. The man was a farmer and has been healthy for most of his life. Gamma-glutamyltranspeptidase level and total calcium level are within normal limits. Upon further questioning, the man denies any abdominal pain, nausea, vomiting, or other gastrointestinal symptoms. His Serum levels show:

- **I. Serum alanine aminotransferase (ALT) 15 U/L**
- **II. Serum alkaline phosphatase 770 U/L**
- **III. Serum aspartate aminotransferase (AST) 26 U/L**
- **IV. Total serum bilirubin 0.8 mg/dL**

But his systemic examination shows slightly diminished hearing and a mild, chronic bilateral tinnitus. The most likely diagnosis is:

1. Osteoclastoma
2. Osteoid osteoma
3. Bone cyst
4. Chondroma
5. Chondrosarcoma
6. Marble bone disease
7. Ganglion cyst
8. Osteitis deformans

Ans. 8. Osteitis deformans

Pagets Disease itself has high Serum Alkaline phosphatase levels

USMLE Case Scenario

A 13-year-old boy has a solitary lesion in his left femur which is exquisitely painful. Pain is described as a persistent discomfort unrelated to activity or rest and is often worse at night. Curiously, pain is relieved for several hours by the use of Nonsteroidal anti-inflammatory drugs. The lesion is composed of a central nidus of closely packed trabeculae of woven bone. Most likely lesion is:

1. Bone cyst
2. Chondroma
3. Chondrosarcoma
4. Osteoid osteoma
5. Enchondromas
6. Marble bone disease
7. Ganglion cyst

Ans. 4. Osteoid osteoma

USMLE Case Scenario

A benign growth of hyaline cartilage lying in the medullary cavity of a bone arising from ectopic cartilaginous rests in the phalanges and metacarpals was noticed by an orthopedician. Radiographically it is seen to be producing a lucent defect with well defined margins and surrounding sclerotic reactive bone is most likely:

1. Osteoclastoma
2. Osteoid osteoma
3. Bone cyst
4. Chondroma
5. Chondrosarcoma
6. Enchondroma
7. Marble bone disease
8. Ganglion cyst
9. Osteitis deformans

Ans. 6. Enchondroma

USMLE Case Scenario

A 15-year-old has a lesion in the metaphyseal end of his distal femur. Areas of lytic bone destruction mixed with areas of reactive and tumor bone formations are seen. This tumor is seen to be rapidly permeating through the overlying cortex into the subperiosteal space. It produces a characteristic appearance of trabecular bone oriented at right angles to the underlying cortical surface.

Most likely tumor diagnosis is:

1. Osteosarcoma
2. Osteoid osteoma
3. Bone cyst
4. Chondroma
5. Chondrosarcoma

Ans. 1. Osteosarcoma

USMLE Case Scenario

A young girl presents with complaints of local pain and swelling in her femur. There is fever, leukocytosis, and an increased erythrocyte sedimentation rate. The radiographic appearance shows the lesion to be occurring in the diaphysis with periosteal elevation. Varying degrees of bone destruction and varying degrees of reactive new bone formation create a wide range of radiographic appearances. Microscopically, the tumor is composed of uniform round cells gathered in nests or cords and separated by thin fibrous septa. The Tumor is positive for glycogen on periodic acid–Schiff.

Most likely cause is:

1. Osteoid osteoma
2. Bone cyst
3. Chondroma
4. Chondrosarcoma
5. Sarcoma

Ans. 5. Sarcoma

I mean Ewings Sarcoma. Sometimes questions are put like this

USMLE Case Scenario

15-year-old boy presented with a mass in the distal femur. X-ray from the lesion showed features of Codman's Triangle and Sun ray appearance. The diagnosis is most likely to be:

1. Osteosarcoma
2. Ewing's sarcoma
3. Osteoclastoma
4. Chondroblastoma

Ans. 1. Osteosarcoma

USMLE Case Scenario

A 72-year-old engineer from Colarado has pain and discomfort in addition to fever, anemia hypercalcemia and renal failure related to extensive skeletal involvement and the abnormal production of immunoglobulins. The lesions would be characteristic of:

1. Myeloma
2. Osteoid Osteoma
3. Bone cyst
4. Chondroma
5. Chondrosarcoma
6. Sarcoma

Ans. 1. Myeloma

USMLE Case Scenario

An obese boy in 2nd decade presents with Pain and with limited Flexion, Abduction of femoral head seen downwards and Posteriorly has:

1. Perthes disease
2. Keinbocks disease
3. SCFE
4. Os good Schalters Disease

Ans. 3. SCFE

USMLE Case Scenario

A 13-year-old boy with a hot, tender swelling arising from diaphysis of bone with characteristic feature of onion skinning has:

1. Myeloma
2. Osteoid osteoma
3. Bone cyst
4. Chondroma
5. Chondrosarcoma
6. Sarcoma

Ans. 6. Ewings Sarcoma

USMLE Case Scenario

A 10-year-old boy with Pain and limp. X-ray shows distorted femoral neck and Head:

1. Perthes disease
2. Keinbocks disease
3. SCFE
4. Os good Schalters disease

Ans. 1. Perthes disease

USMLE Case Scenario

An itching, squeezing pain sensation after amputation that an amputated limb is still attached and functioning with intensely painful sensations is called as:

1. Phantom Limb
2. RDS
3. Myositis Ossificans
4. Sudecks Atrophy
5. Causalgia
6. Allodynia

Ans. 1. Phantom Limb

USMLE Case Scenario

Complex and progressive disease with pain swelling and changes in skin without demonstrable nerve lesions after injury:

1. Phantom Limb
2. Reflex Sympathetic Dystrophy
3. Myositis Ossificans
4. Causalgia
5. Allodynia

Ans. 2. Reflex Sympathetic Dystrophy

USMLE Case Scenario

A boy presents with triad of Lytic bony lesions on skull, diabetes Insipidus and Exomphalos has:

1. Dercums Disease
2. Diidmoad Syndrome
3. Multiple Myeloma
4. Metastasis
5. Hand Schuller Christian Disease

Ans. 5. Hand Schuller Christian Disease

USMLE Case Scenario

A 44-year-old female who is a typist presents to her physician with mild complaints of burning and tingling sensations in the left hand for several months. She is frequently awakened at night by pain in the same hand. The pain is elicited by extreme dorsiflexion of the wrist. Which of the following is the most likely diagnosis?

1. Angina pectoris
2. Ainhum
3. Colles fracture
4. Cubital tunnel syndrome
5. Carpal tunnel syndrome
6. Dupuytren contracture
7. Sudecks dystrophy
8. Fibrositis

Ans. 5. Carpal tunnel syndrome

Carpal tunnel syndrome is a result of compression of the median nerve. Pain, tingling sensations and hypoesthesia in the distribution of the median nerve are the main manifestations. Pain upon percussion on the volar aspect of the wrist (Tinel sign) is characteristic. Carpal tunnel syndrome is most often idiopathic, but may represent a manifestation of underlying disorders such as:

- **Rheumatoid arthritis**
- **Sarcoidosis**
- **Amyloidosis**
- **Acromegaly**
- **Leukemia**

USMLE Case Scenario

An infant presents with failure to thrive, Pancytopenia. Bones are brittle and fracture easily. Infantile Osteopetrosis is the diagnosis. Defect is found in:

1. Osteocytes
2. Osteoblasts
3. Osteoclasts
4. Blood vessels

Ans. 3. Osteoclasts

USMLE Case Scenario

A two-year-old presents with multiple fractures in different stages of healing brought by over concerned parents. Most likely cause is:

1. Osteogenesis imperfecta
2. Sexual abuse
3. Myositis ossificans
4. Battered baby syndrome

Ans. 4. Battered baby syndrome

USMLE Case Scenario

A six-year-old with bilateral and symmetrical fractures and blue sclera. Bones are osteopenic and brittle. Likely cause is:

1. Osteogenesis imperfecta
2. Sexual abuse
3. Myositis ossificans
4. Battered baby syndrome

Ans. 1. Osteogenesis imperfecta

USMLE Case Scenario

A patient with multiple injuries on day 2 detiorates and develops Tachycardia, Tachypnea, ↓PO2 and rash. Most likely cause is:

1. Hemorrhage
2. Embolism
3. Thrombosis
4. Neurogenic shock

Ans. 2. Embolism

USMLE Case Scenario

Meralgia parasthetica is due to the involvement of:

1. Medial cutaneous nerve of thigh
2. Lateral cutaneous nerve of thigh
3. Sural nerve
4. Femoral nerve
5. Obturator nerve
6. Saphenous nerve
7. Iliohypogastric nerve
8. Ilioinguinal nerve

Ans. 2. Lateral cutaneous nerve of thigh

USMLE Case Scenario

Claw hand is caused by lesion involving:

1. Ulnar nerve
2. Median nerve
3. Radial nerve
4. Posterior interosseous nerve

Ans. 1. Ulnar nerve

USMLE Case Scenario

Disorder of the growth plate in which the hypertrophic cartilage is not resorbed and ossified normally resulting in masses of cartilage with disorderly arrangement of the chondrocytes showing variable proliferative and hypertrophic changes and masses located in the metaphyses in close association with the growth plate in children with common sites of involvement are the ends of long bones is a feature of:

1. Myeloma
2. Osteoid osteoma
3. Bone cyst
4. Enchondroma
5. Chondrosarcoma
6. Sarcoma

Ans. 4. Enchondroma

USMLE Case Scenario

A 45-year-old Scandinavian has a family history has a fixed flexion contracture of the hand where the fingers bend towards the palm and cannot be fully extended. Pathology is underlying contractures of the palmar aponeurosis. Most likely condition is:

1. Tenosynovitis
2. Carpal tunnel syndrome
3. Volkmans contracture
4. Ape hand
5. Dupuytren's contracture

Ans. 5. Dupuytren's contracture

USMLE Case Scenario

A drug which is an Activator of calcium sensing receptor in the parathyroid gland (augments feedback inhibition of PTH by Ca^{++}) is:

1. Etidronate
2. Cinacalcet
3. Pamidronate
4. Plicamycin
5. Gallium nitrate

Ans. 2. Cinacalcet

USMLE Case Scenario

In Paget's Disease:

1. Calcium levels ↑, Phosphate levels ↑
2. Calcium levels ↑, Phosphate levels ↓
3. Calcium level ↓, Phosphate levels ↓
4. Calcium levels N, Phosphate levels ↑
5. Calcium levels ↑, Phosphate levels N
6. Calcium levels N, Phosphate levels N

Ans. 6. Calcium levels N, Phosphate levels N

USMLE Case Scenario

A disease is characterized by Deposition of Pyrophosphate crystals with Crystals Rhomboid in shape, positively Birefrigent and Usually large joints affected. Most likely cause is:

1. Psoriatic arthritis
2. Gouty arthritis
3. Alkaptonuria
4. CPPD deposition disease
5. Ankylosing spondylitis

Ans. 4. CPPD deposition disease

USMLE Case Scenario

Indicator of bone formation is:

1. AFP
2. C-telopeptide
3. Deoxypyridinoline (DPD)

4. Tartrate-resistant acid phosphatase
5. Osteocalcin
6. Pyridinium Crosslinks
7. GGT

Ans. 5. Osteocalcin

USMLE Case Scenario

Increased bone density is seen in:

1. Hypervitaminosis B and Hypervitaminosis D
2. Hypervitaminosis C and Hypervitaminosis D
3. Hypervitaminosis E and Hypervitaminosis D
4. Hypervitaminosis A and Hypervitaminosis D
5. Hypervitaminosis B and Hypervitaminosis C
6. Hypervitaminosis A and Hypervitaminosis C

Ans. 4. Hypervitaminosis A and Hypervitaminosis D

USMLE Case Scenario

A patient developed breathlessness and chest pain, on second postoperative day after a total hip replacement. Echocardiography showed right ventricular dilatation and tricuspid regurgitation. What is the most likely diagnosis:

1. Acute MI
2. Pulmonary embolism
3. Hypotensive shock
4. Cardiac tamponade

Ans. 2. Pulmonary embolism

USMLE Case Scenario

A 30-year-old man had road traffic accident and sustained fracture of femur. Two days later he developed sudden breathlessness. The most probable cause can be:

1. Pneumonia
2. Congestive heart failure
3. Bronchial asthma
4. Fat Embolism

Ans. 4. Fat Embolism

USMLE Case Scenario

A 22-year-old young boy presents to a Rheumatology clinic with chief complaints of low back pain for the past 6 months which was accompanied by stiffness of the lower spine. He denies any gastrointestinal or genital infections. Detailed Physical Examination reveals moderate limitation of back motion and tenderness of the lower spine. X-ray films of the vertebral column and pelvic region show flattening of the lumbar curve and subchondral bone erosion involving the sacroiliac joints. Which of the following is the most likely diagnosis?

1. Psoriatic arthritis
2. Gout
3. Caplans syndrome
4. Ankylosing spondylitis
5. Degenerative joint disease
6. Reiter syndrome

7. Seronegative rheumatoid arthritis
8. Still disease
9. Caplans syndrome

Ans. 4. Ankylosing spondylitis

It should be suspected in any young person complaining of chronic lower back pain and confirmed by radiographs or CT scans of sacroiliac joints.

USMLE Case Scenario

Brown Tumor is seen in:

1. Hypothyroidism
2. Hyperthyroidism
3. Hypoparathyroidism
4. Hyperparathyroidism

Ans. 4. Hyperparathyroidism

USMLE Case Scenario

Feature of a bony disease is generalized osteopenia with recurrent fractures and skeletal deformity. Fracture healing however is normal. Fracture in utero may be seen. Laxity of joint ligaments leads to hypermobility. The disease is Identified as Osteogenesis imperfecta. Defect lies in:

1. Elastin
2. Chondroblasts
3. Chondrocutes
4. Osteoblasts
5. Osteocytes
6. Osteoclasts
7. Collagen
8. Fibrillin

Ans. 7. Collagen

USMLE Case Scenario

A nerve of upper limb Supplies Extensor Compartment of Arm and Forearm, traverses Spiral groove and is accompanied by Profunda Brachii vessels is:

1. Ulnar nerve
2. Median nerve
3. Radial nerve
4. Musculocutaneous nerve
5. Posterior interosseous nerve
6. Axillary nerve
7. Suprascapular nerve

Ans. 3. Radial nerve

USMLE Case Scenario

The rotator cuff consists of the tendons of the:

1. Subclavius, infraspinatus, subscapularis and teres major muscles
2. Subclavius, infraspinatus, subscapularis and teres minor muscles
3. Supraspinatus, latismusdorsi, subscapularis and teres minor muscles
4. Supraspinatus, infraspinatus, subscapularis and teres minor muscles

Ans. 4. Supraspinatus, infraspinatus, subscapularis and teres minor muscles

USMLE Case Scenario

Wartenburgs Syndrome is:

1. Entrapment of Sensory branch of Radial nerve as it emerges beneath Brachioradialis proximal to Radial Styloid process
2. Entrapment of motor branch of ulnar nerve as it emerges beneath Brachioradialis proximal to Radial Styloid process
3. Entrapment of Sensory branch of median nerve as it emerges beneath Brachioradialis proximal to Radial Styloid process
4. Entrapment of motor branch of Radial nerve as it emerges beneath Brachioradialis proximal to Radial Styloid process

Ans. 1. Entrapment of Sensory branch of Radial nerve as it emerges beneath Brachioradialis proximal to Radial Styloid process

USMLE Case Scenario

Osteopathia striata is:

1. Marble bone disease
2. Spotted bone disease
3. Stripped bone disease
4. Candle bone disease

Ans. 3. Stripped bone disease

USMLE Case Scenario

Panners disease is:

1. Osteochondritis of lunate
2. Osteochondritis of Metatarsal head
3. Osteochondritis of capitulum
4. Osteochondritis of vertebrae
5. Osteochondritis of patella

Ans. 3. Osteochondritis of capitulum

USMLE Case Scenario

A bony disease is characterized Increased generation and overactivity of osteoclasts and the calcification rate is characteristically increased with increased urinary excretion of small peptides containing hydroxyproline reflects:

1. Myeloma
2. Osteogenesis imperfecta
3. Pagets disease
4. Eosinophilic granuloma
5. Caffeys disease

Ans. 3. Pagets Disease

USMLE Case Scenario

A tumor like lesion which is developmental in origin and hormone dependent. Pathology is replacement of bone by fibrous tissue. X-ray shows 'Ground glass' appearance and 'Chinese lettering of bone. Most likely disease is:

1. Pagets disease
2. Marble bone disease
3. Osteoma
4. Osteoclastoma
5. Dysplasia of fibrous type

Ans. 5. Dysplasia of fibrous type

USMLE Case Scenario

A bony disease is characterized Increased generation and overactivity of osteoclasts and the calcification rate is characteristically increased with increased urinary excretion of small peptides containing hydroxyproline reflects:

1. Myeloma
2. Osteogenesis imperfecta
3. Pagets disease
4. Eosinophilic granuloma
5. Caffeys disease

Ans. 3. Pagets Disease

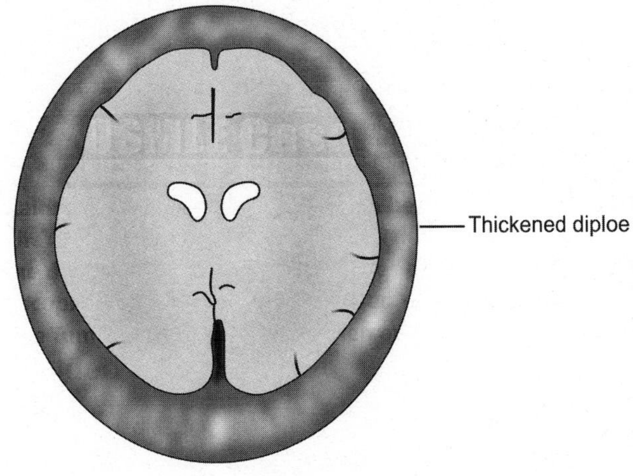

Pagets disease

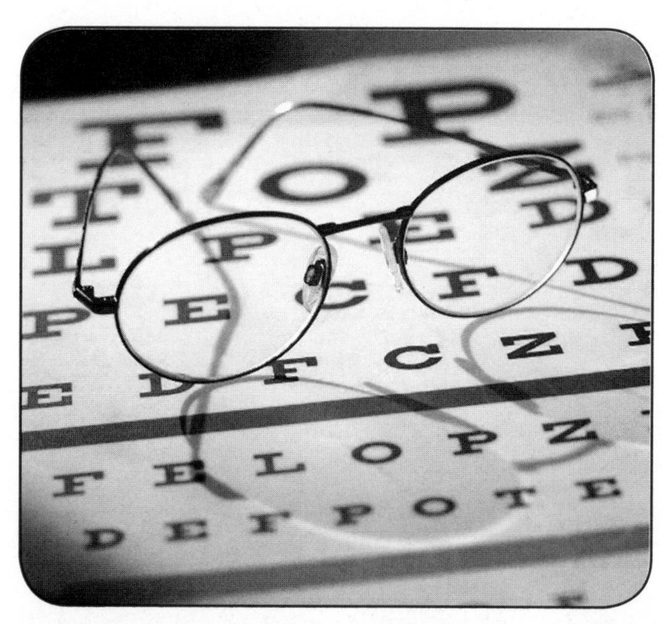

OPHTHALMOLOGY

Ophthalmology 7

Anatomy of Eye

Muscles of eye and their innervations

- The **'Extorter'** of Eye Ball is **Inferior Oblique and Inferior Rectus**
- The **'Intorter'** of Eye ball is **Superior Oblique and Superior Rectus**
- Action of Superior oblique is **Abduction, Intorsion and depression**
- Dilator Pupillae dilates pupil and is supplied by **Sympathetics**
- Sphincter Pupillae constricts pupil and is supplied by **Parasympathetics**

LR_6SO_4

- Lateral Rectus is supplied by **6th Cranial Nerve** (Abducent)
- Superior Oblique is supplied by **4th Cranial Nerve** (Trochlear)
- Rest other ocular muscles are supplied by **3rd Cranial Nerve** (Occulomotor)
- Levator palpabrae superior is supplied by 3rd caranial nerve
- Muscle attached to posterior tarsal margin: **Mullers muscle**
- Third nerve gets affected in a variety of syndromes of Midbrain such as:
  - **Benedict's Syndrome**
  - **Claude's Syndrome**
  - **Weber's Syndrome**
  - **Nothnagel's Syndrome**

Trigeminal nerve (Fifth Cranial nerve) is involved in **afferent pathway of corneal reflex**

Gems about Pupil

- Sphincter pupillae is a circular **'constrictor muscle'** innervated by **Parasympathetic** Nervous system
- Dilator Pupillae is a **'radial dilator'** innervated by **Sympathetic** Nervous system
- Pupillary inequality is called **'Anisocoria'**
- **III Nerve lesion** causes **dilated pupil, Ptosis**
- **Horners' syndrome causes constricted pupil**
- **Argyl Robertson Pupil:** Small pupils, irregular in shapes which do not react to light but react to accommodation. (**ARP: Accomdation Reflex present)**
- **Marcus Gunn Pupil (Pupillary Escape):** Illumination of one eye normally produces constriction. In case light source is swung from eye to eye, affected pupil may **'paradoxically' dilate. (Marcus Gunn Pupil) (Defect anterior to optic chiasma)**
- **Aides Pupil:** It is dysfunction of constrictor muscle and hence does not respond to light or to accommodation **(Tonic pupil)**

Cornea

- **The cornea is quite unlike most tissues in that it is perfectly transparent**
- **The epithelium** consists of a thin layer of **nonkeratinized stratified squamous**

- Corneal epithelium is **very thin** (only a few cells thick)
- Corneal epithelium lies flat against the underlying substantia propria.
- There is **absence of connective tissue** papillae
- **The Basement membrane** between corneal epithelium and substantia propria is exceptionally thick and is called **Bowman's membrane**
- **The substantia propria** of the cornea is mostly collagen and ground substance, with fibroblasts as the most common cell type
- Collagen of the cornea is organized into extremely **regular layers**. All the collagen fibers in one layer arranged in parallel, and alternating layers run in different directions
- Corneal connective tissue has no blood vessels
- Even though cells of the cornea are not very active metabolically, they still need oxygen and nutrients
- As long as the cornea is in direct contact with air, oxygen can be absorbed directly
- Nutrients can diffuse into cornea from aqueous humor. **(avascular coat)**
- Cells of corneal connective tissue are limited to fibroblasts
- **There is** no immune-system component; hence the relative ease with which corneal tissue can be transplanted without need for careful tissue typing
- **Descemet's membrane** is a thick basal lamina made of elastic fibers over endothelium
- **Corneal endothelium** is simple squamous epithelium present below Descemet's membrane. Corneal epithelium contains **free nerve endings**. Since pain seems to be the only sensation of cornea.

Layers of Retina

- Retinal pigment epithelium (RPE)
- Layer of rod and cone cells outer segments
- Outer limiting membrane
- Outer nuclear layer
- Outer plexiform layer
- Inner nuclear layer
- Inner plexiform layer
- Ganglion cell layer
- Nerve fiber layer
- Internal limiting membrane

The 'Medial Longitudinal Fasciculus'

The Medial longitudinal fasciculus (MLF) connects the

- **Oculomotor (III)**
- **Trochlear (IV)**
- **Abducens (VI) nuclei**

It is essential for **conjugate gaze**

'Alesion in the MLF will result in the inability to medially rotate (adduct) the ipsilateral eye on attempted lateral gaze.' (**Intranuclear ophthalmoplegia INO**)

However, a lesion of the motor fibers of the right oculomotor nerve would also leads to the same symptoms. The way to truly distinguish between an INO from a lesion of the medial rectus muscle or a lesion of the motor fibers of CN III is to determine whether the patient can converge her eyes. If the innervation of the medial rectus muscle is interrupted the patient will not be able to move the ipsilateral eye medially for either conjugate or dysconjugate (convergence) movements. **However, if the lesion is in the MLF this would only affect conjugate movement and not convergence.**

Important Membranes in Ophthalmology

Bowman's Membrane	**'Anterior' limiting membrane of Cornea**
Descemet's Membrane	**'Posterior' limiting membrane of Cornea**
Bruch's Membrane	**Pigment membrane in Retina**
Elsching's Membrane	**Astroglial membrane covering Optic Disk**

Important Glands in Ophthalmology

• Glands of **Zeis**	• **Sebaceous** glands
• Glands of **Moll**	• **Modified sweat** glands
• Glands of **Krause and Wolfring**	• **Accessory Lacrimal** glands

Structures Passing Through 'Inferior Orbital Fissure'

- **Maxillary division** of Trigeminal nerve
- **Infraorbital artery**
- **Zygomatic nerve**
- **Branches of inferior ophthalmic vein**

'The Annulus of Zinn', also known as the 'Annular tendon' or 'Common Tendinous Ring'

It is a ring of fibrous tissue surrounding the optic nerve at its entrance at the apex of the orbit? It is the origin for five of the six extraocular muscles

Annulus of Zinn (Annulus communis tendinis) is seen to transmit: **(NAO)**

- **Occulomotor nerve**
- **Nasociliary nerve**
- **Abducent nerve**

Structures Passing Through 'Superior Orbital Fissure' are

Live Free To See No Insult At All

- **Lacrimal Nerve**
- **Frontal Nerve**
- **Trochlear Nerve**
- **Superior Ophthalmic Vein**
- **Nasociliary Nerve**
- **Inferior Ophthlamic vein**
- **Abducent Nerve**

Structures Passing Through 'Optic Canal'

Structures passing through **'Optic Canal'**

- **Optic nerve and ophthalmic artery**

'Optic Nerve Glioma'

- Causes **gradual, painless loss of vision**
- A tumor of **first decade of life**

Associated with
- **Optic atrophy**
- **Papilledema**
- **Neurofibromatosis**

Embryology of Eye (Very Important Topic for PG examinations)

Mesoderm	Surface ectoderm	Neuroectoderm
Sclera	Corneal epithelium	Epithelium of iris and ciliary body
Choroid	Conjunctival epithelium	Muscles of iris (constrictor pupillae and dilator pupillae)
Corneal stroma and endothelium	Lens	**Retinal pigment epithelium**
Iris **stroma and endothelium**	Lacrimal and tarsal glands	**Optic** vesicle
Blood vessels		**Optic** nerve
Muscles **except iris muscles**	**L2 C2**	Part of vitreous
But only smooth muscles of iris are derived from mesoderm		
Part of vitreous		

Important Milestones in development of Eye

- Eye of newborn is **'Hypermetropic'** by 2 – 3D
- Myelination of optic nerve is **complete at birth**
- Orbit is **divergent**
- At 6 weeks **Fixation reflex** is apparent
- At 2 – 4 months is **critical period** for development of fixation reflex
- During **Ist 6 months** binocular single vision develops
- Binocular vision has important role in-**depth perception**
- At **6 – 8 months depth perception** develops

Angles of Eye

- **Alpha angle:** Between visual axis and optical axis
- **Kappa angle:** Between puppilary axis and visual axis
- **Visual angle:** Angle subtended by object at nodal point of lens

Ophthalmological Tests

Direct Ophthalmoscopy	Indirect Ophthalmoscopy
Condensing lens **not required**	Condensing lens **required**
Examination **close** to patient	Examination at a **distance**
Image is **virtual and erect**	**Image is real and inverted**
Magnification is **15 times**	Magnification **is 5 times**
Stereopsis **absent**	Stereopsis **present**
Area of field in focus **is 2 disk diopters**	Area of field in focus **is 8 disk diopters**
Examination through hazy media **not possible**	Examination through **hazy media possible**
Illumination **not so bright**	Illumination **bright** is done for **examination of periphery of retina** up to orra seratta.

Various other Important Tests

- **Keratometry**: Measures **Curvature** of Cornea
- **Pachymetry**: **Thickness** of cornea
- **Campimetry**: Measures field of vision
- **Electronystatogram**: Graph of movement of eye
- **Anomoloscope** detects **color blindness**
- **Retinoscopy: Objective assessment of refractive state of eye**

Tonometry measures IOP

Tonography measures rate of fall in IOP from which facility of aqeous outflow is measured

- **Gonioscopy measures angle of anterior chamber**
- **Best type tonometry is applanation tonometry**
- **Arden ratio is seen in EOG**

Macular Function is tested by

- **Indirect slit lamp biomicroscopy**
- **Photo stress test**
- **Two point discrimination test (card board test)**
- **Amsler grid test**
- **Maddox rod test**
- **Entopic view test**
- **LASER interferometry**

Visual Tests Done in Infants

- **Visual evoked potentials**
- **Teller acuity tests**
- **Cardiff acuity tests**
- **Visual acuity by Landolts rings**

- **Swinging flash light test** tests: Pupil
- **Snellens chart tests**: Vision
- **Retinoscopy** detects errors of refraction

Important Points about Lids

- **Internal hordeolum: acute inflammation of 'Zeis glands.'**
- **Chalazion is chronic inflammation of 'Meibomian gland'**
- **'Recurrent'chlazion is predisposed to sebaceous cell carcinoma**
- **'Basal cell carcinoma' is the most common type of lid carcinoma**
- **Adhesion of margins of two lids is called Ankyloblepharon.**

Congenital Chronic Dacrocystitis

- Failure of nasolacrimal duct to open into inferior meatus of noseleads to dacrocystitis
- Presents with
- **Epiphora (abnormal tear overflow)**

- **Regurgitation of pus**
- Treated by: **Massage over Lacrimal sac, Lacrimal syringing, Probing, Intubation with silicone tube, Dacrosystorhinostomy**
- **Dacrocystectomy**
- **Conjunctivocystorhinostomy**

Field Defects

'Visual Field Defects'

The main points for the exam are:

- Left homonymous hemianopia means visual field defect to the left, i.e. lesion of right optic tract
- Homonymous quadrantanopias: **PITS** (Parietal-Inferior, Temporal-Superior)
- Incongruous defects = optic tract lesion; congruous defects= optic radiation lesion or occipital cortex

Homonymous Hemianopia

- **Incongruous defects: Lesion of optic tract**
- **Congruous defects: Lesion of optic radiation or occipital cortex**
- **Macula sparing: Lesion of occipital cortex**

Homonymous Quadrantanopia

- Superior: Lesion of temporal lobe
- Inferior: Lesion of parietal lobe
- Mnemonic = PITS (Parietal-Inferior, Temporal-Superior)

Bitemporal Hemianopia

- Lesion of **optic chiasm**
- **Upper quadrant defect > lower quadrant defect = inferior chiasmal compression**, commonly a pituitary tumor
- **Lower quadrant defect > upper quadrant defect = superior chiasmal compression**, commonly a craniopharyngioma.

Cranial Nerve II (OPTIC Nerve)

- It is the nerve of **Vision**
- It is **not a true nerve** but basically a **diverticulum of the brain** or a tract of the C N S
- It is **covered by the meninges** and hence any infection can spread directly to the brain
- The optic nerve has **no neurilemma** sheath and once damaged it **cannot regenerate**
- It leaves the orbit through the **Optic Canal**.

The complete optic pathway has:

1. A receptor
2. A pathway to the Thalamus
3. A nucleus in the Thalamus
4. A radiation from the thalamus to the Cortex
5. A sensory area in the Cortex

The receptors are the **rods and cones of the retina** and the thalamic nucleus for vision is the **lateral geniculate body**.

Functionally, the retina is composed of 3 elements, i.e. three neurones carry the impulses in the retina 'Itself', these are:

1. **The receptor cells (The rods and cones)**
2. **The bipolar nerve cells**
3. **The ganglion cells**

- The **rods and cones** synapse with the bipolar cells (in the retina)
- The **bipolar cells** synapse with the ganglion cells (in the retina also)
- The **axons of the ganglion cells** from the **optic nerve** which contains nasal and temporal fibers.

- The optic nerves pass to the **optic chiasma** (which lies immediately in front of the pituitary gland)
- The **nasal fibers of the optic nerve cross to the opposite side while the temporal fibers remain on the same side**
- The part of the visual pathway which passes backwards from the chiasma is called the **optic tract**
- Each optic tract carries **«temporal» fibers of its «own» side and «nasal» fibers from the «opposite» side**
- Most of the fibers of the optic tract end in the **lateral geniculate body** while some fibers leave the optic tract to end in the superior colliculus of the midbrain and in the **pretectal nucleus.**

The fibers of the optic tract which reach the superior Colliculus and the pretectal nucleus are concerned with the light reflex (i.e. narrowing of the pupil in response to excess light) while those fibers of the optic tract which reach the **lateral geniculate body** from part of the visual pathway which will reach the visual cortex

The optic radiation (or the geniculo-calcarine tract) [The pathway from the lateral geniculate body to the visual area of the cortex]

The lateral geniculate body (LGB) is the thalamic center for vision

The axons of the cells of the LGB form the **«optic radiation»** which passes in the internal capsule to reach to the **«striate area» or the Area 17 or the Visual Area in the occipital lobe**

The optic radiation has fibers running downwards and forwards

The visual area

The **«Visual Area»** surrounds the calcarine fissure on the medial surface of the occipital lobe. It is formed of the **cuneus** and the **lingual gyrus.**

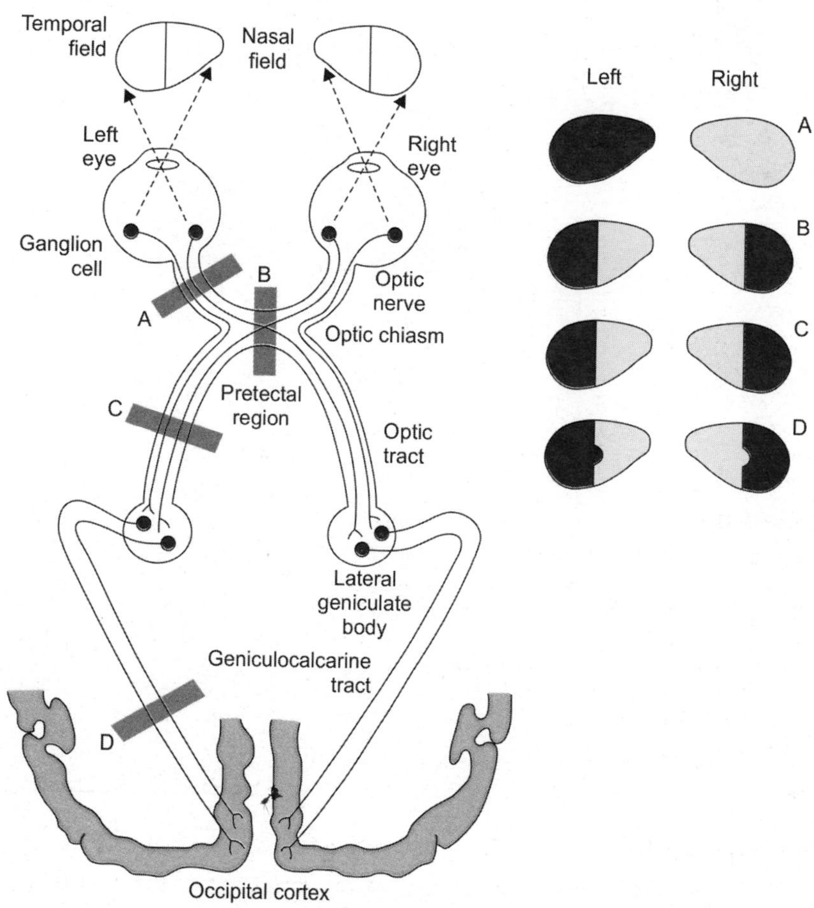

Lesions of optic pathway

- Destruction to one **optic nerve** → **blindness** in the corresponding eye
- Lesion to the middle part of the optic **chiasma** is produced usually from a rumor of the pituitary gland (which lies very close to the optic chiasma). The nasal fibers of the optic nerve which decussate in the chiasma are destroyed and visual impulses from the nasal halves of each retina cannot pass to the optic tract; this means that there will be a **defect in the temporal field of each eye** (a condition called **Bitemporal hemianopia**); in this case the left eye does not see images in the left ½ if its field and the right eye does not see images in the right ½ of its field
- A **lesion of the optic tract** interrupts fibers from **one half of each retina**. If the left tract is destroyed, visual function will be lost in the left halves of both retinas. In this case there is **blindness for objects in the right ½ of each field of vision**; this condition is called **right homonymous hemianopia**. In spite of the fact that one optic tract may be completely interrupted, vision is sometimes preserved in small area (the area of the macula) which is the center of fixation of the eye
- A lesion which destroys the **left optic radiation Ú right homonymous hemianopia** (as in case of lesion of the left optic tract).

- **Destruction of area 17 causes blindness.**
- **Destruction of area 18: Patient can see but cannot recognize what he sees. This is called as 'Mind blindness'**
- **Destruction of area 19: Patient may be able to recognize objects but cannot recall their meaning. This is called 'Word Blindness'.**

The Pituitary Tumor Compressing the Optic Chiasma

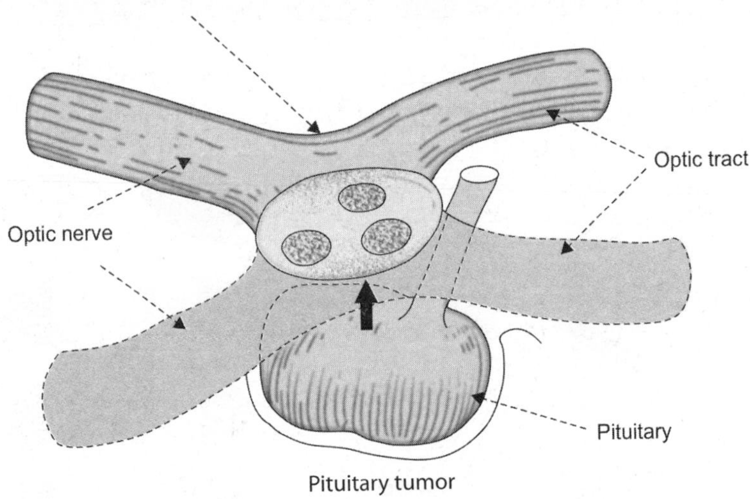

Pituitary tumor

VISION

Color Vision is tested by

- **Ishihara plates**
- **Hardy rand Rittler plates**
- **Edridge green lantern test**
- **City university test**
- **Farnsworth Munsell 199 hue test**
- **Nagels anamoloscope**
- **Holmgrens wool test**

Important Basic Terminology

- **Amaurosis** is complete loss of sight
- **Amblyopia** is partial loss of sight

- **Nyctalopia** is night blindness
- **Hamarlopia** is day blindness
- **Achromatopsia** is color blindness
- **Protanomalous** is **defective** red color appreciation
- **Dueteranomalous** is **defective** green color appreciation
- **Tritanomalous** is **defective** blue color appreciation
- **Protanopia** is complete red color blindness
- **Deuteronopia** is complete green color blindness
- **Tritanopia** is complete blue color blindness

Amaurosis

This term refers to a **'transient ischemic attack of the retina.'**

- Because neural tissue has a **high rate of metabolism**, interruption of blood flow to the retina for more than a few seconds results in **transient monocular blindness**, a term used interchangeably with amaurosis fugax
- Patients describe a rapid fading of vision like a **curtain descending**, sometimes affecting only a portion of the visual field
- Amaurosis fugax usually **occurs from an embolus** that becomes stuck within a retinal arteriole
- **Ophthalmoscopy** reveals zones of **whitened, edematous retina** following the distribution of branch retinal arterioles
- Complete occlusion of the central retinal artery produces arrest of blood flow and a milky retina with a **cherry-red fovea**
- Emboli are composed of either **cholesterol (Hollenhorst plaque)**, calcium, or platelet-fibrin debris
- The most common source is an atherosclerotic plaque in the **carotid artery or aorta**, although emboli can also arise from the heart, especially in patients with diseased valves, atrial fibrillation, or wall motion abnormalities
- Retinal arterial occlusion also occurs rarely in association with **retinal migraine, lupus erythematosus, anticardiolipin antibodies, anticoagulant deficiency states (protein S, protein C, and antithrombin III deficiency), pregnancy, intravenous drug abuse, blood dyscrasias, dysproteinemias, and temporal arteritis**
- Amaurosis fugax **warns of a patient at high-risk for stroke**
- Marked systemic hypertension causes sclerosis of retinal arterioles, splinter hemorrhages, **focal infarcts of the nerve fiber layer (cotton-wool spots)** and **leakage of lipid and fluid (hard exudate)** into the macula. In hypertensive crisis, sudden visual loss can result from vasospasm of retinal arterioles and consequent retinal ischemia. In addition, acute hypertension may produce visual loss from ischemic swelling of the optic disk.

OPTIC REFLEXES

The Light Reflex

(Constriction of the pupil in response to excess light)

This is a **'protective'** reflex: **the pupil becomes narrow to prevent excess light from injuring the rods and cones in the retina**

Types: There are 2 types of light reflex — **Direct and Indirect**

Direct Pupillary Reflex:

Light falls on the right eye → constriction of the right pupil

indirect Pupillary Reflex: (Consensual light reflex)

Light falls on the right eye → constriction of the left pupil.

Pathway of the Light Reflex

- **Excess light → RETINA → optic nerve → optic chiasma → optic tract**
- Some fibers leave the optic tract to reach the **PRETECTAL NUCLEUS** (which is part of the superior colliculus in Man). Each pretectal nucleus sends fibers to the Edinger-Westphal (EW) part of the oculomotor nucleus of the two sides.

- Edinger-Westphal parts of the oculomotor [III] nucleus of the **Rt and Lt** sides → (preganglionic fibers) in the oculomotor [III] nerves (of both sides) → the ciliary ganglia (on both sides)
- Each ciliary ganglion → (postganglionic fibers) in the short ciliary nerves → sphincter pupillae muscle → constriction of the pupil.

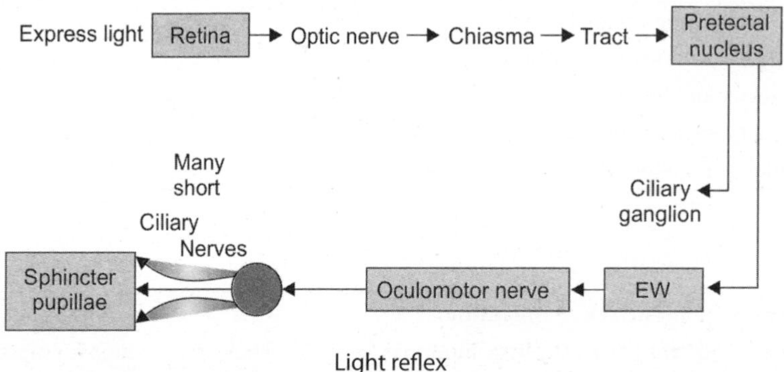

Light reflex

Accommodation Reflex

- An object placed 6 meters or more from the eye considered a 'far' object and light rays falling on the eye from it are parallel and are brought to focus on the retina. This is vision **'at rest'**
- A 'near' object is placed nearer than 6 meters from the eye (e.g. a book). Light rays falling on the eye from a near object are divergent. In order to bring them to focus on the retina the **LENS MUST INCREASE ITS THICKNESS** to have a stronger refractive power. This is called accommodation. In order for the lens to increase its thickness, the ciliary muscle must contract; contraction of the ciliary muscle → **relaxation of the suspensory ligament of the lens** → thicker and more powerful lens.

Pathway of Accommodation

- **Light from a near object → RETINA → optic nerve → optic chiasma → optic tract → Lateral geniculate body (LGB) → optic radiation → AREA 17 of the occipital cortex**
- The first picture which falls on the eye does not fall in focus on the retina so the first picture which reaches the visual cortex is blurred (not seen clearly). Area 17 now sends signal to area 19
- In order to make the picture fall on the retina area 19 sends signal to the **superior colliculus** (in the midbrain) **(by way of the occipitotectal tract)**. The superior colliculus then sends orders to **Edinger-Westphal nucleus** of the third nerve → **contractions of the ciliary muscle → relaxation of the suspensory ligament → thicker and more powerful lens → picture NOW falls in focus on the retina** can be seen clearly when it reaches the visual area.

Why does a student who studies for a long-time become tired?

This is because he is contracting three sets of his muscles:

1. **Contracting the ciliary muscle of both eyes (i.e. accommodation)**
2. **Contracting the medial rectus of both eyes at the same time (i.e. convergence)**
3. **Contracting the constrictor pupillae of both eyes (to prevent spherical aberration) and to see clearly**

Corneal Reflex

Light touching of the cornea or conjunctiva results in blinking of the eyelids

On touching the cornea **afferent impulses from the cornea or conjunctiva** travel through the **ophthalmic division of the trigeminal nerve** to the sensory nucleus of the trigeminal nerve. Internuncial neurons connect with the motor nucleus of the facial nerve on both sides through the medial longitudinal fasciculus. The **facial nerve which carries the efferent impulses** supplies the orbicularis oculi muscle, which causes closure of the eyelids.

- **Rods are more sensitive to light**
- **Cones,** on the other hand, are sensitive to specific wavelengths of light allowing you to **discern colors**

The Fovea is a small shallow depression in the central region of the eye located such that:

- Most of the incident light collected by the cornea and lens is focused onto this region
- Most of the inner layers of the retina are markedly reduced or absent and what dominates is a layer of photoreceptors
- **Composed entirely of cone cells** for very **fine discrimination of colors and details**
- Retinal vessels are also absent in the region of the fovea. It is most sensitive part of eye.

Disorders of Cranial Nerves Related to Eye

The Third (Oculomotor) Nerve Palsy

It supplies all extraocular muscles except the superior oblique and the lateral rectus

Complete paralysis results in:

- **External ophthalmoplegia** in a **complete lesion** inability to move the eye upward, inward and downward
- **External Squint:** The eye is deviated laterally and downwards due to the unopposed action of the lateral rectus and superior oblique
- **Diplopia:** A person sees double
- **Ptosis:** Drooping of the upper eyelids due to paralysis of levator palpabrea superioris
- **Dilated nonreactive pupil** due to paralysis of the sphincter pupillae
- The **pupil also shows no reaction to light** (direct or consensual), or to accommodation
- **Puppilary sparing** is seen in diabetes mellitus.

The Fourth (Trochlear) Nerve Palsy

- There is weakness or paralysis of the **superior oblique muscle which normally moves the eye downwards and inwards**
- **Result:** Defective depression of the adducted eye. The patient is unable to look at his shoulder
- **Symptom presentation: DIPLOPIA** (double vision), **when looking downwards,** e.g. when reading or descending the stairs. The head may tilt to the opposite side to minimize the diplopia.

The Sixth (Abducent) Nerve Palsy

The sixth nerve supplies the **lateral rectus which normally rotates the eye laterally**

Its paralysis causes:

- **Internal Squint:** The eyeball is turned inwards due to unopposed adduction of the medial rectus
- **Diplopia,** which is maximum on **looking outwards**
- **Limitation of abduction** of the corresponding eye.

- **Arygyll Robertson Pupil**

This consists of:

- **Constriction of the pupil (meiosis), which fails to dilate completely with mydriatics**
- **Irregularity of the pupil**
- **Absence of light reflex, but normal accommodation reflex. This combination is diagnostic of the condition**
- **It is especially seen in Syphilis of the Nervous System (NEURO SYPHILIS).**

Adie's Tonic Pupil

- **The pupil is dilated in one eye**
- **Loss of light reflex (direct and consensual)**
- **The condition is benign and is seen in healthy individuals (mostly females)**

Horner's Syndrome

This results from paralysis of the sympathetic fibers at any site along its long course in the head, in the neck or mediastium as a result, e.g. of neoplasm or trauma. It consists of:

- **Ptosis**, which is partial: The lid may be slightly raised voluntarily
- **Enophthalmos**
- **Miosis**: Fixed construction, i.e. does not dilate on shading the eye
- **Anhydrosis**: Loss of sweating on ipsilateral half of head and face when the lesion is proximal to sympathetic fiber separation along the external carotid
- **Loss of the ciliospinal reflex**

Causes:

- Brainstem (vascular-syringobulbia)
- Cervical cord (glioma- syringobulbia)
- Damage to C8, T1
- Cervical sympathetic chain damage by: pancoast tumor of lung.

Remember Important Points about Nerves Supplying Eye

- **The sixth cranial nerve innervates the lateral rectus muscle**
- **Palsy of Abducens nerve produces horizontal diplopia, worse on gaze to the side of the lesion**
- **Foville's syndrome** following **'Dorsal pontine injury'(VI, VII) CN**
- Includes **lateral gaze palsy VI**
- **Ipsilateral facial palsy** and **VII**
- Contralateral hemiparesis incurred by damage to descending corticospinal fibers
- **Millard-Gubler syndrome** following **'Ventral pontine injury'** is similar, except for the eye findings. There is lateral rectus weakness only, instead of gaze palsy, because the abducens fascicle is injured rather than the nucleus
- **Infarct, tumor, hemorrhage, vascular malformation, and multiple sclerosis are the most common etiologies of brainstem abducens palsy**
- **In the cavernous sinus, the nerve can be affected by carotid aneurysm, carotid cavernous fistula, tumor (Pituitary adenoma, meningioma, nasopharyngeal carcinoma), herpes infection and Tolosa-Hunt syndrome**
- **Unilateral or bilateral abducens palsy is a classic sign of raised intracranial pressure**

Oculomotor Nerve: The third cranial nerve innervates the medial, inferior, and superior recti; inferior oblique; levator palpebrae superioris; and the iris sphincter

Total palsy of the oculomotor nerve causes **ptosis, a dilated pupil, and leaves the eye 'down and out'** because of the unopposed action of the lateral rectus and superior oblique

Injury to structures surrounding fascicles of the oculomotor nerve descending through the midbrain has given rise to a number of classic eponymic designations

- **Nothnagel's syndrome**, injury to the superior cerebellar peduncle causes **ipsilateral oculomotor palsy and contralateral cerebellar ataxia**
- **Syndrome**, injury to the red nucleus results in **ipsilateral oculomotor palsy and contralateral tremor, chorea and athetosis**
- **Claude's syndrome** incorporates features of **both the aforementioned syndromes**, by injury to both the red nucleus and the superior cerebellar peduncle
- **Weber's syndrome**, injury to the cerebral peduncle causes **ipsilateral oculomotor palsy with contralateral hemiparesis**

Trochlear Nerve: The fourth cranial nerve originates in the midbrain, just caudal to the oculomotor nerve complex

- Fibers exit the brainstem dorsally and cross to innervate the contralateral superior oblique
- The principal actions of this muscle are to **depress and to intort the globe**
- **Supplies superior oblique muscle**
- A palsy therefore results **in hypertropia and excyclotorsion**
- The **'head tilt test'** is a cardinal diagnostic feature

- **Blepharitis:** This refers to **inflammation of the eyelids**. The most common form occurs in association with **acne rosacea or seborrheic dermatitis.**
- **A chalazion** is a **painless, 'granulomatous inflammation of a meibomian gland** that produces a pealike nodule within the eyelid. It can be incised and drained, or injected with glucocorticoids
- **Recurrent chalazion might indicate malignant transformation. (sebaceous cell carcinoma)**
- Basal cell, squamous cell, or meibomian gland carcinoma should be suspected for any **'nonhealing, ulcerative lesion' of the eyelids**
- **Basal cell carcinoma:**
  - **It is the most common tumor of eyelid**
  - **Lower lid is the most common site**

Found in association with

- **Xeroderma pigmentosa**
- **Gorlin Goltz syndrome**

Ptosis

'Ptosis': Drooping of upper eyelids

Tylosis: hypertrophy and drooping of eyelids

- **Blepharoptosis:** This is an abnormal drooping of the eyelid. Unilateral or bilateral ptosis can be congenital, from dysgenesis of the levator palpebrae superioris, or from abnormal insertion of its aponeurosis into the eyelid
- **Mechanical Ptosis:** This occurs in many **elderly patients from stretching and redundancy of eyelid skin and subcutaneous fat (dermatochalasis).** The extra weight of these sagging tissues causes the lid to droop. Enlargement or deformation of the eyelid from infection, tumor, trauma or inflammation also results in ptosis on a purely mechanical basis
- **Aponeurotic Ptosis:** This is an **acquired dehiscence or stretching of the aponeurotic tendon, which connects the levator muscle to the tarsal plate of the eyelid**. It occurs commonly in older patients, presumably from **loss of connective tissue elasticity**. Aponeurotic ptosis is also a frequent sequela of eyelid swelling from infection or blunt trauma to the orbit, cataract surgery, or hard contact lens usage
- **Myogenic Ptosis:** The causes of myogenic ptosis include **myasthenia gravis** and a number of rare myopathies that manifest with ptosis
- **In the Kearns-Sayre variant**, retinal pigmentary changes and abnormalities of cardiac conduction develop. Peripheral muscle biopsy shows characteristic 'ragged-red fibers.'
- **Oculopharyngeal dystrophy** is a distinct autosomal dominant disease with onset in middle age, characterized by ptosis, limited eye movements, and trouble swallowing
- **Myotonic dystrophy**, another autosomal dominant disorder, causes ptosis, ophthalmoparesis, cataract, and pigmentary retinopathy. Patients have muscle wasting, myotonia and frontal balding and cardiac abnormalities
- **Neurogenic Ptosis:** This results from a lesion affecting the innervation to either of the two muscles that open the eyelid: Muller's muscle or the levator palpebrae superioris
- **In Horner's syndrome**, the eye with ptosis has a smaller pupil and the eye movements are full
- **Patient with nonretractable ptosis gets corrected due to action like mimicking, chewingin marcus gunn jaw winking syndrome**
- **In oculomotor nerve palsy**, the eye with the ptosis has a larger, or a normal, pupil. If the pupil is normal but there is limitation of adduction, elevation, and depression, a pupil-sparing oculomotor nerve palsy is likely
- **Corrected by Blaskowicks operation.**

Horner's Syndrome

- **Ptosis**
- **Miosis**
- **Anhydrosis**

- **Loss of ciliospinal reflex**
- **Treated by Fasanella-Servat operation**

Cavernous Sinus Thrombosis: Features

Infection from nose, sinuses, orbits or pharynx with high fever, chills and
- **Ptosis**
- **Proptosis**
- **Chemosis**
- **Loss of accommodation and loss of puppilary reflex**
- **Dilated pupil**
- **Diplopia**
- **Engorged retinal veins**

Swellings in Relation to Eye

• **Dermoid cyst**	• Located subcutaneously a long embryonic lines of closure
• **Capillary hemangioma**	• Most common tumor of orbit and periorbital areas in **childhood**
• **Orbital pseudotumor**	• Enlargement of extraoccular muscles
• **Cavernous hemangioma**	• Most common benign orbital tumor. Most common in second to fifth decade.

REFRACTIVE ERRORS

Myopia

- Myopia is **short sightedness**
- Rays of light focused **in front** of retina
- **Big eyeball is seen**
- Corrected by **concave lens**
- **Deep** anterior chamber
- Patient squeezes eyes to see distant things clearly
- **Myopic crescents (on temporal side)**
- **Foster Fuchs spots**
- **Cystoid Degeneration**
- **Lattice and Snail track degeneration**
- **Peripheral retinal degeneration**
- **Posterior staphyloma**

Surgeries for Myopia

- **Radial keratotomy (SMALL DEGREE)**
- **Photorefractive keratotomy**
- **Automated lamellar keratectomy**
- **Soft contact lens**
- **LASIK**
- **LASEK**
- **Intracorneal rings**
- **Clear lens extraction**

Hypermetropia

- It is **long sightedness**
- Rays of light focused **behind retina**
- Corrected by **convex Lens**
- **Shallow** anterior chamber
- Eyeball and cornea are **small**

Presbyopia

- Not an error of refraction
- Weakness of ciliary muscles, ligaments
- Loss of elasticity of lens capsule
- Condition of **physiological insufficiency of accommodation**
- **Loss of power of accommodation is seen**
- Physiological change appropriate for age
- Treatment is **convex lens**

Astigmatism

- It is **spherical aberration**
- Due to **irregular curvature of cornea**
- Corrected by **convex lens**

Aphakia

It is **absence of crystalline lens**

- Eye becomes **hypermetropic**
- **Accommodation is lost**
  - **Deep anterior chamber**
  - **Jet black pupil**
- **Iridodenesis**
- **Purkinje image test show only two test images**
- **Post chamber IOL** is the treatment of choice
- **Spectacles are prescribed to patient of aphakia after 6 weeks of surgery**

Important Facts

- ↑ **inter pupillary** distance: **Hypertelorism**
- ↓ **inter pupillary** distance: **Hypotelorism**
- ↑ **inter canthal** distance: **Telecanthus**

- **Convergent squint (esotropia)** is due to 6th nerve palsy
- **Divergent squint (exotropia)** is due to 3rd nerve palsy
- **In paralytic squint** primary deviation < secondary deviation
- **Inconcomitant squint** primary deviation = secondary deviation

Nystagmus

- **Down beat Nystagmus** is seen in cerebellar/brainstem lesions, multiple sclerosis, alcohol, anticonvulsants and lithium intoxication
- **Upbeat Nystagmus** is seen in **pontine lesions**
- **Vestibular Nystagmus** is seen in **Menier's disease, Vestibular lesions**
- **Rotatory Nystagmus: Miners Nystagmus**

Anisokenia: Difference in **image size. (USE CONTACT LENS)**
Anisometropia: Difference in **refraction of two eyes**
Anisocoria: Difference in **pupil size of two eyes**

Conjunctiva

Conjunctivitis and most frequently asked questions

- **Hemorrhagic Conjunctivitis:** Enterovirus adenovirus coxsackie virus
- **Acute purulent conjunctivitis** Staph, aureus
- **Phylenticular conjunctivitis:** Tuberculosis, staph aureus
- **Giant papillary conjunctivitis**: Contact lens
- **Acute membranous conjunctivitis**: Cornyebacterium diphtheriae, streptococcus hemolyticus
- **Acute follicular conjunctivitis**:Chlamydia trachomatis
- **Epidemic keratoconjunctivitis Pharyngo Conjunctival fever**: Adenovirus
- **Granulomatous conjunctivitis**: Granulomatous diseases
- **Angular conjunctivitis**: Moraxella

Phylenticular Conjunctivitis

- **Type IV hypersensitivity reaction**
- **Due to staph aureus (MC) and tuberculous protein**
- **Koeppes nodule**
- **Busaca nodules are manifestations**
- **MC allergic manifestation is Koppes nodule**
- **Phylycten is hence due to endogeneous causes**
- **Doc : Topical steroids**

Spring Catarrh

- **Recurrent, bilateral conjunctivitis**
- **Horner Trantas spots on bulbar conjunctiva**
- **More common in summer not spring**
- **Burning and itching are common**
- **Cobble stone appearance of palpebral conjunctiva**
- **Pseudogerentoxon with cuspid bow appearance**
- **Papillary hypertrophy**
- **Type 1 Hypersensitivity**
- **Maxwell lyon sign (stringy, ropy discharge)**
- **Shield ulcer**
- **DOC: steroids**

Trachoma

- Trachoma is a **chronic Keratoconjunctivitis** affecting conjunctiva and cornea simultaneously
- It is caused by **Chlamydia Trachomatis11 Serotypes (A-K)**
- It is one of the leading causes of preventable blindness.

- **Unhygienic conditions** predispose
- Incubation period of trachoma varies **from 5–21 days**
- Trachoma is characterized by presence of follicles which contain Histiocytes, lymphocytes and large multinucleated cells called **'Leber cells'**
- Trachoma is characterized by presence of **Limbal follicles or 'Herberts Pits'** formed on the cornea near the limbus
- **Conjunctival scarring** may be present in the form of irregular or stellate present in sulcus subtarsalis called **'Art is line.'**
- **'Pannus'**: Infiltration of cornea with vascularization is a feature
- **SAFE strategy (Surgery, antibiotics, facial cleanliness, environmental improvement**
- **DOC: Tetracycline.**

Pinguecula:

- It is a **small, raised conjunctival nodule** at the temporal or nasal limbus. In adults such lesions are extremely common and have little significance, unless they become inflamed **(pingueculitis)**
- It is hyaline infiltration and elastotic degeneration

Pterygium:

- Resembles a pinguecula but has **crossed the limbus to encroach upon the corneal surface**. Removal is justified when symptoms of irritation or blurring develop, but recurrence is a common problem
- **It is elastotic degeneration with proliferation of vascularized granulation tissue**
- **Stocker's line is seen**
- **Mitomycin, thiotepa and β irradiation are used for treatment.**

Glaucoma

- Aqueous humor is produced by **ciliary processes**. At the rate of 2 µl/min
- Aqueous humor has **less protein** than plasma
- It **maintains IOP. (Intraocular pressure)**
- It provides **substrates and removes metabolites from cornea**
- It flows from posterior chamber to anterior chamber
- **Carbonic anhydrase** is important in aqueous humor production
- **Conventional outflow** is main pathway and uveoscleral outflow is minor pathway

USMLE Case Scenario

A 66-year-old man comes to the emergency department complaining of nausea, vomiting, and a severe headache. Last night he awoke with severe pain, and his family brought him to the nearest emergency room. He has never suffered symptoms like this in the past. His headache is mainly retro-orbital, and much of his pain actually seems to originate in his left eye. On examination, the man shields his left eye with his hand. The eye is markedly red and infected and the cornea appears hazy. The pupil is mid-dilated and minimally reactive to light. The right eye appears normal. Visual acuity tested with a Snellen chart is 20/40 OD and 20/200 OS. Which of the following is the most likely location of this patient's lesion?

1. Conjunctiva
2. Cornea
3. Iris
4. Lens
5. Retina

Ans. 3. Iris

This patient has a classic presentation of acute angle closure glaucoma.

'Congenital Glaucoma'

- **Boys effected** more
- Bilateral

- Blepharospasm
- **Big, (Buphthalmos) 'ox eyes', Large cornea**
- Blue eyes
- Presents as photophobia
- Hazy frosted glass cornea due to edema with Habbs striae. **'Habbs striae are due to breaks in descemet's membrane where corneal opacities appear as lines with double contours'**
- Lens flattened anteroposteriorly
- Deep anterior chamber.
- **Goniotomy** or **Trabeculotomy** is used for treatment.
- **Trabeculectomy** is considered in case of failure of above procedures
- **Trabeculotomy and trabeculectomy (Combined)** is preferential method of choice
- **'Hereditary glaucoma' is due to optineurin abnormality.**

'Secondary' Congenital Glaucoma is associated with

- Aniridia
- Neurofibromatosis
- Sturge Weber syndrome
- Rubella
- Mesodermal dysgenesis

Megalocornea:

- Defined as **diameter of cornea > 11.7 mm at birth or > 13 mm at age 2 years**
- Cornea usually clear with normal thickness and vision
- **Usually bilateral** and **nonprogressive**
- Associated with **Marfan's syndrome**

Primary Open Angle Glaucoma

- Mostly asymptomatic or **progressive painless** loss of vision
- Difficulty in near work and frequent change of presbyopic glasses
- Mild headache or eye ache
- **Optineurin gene** and **MYOC gene** are implicated in pathogenesis
- **Classical Triad** is **↑IOP, classic Field defects, Cupping of optic disk**

Visual Field Defects in Glaucoma are

- **Barring of blind spot. (early)**
- **Paracentral scotoma in Bjerrum's area or arcuate area**
- **Seidels scotoma**
- **Arcuate or bjerrums scotoma**
- **Roenne's nasal step**
- **Tubular vision**
- **Total blindness**

Optic Disk Changes in Glaucoma are

- Oval cup, Asymmetric cup or Large cup
- Splinter hemorrhages
- Pallor of cup
- Atrophy of retinal nerve fiber layer
- Pallor of disk
- Bayoneting sign, Lamellar dot sign

Ist line treatment is: **Timolol**
Argon LASER Trabeculoplasty is done in open angle glaucoma

ANGLE CLOSURE GLAUCOMA

Predisposing Factors

- **Shallow anterior chamber**
- **Anterior dislocation of iris-lens diaphragm**
- **Small corneal diameter**
- **Hypermetropia**

- More common in females
- Dilatation of pupil in dimlight
- Atropine, mydriatics worsen the condition
- May present as painful red eye with headache, nausea vomiting

Features (In Increasing Order of Severity and Progression)

- Narrow angle, shallow anterior chamber
- IOP ↑with pupil dilated
- **Sudden onset severe pain in eye** with nausea, vomiting, progressive loss of vision, photophobia, lacrimation
- **Pupilis semi dilated, vertically oval and fixed**
- It is **nonreactive** to light and accommodation
- Eye becomes **painful, irritable and completely blind**
- **In acute congestive stage of PACG pilocarpine is the 'initial DOC'**
- **Laser iridotomy** and **surgical iridectomy** are procedures of choice
- The **fellow eye** requires **prophylactic peripheral iridotomy and surgical iridectomy**
- **PPP** (Painful, Pilocarpine, Peripheral iridotomy)

Neovascular Glaucoma

Usually associated with neovascularization of Iris **(Rubeosis iridis).** Seen in association with:

- Diabetic retinopathy
- Eales disease
- CRVO
- Sickle cell retinopathy
- CRAO
- Intraocular tumors
- Intraocular inflammation
- Treated by **Pan Retinal Photocoagulation**

Steroid Induced Glaucoma:

The steroid **most likely** among the choices to cause steroid induced glaucoma on topical application is **Betamethasone**

Five to Six percent of people on Betamethasone develop increased IOP after 4 to 6 weeks

This condition is more in people with:

- **Primary open angle glaucoma**
- **Ist degree relative**
- **Diabetes Mellitus**
- **High Myopes**

Drugs used in treatment of glaucoma:

Acetazolamide is a carbonic anhydrase inhibitor used in treating glaucoma

Mannitol is also used as an **IV** Solution used in treating glaucoma

Other drugs used in glaucoma are:

- **Topical Pilocarpine 2%**
- **Topical Timolol**
- **Topical Dorzolamide**
- **Topical Brinzolamide**
- **Atropine is contraindicated in glaucoma**

Pigmentary glaucoma

- It is a form of **open angle glaucoma** with **AD pattern of inheritance** with **pigment disruption of iris and deposition in anterior chamber**
- Corneal pigmentation **(Krukenbergs spindle)** is a feature.

- **Medical therapy** (Topical beta blockers are the drugs of choice.) Timolol, betaxolol, cartelol
- **Carbonic anhydrase inhibitors (acetazolomide, dorzolamide)**
- **Acetazolomide is used orally not topically**
- **Prostaglandin analogues (latanoprost)**
- **Pilocarpine and adrenergic agents. (Epinephrine and Dipivefrine)**
- Atropine is **contraindicated**
- **Timolol is a beta blocker**
- **Argon or diode laser trabeculoplasty and trabeculectomy are surgical options**

Dorzolamide is a carbonic anhydrase inhibitor

- It is an anti-glaucoma agent and topically applied in the form of eye drops
- **Side effects**: Ocular burning, stinging, or discomfort immediately following ocular administration

Superficial punctate keratitis, signs and symptoms of ocular allergic reaction, conjunctivitis and lid reactions blurred vision, eye redness, tearing, dryness, and photophobia. Other ocular events and systemic events were reported infrequently, including headache, nausea, asthenia/fatigue; and, rarely, skin rashes, urolithiasis and iridocyclitis

It is a sulfonamide and, although administered topically, is absorbed systemically. Therefore, the same types of adverse reactions that are attributable to sulfonamides may occur with topical administration

- Fatalities have occurred, although rarely, due to severe reactions to sulfonamides including Stevens-Johnson syndrome, toxic epidermal necrolysis, fulminant hepatic necrosis, agranulocytosis, aplastic anemia and other blood dyscrasias
- Sensitization may recur when a sulfonamide is readministered irrespective of the route of administration. If signs of serious reactions or hypersensitivity occur, discontinue the use of this preparation. Dorzolamide hydrochloride is an **inhibitor of human carbonic anhydrase II.**

Brinzolamide Ophthalmic Suspension

One percent, the most frequently used

Reported adverse events associated with were

- Blurred vision and bitter

- Sour or unusual taste
- Blepharitis, dermatitis, dry eye, foreign body sensation
- Headache, hyperemia, ocular discharge, ocular discomfort, ocular keratitis, ocular pain, ocular pruritus and rhinitis were reported.

- **Carbonic anhydrase (CA)** is an enzyme found in many tissues of the body including the eye. It catalyzes the reversible reaction involving the hydration of carbon dioxide and the dehydration of carbonic acid.
- In humans, carbonic anhydrase exists as a number of isoenzymes, the most active being carbonic anhydrase II (CA-II), found primarily in red blood cells (RBCs), but also in other tissues.
- Inhibition of carbonic anhydrase in the ciliary processes of the eye decreases aqueous humor secretion, presumably by slowing the formation of bicarbonate ions with subsequent reduction in sodium and fluid transport. The result is a reduction in intraocular pressure (IOP).

- **Latanoprost is a prostaglandin F2 analog that is believed to reduce IOP by increasing the outflow of aqueous humor. It is indicated for lowering**
- **IOP in patients with open-angle glaucoma and ocular hypertension who are intolerant to other agents.**

Lens Associated Glaucoma

- **Phacomorphic glaucoma**: Lens swells and obliterates the angle
- **Phacolytic glaucoma:** Lens dissolution escapes into aqueous
- **Phactopic glaucoma:** Iris becomes firmly contracted over posterior surface of lens.

Eponym Glaucoma's

- **Hundred day glaucoma:** Neovascular glaucoma
- **Hypersecretory glaucoma:** Epidemic Dropsy
- **Ghost cell glaucoma:** Vitreous Hemorrhage
- **Angle recession glaucoma:** Blunt trauma
- **Glaucoma Fleckens:** After Acute congestive glaucoma
- **Malignant glaucoma:** Ciliary block glaucoma

Cornea

- **Dendritic ulcers** are pathogonomic **of herpes simplex virus**
- **Acanthameba** causes **pseudodendritic corneal ulcers**
- **Decreased corneal sensation** is a feature

Band shaped keratopathy in cornea is due to deposition of calcerous salts after hyaline infiltration

Seen in:

- **Chronic uveitis**
- **Hyperparathyroidism**
- **Vitamin D toxicity**
- **Sarcoidosis**

Keratoconus

Keratoconus is protrusion of central part of cornea with thinning

Corneal nerves visible

Seen in association with

- Downs

- Turner's
- Ehler-Danlos
- Marfan's
- Osteogenesis imperfecta
- Mitral valve prolapsed
- Features:
  - **Munson's sign**
  - **Fleischer ring**
  - **Vogt lines**
  - **Oil droplet reflex are seen**

Vitamin A deficiency affects cornea: Causes

- Night blindness
- Bitots spots
- Conjunctival xerosis
- Corneal ulceration/Keratomalacia
- Corneal scar
- Xerophthalmic fundus

Kindly Know the Clinical Associations

• **Satellite lesions, dry corneal ulcer**	Fungal corneal ulcer
• **Dalen Fuchs nodules**	Sympathetic ophthalmitis
• **Dendritic ulcer**	Herpes simplex
• **Snow ball opacities in vitreous**	Pars planitis, sarcoid, Amyloidosis, candidiasis, lyme disease
• **Fleischer ring, Munson's sign, Vogt line**	Keratoconus
• **Habbs straie**	Buphthalmos

Epiretinal Membrane

- This is a fibrocellular tissue that grows across the **inner surface of the retina, causing metamorphopsia and reduced visual acuity from distortion of the macula**
- With the ophthalmoscope one can see a **crinkled, cellophane-like membrane** on the retina. Epiretinal membrane is most common in patients over 50 years of age and is usually unilateral
- Most cases are **idiopathic, but some occur as a result of hypertensive retinopathy, diabetes, retinal detachment, or trauma**
- When visual acuity is reduced to the level of about 6/24 (20/80), vitrectomy and surgical peeling of the membrane to relieve macular puckering are recommended. Contraction of an epiretinal membrane sometimes gives rise to a macular hole.
- Vitrectomy may improve visual acuity in some patients with macular hole. Fortunately, fewer than 10% of patients with a macular hole develop a hole in their other eye.

Important Indices

- **Power of lens: +16 D**
- **Power of cornea: + 44 D cornea is the most important refractive surface of eye**
- **Power of eye: + 60 D**
- **Refractive index of air: 1**
- **Refractive index of aqueous humor: 1.33**
- **Refractive index of vitreous humor: 1.33**

- **Refractive index of cornea: 1.37**
- **Refractive index of lens: 1.39**
- **Respiratory coefficient of lens: 1**
- **Equatorial diameter of lens: 9 mm**
- **Maximum refractive power is in center of lens**

Lens

- Lens is **avascular**
- Lens has **no nerve supply**
- Lens derives nutrition from **aqueous humor, perilimbal capillaries and oxygen in air**
- Lens **thicker anteriorly than posteriorly**
- Oldest cells are present in **center** and youngest cells in periphery
- **Crystallins** and **Major intrinsic protein MIP 26** enhance lens transparency
- Glutathione, peroxidase, catalase, ascorbic acid, α tocopherol and β carotene are protective against free radicals.

Cataracts

Majority are age related and due to UV light

Systemic causes:

- DM, Hypoglycemia, Hypocalcemia, Galactosemia, Hypothyroidism, Hypoparathyroidism, Alport's, Down's Syndrome, Dystrophia myotonica, Lowe's syndrome, Wilson's Disease
- Steroids, Chloroquin, Amidarone, Busulfan, Chlorambucil, Copper, Gold, Iron
- Infection (Congenital rubella, CMV, Toxoplasmosis)
- Smoking, HTN, Diabetes mellitus

Ocular causes:

- Trauma
- Radiation
- High myopia
- Atopic dermatitis, Icthyosis, Rothmund's Syndrome, Wener's syndrome (Dermatological causes)
- Cataract is **the most common cause of blindness** in India.

Typical Features of Various Cataracts are

• **Diabetes**	Snow flake cataract
• **Galactosemia**	Oil drop cataract
• **Wilson's disease**	Sunflower cataract
• **Infrared**	Glass workers cataract
• **Atopic Diseases**	Syndermatotic cataract
• **Myotonic Dystrophy**	Christmas tree pattern
• **Trauma**	Rossette cataract
• **Shield cataract**	Atopic dermatitis

- **MC congenital cataract Punctate/Blue Dot cataract**
- **MC cataract in adults Cortical cataract**
- **MC visually significant congenital cataract Zonular/Lamellar cataract**
- **Nuclear cataract Associated with Rubella infection**
- **Coronary cataract Develops at puberty**

Complicated Cataract

- Complicated Cataract: Refers to opacification of the lens **secondary to other intraocular disease**
- The opacity in complicated cataract is **irregular in outline** and variable in density
- A slit lamp examination shows **'Bread Crumb appearance'**
- A characteristic sign is the appearance of iridescent colored particles so called **'Polychromatic lusture'** of reds, greens and blues
- Posterior subcapsular cataract is visually handicapping and presents as marked diminution of vision
- Here patient sees better in dark.

Posterior **Hyperplastic Primary Vitreous** Cataract:

- It is due to **embryological persistence** of Vitreous and Hyaloid
- Almost always **unilateral**
- Associated with **glaucoma, cataract, microphthalmos**
- Does not calcify
- It is a feature of **Patau syndrome**
- It is associated with a **poor visual prognosis**

Lamellar cataract is also called as **zonular or perinuclear cataract**

Bilateral lamellar cataracts account for **50% of visually significant cataracts**

They are associated **with Malnutrition and hypoparathyroidism**

- Linear opacities like spokes of wheel called **riders** are a feature.

Cataract Surgeries

- **ICCE: (Intracapsular cataract extraction): Whole lens removed with intact capsule**
- **ECCE: (Extracapsular cataract extraction): Lens removed, capsule left behind**
- **Phecoemulsification: Whole lens removed with intact capsule**
- **Phecoemulsification: Emulsifies lens nucleus and cortex by ultrasonic vibration**

After cataract is opacity persisting or developing after ECCE

- **Sommering's Ring** is a feature
- **Elschnig's Pearls** are a feature
- **Nd-Yag LASER capsulotomy** is done

Lens Dislocation:

- **Inferior**: Homocystinuria
- **Superior**: Marfans
- **(Superotemporal)**
- **Forward**: Marchesani Weil Syndrome, Trauma, Hypermature cataract, Ehler-Danlos syndrome also cause lens Dislocation

- **Anterior lenticonus:** Anterior conical projection of center of lens. **(Alport's Syndrome)**
- **Posterior lenticonus:** Posterior conical projection of center of lens. **(Lowe Syndrome)**
- **Microspherophakia:** Instead of normal biconvex shape, lens is spherical. **(Marfan's Syndrome)**
- **Ectopia Lens:** Subluxation of Lens, **(Marfan's, Familial, Ehler-Danlos Syndrome, Trauma)**

- **Hard lens** is made of **PMMA (Polymethyl methacrylate)**
- **Soft lens** is made of **HEMA (Hydroxy methyl methacrylate)**
- **Modern IOL** are made of silicon, acrylic acid

Contact Lens

- **MC infection** is **pseudomonas infection**
- Most common predisposing factor for **acanthameba** is use of contact lens
- Other complications related to use of contact lens:
  - **Over wear syndrome**
  - **Giant papillary conjunctivitis**
  - **Allergic conjunctivitis**

Papilledema

Causes: Raised ICT:
- ICSOLS (Intracranial space occupying lesions), Postcranial fossa tumors
- Intracranial infections (Cavernous sinus Thrombosis, cerebral abscess)
- Malignant Hypertension, Toxemia of pregnancy
- Pseudotumor cerebri **(Tetracycline, Nalidixic acid, OCP, Vitamin A.)**
- **Foster Kennedy Syndrome** (Optic atrophy on same side and papilledema on other side)

- **Clinical features:**
- Headache, nausea, Projectile vomiting
  - **Painless, Progressive loss of vision**
  - **Amourosis fugax**
  - **Enlargement of blind spot**
  - Progressive contraction of visual field
  - Visual acuity and puppilary reaction remain normal until optic atrophy occurs
  - Leads to postneuritic ophthalmopathy

- Axonal swelling
- Stasis of axoplasmic flow
- Extracellular edema are a feature

- **Blurring of margins of optic disk**
- **Hyperemia of disk**
- **↓Physiological cup**
- **Venous pulsations absent. Flame shaped and punctuate hemorrhages**
- **Elevated disk (mushroom/dome shaped)**
- **Cotton wool spots**
- **Macular fan**

Papillitis/Optic Neuritis

Causes: Idiopathic plus:
- Multiple sclerosis, Devices disease, Leucodystrophies, Postviral infections, Vitamin B complex deficiency
- Diabetes
- Syphilis
- Drugs: Quinine, Chloroquine, Ethambutol, digitalis, INH, NSAIDS, Tobbaco, alcohol, arsenic
- Pseudopapillitis is seen in hypermetropia.

Features:
- (Monocular) unilateral decrease in visual acuity over hours or days
- Poor discrimination of colors, 'Red Desaturation'
- Inflammation of optic nerve
- Pain worse on eye movement
- Relative afferent pupillary defect/Marcus Gun pupil (EARLY)
- Full afferent puppilary defect is seen in optic nerve lesion.

Defects:
- **Defective** contrast sensitivity
- **Decreased** color vision
- **Defective** depth perception of moving objects **(Pulfrich phenomenon)**
- Worsening of symptoms with exercise **(Uhthoff Phenomenon)**
- Visual evoked potentials show **latency and delay in amplitude**

Toxic Optic Neuropathy

This can result in acute visual loss with bilateral optic disk swelling and central or cecocentral scotomas. Such cases have been reported to result from exposure to **ethambutol, methyl alcohol (moonshine), ethylene glycol (antifreeze), or carbon monoxide**

Many agents have been implicated as a cause of toxic optic neuropathy, but the evidence supporting the association for many is weak. The following is a partial list of potential offending drugs or toxins:
- **Disulfiram, ethchlorvynol**
- **Chloramphenicol**
- **Amiodarone**
- **Monoclonal anti-CD3 antibody**
- **Ciprofloxacin**
- **Digitalis**
- **Streptomycin**
- **Lead, arsenic, thallium**
- **D-penicillamine**
- **Isoniazid, emetine**
- **Sulfonamides**

Deficiency states, induced either by **starvation, malabsorption, or alcoholism,** can lead to insidious visual loss.

Remember: Clinical Ophthalmology

- **<u>Optic neuritis</u> is inflammation of optic nerve**
- **<u>Pappilitis</u> is inflammation affecting optic nerve head**
- **<u>Neororetinitis</u> is pappilitis+ inflammation of retinal nerve fiber layer**
- **<u>Optic atrophy</u> is degeneration of optic nerve fibers**
- **<u>Primary</u> optic atrophy is characterized by chalky white disk with sharp clearly defined margins and deep cup**
- **<u>Secondary</u> optic atrophy is characterized by dirty/grey disk with blurred margins and obliterated cup**
- **<u>Wolfram syndrome</u> is Hereditary optic atrophy**
- **<u>DIDMOAD</u> syndrome is diabetes mellitus, diabetes Insipidus, optic atrophy and deafness**
- **<u>Foster Kennedy syndrome</u> is optic atrophy on side of lesion and papilledema on opposite side**
- **<u>Pseudo Foster Kennedy syndrome</u> is unilateral papilledema associated with ↑ICT**
- **<u>Leber's</u> hereditary <u>optic neuropathy</u> (LHON) is bilateral optic neuritis transmitted as mitochondriopathy**
- **<u>Morning glory syndrome</u> is malformation of optic disk, absence of lamina cribrosa**
- **<u>De Morsier syndrome</u> is optic nerve hypoplasia+absence of corpus callosum +absence of septum pellucidium.**

Macular Degeneration

- This is a major cause of **gradual, painless, bilateral central visual loss in the elderly**
- It occurs in a **nonexudative (dry) form and an exudative (wet) form**
- **The nonexudative process** begins with the accumulation of extracellular deposits, called **drusen,** underneath the retinal pigment epithelium
- **Exudative macular degeneration**, which develops in only a minority of patients, occurs when neovascular vessels from the choroid grow through defects in Bruch's membrane into the potential space beneath the retinal pigment epithelium
- **Leakage from these vessels produces elevation of the retina and pigment epithelium, with distortion (metamorphopsia) and blurring of vision**
- **Verteporfin**
- Verteporfin is indicated for **treatment of age-related macular degeneration in patients with predominantly classic subfoveal choroidal neovascularization**
- Verteporfin is a **photosensitizing agent** composed of two isomers
- It **accumulates preferentially in neovasculature, including choroidal neovasculature**
- Activation of verteporfin by **nonthermal light** (689 nanometers wavelength) in the presence of oxygen generates highly reactive, short-lived singlet oxygen and reactive oxygen radicals
- The activated particles cause local damage to neovascular endothelium and subsequent vessel occlusion
- Damaged endothelium releases procoagulant and vasoactive factors causing platelet aggregation, fibrin clot formation, and vasoconstriction
- These factors contribute to the temporary occlusion of choroidal neovascularization
- **Distribution:** Verteporfin is transported in the plasma primarily by lipoproteins.

Cherry Red Spot

- CRAO
- Berlin's edema
- Metachromatic dystrophy
- Niemann Pick disease
- Taysachs disease
- Sandhoffs disease
- Quinidine toxicity
- Sarcoidosis

- **Fleischer's ring**: Keratoconus
- **Pterygium**: Stockers line
- **Ferry's line:** Filtering Bleb
- **Kayser Fleischer Ring**: Wilson's Disease
- **Krukenberg's Spindle**: Pigment dispersion syndrome

Lish nodules

- Are **melanocytic hamartomas of Iris**
- They are **not** seen on naked eye examination
- They are seen on **slit lamp examination**
- They are seen in Neurofibromatosis (von Recklinghausen's disease)

Fundoscopy:

- **Chloroquine toxicity: Bulls Eye Maculopathy**
- **CMV Retinitis: Pizza fundus, Tomato Ketchup Retinopathy**
- **CRAO: Cattle trucking appearance**

- **CRVO: Blood and Thunder fundus**
- **Morning glory appearance: Optic disk coloboma**
- **Bony spicule pigmentation: Retinitis Pigmentosa**
- **Salt and pepper fundus: Congenital syphilis, Rubella**
- **Tesselated fundus: Myopia, Retinitis pigmentosa**
- **Mulberry appearance: Tuberous sclerosis**

Uveal Tract

Episcleritis

- It is an **inflammation of the episclera**, a thin layer of connective tissue between the conjunctiva and sclera
- Episcleritis resembles conjunctivitis but is a **more localized process and discharge is absent**
- Most cases of episcleritis are idiopathic, but some occur in the setting of an autoimmune disease

Scleritis

- Refers to a **deeper, more severe inflammatory process**, frequently associated with a connective tissue disease such as
- **Rheumatoid arthritis**, (MC)
- **Lupus erythematosus, polyarteritis nodosa, Wegener's granulomatosis, or relapsing polychondritis**
- The inflammation and thickening of the sclera can be diffuse or nodular
- In anterior forms of scleritis, the globe assumes a violet hue and the patient complains of severe ocular tenderness and pain
- With posterior scleritis the pain and redness may be less marked, but there is often proptosis, choroidal effusion, reduced motility and visual loss
- Episcleritis and scleritis should be treated with **NSAIDs**
- If these agents fail, **topical or even systemic glucocorticoid therapy** may be necessary, especially if an underlying autoimmune process is active.

Uveitis

Involving the anterior structures of the eye, this is called iritis or iridocyclitis

The diagnosis requires slit-lamp examination to identify inflammatory cells floating in the aqueous humor or deposited upon the corneal endothelium (keratic precipitates)

Circum ciliary congestion

Cells and flare in aqueos are a feature.

Acute Anterior Uveitis

Presents with

- Deep anterior chamber with
- Miotic
- Sluggishly reacting pupil and
- Hazy cornea due to keratitic precipitates
- **Occlusio pupillae** due to organization of exudates across pupillary area, ectropion and **festooned pupil**

Anterior uveitis develops in

- **Sarcoidosis**
- **Ankylosing spondylitis**
- **Juvenile rheumatoid arthritis**
- **Inflammatory bowel disease**
- **Psoriasis**

- **Reiter's syndrome**
- **Behcet's disease**

It is also associated with **herpes infections, syphilis, Lyme disease, onchocerciasis, tuberculosis and leprosy.**

- Treatment is aimed at reducing inflammation and scarring by judicious use of **topical glucocorticoids**. Dilation of the pupil by atropinereduces pain and prevents the formation of synechiae
- **'Secondary glaucoma'** is the **most common complication of recurrent anterior uveitis**
- **'Pilocarpine'** and other cholinergics are **contraindicated**
- **'Steroids' are the drug of choice** followed by mydriatics

Posterior Uveitis

This is diagnosed by **observing inflammation of the vitreous, retina, or choroid on fundus examination**. It is more likely than anterior uveitis to be associated with an **identifiable systemic disease**

Posterior uveitis is a manifestation of autoimmune diseases such **as:**

- **Sarcoidosis**
- **Behçet's disease**
- **Vogt-Koyanagi-Harada syndrome**
- **Inflammatory bowel disease**

It also accompanies diseases such **as toxoplasmosis, onchocerciasis, cysticercosis, coccidioidomycosis, toxocariasis and histoplasmosis**; infections caused by organisms such as Candida, Pneumocystis carinii, Cryptococcus, Aspergillus, herpes, and cytomegalovirus; and other diseases such as syphilis, Lyme disease, tuberculosis, cat-scratch disease, Whipple's disease, and brucellosis

In multiple sclerosis, chronic inflammatory changes can develop in the extreme periphery of the retina (pars planitis or intermediate uveitis).

'Hypopyon associated with uveitis' is seen in

- Ankylosing spondylitis
- Behçet's syndrome
- Reiter syndrome
- Inflammatory Bowel diseases
- Sarcoidosis
- Trauma
- Herpes simplex virus

Features of Pauci articular JRA:

- It is the **most common type** and accounts for 60% cases
- **Involves < 4 joints**
- Rheumatoid factor **is negative**
- Risk of developing **chronic uveitis is highest**. Especially with ANA positivity, early onset and HLA DR 5 positivity
- In **poly articular** JRA Uveitis occurs in only 5% cases
- In systemic JRA, Uveitis is rare.

Vogt-Koyangi-Harada Syndrome

A disease of melanocyte containing tissue. (Soon)

- **Skin Changes:** Vitiligo, Alopecia, Poliosis
- **Occular Changes:** Uveitis, Retinal detatchment, Depigmented fundus, Dalen fuchs nodules
- **Otological Changes:** Deafness, Vertigo, Tinitus
- **Neurological Changes:** Meningitis, Encephalitis

Sympathetic Ophthalmitis

- **Bilateral granulomatous panuveitis**
- **Ciliary body is injured**
- After **penetrating trauma in ciliary region. (Dangerous zone)**
- **Keratatic precipitates or retrolental flares are IST signs**
- Traumatized eye is **'Exciting eye'**
- Fellow eye is **'Sympathizing eye'**
- **Keratitic precipitates are seen early**
- **'Dalen Fuchs nodule'** are characteristic
- **Early excision of injured eye** is the best prophylactic measure
- **Steroids** (Systemic) followed by topical steroids and cycloplegics are used for treatment
- **Example: Difficulty in reading in one eye after sustaining an injury in other eye after 3 to 4 weeks.**

EYE Tumors

- MC **intraocular** malignancy in children: Retinoblastoma
- MC tumor of orbit/periorbitin children: Capillary hemangioma
- MC **primary orbital malignancy** in children Rhabdomyosarcoma
- MC cause of orbital metastasis in children: Neuroblastoma
- MC benign orbital tumor in adults: Cavernous hemangioma
- MC eyelid tumor is: BCC
- MC tumor of lacrimal glands: Benign mixed tumor

Retinoblastoma

- Retinoblastoma develops from **'Neuroectoderm'** from **'Photoreceptor cells'** of Retina. **(Primitive Neuroectodermal Tumor)**
- **There is mutation of Rb gene which is a tumor suppressor gene**
- Retinoblastoma metastasizes to brain via **optic nerve**
- Retinoblastoma is **bilateral in 30–40 % of cases**
- Majority of cases of Retinoblastoma are **sporadic** (85–95%)
- Only a minor are familial
- Familial ones are usually bilateral
- The gene for Retinoblastoma is located on **chromosome 13**
- **Knudson Hypothesis applies to Retinoblastoma**
- Pathological features of Retinoblastoma are:
  - **Flexner Wintersteiner Rosettes**
  - **Homer Wright Rosettes**
  - **Pseudorosettes**
  - **Flurettes**

- The most common manifestation of Retinoblastoma is **Amauratic cats eye reflex or 'Leukocoria' (Do not confuse with Leukorrhea)**
- Metastasis in the form of Orbital invasion, Invasion of regional Lymph nodes, Invasion of Brain, Meninges, bone marrow, is common
- Treatment of Retinoblastoma depends **on size**
- Diffuse Retinoblastoma is treated with **Ennucleation**
- **Ennucleation** Removal of **eye ball with portion of Optic Nerve** from Orbit
- **Small tumors are removed by Brachytherapy**
- Enlargement of Orbit and Orbital canal is a feature
- Treatment of **metastatic disease** is chemotherapy

- Treatment of **bilateral disease** is chemotherapy
- Malignancies associated with Retinoblastoma are:
  - **Pinealoblastoma (MC)**
  - **Osteosarcoma**
  - **Malignant Melanoma**
  - **Soft tissue tumors**
  - **Brain tumors**

Malignant Melanoma

- It is commonest intraocular primary malignant tumor in adults
- It involves vortex veins.

Orbital Pseudotumor

- This is an **idiopathic, inflammatory orbital syndrome**
- Symptoms are **pain, limited eye movements, proptosis and congestion**
- Imaging often shows **swollen eye muscles (orbital myositis) with enlarged tendons**
- The **Tolosa-Hunt syndrome** may be regarded as an extension of orbital pseudotumor through the superior orbital fissure into the cavernous sinus
- Biopsy of the orbit frequently yields **nonspecific evidence of fat infiltration by lymphocytes, plasma cells and eosinophils**
- A dramatic response to a therapeutic trial of **systemic glucocorticoids** indirectly provides the best confirmation of the diagnosis.

Retinal Detachment

- It is separation of neurosensory retina from retinary pigment epithelium
- RD is of three types:
  a. **Rhegmatogenous**: Formation of hole in retina
  b. **Exudative**: Retina pushed from bed by fluid accumulation
  c. **Tractional**: Mechanical detachment

Causes:
  - Myopia
  - Trauma, cataract surgery
  - Hypertension
  - Malignant neoplasms of eye
  - Penetrating trauma
  - Diabetes
  - Eales disease
  - Toxemia of pregnancy predispose to RD
  - Photopsia, floaters **(muscae volitantes)** are present
  - Vitreous shows **Tobacco dusting** which is also called as **'Shafer's Sign'**
  - **Indirect ophthalmoscopy is the investigation of choice**
  - Primary aim of RD surgery is **closure of break.**

Retinitis Pigmentosa

This is a general term for a disparate group of rod and cone dystrophies characterized by progressive night blindness (**nyctalopia**)

- **Visual field constriction with a ring scotoma**
- **Loss of acuity**

- **An abnormal electroretinogram (ERG)**
- It occurs sporadically or in an **autosomal recessive, dominant, or X-linked pattern**
- **Irregular black deposits of clumped pigment in the peripheral retina, called bone spicules**
- Most cases are due to a mutation in the gene for rhodopsin, the rod photopigment, or in the gene for peripherin, a glycoprotein located in photoreceptor outer segments
- There is no effective treatment for retinitis pigmentosa. Vitamin A (15,000 IU/day) slightly retards the deterioration of the ERG but has no beneficial effect upon visual acuity or visual fields
  - Some forms of retinitis pigmentosa occur in association with rare, hereditary systemic diseases **(olivopontocerebellar degeneration)**
  - **Bassen-Kornzweig disease**
  - **Kearns-Sayre syndrome**
  - **Refsum's disease**

Central Serous Retinochoriodopathy

- It is a disease which may have **short course** and **recover spontaneously**
- It is spontaneous detachment of **neurosensory retina** in macular region with or without retinal pigment epithelium detachment
- Typically affects younger **20–40 years age** group with **type a personality**
- Presents with **sudden painless loss of vision, scotomas, micropsia and metamorphosia**
- Ophthalmoscopy reveals:

Mild elevation of macular area

Absent or distorted foveal reflex

- **Fluorescein Angiography Shows**
  - **Inkblot or enlarging dot pattern**
  - **Smoke stack pattern**
  - **Mushroom or umbrella configuration**
- Treatment is **reassurance** for spontaneous recovery or **Argon Laser photocoagulation**

Parinaud's Syndrome

It is a distinct **supranuclear** vertical gaze disorder from damage to the posterior commissure

It is a classic sign of hydrocephalus from aqueductal stenosis

Pineal region tumors (germinoma, pineoblastoma), cysticercosis, and stroke also cause Parinaud's syndrome

Features Include:

- **Loss of upgaze (and sometimes downgaze)**
- **Convergence-retraction nystagmus on attempted upgaze**
- **Downwards ocular deviation ('setting sun' sign)**
- **Lid retraction (Collier's sign)**
- **Skew deviation**
- **Pseudoabducens palsy**
- **Light-near dissociation of the pupils**

Disorders of vertical gaze, especially downwards saccades, are an early feature of progressive supranuclear palsy, Parkinson's disease, Huntington's chorea, and olivopontocerebellar degeneration.

Herpes Zoster

- Herpes zoster from reactivation of latent varicella **(chickenpox)** virus causes **a dermatomal pattern of painful vesicular dermatitis**
- Ocular symptoms can occur after zoster eruption in any branch of the trigeminal nerve but are particularly common when vesicles form on the nose, reflecting **nasociliary (V1) nerve involvement (Hutchinson's sign)**.

- **Herpes zoster ophthalmicus** produces corneal dendrites, which can be difficult to distinguish from those seen in herpes simplex
- Stromal keratitis, anterior uveitis, raised intraocular pressure, ocular motor nerve palsies, acute retinal necrosis, and postherpetic scarring and neuralgia are other common sequelae
- Herpes zoster ophthalmicus is treated with antiviral agents and cycloplegics. In severe cases, glucocorticoids may be added to prevent permanent visual loss from corneal scarring.

Tunnel Vision

Tunnel vision is the **concentric diminution of the visual fields**

Causes:

- Papilledema
- Glaucoma
- Retinitis pigmentosa
- Choroidoretinitis
- Optic atrophy secondary to tabes dorsalis
- Hysteria

Factitious (Functional, Nonorganic) Visual Loss

- Claimed by **hysterics or malingerers**
- Malingerers comprise the vast majority, seeking sympathy, special treatment, or financial gain by feigning loss of sight
- The diagnosis is suspected when the
  - **History is atypical**
  - **Physical findings are lacking or contradictory**
  - **Inconsistencies emerge on testing**
  - **Secondary motive can be identified**

Optic Disk Drusen

- These are **refractile deposits** within the **substance of the optic nerve head**
- They are unrelated to drusen of the retina, which occur in age-related macular degeneration. Their diagnosis is obvious when they are visible as glittering particles upon the surface of the optic disk
- However, in many patients they are hidden beneath the surface, producing **an elevated optic disk with blurred margins that is easily mistaken for papilledema**
- **Ultrasound or CT scanning** are sensitive for detection of buried optic disk drusen because they contain calcium
- In most patients, optic disk drusen are an **incidental, innocuous finding,** but they can produce visual obscurations
- On perimetry they give rise to **enlarged blind spots and arcuate scotomas** from damage to the optic disk
- With increasing age, drusen tend to become more exposed on the disk surface as optic atrophy develops. **Hemorrhage, choroidal neovascular membrane, and AION are more likely to occur in patients with optic disk drusen.**

Anterior Ischemic Optic Neuropathy (AION)

- **AION** is segmental infarction of **anterior part of optic nerve.** (Fragment the word AION)
- It results from infarction of **short posterior ciliary arteries**
- It may occur as a result of atherosclerosis. In association with giant cell arteritis, anemia, collagen vascular disorders, migrane, malignant Hypertension
- There is sudden visual loss
- Visual fields show **altitudnal hemianopia** usually inferior or superior
- Treatment is by high dose corticosteroids.

Diabetic Retinopathy

- Diabetic retinopathy is the **most common cause of blindness** in adults aged 35–65 years old. **Hyperglycemia** is thought to cause increased retinal blood flow and abnormal metabolism in the retinal vessel walls. This precipitates damage to endothelial cells and pericytes
- Endothelial dysfunction leads to increased vascular permeability which causes the characteristic exudates seen on fundoscopy
- **Pericyte dysfunction** predisposes to the formation of microaneurysms
- Neovascularization is thought to be caused by the production of growth factors in response to retinal ischemia
- Person with NIDDM should have ophthalmic examination as early as possible
- Person with IDDM should have fundus examination five years after diagnosis definitely
- **INCIDENCE increases with disease duration.**

Background retinopathy:
- Microaneurysms (dots)
- Blot hemorrhages (< = 3)
- Hard exudates

Preproliferative retinopathy:
- Cotton wool spots (soft exudates; ischemic nerve fibers)
- Blot hemorrhages
- Venous beading/looping
- Deep/dark cluster hemorrhages
- More common in Type I DM, treat with laser photocoagulation

Proliferative retinopathy:
- Retinal neovascularization may lead to vitrous hemorrhage
- Fibrous tissue forming anterior to retinal disk
- More common in Type I DM, 50% blind in 5 years

Maculopathy:
- Based on location rather than severity, anything is potentially serious
- Hard exudates and other 'background' changes on macula
- More common in Type II DM

Ophthalmologic Disease in HIV infections
- Ophthalmologic problems occur in **approximately half of patients** with advanced **HIV infection**
- The most common abnormal findings on funduscopic examination are **cotton-wool spots**. (Hard white spots that appear on the surface of the retina and often have an irregular edge.)
- They represent **areas of retinal ischemia secondary to microvascular disease**
- One of the most devastating consequences of **HIV** infection is **CMV retinitis**
- The majority of cases of CMV retinitis occur in patients with a **CD4 + T cell count < 50/μL**
- Therapy for CMV retinitis consists of **intravenous ganciclovir or foscarnet, with cidofovir as an alternative**
- Both **HSV and varicella zoster virus** can cause a **rapidly progressing, bilateral necrotizing retinitis** referred to as the **'Acute Retinal Necrosis Syndrome'**.

EYE in Thyroid Diseases

Hyperthyroidism is blessed with lots of eye signs. Important ones are:

Lid retraction: Dalrymple sign
Lid lag: von Grafes sign
Infrequent blinking: Stellwag sign
Poor convergence: Mobius sign

Tremor of closed lids: Rosenbach sign
Extraocular muscle palsy: Ballet's sign
Audible bruit over closed eye: Riesman's sign
Unequal puppilary dilatation: Knie sign
Increased lid pigmentation: Jellinek sign

- **Other features:**
- **External ophthalmoplegia**
- **Proptosis**
- **Exophthalmos**
- **Large extraocular muscles**
- **Myopathy**
- **Inferior rectus is the muscle mc involved**

Guanetidine is used in treatment of thyroid ophthalmopathy.

Pupil in Various Conditions

- **Acute Conjunctivitis: Normal**
- **Acute Iridocyclitis: Miotic (small) and sluggishly reacting**
- **Acute Glaucoma: Dilated and Fixed.**

Sjögren's Syndrome

Dry eye or **Keratitis Sicca** or **Aqueous deficiency dry eye** occurs in **'Sjögren's syndrome'**. Mucosal involvement is widespread and clinical manifestations include

- **Dry mouth**
- **Dry nose**
- **Dry eyes**
- **Dry skin**
- **Dry throat**
- **Dry sex (vaginal involvement)**
- Both dry eye and dry mouth is a feature of Sjögren's syndrome
- This occurs as a result of **decreased function of lacrimal glands**
- Cornea will be thickened and there will decrease visual acuity
- Most common cause includes Sjögren's syndrome and sometimes Rheumatoid arthritis and SLE Produce similar conditions.

Other Important Causes of 'Aqueous Deficiency Dry Eye' are

- Aplasia, Injury of Lacrimal glands
- Aplasia of Trigeminal Nerve
- Medications: Antihistaminics, anticholinergics, beta blockers
- Sjögren's syndrome, Riley Day syndrome
- Mucin deficiency: Steven Johnson's Syndrome, Trachoma, Burns, Pemphigoid, Vitamin A deficiency
- **Remember:**
- **Tears are produced in newborn after 4 weeks**
- **Tear film has 3 layers**

Test used for detection of Dry eye syndrome is Schirmer's test

Hypertensive Retinopathy

Characteristic changes seen with hypertensive retinopathy include:

- Narrowing of the aterioles due to smooth muscle contraction, hyperplasia, or fibrosis
- Abnormalities (apparent 'nicking') where the arterioles and venules cross; called 'A-V nicking'
- Increased tortuosity of blood vessels as they spread out over the retina.

The Keith-Wagner and Barker (KWB) classification system evaluates the retinal changes seen with hypertension.

- **Group 1 changes**: Increased light reflex from the arterioles; moderate arteriolar narrowing; focal narrowing.
- **Group 2 changes**: To the above changes, add A-V crossing changes; arterioles are reduced to about half size.
- **Group 3 changes**: To the above changes, add cotton wood spots; hemorrhages.
- **Group 4 changes**: To the above changes, add papilledema.

Important Signs

- **Gunn's sign:** Crossing of artery over vein with compression of underlying vein
- **Gvist's sign**: Increased tortuosity of small venules surrounding maculae
- **Siegrist sign**: Hyperpigmented flecks and choridal vessels arranged in radial fashion in Hypertension and Temporal arteritis
- **Salus Sign:** Venous deflection
- **Bonnet's sign**: It is right angled deflection of vein under artery

Leber's Hereditary Optic Neuropathy (LHON)

- LHON typically presents with **painless, subacute, bilateral visual loss with central scotomas and dyschromatopsia**
- **Mitochondrial** disease
- **Males** are affected three to four times more commonly than females.

River blindness is due to:

- **Oncerchiasis volvolus**
- **Transmitted by black fly**
- **Mazotti test is helpful in diagnosis**
- **Ivermectin is drug of choice.**

Evisceration

It is removal of contents of eyeball leaving behind the sclera

Indications are:

- **Panophthalmitis**
- **'Frills excision' is done for pan ophthalmitis**
- Bleeding anterior staphyloma

Expulsive Choroidal hemmorhage

Enucleation:

It is removal of eye ball with a part of optic nerve from the orbit

Indications are:

- Retinoblastoma in children
- Malignant melanoma in adults
- Sympathetic ophthalmitis
- Endophthalmitis (DOES NOT INVOLVE SCLERA)
- Pthisis bulbi
- Blind and disfigured eye
- Blind eye
- **Contraindicated in panophthalmitis**

Trauma to Orbit

- **Blowout #**: isolated comminuted # of orbital floor and medial wall. **'Hanging drop' or 'Tear drop' sign on Waters view**
- Orbital hematoma, caroticocavernous fistula
- Iridodialysis
- Subluxation/dislocation of lens
- Rosette cataract
- **Vossius ring (Lens concussion)**
- Macular edema/hole
- **Commotio retinae (Berlin's edema)** milky white cloudiness involving posterior pole with cherry red spot in foveal region. **(concussion injury)**
- **Optic nerve evulsion**
- Globe rupture
- **Bilateral** black eye **(Panda eye/Raccoon eye)**
- Unilateral Black eye
- Berlins edema
- **D shaped pupil is seen in IRIDODIALYSIS**

Chloroquine and Eye Ocular Manifestations

- **Keratopathy**
- **Retinal toxicity**
- **Blurred vision**
- **Corneal deposits**
- **Optic atrophy**

Important Questions asked in Previous Examinations (Repeated Multiple Times)

- **Retinopathy of Prematurity** Oxygen
- **Bulls Eye Maculopathy** Chloroquine
- **Nystagmus** Phenytoin
- **Optic Neuritis** Ethambutol
- **Posterior Subcapsular Cataracts** Steroids
- **Corneal deposits** Amiodarone
- **Blue Vision (Cyanopsia)** sildenafil
- **Yellow Vision (Xanthopsia)** Digitalis
- **Whorled keratopathy** Amidarone

Mydriatics

- **Tropicamide:** Quickest and shortest
- **Phenylephrine**: No cycloplegia
- **Atropine**: Used as an ointment in children
- **Commonest complication of topical steroids: Glaucoma**
- Drug used for **blepharospasm: Botulinium toxin**

Associations Asked

- **Candle wax spots**: Sarcoidosis
- **Fleischer ring**: Keratoconus
- **Arlt's line**: Trachoma

- **Sago grains**: Trachoma
- **Roth's spots**: Bacterial endocarditis
- **Epibulbar dermoids**: Goldenhars syndrome
- **Dalen Fuchs nodules**: Sympathetic ophthalmitis
- **Scintillating scotoma**: Migraine
- **Ring scotoma**: Retinitis pigmentosa
- **Angioid streaks**: Pseudoxanthoma elasticum
- **KF ring**: Wilson's disease
- **Schwalbe's ring**: Descemet's membrane
- **Arcus senilis**: Old Age

USMLE Case Scenario

Ophthalmoscopic examination of a 7-year-old child from Washington DC demonstrates a retinal angioma. This finding should raise the possibility of which of the following syndromes?

1. Neurofibromatosis type I
2. Neurofibromatosis type II
3. Tuberous sclerosis
4. von Hippel-Lindau disease

Ans. 4. von Hippel-Lindau disease

USMLE Case Scenario

A 22-year-old male from New York presents with adenoma sebaceum of the skin and cortical tubers. The person is most probably having:

1. Neurofibromatosis type I
2. Neurofibromatosis type II
3. Tuberous sclerosis
4. von Hippel-Lindau disease

Ans. 3. Tuberous sclerosis

USMLE Case Scenario

A 3-year-old child with mental retardation, seizures and facial angiofibromas develops repeated episodes of syncope. Echocardiogram reveals a mass in the left ventricle producing intermittent obstruction. Pathologic examination of the resected mass demonstrates a cardiac rhabdomyoma. Which of the following lesions would this patient most likely also have?

1. Acoustic neuromas
2. Berry aneurysm
3. Cortical tubers
4. Neurofibromas

Ans. 3. Cortical Tubers

The disease is Tuberous Sclerosis

USMLE Case Scenario

A recurrent bilateral conjunctivitis occurring with the onset of hot weather in young boys with symptoms of burning, itching and lacrimation with polygonal raised areas in the palpebral conjunctiva is:

1. Trachoma
2. Phlyctenular conjunctivitis
3. Mucopurulent conunctivitis
4. Vernal keratoconjunctivitis

Ans. 4. Vernal keratoconjunctivitis

USMLE Case Scenario

In von Hippel-Lindau Syndrome the retinal vascular tumors are often associated with intracranial hemangioblastoma. Which one of the following regions is associated with such vascular abnormalities in this syndrome?

1. Optic radiation
2. Optic tract
3. Cerebellum
4. Pulvinar

Ans. 3. Cerebellum

USMLE Case Scenario

The mother of a one and a half year old child gives history of a white reflex from one eye for the past 1 month. On computed tomography scan of the orbit there is calcification seen within the globe. The most likely diagnosis is:

1. Congenital cataract
2. Retinoblastoma
3. Endophthalmitis
4. Coats disease

Ans. 2. Retinoblastoma

USMLE Case Scenario

A patient complains of pain both eyes with congestion. Blurring of vision, photophobia and mucopurulent discharge since one day. Many cases have been reported from the same community. The causative agent is probably:

1. Adenovirus
2. Enterovirus 70
3. Herpes simplex
4. ECHO virus

Ans. 2. Enterovirus 70

USMLE Case Scenario

A 55-year-old female comes to the eye casualty with history of severe eyes pain, redness and diminution of vision. On examination the visual acuity is 6/60, there is circumcorneal congestion, corneal edema and a shallow anterior chamber. Which of the following is the best drug:

1. Atropine ointment
2. IV Mannitol
3. Ciprofloxacin eyes drops
4. Betamethasone eyes drops
5. Moxifloxacin drops
6. Timolol

Ans. 2. IV Mannitol

USMLE Case Scenario

Pterygium is:

1. A vascular anomaly
2. A connective tissue degeneration
3. An inflammatory condition
4. Associated with vitamin A deficiency

Ans. 2. A connective tissue degeneration

USMLE Case Scenario

Chalazion of lid is:

1. Caseous necrosis
2. Chronic nonspecific inflammation
3. Chronic lipogranulomatous inflammation
4. Liposarcoma

Ans. 3. Chronic lipogranulomatous inflammation

USMLE Case Scenario

The afferent pathway for light pupillary reflex is:

1. Trigeminal nerve
2. Optic nerve
3. Abducent nerve
4. Ciliary nerve
5. Trochlear nerve
6. Facial nerve

Ans. 2. Optic nerve

USMLE Case Scenario

A 56-year-old man has painful weeping rashes over the upper eyelid and forehead for the last 2 days along with ipsilateral acute punctate keratopathy. About a year back, he had chemotherapy for non-Hodgkin's lymphoma. There is no other abnormality. Which of the following is the most likely diagnosis?

1. Impetigo
2. Systemic Lupus Erythematosus
3. Herpes Zoster
4. Pyoderma gangrenosum
5. Pox virus infection

Ans. 3. Herpes Zoster

USMLE Case Scenario

Which of the following drugs is contraindicated in a patient with history of sulfa allergy presenting with an acute attack of angle closure glaucoma:

1. Glycerol
2. Acetazolamide
3. Mannitol
4. Latanoprost

Ans. 2. Acetazolamide

USMLE Case Scenario

An elderly male with heart disease presents with sudden loss of vision in one eye; examination reveals cherry red spot; diagnosis is:

1. Central retinal vein occlusion
2. Central retinal artery occlusion
3. Amaurosis fugax
4. Acute ischemic optic neuritis

Ans. 2. Central retinal artery occlusion

USMLE Case Scenario

Eye is deviated laterally and downwards; patient is unable to look up or medially; likely nerve involved is:

1. Trochlear
2. Trigeminal
3. Oculomotor
4. Abducent

Ans. 3. Oculomotor

USMLE Case Scenario

A patient has a miotic pupil, IOP = 25, normal anterior chamber, hazy cornea and a shallow anterior chamber in fellow eye. Diagnosis is:

1. Acute anterior uveitis
2. Acute angle closure glaucoma
3. Acute open angle glaucoma
4. Senile cataract

Ans. 1. Acute anterior uveitis

USMLE Case Scenario

A 55-year-old diabetic presents with sudden loss of vision and onset of floaters. Fundus is difficult to visualize. Most likely diagnosis is:

1. CRAO
2. CRVO
3. Viterous hemmorhage
4. ARMD

Ans. 3. Viterous Hemmorhage

USMLE Case Scenario

A 45-year-old presents with pain, photophobia and blurred vision. There are Dendritic ulcers on the cornea. Most likely diagnosis is:

1. Herpes simplex keratitis
2. Herpes zoster ophthalmicus
3. Fungal keratitis
4. Bacterial retinitis

Ans. 1. Herpes simplex keratitis

USMLE Case Scenario

A 25-year-old male gives history of sudden painless loss of vision in one eye for the past 2 weeks. There is no history of trauma. On examination the anterior segment is normal but there is no fundal glow. Which one of the following is the most likely cause?

1. Vitreous hemorrhage
2. Optic atrophy
3. Developmental cataract
4. Acute attack of angle closure glaucoma

Ans. 1. Vitreous hemorrhage

USMLE Case Scenario

A 44-year-old has intermittent episodes of Bladder incontinence and leg weakness. He presently complains of painful eye movements and blurry vision optic disk is swollen. The most likely diagnosis can be:

1. Myasthenia gravis
2. Parkinsonism
3. Multiple sclerosis
4. Lewy body disease
5. Pick's disease
6. Coat's disease
7. Eale's disease
8. TIA

Ans. 3. Multiple sclerosis

USMLE Case Scenario

Dangerous zone of eye refers to:

1. Sclera
2. Retina
3. Optic nerve
4. Ciliary body
5. Limbus

Ans. 4. Ciliary body

USMLE Case Scenario

Typically bilateral inferior lens subluxations of the lens are seen in:

1. Marfan's syndrome
2. Homocystinuria
3. Hyperinsulinemia
4. Alkaptonuria
5. Cystinosis
6. Ocular trauma

Ans. 2. Homocystinuria

USMLE Case Scenario

Spontaneous subconjunctival hemorrhage is a:

1. Benign condition
2. Malignant condition
3. Medical emergency
4. Surgical emergency

Ans. 1. Benign condition

USMLE Case Scenario

A 66-year-old presents to emergency with sudden onset severe pain, blurring vision in right eye. Examination reveals decreased visual acuity with shallow cornea, hazy cornea in the same eye. Eye has a stony hard consistency. Likely diagnosis is:

1. Keratitis
2. Uveitis
3. Conjunctivitis
4. Glaucoma

Ans. 4. Glaucoma

USMLE Case Scenario

A 10-year-old boy presents with severe itching of the eye and a ropy discharge. His symptoms aggravate in summer season. Most likely diagnosis is?

1. Trachoma
2. Vernal keratoconjunctivitis
3. Acute conjunctivitis
4. Blepharitis

Ans. 2. Vernal keratoconjunctivitis

USMLE Case Scenario

A 66-year-old diabetic and hypertensive presents with cupping of optic disk and constricted peripheral vision on visual examination. Most likely diagnosis is:

1. Cataract
2. Glaucoma
3. Macular degeneration
4. Diabetic retinopathy

Ans. 2. Glaucoma

USMLE Case Scenario

A young man aged 30 years, presents with difficulty in vision in the left eye for the last 10 days. He is immunocompetent, a farmer by occupation, comes from a rural community and gives history of trauma to his left eye with vegetative matter 10–15 days back. On examination, there is an ulcerative lesion in the cornea, whose base has raised soft creamy infiltrate. Ulcer margin is feathery and hyphate. There are a few satellite lesions also. The most probable etiological agent is:

1. Acanthameba
2. Corynebacterium diphtheriae
3. Fusarium
4. Streptococcus pneumonia

Ans. 3. Fusarium

USMLE Case Scenario

A 4-year-old boy comes for ophthamological examination. He presents with bilateral white reflex retina is not visualized properly. Most likely cause is:

1. Congenital cataract
2. Congenital glaucoma
3. Retinoblastoma
4. Optic glioma

Ans. 1. Congenital cataract

USMLE Case Scenario

A 33-year-old hypertensive presents with sudden loss of vision describing as curtain falling down. Fundoscopy reveals edematous whitened retina along retinal arterioles. Most likely diagnosis is:

1. CRAO
2. CRVO
3. Amaurosis fugax
4. Viterous hemorrhage

Ans. 3. Amaurosis fugax

USMLE Case Scenario

A 22-year-old female has a clinical presentation of central scotoma, afferent puppilary defect and altered color perception and decreased visual acuity. The most likely diagnosis can be:

1. Orbital cellulitis
2. Optic neuritis
3. Open angle glaucoma
4. Keratitis

Ans. 2. Optic neuritis

USMLE Case Scenario

Visual loss with Pale retinal lesions with central retinal necrosis in an immunocompromised patient having eye pain is most likely due to:

1. HSV Virus
2. CMV Virus
3. EBV Virus
4. CMV Virus

Ans. 1. HSV Virus

USMLE Case Scenario

A 34-year-old female from New Orleans presents with dendriform ulcers, rash on tip of nose and forehead and chemosis of conjunctiva. Most likely diagnosis is:

1. HSV Keratitis
2. Herpes zoster ophthalmicus
3. Bacterial keratitis
4. Trigeminal neuralgia

Ans. 2. Herpes zoster ophthalmicus

USMLE Case Scenario

A 30-year-old man came to the outpatient department because he had suddenly developed double vision. On examination it was found that his right eye when at rest was turned medially. The most likely anatomical structures involved are:

1. Medial rectus and superior division of oculomotor nerve
2. Inferior oblique and inferior division of oculomotor nerve
3. Lateral rectus and abducent nerve
4. Superior rectus and trochlear nerve

Ans. 3. Lateral rectus and abducent nerve

USMLE Case Scenario

An immunocompromised hypertensive patient with diminished vision presents with yellowish white patches of retinal opacification with hemorrhages on retinal surface. Most likely diagnosis is:

1. Ocular toxoplasmosis
2. Retinal hemorrhage
3. CMV retinitis
4. Herpes zoster ophthalmicus

Ans. 3. CMV retinitis

USMLE Case Scenario

In a case of hypertensive uveitis, most useful drug to reduce intraocular pressure is:

1. Pilocarpine
2. Latanosprost
3. Physostigmine
4. Dipivefrine

Ans. 2. Latanosprost

USMLE Case Scenario

A patient having glaucoma develops blepharoconjunctivitis after instilling some antiglaucoma drug. Which of the following drug can me responsible for it:

1. Timolol

2. Latanoprost
3. Dipiverine
4. Pilocarpine

Ans. 1. Timolol

USMLE Case Scenario

You have been referred a midle-aged patient to rule out open angle glaucoma. Which of the following findings will help in the diagnosis:

1. Cupping of the disk
2. Depth of anterior chamber
3. Visual acuity and refractive error
4. Angle of the anterior chamber

Ans. 1. Cupping of the disk

USMLE Case Scenario

A male patient with a history of hypermature cataract presents with a 2-day history of ciliary congestion, photophobia, blurring of vision and on examination has a deep anterior chamber in the right eye. The left eye is normal. The diagnosis is:

1. Phakomorphic glaucoma
2. Phakolytic glaucoma
3. Phakotoxic glaucoma
4. Phakoanaphylactic uveitis

Ans. 4. Phakoanaphylactic uveitis

USMLE Case Scenario

A 60-year-old male patient operated for cataract 6 months back now complains of floaters and sudden loss of vision. The diagnosis is:

1. Vitreous hemorrhage
2. Retinal detachment
3. Central retinal artery occlusion
4. Cystoid macular edema

Ans. 2. Retinal detachment

USMLE Case Scenario

A 12-year-old boy presents with recurrent attacks of conjunctivitis for the last 2-years with intense itching and ropy discharge. The diagnosis is:

1. Vernal conjunctivitis
2. Phlyctenular conjunctivitis
3. Trachoma
4. Viral conjunctivitis

Ans. 1. Vernal conjunctivitis

USMLE Case Scenario

A 25-year-old lady presents with severe sudden onset of pain, corneal congestion, photophobia and deep anterior chamber in the right eye. The left eye is normal. X-ray pelvis shows sacroiliitis. The diagnosis is:

1. Anterior uveitis
2. Posterior uveitis
3. Intermediate uveitis
4. Scleritis

Ans. 1. Anterior uveitis

USMLE Case Scenario

A neonate, 30 days old, presented with excessive lacrimation and photophobia. He has a large and hazy cornea. His both lacrimal duct systems are normal. The diagnosis is:

1. Megalocornea
2. Keratoconus
3. Congenital glaucoma
4. Hunter's syndrome

Ans. 3. Congenital glaucoma

USMLE Case Scenario

A patient has normal anterior chamber and hazy cornea in one eye and shallow anterior chamber and miotic pupil in fellow eye. The diagnosis is:

1. Endophthalmitis
2. Acute congestive glaucoma
3. Chronic simple glaucoma
4. Acute anterior uveitis

Ans. 4. Acute anterior uveitis

USMLE Case Scenario

A 30-year-old patient with history of recurrent headache was sent for fundus evaluation. He was found to be having generalized arterial attenuation with multiple cotton wool spots and flame shaped hemorrhages in both eyes. The most likely cause is:

1. Diabetic retinopathy
2. Hypertensive retinopathy
3. Central retinal artery occlusion
4. Temporal arteritis

Ans. 2. Hypertensive retinopathy

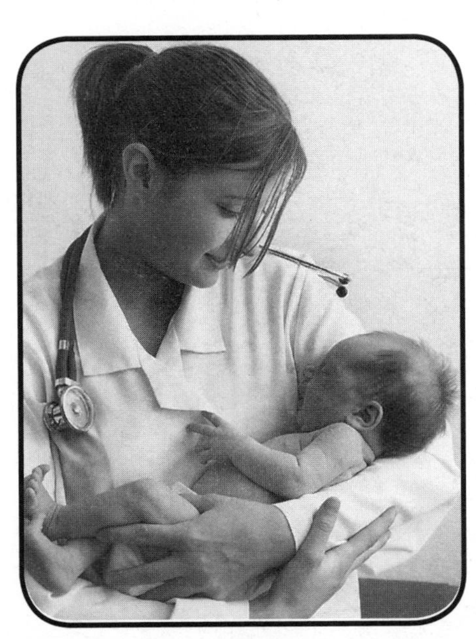

OBSTETRICS AND GYNECOLOGY

Obstetrics and Gynecology 8

Remember Basic Facts

- **Fertilization occurs in 'Ampulla' of fallopian tubes**
- **Sperm binds with 'Secondary' oocyte**
- **'Zona pellucida' must degenerate before implantation occurs**
- **'Implantation' occurs in posterosuperior wall of uterus**
- **Endometrium of pregnant uterus is called 'Decidua'**
- **Deciduas basalis is part of deciduas in contact with blastocyst**
- **Deciduas capsularis is part of deciduas covering the ovum**
- **Deciduas parietalis is the rest of deciduas outside the implantation area**

Important Events Following Fertilization

• 0 hour	• Fertilization
• 30 hours	• 2 cell stage (Blastomeres)
• 40–50 hours	• 4 cell stage
• 72 hours	• 12 cell stage
• 96 hours	• 16 cell stage. (Morula) enters the uterine cavity
• 5th day	• Blastocyst
• 6–7th day	• Zona pellucida disappears, Interstitial implantation occurs
• 9th day	• Lacunar period; Endometrial vessels tapped
• 10–11th day	• Implantation completed
• 13th day	• 'Primary' villi
• 16th day	• 'Secondary' villi
• 21st day	• 'Tertiary' villi
• 21–22nd day	• Fetal heart. Fetoplacental circulation

Placenta: Frequently asked Questions

• **Biscoidal placenta**	• Placenta has two disks
• **Lobed placenta**	• Placenta divides into lobes
• **Diffuse placenta**	• Chorionic villi persist all around the blastocyst
• **Placenta succenturaita**	• Small part of placenta separated from the rest
• **Fenestrated**	• Placenta has hole in center
• **Circumvallate**	• Edge of placenta is covered by circular fold of deciduas

According to 'Umbilical Cord' Attachment

- **Marginal:** Marginal as well as battle dore placenta refers to placenta with cord attached to margins
- **Furcate:** Blood vessels divide before reaching the placenta
- **Velemantous insertion:** Blood vessels are attached to amnion where they ramify before reaching the placenta

Placentation in Humans is an Important PG Topic

- In humans implantation is **Interstitial**
- Human placenta is **Hemochorial**
- Human placenta is **6 to 8 inches** in diameter
- Human placenta weighs about **500 gms**
- Human placenta has a surface area of **14 m^2**
- Human placenta has **60 to 100 fetal cotlydens**
- Human placenta has **15 to 20 maternal Cotyledons**
- Zone of fibrinoid degeneration where trophoblast and decidua meet is called **Nitbauchs layer**

- Oogonia are derived from: **yolk sac**
- Zygote reaches uterine cavity as **16 celled stage**
- Commonest site of fertilization is: **ampulla**
- Placental circulation is established on **17th day of fertilization**
- Placenta has **2 arteries, onze vein**
- **Folds of Hoboken** are a feature of umblical cord

- **Placenta accerta:** Placenta directly anchored to Myometrium without intervening deciduas
- **Placenta incerta:** Placenta invades muscle bundle
- **Placenta percerta:** Placenta invades serosa. Treated by hysterectomy
- **Absence of deciduas basalis** is seen
- **Absence of nitbauchs fibrinoid layer** is seen

Hormones of Placenta

Protein Hormones:

- **Human Chorionic Gonadotrophin (HCG)**
- **Human Placental Lactogen (HPL)**
- **Human Chorionic Thyrotrophin (HCT)**
- **Human Chorionic Corticotrophin (HCC)**
- **Pregnancy specific Beta-1 Glycoprotein**

Steroid hormones:

- **Estrogens: Estriol, Estradiol and Estrone**
- **Progesterone**

Human Chorionic Gonadotrophin (HCG)

- **'Glycoprotein'**
- 2 subunits
- **Alpha Subunit____'Hormone nonspecific'**
- **Beta Subunit______Hormone 'specific'**
- Alpha Subunit is **chemically similar to LH, FSH and TSH**

- **Beta Subunit** is relatively **unique** to HCG
- Synthesized by the **syncytiotrophoblast**
- Secreted into the blood of both mother and fetus
- Half-life is about **1.5** day
- By RIA, it can be detected in the maternal serum or urine as early as **8 to 9** days following Ovulation
- The **doubling time** of HCG in plasma is **about 2** days
- The blood and urine levels reach maximum ranging **100 IU and 200 IU/ml**
- HCG **disappears** from the circulation within **2 weeks** following delivery

Human Placental Lactogen (HPL)

- Also known as **human chorionic somatotrophin**
- Synthesized by **Syncytiotrophoblast** Promotes **growth hormone (GH) release** and insulin Secretion but **decreases** insulins peripheral effects, Liberates maternal fatty acids so sparing maternal glucose use **i.e. Insulin resistance** (Seen during pregnancy)
- Stimulates mammary growth and maternal **casein, lactalbumin and lactoglobulin** production
- Values of **HPL < 5 mg/ml after the 35 weeks** indicate the possibility of **fetal distress**

Pregnancy Specific ß-1 Glycoprotein

- Produced by the **trophoblast**
- Detected in maternal serum as early as **7 day after ovulation**
- Used as a **specific test** of pregnancy

Estrogen

- Produced by the **Syncytiotrophoblast**
- Its synthesis depends much on the precursor derived mainly from the fetus
- In late pregnancy, **estriol** is the most important estrogen
- Estrogen increases the secretion and ciliary beating in fallopian tubes
- Estrogen changes the cuboidal lining of vagina to stratified
- Estrogen changes the breakdown of glycogen into lactate in vagina
- Estrogen initiates **breast development**
- Estrogen causes **early epiphyseal closure**
- Estrogen causes **water retention**

Progesterone

- Produced by **Syncytiotrophoblast**
- Chief hormone of **Corpus luteum**
- After delivery, its level decreases rapidly and is **not** detectable **after 24 hours**

Amniotic Fluid

• **Green colored**	• Fetal distress
• **Golden colored**	• Rh Incompatibility
• **Saffron colored**	• Postmaturity
• **Dark brown**	• IUD

Amnoicentesis

- Done in:
- Pregnancy above the age of **35 years** (Chance of **Downs Syndrome**)
- **A previous** child with chromosomal abnormalities (e.g. **Autosomal Trisomy**)
- X-linked genetic recessive disorders
- To detect **inborn errors** of metabolism

Investigation to be done:
- **Culture of the desquamated fetal cells in the amniotic fluid**
- **Chromosomal study of the desquamated fetal cells in the amniotic fluid**
- **Fetal sex is determined by karyotyping of cultured amniotic cells**
- Other related **points to be remembered**
- Fetal serum also contains AFP in a concentration **150 times** that of maternal serum
- **Acetyl cholinesterase levels** in amniotic fluid is **more specific** than AFP in predicting Neural tube defects

Therapeutic Indications

First Half of Pregnancy:
- Induction of **abortion** (Instillation of chemicals, e.g. **hypertonic saline, urea, prostaglandin)**
- Repeated **decompression** of the uterus in **acute hydramnios**

Second Half of Pregnancy:
- **Decompression** of uterus in unresponsive cases of **chronic hydramnios**
- To give intrauterine fetal **transfusion** in severe hemolysis following Rh-isoimmunization

Preferred Sites for Amniocentesis

Early Months:1/3rd of the way up the **uterus from symphysis pubis**

Later Months:
- **Trans-isthmic suprapubic** approach after lifting the presenting part **OR**
- Through **the flanks** in between the fetal limbs **OR**
- Below **the umbilicus** behind the neck of the fetus

Other points to be remembered
- A **20–22** gauze **spinal needle** is used
- **Length** of needle **is 4" (inches or 10 cm)**
- Amount to be collected for diagnostic purposes is **10 ml**

Precautions for amniocentesis
- **Prior USG localization** of placenta to prevent fetomaternal bleeding
- Prophylactic administration of **100 microgram of anti-D Ig** in Rh-negative nonimmunized mother

Hazards of Amniocentesis

Maternal Complications
- Infection
- Hemorrhage (placental or uterine injury)
- Premature rupture of the membranes
- Premature labor

Fetal Complications

- Trauma
- Fetomaternal hemorrhage
- Triple test was devised to increase sensitivity for pick-up rates of down's syndrome

↑Maternal Serum Alpha Fetoprotein Levels

Maternal Conditions	Fetal Conditions
• Neural tube defects	• Low weight
• Gastrochisis, Exomphalos	• Hepatocellular Ca
• Renal agenesis, Posterior urethral valves	• SLE
• Amniotic band disruption	
• IUGR	
• Osteogenesis imperfecta	
• Placental tumors	
• Umbilical cord tumors	
• Sacrococcygeal teratoma	
• Cystic hygroma	
• Twins	

↓Maternal Serum Alpha Fetoprotein Levels

- Down's syndrome
- Cystic fibrosis
- Hydrocephalus
- Increased maternal weight
- Overestimated gestational age

Triple Test

- **It includes:**
- **HCG**
- **Estriol**
- **Alpha fetoprotein (Maternal)**

In Down's Syndrome:		
HCG↑	**AFP↓**	**Estriol ↓**
In Edward's syndrome:		
HCG↓	**AFP↓**	**Estriol ↓**

Quadruple Test is done for Down's Syndrome

It involves Triple Test Plus Inhibin

- **Alpha fetoprotein**
- **HCG**
- **Estriol**
- **Inhibin**

Chorionic Villus Sampling

- **10–12 weeks preferebally**
- **Done transcervically: 10–12 weeks**
- **Done transabdominally: 10 weeks to term**
- **Done before 10 weeks results in oromandibular limb defects**
- **Slightly higher risk of fetal loss**

- **Chorionic villus sampling: 10–12 weeks**

Done before 10 weeks results in oromandibular limb defects

- **Amniocentesis: 14–16 weeks**
- **Percutaneous umblical blood sampling: 18 weeks**
- **Fetoscopy: 16–20 weeks**

USMLE Case Scenario

A 46-year-old woman from New Texas, gravida 4, para 3, at 8 weeks' gestation comes to the physician for her first prenatal visit. She has mild nausea and vomiting but no other complaints. Her obstetric history is significant for three full-term, normal vaginal deliveries of normal infants. She has no medical or surgical history and takes no medications. Physical examination reveals an 8-week-sized uterus, but is otherwise unremarkable. She wishes to have chromosomal testing of the fetus and wants to have chorionic villus sampling performed. Compared with amniocentesis, chorionic villus sampling may place the patient at greater risk for which of the following?

1. Fetal Down's syndrome
2. Fetal open neural tube defects
3. Maternal sepsis
4. Mid-second-trimester abortion
5. Fetal limb defects
6. Diabetes
7. Hypertension

Ans. 5. Fetal limb defects

Associations of Oligohydramnios and Polyhydramnios

Oligohydramnios	Polyhydramnios
• Renal agenesis	• Esophageal atresia
• Multicystic dysplastic kidneys	• Duodenal atresia
• Amnion nodosum	• Diabetes **mellitus** not Insipidus
• IUGR	• Multiple pregnancy
• Postmaturity	• Open neural tube defects
• Premature rupture of membranes	• Chorioangioma placenta
• Posturethral valves	
• AF index < 5	

Doppler Flow

- Peak velocity of blood flow occurs **during systole**
- Small amount of blood flow occurs in diastole
- S/D ratio assessments are used

Abnormal flows:

- **Absence of blood flow**

- **Reverse flow**
- **Notching of wave form at end of systole**

Abnormal flows cause:

- IUGR
- Fetal distress

Remember

- Cardiac activity of fetus seen by USG at: **6 weeks**
- **Anencephaly is the earliest** fetal anomaly detected by USG
- External genitalia earliest diagnosed by USG at: **10 weeks**
- Fetal respiratory movements occur at: **12 weeks**
- Fetal bradycardias **less than 120 bpm for 15 minutes** period of continuous monitoring
- Fetal scalp **pH <7.2 is abnormal.**

Fetal Scalp Sampling (FSS)

- It is a method of fetal assessment that is used during labor and delivery to obtain fetal blood for pH assessment
- Normal labor and delivery is characterized by a lowering of the fetal pH as the labor progresses
- However, most fetuses tolerate labor and delivery without a dangerous drop in pH (i.e. an acidosis that will result in organ damage)
- When the fetal heart rate tracing is not reassuring, FSS can be used to determine the acid-base status of the fetus, which will help with management of the labor
- **If the pH is > 7.25** then the patient may be managed expectantly with continued observation of the labor and the fetal heart rate
- **If the pH is between 7.20 and 7.25** the FSS should be repeated in 15 to 30 minutes
- **If the pH is < 7.20**, steps should be taken to bring about delivery. Acidemia likely to cause damage to the fetus appears to occur at values < 7.00. However, by using a cutoff of 7.20, there is a margin for error to protect the fetus. This fetus has fetal scalp blood pHs of 7.04, 7.05, and 7.06. This level of acidemia is considered an indication for immediate delivery.

Crown Rump Length

- Crown Rump Length is an accurate parameter used to calculate gestational age in the first trimester **especially during 5–15 weeks**
- CRL is **linear measure of longest axis**
- Usually three images are taken on USG and maximum length is used as the final CRL
- Other parameters such as BPD, Femur length, Abdominal or head circumference are less accurate initially
  - **CRL at 1 month: 5 mm**
  - **CRL at 2 month: 30 mm**
  - **CRL at full term: 300 mm**

NORMAL PREGNANCY

Total Duration: 280 days

Gravidity	**Total number of previous pregnancies (normal or abnormal)**
Parity	**State of having given birth to an infant or infant weighing 500 gms or more dead or alive**
Immature infant	**Weighing <1000 gms and completed < 28 weeks**
Premature infant	**Weighing >1000 gms and completed > 28 weeks**
Low birth weight	**Live born infant weighing 2500 gms or less**
Mature infant	**Live born infant completed 38 weeks of gestation and weighing more than 2500 gms**
Postmature infant	**Live born infant completed 42 weeks of gestation or more**

'Presumptive' Manifestations of Pregnancy

- **Amenorrhea**
- **Nausea and vomiting**
- **Breast tenderness**
- **Quickening (first Perception of fetal movements) at 18 to 20 weeks in primi, 14 to 16 weeks in multigravida**
- **Bladder irritability, frequency and nocturia**

'Changes' in Pregnancy are

Hemodynamic changes

- Increased cardiac output
- Increased blood volume
- Increased plasma volume
- Increased pulse rate
- Compression of superior vena cava (supine hypotension syndrome) in 3rd trimester
- Decreased peripheral vascular resistance
- Decreased pulmonary vascular resistance
- Decreased arterial BP

Integumentary System

- ↑Pigmentation of aerola
- Chloasma
- Linea Nigra (On Abdomen in midline)
- Spider angioma
- Palmar erythema
- Stria gravidarum

Respiratory System

- **↓TLC, FRC, RV**
- **↑Tidal volume**
- **↑Minute ventilation**
- **↑O_2 requirements**

Genitourinary System

- **↑Urinary frequency**
- **↑UTI, Pyelonephiritis**
- **Glycosuria**

Other Changes

- ↑Incidence of **Carpal Tunnel Syndrome**
- ↑Total Thyroxine and ↑Thyroxine binding globulin levels. **Normal TSH**
- ↑Incidence of **Gallstones, GERD** (Reflux)
- ↑Renal blood flow, ↑GFR

Pregnancy Causes Increase in Concentrations of

- **↑Globulin**
- **↑Fibrinogen**

- ↑Transferrin
- ↑Leukotrienes

Fetal Growth is predominantly by

- IGF 1
- Insulin
- Growth factors

'Signs'of Pregnancy

- Chadwick's sign: Congestion of pelvis causes bluish/purplish hue of vagina/cervix
- Leukorrhea: Non fern pattern of cervical mucus
- Goodells sign: Cyanosis and softening of cervix
- Ladin's sign: Softening of uterus in anterior midline
- Hegar's sign: Compressibility of isthmus on bimanual examination
- Mc Donald's sign: Uterus becomes flexible at uterocervical junction
- von Frendwal's sign: Irregular softening of fundus at site of implantation
- Piskacek's sign: Softening of cervix with lateral implantation
- Osianderr's sign: Pulsations in lateral vaginal fornix
- Palmer's sign: Rythmic contractions of uterus
- Weinberg sign: Abdominal pregnancy

Probable Manifestations of Pregnancy

- Abdominal enlargement
- Uterine contractions (painless uterine contractions: Braxton Hicks contractions)
- Uterine ballotment
- Uterine souffle

Pseudocyesis

- Patient having an intense desire for pregnancy and develops symptoms of pregnancy
- No FHS
- No USG documentation of gestational sac
- Refer to pshyciatrist

X-ray Evidence of Fetal Death

- Overlapping of skull bones–Spadling sign
- Gas in Aorta-Roberts sign
- ↑Curvature of fetal spine
- Angulation of spine

True labor	False labor
• Regular uterine contractions • Effacement and dilatation of cervix occur	• Irregular uterine contractions • Effacement and dilatation of cervix do not occur

- **Ideal number of antenatal visits: 12–14**
- **Minimum number of antenatal visits: 3**

- **Total duration: 280 days**
- **Quickening occurs at 20 weeks in primi, 18 weeks in multi**
- **Earliest detection of pregnancy by USG is by: gestational sac**
- **Pregnancy is confirmed by:**
  - **FHR**
  - **FM**
  - **Fetal sac on USG**
- **TVS detects gestational sac at 14 days after ovulation**
- **Fetal parts can be detected by X-ray at: 16 weeks**

Important Terms Frequently asked

- **Fetal presentation: Designates fetal parts which lie over the inlet**
- **Fetal lie: Refers to relation of long axis of fetus to long axis of mother**
- **Fetal position: Relationship of point of direction of presenting part to one of the four quadrants of maternal pelvis**

Pelvis

- Normal female pelvis is **Gynecoid pelvis**
- Most common type of pelvis is **Gynecoid pelvis**
- Transverse diameter is more than AP Diameter in **Gynecoid pelvis**

- Transverse diameter is more than AP Diameter in **Platypelloid pelvis**
- Flat type of pelvis is **Platypelloid pelvis**
- Least common type of pelvis is **Platypelloid pelvis**
- Engagement occurs by asyncitilism in **Platypelloid pelvis**

- Male type/Wedge shaped pelvis is **Android pelvis**
- All diameters are reduced in **Android pelvis**
- **Engagement is delayed** in **Android pelvis**
- **Deep transverse arrest/Persistent occipitoposterior position** is common in **Android pelvis**
- **Dystocia dystrophia syndrome is seen in Android pelvis**

- Ape like pelvis is **Anthropoid pelvis**
- Non rotation/Face to pubis delvery is common in **Anthropoid pelvis**
- Only pelvis with AP diameter > transverse diameter is **Anthropoid pelvis**
- **Face to pubis delivery** is common in **Anthropoid pelvis**

- **Shortest diameter of pelvic inlet** is obstretic conjugate
- **Most important diameter during labor is** interspinal diameter of outlet
- **Shortest diameter of fetal skull is Bitemporal**
- **Largest diameter of fetal skull is submentovertical**

• Engaging Diameter	• Presentation
• Suboccipitobregmatic	• Vertex
• Suboccipitofrontal	• Vertex

• **Occipitofrontal**	• **Vertex**
• **Mentovertical**	• **Brow**
• **Submentovertical**	• **Face**
• **Submentobregmatic**	• **Face**
• **Inlet contraction**	• **If AP diameter is 10 cms or less**
• **Mid pelvic contraction**	• **If inter ischial diameter is < 9.5 cms**
• **Mid pelvic contraction**	• **Prominent ischial spines, converging pelvic walls**
• **Outlet contraction**	• **Intertuberous diameter is 8 cms or less**

- **When saggital suture is midway between pubic and sacrum: Synclitism**
- **When saggital suture deviates from midline: A synclitism**
- **Commonest type of vertex presentation: LOA (left occipito anterior)**
- **Commonest presentation: Cephalic**
- **Commonest presenting part: Vertex**

Bishops Scoring

It is used for labor

Bishops scoring includes:

- **Dilatation of cervix**
- **Effacement of cervix**
- **Consistency of cervix**
- **Position of cervix**
- **Station of head**

Bishops score > 6 indicates beginning of labor.

Labor

- Graphical representation of stages of labor is **partogram**
- Assessment of labor is **best done** by Partogram
- **Graph showing relationship between cervical dilatation and labor is cervicograph**
- Cervical ripening is **mainly due to PGE_2**
- **Sensitivity of uterine musculature is ↑ by: estrogen**
- Cervical ripening is done by **PGE_2, oxytocin, misoprostol**

	Primi	Multi
Ist stage labor • **Onset of labor-dilatation of cervix** • **8–10 hours in primi** • **6–8 hours in multi gravid**	• **6–20 hours**	• **2–10 hours**
2nd stage labor • **From full dilatation of cervix–complete birth of baby** • **Not more than 2 hours usually**	• **30 minutes–3 hours**	• **5–30 minutes**
3rd stage labor • **Birth of infant to delivery of placenta**	• **0–30 minutes**	• **0–30 minutes**

Signs of Placental Separation

- **Gush of blood**
- **Lengthening of cord**
- **Uterus becomes globular**
- **Fundal height increases**

Cardinal Movements of Labor

- Engagement (In relation to BPD)
- Descent
- Flexion
- Internal rotation
- Extension
- Restitution
- External rotation
- Expulsion

Trial of Labor

Indications: Minor CPD

Contraindications:

- Elderly primi
- Major CPD (disproportion)
- Severe PET
- Previous cesarean
- Malpresentation
- Outlet contraction

Postdecidual Secretions: Lochia

• **Lochia rubra**	• **1–4 days usually**	• **Reddish**
• **Lochia serosa**	• **5–9 days**	• **Yellowish**
• **Lochia alba**	• **10–15 days**	• **Pale white**

- **Puerperium is 6 weeks period after delivery**
- **Uterus becomes a pelvic organ 2 weeks after delivery**
- **Involution of uterus is complete by: 6 weeks**

• **Mc site of puerpereal infection**	• **Placental site**
• **Mc manifestation of purpureal infection**	• **Endometritis**
• **Mc cause of puerpereal infection**	• **Streptocococcus**
• **Mc route of puerpereal infection spread**	• **Direct spread**

Bandl's Ring

- **Retraction ring**
- **Seen in CPD, malpresentation**

- **Average pressure** of uterine contractions during first stage of labor: **30 mm Hg** immediately following delivery, height of uterus corresponds to 20 weeks
- Graph showing relationship **between cervical dilatation and duration of labor is called cervicograph**
- **Assessment of labor** is best done by **Partogram**
- Pressure inside uterus during **second stage of labor is 100–120 mm Hg**
- **Precipitate labor is labor occurring in less than 2 hours**

'Preterm Labor'

It is defined as labor occurring before 37 completed weeks of gestation
Differentiate from premature baby: < 38 weeks
Prediction of preterm labor:

- Symptoms of preterm labor
- Uterine contraction greater than 4 per hour
- Cervical length **less than 2.5 cm**
- **U shaped cervix is indicative**
- Presence of fibronectin in vaginal discharge between **24 and 36 weeks**
- Bishops score greater than 4
- Cervical dilatation greater than 2 cm and effacement 80%
- Vaginal bleeding
- Prior preterm

Causes of preterm labor are:

- **Chorioamnionitis**
- **Bacterial vaginosis**
- **Previous history**
- **Recurrent UTI**
- **Smoking**
- **Low socioeconomic and nutritional status**
- **Uterine anomalies**
- **Medical and surgical illnesses**
- **Cervical incompetence**
- **Increased amniotic fluid IL-6 levels and Neoptrin are considered as markers of preterm labor**

Tocolytics

These are drugs used to **arrest premature labor**
Important Tocolytics are:

- Beta mimetics: **Ritodrine, Salbutamol, Isoxsuprine**
- Oxytocin antagonists: Atosiban
- Magnesium Sulfate
- Nifedepine
- Glyceryl Trinitrate
- Progesterone
- Diazoxide
- Ethyl Alchohol
- Atropine
- PG inhibitors: Indomethacin, Sulindac

Abortion

• **Threatened abortion**	Os closed
• **Inevitable abortion**	Os open
• **Incomplete abortion**	Patulous os
• **Complete abortion**	Os closed with expulsion of gestational sac

Septic Abortion

- **Any abortion with clinical evidence of infection of uterus or its contents**
- **Rise of temp at least 100 °F for at least 24 hours**
- **Presence of offensive/purulent vaginal discharge**
- **Presence of evidence of pelvic infection**
- **Most commonly follows illegal abortion**
- **Infection is polymicrobial**

Tests Done for Recurrent Abortions

- Complete blood counts
- Lupus anticoagulant
- Anticardiolipin antibody level
- TSH level
- Luteal phase endometrial biopsy
- Hysterosalpingography
- Karyotyping (most important)
- **Not TORCH Infections**

- Abortion is expulsion of **fetus less than 500 gms/before 20 weeks**
- MTP is **legal up to 20 weeks**
- **First trimester abortions are** mainly due to (SAME)
  - **Chromosomal aberrations**
  - **Embryonic defect**
  - **Germ cell defect**
  - Ovofetal factor
- **Commonest cause of first trimester abortions is trisomy**
- **Among trisomies commonest to cause abortion is Trisomy 16**
- **Blighted ovum is avascular villi**
- **Second trimester abortions** are mainly due to **incompetent cervix**
- **Cervical incompetence** is treated by: **Shirodkars procedure, Mc Donalds procedure, Wurms procedure**
- **Induction of mid trimester abortions** is usually done by: **intra-amniotic saline, intra-amniotic prostaglandins, hysterotomy**
- **Best method** of Induction of **mid trimester abortions** is by: **intra-amniotic prostaglandins**
- **Female with recurrent abortions and ↑APTT** is most likely having: **antiphospholipid antibody syndrome**
- **Dose of anti D** following **first trimester abortion is: 50 μg**

Ectopic Pregnancy

- **A young girl with 8 weeks ammenorrhea comes in shock. Likely diagnosis is: ectopic**
- **A young girl with 6 weeks ammenorrhea presents with mass abdomen, USG shows empty uterus. Likely diagnosis is: ectopic**
- **A young girl with 6 weeks ammenorrhea comes with pain abdomen USG shows fluid in pouch of douglas Aspiration yields dark colored fluid failing to clot. Likely diagnosis is: ruptured ectopic**

It is associated with:

- **Tubal diseases (commonest)**
- **Endometriosis**
- **PID**
- **Tuberculosis**
- **IUCD**
- **Following Tubal procedures Congenital tubal anomalies**
- **Progastasert**
- **Most common feature** of ectopic is **abdominal pain**
- Most reliable indicator of ectopic gestation is **no gestational sac in USG**
- Expelled products in ectopic originate from: **decidua vera**
- Medical treatment of ectopic pregnancy is by: **methotrexate, actinomycin-D, mifeprestone, prostaglandins**
- **STUDOFORD CRITERION** is for primary abdominal pregnancy
- **Laproscopy** is the best investigation for diagnosis
- **Commonest type which ruptures is: Isthmic**
- **Transvaginal USG** and HCG levels are also used

Bagel sign: It is a sign of ectopic pregnancy in Ultrasonography

It is a hyperechoic ring around gestational sac in adenexal region

Blob sign is in homogenous mass adjacent to ovary or moving separate from ovary. It is a gestational sac without cardiac activity

SALPINGOSTOMY FOR unruptured tubal pregnancy **(Tubes to be preserved)**

SALPINGECTOMY FOR ruptured tubal pregnancy with no desire for future pregnancy

Indications of Medical Management of ECTOPIC PREGNANCY

- **Hemodynamic stability**
- **Gestational sac not more than 4 cms**
- **Serum HCG level not more than 10000 μl**
- **Willing for follow-up**
- **No evidence for acute intra-abdominal hemorrhage**
- **Preferably absent fetal cardiac activity**

Arias Stella Reaction

It is typical adenomatous change of endometrial glands

- Loss of polarity of cells
- Hyperchromatic nuclei
- Vacuolated cytoplasm

- Occasional mitosis
- It occurs in 10–15% cases of ectopic pregnancy
- It is because of progesterone influence

Post-term Pregnancy

- **Post-term pregnancy is characterized by:**
- **Wrinkled skin appearance**
- **Overgrown nails**
- **Absence of Vernix caseosa**
- **'Scanty saffron colored meconium and subsequent oligohydramnios'**
- **Placental calcification**
- **Hypoxia and RDS**
- **Polycythemia**
- **Hypoglycemia**
  - **Golden colored meconium: Rh incompatibility**
  - **Saffron colored meconium: Postmaturity**
  - **Dark brown meconium: IUD**

Hydatid Mole

- Molar pregnancy is an abnormal form of pregnancy, characterized by the presence of a hydatidiform mole **(or hydatid mole, mola hytadidosa)**
- Molar pregnancy comprises two distinct entities, **partial and complete moles**
- **Complete moles** have no identifiable embryonic or fetal tissues and arise when an empty egg with no nucleus is fertilized by a normal sperm
- **Partial mole** occurs when a normal egg is fertilized by two spermatozoa. Hydatidiform moles may develop into choriocarcinoma
- **Caused by triploidy**

Causes persistent GTD

- A hydatidiform mole is a pregnancy/conceptus in which the placenta contains **grapelike vesicles** that are usually visible with the naked eye. The vesicles arise by distention of the chorionic villi by fluid. When inspected in the microscope, **hyperplasia of the trophoblastic tissue** is noted. If left untreated, a hydatidiform mole will almost always end as a **spontaneous abortion**
- Hydatidiform moles are a common complication of pregnancy, occurring once in every 1000 pregnancies in the US, with much higher rates in **Asia**
- Blood tests will show **very high levels of human chorionic gonadotropin (hCG)**
- The diagnosis is strongly suggested by ultrasound (sonogram), but **definitive diagnosis requires histopathological examination**. The mole grossly resembles a bunch of grapes ('cluster of **grapes' or 'honeycombed uterus' or 'snow-storm')**
- There is **increased trophoblast proliferation** and enlarging of the chorionic villi. Angiogenesis in the trophoblasts is impared as well
- **Sometimes symptoms of hyperthyroidism** are seen, due to the extremely high levels of hCG, which can mimic the normal Thyroid-stimulating hormone (TSH)
- Hydatidiform moles should be treated by **evacuating the uterus by uterine suction or by surgical curettage** as soon as possible after diagnosis, in order to avoid the risks of choriocarcinoma. Patients are followed up until their serum human chorionic gonadotrophin (hCG) level has fallen to an undetectable level
- Invasive or metastatic moles (cancer) may require chemotherapy and often respond well to **methotrexate.** The response to treatment is nearly 100%.

Complications of H. Mole

- Hemorrhage and shock due to separation of vesicles from its attachment to deciduas
- Massive intraperitoneal hemorrhage
- Sepsis
- Perforation of uterus
- Preeclampsia with convulsions
- Acute pulmonary insufficiency due to pulmonary embolism
- Thyroid storm
- Development of choriocarcinoma

Nut Shell

- **Large for date uterus**
- **Chromosome configuration is: 46XX**
- **Excessive nausea/vomiting**
- **Early onset PET**
- **Absent fetal heart**
- **Grape like vesicles per vaginum**
- **Bilateral theca leutin cysts associated**
- **High HCG**
- **Snow storm appearance on USG**
- **Investigation of choice to diagnose H mole is USG**
- **Confirmation of diagnosis is by vaginal examination**
- **Evacuate by suction evacuation**
- **Immediate complication of evacuation of H mole is bleeding**

Associations:

- **PIH**
- **Thyrotoxicosis**
- **Hyperemesis**

- **Commonest complication of H mole is sepsis**
- **Imaging technique of choice for diagnosing H. mole is USG**
- **Chromosomal configuration in H. mole is 46 XX**
- **Treatment of choice in H. mole is suction evacuation**
- **In a female of age 40 and above with h. mole and completed family treatment of choice is total hysterectomy**
- **Immediate complication of H. mole is bleeding**
- **Hydropic degeneration of villi is histological characteristic of H. mole**
- **Most common gestational trophoblastic disease following H. mole is: invasive mole**
- **Molar pregnancy is usually diagnosed in First trimester**

Sarcoma Botyrides

- Sarcoma botyrides is **anembryonal rhabdomyosarcoma**
- **Mesenchymal in origin**
- **Readily bleeds on touching**
- Tumor cells resemble **Tennis racket**
- Presents as **grape like mass buldging through vaginal orifice**
- **Locally invasive**
- **Chemoradiation** is treatment of choice

Twinning

- **Negroes** have the highest rate of twinning
- **Hellin's law** indicates chances of twinning
- **Most common** types of twins are **both vertex**
- **Superfecundation** is fertilization of two ova released at same time by sperms released at **two different occasions of sexual intercourse**
- **Siamese twins** have **highest mortality**
- **Thoracophagus** is the most common type of **conjoined twins**
- **A double headed monoster** is called **dicephalous**
- **Twin peak sign is seen in diamniiotic dichorionic twins**
- **In multiple fetal pregnancy fetal reduction is done by: Potassium chloride**
- **Most common cause of perinatal mortality in twins is prematurity**
- **Twin pick sign is seen in dichorionicity**

- **Siamese/conjoined twins: Twins fused to each other**
  - **Thoracophagus: Fused in region of thorax**
  - **Ischiophagus: Fused in region of pelvis**
  - **Pyophagus: Fused in region of back**
  - **Craniophagus: Fused in region of head**
- **Superfecundation: Fertilization of two different ova released in same cycle**
- **Superfetation: Fertilization of two ova released in two different cycles**

Anencephaly

- Associated with:
  - **Face presentation**
  - **Hydramnios**
  - **Postmaturity**
  - **Prematurity**
- Best diagnosed by USG at **10 to 12 weeks**

MALPRESENTATIONS

Breech

- Most common cause of breech is **prematurity**
- Most common type of breech is **frank breech**
- **Engagement occurs earliest** in **frank breech**
- Mortality in breech is mainly due to **intracranial hemorrhage**
- Commonest position **is left sacroanterior**
- Engaging diameter is **bitrochanteric**
- Head is borne by **flexion**

Delivery of head is by:
- **Burns Marshall Method**
- **Maureciau-smeille-veit method**
- **Pipers forceps**

Extended legs: **Pinards Maneuver**
Extended arm: **Lovests Maneuver**
Prematurity, congenital anomalies and birth asphyxia are the main causes of perinatal mortality

Most unfavorable presentation is Mentoposterior

USMLE Case Scenario

A 35-year-old woman from Washington, gravida 4, para 3, at 38 weeks' gestation comes to the labor and delivery ward after noticing a sudden gush of fluid from the vagina. After the gush of fluid, she has had increasing contractions. Speculum examination shows clear fluid in the vagina that is nitrazine positive. Cervical examination by O/G Specialist shows that the patient is 5 cm dilated, with the fetal face presenting in a mentum anterior position. External uterine monitoring shows that the patient is contracting every 2 minutes and external fetal monitoring shows that the fetal heart rate 146/ s and reactive. Which of the following is the most appropriate next step in management?

1. Expectant management
2. Adminster oxytocin
3. Adminster ergometrine
4. Forceps delivery
5. Vacuum delivery
6. Cesarean section
7. Wait for complications

Ans. 1. Expectant management

This patient has a face presentation. It is a case of a fetus in labor is as an occiput presentation. A vaginal delivery is possible when the fetus is in a mentum anterior position

Shoulder Dystocia

- **Impaction of anterior shoulder of fetus against symphysis pubis after fetal head has been delivered**
- Occurs when breadth of shoulders is greater than BPD
- **Risk factors are:**
  - **Diabetes**
  - **Obesity**
  - **Post-term baby**
  - **Excessive weight gain in pregnancy Approach is:**
- **Apply suprapubic pressure**
- **Legs in flexion (Mc Robert's maneuver)**
- **Woods procedure**
- **Release posterior shoulder**
- **Manual corckscrew**
- **Episiotomy**
- **Rollover**

Turtle sign positive: Head delivers but retracts against symphisis pubis

Complications: Erbs palsy, klumpkes palsy#clavicle, humerus, spine, PPH (injury to perineum), Fetal hypoxia

Treatment

- **Cleidotomy**
- **Zanavelli maneuver: Replacement of fetus to uterine cavity and cesarean section**
- **Symphisiotomy**

Rh Incompatibility

- **Immune hydrops**
- **Father Rh+, mother Rh-, fetus Rh+**
- **Ist child escapes usually**

Can have adverse effects on baby as well as mother such as:

- Preeclampsia
- Polyhydramnios
- Big baby
- Hypofibrinogenemia
- PPH
- Maternal syndrome: Generalized edema, proteinuria, pruritis

- **Immune Hydrops in fetus**
  - **Pericardial effusion**
  - **Large placentas**
  - **Skin edema Earliest sign on USG**
  - **Ascites**
- **Icterus neonatorum gravis in fetus**
- **Hemolytic anemias in fetus**

- Anti D immunoglobulin should be given within **72 hours of delivery**
- **300 μg following delivery**
- **50 μg following abortion**
- **Prognosis depends on serum bilirubin**
- **Immediate cord ligation is done**
- **Fetomaternal transfusion is detected by: Kleihauer Betke test**

Diabetes and Pregnancy

- The metabolic changes are accompanied by maternal insulin resistance, caused in part by placental production of steroids, a growth hormone variant and **placental lactogen**
- Pregnancy complicated by diabetes mellitus is associated with **higher maternal and perinatal morbidity and mortality rates**
- **Folate supplementation reduces the incidence of fetal neural tube defects, which occur with greater frequency in fetuses of diabetic mothers**
- In addition, optimizing **glucose control during key periods of organogenesis** reduces other congenital anomalies including **sacral agenesis, caudal dysplasia, renal agenesis, and ventricular septal defect**
- Once pregnancy is established, **glucose control should be managed more aggressively** than in the nonpregnant state
- **Fetal macrosomia is associated with an increased risk of maternal and fetal birth trauma. Pregnant women with diabetes have an increased risk of developing preeclampsia, and those with vascular disease are at greater risk for developing intrauterine growth restriction, which is associated with an increased risk of fetal and neonatal death**
- Because of **delayed pulmonary maturation** of the fetuses of diabetic mothers, **early delivery should be avoided** unless there is biochemical evidence of fetal lung maturity
- All pregnant women should be screened for gestational diabetes unless they are in a low-risk group
- Pregnant women with gestational diabetes are at **increased risk of preeclampsia**, delivering infants who are large for their gestational age, and birth lacerations.

Their fetuses are at risk of hypoglycemia and birth trauma (Brachial Plexus) injury

• **Maternal Complications**	• **Fetal Complications**
• Abortion	• Fetal macrosomia
• Infections	• Neonatal malformations (CVS and Neural Tube defects)
• Preeclampsia	• Renal Agenesis
• Hydramnios	• Hypoglycemia • Hypomagnesemia • Hypocalcemia
• Maternal Distress	• RDS
• Increased complications of labor • Shoulder Dystocia • PPH • Perineal Injuries	• Hyperviscosity Syndrome • Hyperbilirubinemia • Hypertrophic Cardiomyopathy • Polycythemia • Erbs, Klumpkes palsy

Heart Disease and Pregnancy

MS: (Mitral Stenosis and Pregnancy)

- Most common heart disease associated with pregnancy
- This is the **valvular disease most likely to cause death during pregnancy**
- The pregnancy-induced increase in blood volume and cardiac output can cause pulmonary edema in women with mitral stenosis
- Pregnancy associated with long-standing mitral stenosis may result in **pulmonary hypertension. Sudden death** has been reported when hypovolemia has been allowed to occur in this condition
- Pregnant women with mitral stenosis are at **increased risk for the development of atrial fibrillation and other tachyarrythmias**
- **Medical management** of severe mitral stenosis and atrial fibrillation with **digoxin and beta blockers is recommended**
- **Balloon valvulotomy** can be carried out during pregnancy.

Mitral Regurgitation and Aortic Regurgitation. These are **both generally well tolerated** during pregnancy

- The pregnancy-induced decrease in systemic vascular resistance reduces the risk of cardiac failure with these conditions
- As a rule, mitral valve prolapse does not present problems for the pregnant patient and aortic stenosis, unless very severe, is also well tolerated. In the most severe cases of aortic stenosis, limitation of activity or balloon valvuloplasty may be indicated

- For women with artificial valves contemplating pregnancy, it is important that **warfarin be stopped and heparin initiated prior to conception**
- **Warfarin therapy** during the first trimester of pregnancy has been associated with **fetal chondrodysplasia punctata**. In the second and third trimester of pregnancy, warfarin may cause **fetal optic atrophy and mental retardation.**

- **Aortic stenosis** carries **worst prognosis** in pregnancy
- **Highest mortality** in pregnancy is seen in Eisenmengers complex
- Maximum strain on heart during parturition occurs in **immediate postpartum period**
- **Diastolic murmur** is a feature of heart disease in pregnancy
- **Absolute indications for termination:**
  - **Primary pulmonary hypertension**
  - **Eisenmengers syndrome**
  - **Pulmonary venoocclusive disease**

HIV and Pregnancy

HIV can be transmitted in pregnancy:
- **During delivery (most common)**
- **In utero**
- **During breastfeeding**

Highest risk is associated with:
- **High maternal viral load**
- **Low CD 4 T cell count**
- **Chorioamnionitis**
- **Vitamin A deficiency**

Lower risk is associated with
- **LSCS**
- **Antiretroviral prophylaxis (Zidovudine)**
- **Avoiding breastfeeding**
- **Vitamin A prophylaxis**
- **Intrapartum nevirapine**

Hypertension in Pregnancy

Pregnancy induced HTN:
Predicted by:
- **Rolling over test done at 20 weeks**
- **Serum uric acid ↑**
- **Weight gain > 2 kg/month**
- **Earliest sign is ↑ BP**

- **Preeclampsia: Hypertension+proteinuria+edema**
- **Hypertension with proteinuria in a previously normotensive and nonproteinuric patient.**
- **Mild preeclampsia: Systolic BP > 140 or Diastolic BP > 90 mm Hg on two or more occasions and proteinuria > 300 mg/24 hours.**
- **Severe preeclampsia: Systolic BP >160 or Diastolic BP >110 mm Hg on two or more occasions and proteinuria > 5 gms/24 hours**
- **Eclampsia is preeclampsia+convulsions**
- **Imminent eclampsis is heralded by:**
  - Headache
  - Blurring of vision
  - Epigastric pain
  - Brisk deep tendon reflexes
  - Diminished urinary output
- **Delivery of fetus is the definitive treatment**

- **Control of hypertension** is the most important factor in management of preeclampsia
- Eclampsia is **preeclampsia+convulsions**
- Eclampsia is mostly seen **antepartum**
- Causes of convulsions in eclampsia are **cerebral anoxia**
- PIH is **hypertension developing after 20 weeks of pregnancy**
- **Giants roll over test** is done in PIH at **28 to 32 weeks**
- **Rapid gain in weight is the earliest sign** of PIH

- In pregnancy induced hypertension, sudden loss of vision is due to Retinal detachment
- **Magnesium sulfate is effective in eclampsia**
- **Mg sulfate toxicity is monitored by: Urinary output, knee jerk, respiratory rate**

Complications of preeclampsia are:

- Cerebral hemorrhage
- Pulmonary edema
- ARF

Drugs considered safe in pregnancy are:

- **Hydralazine and Methyldopa**
- The drug of choice for **'Hypertension'** in pregnancy is Methyldopa
- The drug of choice for **'Hypertensive crisis'** in Pregnancy is Hydralazine
- The drug of choice for **'SEVERE preeclampsia'** in Pregnancy is Labetelol
- The drug of choice to control **'seizures'** in pregnancy is Magnesium sulfate
- ACE inhibitors are absolutely contraindicated in pregnancy

HELLP Syndrome

- **The HELLP** (hemolysis, elevated liver enzymes, low platelets) syndrome
- Microangiopathic hemolysis occurs
- AST↑
- LDH↑
- Acute fatty liver of pregnancy, cholestasis of pregnancy, eclampsia, and the **HELLP** syndrome (can be confused with viral hepatitis during pregnancy)

ANTEPARTUM HEMORRHAGE

Placenta Previa

Abnormal implantation of placenta usually near cervical os

Risk factors:

- **Prior cesarean**
- **Grand multipara**
- **Multiple gestations**
- **Prior placenta previa**

- Painless
- No tenderness
- Soft uterus
- No uterine irritability
- Malpresentation
- FHR normal usually
- Coagulopathy uncommon

Abruptio Placenta

Premature separation of a normally placed placenta

Risk factors:

- **Hypertension**
- **Trauma to abdomen**
- **Smoking**
- **Cocaine use**

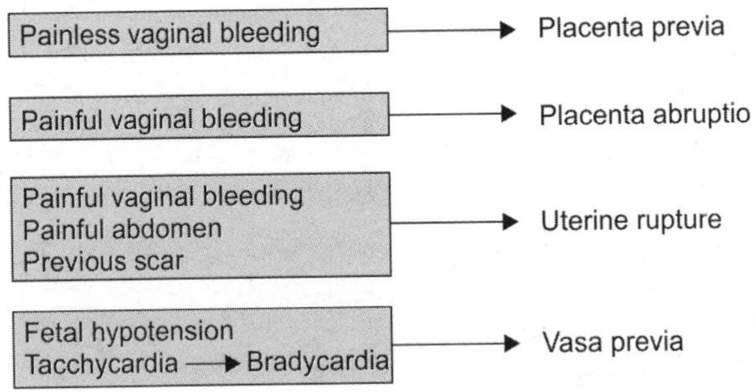

- Painful
- Tenderness
- Increased uterine tone
- Uterine irritability
- Malpresentation none usually
- FHR abnormal usually
- Coagulopathy common

Vasa Previa

- Fetal vessels crossing cervical os
- Associated with **velemantous cord insertion**
- Higher incidence in twins
- **Painless vaginal bleeding + fetal distress**
- **APT test + look for nucleated cells in cord blood by wrights stain**
- **Emergency cesarean** is TOC

PPH

- **'Any amount of bleeding from or into the genital tract following birth of baby until the end of puerperium which adversely affects the general condition of the patient evidenced by rise in pulse rate and falling BP is called PPH.'**
- Commonest cause of PPH is: Atonic uterus

Due to Atonic Uterus:

- Grand multipara
- Overdistension of Uterus
- Malnutrition and Anemia
- APH

- Prolonged labor
- Uterine malformation
- Mismanaged third stage
- Constriction ring

Due to Trauma:

- Instrumental delivery, (cervical lacerations)
- Face to pubis delivery
- Precipitate labor
- Macrosomia

Due to Blood coagulopathies:

- Abruption
- Sepsis
- IUD
- HELLP Syndrome

- **PPH** occurs when blood loss is **> 500 cc**
- **Atonic uterus** is more common in **multipara**
- Drugs used for PPH are: **Misoprostol, carboprost, methergine, ergometrine**
- **B-lynch suture is applied on uterus**

- **Placenta accerta: Chorionic villi attached to superficial myometrium**
- **Placenta incerta: Villi invade myometrium**
- **Placenta percerta: Villi penetrate full thickness of myometrium up to serosa**

Heterotopic or Heterotopic Pregnancy

- Heterotopic or heterotopic pregnancy **is rare**, but the incidents of it are **on the rise**
- Heterotopic pregnancy is a multiple pregnancy with **one embryo viably implanted in the uterus and the other implanted elsewhere as an ectopic pregnancy**
- This type of pregnancy does occur very rarely in natural conception, at the rate of 1 in 30,000
- However, **in pregnancies conceived through assisted reproduction (ART, GIFT, IVF),** the rate of heterotopic pregnancies jumps to as many as 1 in 100 pregnancies
- Today's rate of heterotopic pregnancies has increased dramatically partly due to a rise in **pelvic inflammatory disease (PID)** and partly due to a number of other issues. **Previous pelvic surgery, congenital or acquired abnormalities of the uterine cavity and fallopian tubes may contribute to the condition, as does tubal microsurgery, drug ovulation stimulation, and ART**
- When it comes to women who have undergone IVF (in vitro fertilization), the rise in occurrence is largely due to the transfer of multiple embryos to the uterus
- When **more than five embryos are implanted**, the risk of heterotopic pregnancy increases from 1 in 100 to 1 in 45.

Uterine Inversion

- **Inside out turning of uterus**
- **Results from mismanaged third stage of labor**
- **Patient presents with intense shock**
- **On examination of abdomen, fundus of uterus cant be felt**
- **Hemorrhage (mc), neurogenic shock, pulmonary embolism, uterine sepsis and subinvolution are complications**

Idiopathic Cholestasis of Pregnancy

- Usually in last **(3rd) trimester**
- Slight jaundice
- Generalized pruritis is the commonest symptom, often severe
- Disease recurs in next pregnancies
- Marked
  - **↑In alkaline phosphatase**
  - **↑ALT**
  - **↑AST**
  - **↑Bile acids**
  - **↑Bilirubin**
  - **↑GTT Liver biopsy is the test of choice**
  - **Uresodoxycholic acid is used in treatment**
  - **UROSIDOL is used for treatment**

Antiphospholipid Antibody Syndrome

- Autoimmune disorder
- Due to **lupus anticoagulant/anticardiolipin antibody**
- Predominantly **venous thrombosis**
- Associated with **recurrent fetal loss**
  - **↑ PT**
  - **↑ PTT**
  - **↑ Kaolin clotting time**
  - **↑ Dilute Russell viper venom time**

Monitoring of Growth Restricted Fetus

The tests useful for monitoring of Growth restricted fetus are:

- **Biophysical profile**
- **Cardiotocography**
- **Umbilical artery Doppler**

NST: Nonstress Test

- It is determination of fetal heart rate (FHR) tracing using Doppler to assess FHR and its relationship to fetal movements
- It is indicated in uteroplacental insufficiency/fetal distress
- Normal result is called **reassuring NST**: at least 2 accelerations of FHR >15 beats per minute lasting >15 seconds in 20 minutes
- Abnormal result is called **non reassuring NST**: < 2 accelerations of FHR >15 beats per minute lasting >15 seconds in 40 minutes
- In case of non reassuring **NST do BPP**

FHR

Normal Pattern

- Base line heart rate: 120–160 bpm
- Base line variability: 5–25 bpm
- Two accelerations in 20 minutes
- No deceleration

Abnormal Pattern

- Unexplained tachycardia
- Unexplained bradycardia
- Base line variability < 5 bpm
- Repetitive early or variable decelerations
- Repetitive late decelerations
- Sinusoidal pattern

Deceleration

- Early deceleration: Head compression
- Late deceleration: Placental insufficiency
- Variable deceleration: Cord compression

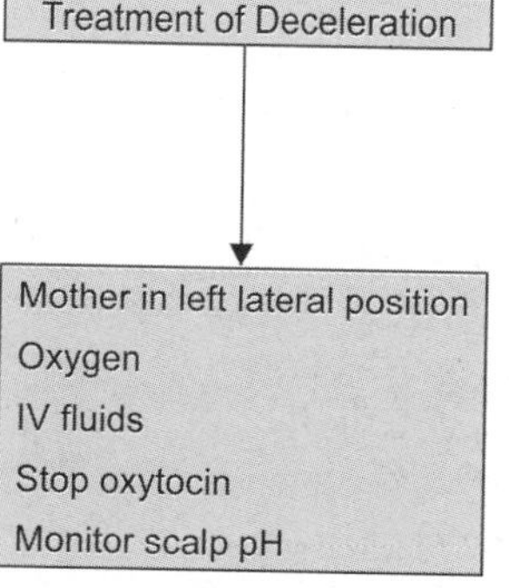

Treatment of deceleration

The biophysical profile (BPP) is a noninvasive test that predicts the presence or absence of fetal asphyxia and, ultimately, the risk of fetal death in the antenatal period. When the BPP identifies a compromised fetus, measures can be taken to intervene before progressive metabolic acidosis leads to fetal death.

The BPP combines data from 2 sources (i.e. ultrasound imaging and fetal heart rate [FHR] monitoring). Dynamic realtime B-mode ultrasound is used to measure the amniotic fluid volume (AFV) and to observe several types of fetal movement. The FHR is obtained using a pulsed Doppler transducer integrated with a high-speed microprocessor, which provides a continuously updated reading

Originally described by **Manning and colleagues**, the BPP has become a standard tool for providing antepartum fetal surveillance. The BPP integrates 5 parameters to yield a biophysical profile score (BPS) and includes:

- **The nonstress test (NST)**
- **Ultrasound measurement of the AFV, (Amniotic fluid volume)**
- **Fetal breathing movements**
- **Fetal body movements and**
- **Tone**

The BPP allows 2 points for each parameter that is present, yielding a maximum score of 10

- **Reassuring score is 8–10**
- **< 6 is fetal distress.**

USMLE Case Scenario

A 22 -year-old primigravida at 31 weeks of gestation has a blood pressure of 162/112 mm Hg, serum total bilirubin level (2.8 mg/dL), serum alanine aminotransferase level of 155U/L and platelet count of 72,000/mm^3. She is hospitalized for observation and electronic fetal heart rate monitoring of the following, the Most ominous sign of fetal distress during monitoring would be: Late decelerations

Cardiotocography

- Monitoring the baby's heartbeat is one way of checking babies' well-being in labor. By listening to, or recording the baby's heartbeat, it is hoped to identify babies who are hypoxic and who may benefit from cesarean section or instrumental vaginal birth
- The heartbeat can also be checked continuously by using a **CTG machine**
- This method is sometimes known as **electronic fetal monitoring (EFM)** and produces a paper recording of the baby's heart rate and their mother's labor contractions.

Risk Factors for Neural Tube Defects (NTD)

- Family history of NTD
- Insufficient folate
- Maternal diabetes
- Maternal use of antiepileptics

Chorioamnionitis

- Fever+maternal tachycardia
- Uterine tenderness
- Foul odor of amniotic fluid
- Leukocytosis

Complications are: Premature rupture of membranes

- Premature labor
- Endometritis
- Parametritis
- Abruptio placenta

Vaginal delivery is the mainstay of treatment

Neonatal Sepsis

Sepsis is asystemic response to infection. In newborns it can be classified as early onset, occurring in the first week of life, and late onset, occurring between 8 and 28 days. Risk factors for neonatal sepsis include:

- Maternal infection during pregnancy (urinary tract infection, chorioamnionitis), prematurity and prolonged rupture of membranes
- **Common organisms causing sepsis in the newborn are:**
  - **Group B streptococci**
  - **Escherichia coli**
  - **Listeria**
- Viral causes can be herpes simplex virus and enteroviruses
- Signs and symptoms of neonatal sepsis are nonspecific, such as grunting, tachypnea, cyanosis, poor feeding, irritability, apnea, bradycardia, jitters, tremors, and seizures
- Newborns do not always develop fever, and hypothermia may be a presenting sign
- A bulging fontanelle may be palpated on physical exam, but there is rarely nuchal rigidity
- Laboratory studies should include a complete blood count, lumbar puncture, and blood and urine cultures, as well as cultures of any visible lesions or drainage.

Remember

- **ACE inhibitors are contraindicated in pregnancy**
- **Yellow fever vaccine is contraindicated in pregnancy**

- **Propyl thiouracil is drug of choice** among antithyroid drugs in pregnancy
- **INH is safe** in pregnancy
- **Streptomycin** is **not given** in pregnancy
- **Primaquine** is **contraindicated** in pregnancy
- **Valproic acid** in pregnancy causes **Neural tube defects**

- **Alcohol: Fetal alcohol syndrome**
- **Warfarin: Fetal warfarin syndrome**
- **Phenytoin: Fetal hydantoin syndrome**
- **Tetracycline: Discoloration of teeth**

- Methotrexate is **unsafe in pregnancy**
- **Propothiouracil is safe** in pregnancy
- Varicella can cause **focal skin lesions and hypoplastic limbs**

- **Couvelaire uterus** seen in: Abruptio placenta
- **Rule of Hasse**: Determines age of fetus
- **Banana and lemon sign:** Seen in neural tube defects
- **Hartmans sign** is implantation bleeding
- **Chemical pregnancy** means positive beta HCG, Negative gestational sac

Causes of Symmetrical Enlargement of Uterus

- Pregnancy
- Submucous or Intramural (Solitary) fibroid
- Adenomyosis
- Myohyperplasia
- Pyometra
- Hematometra
- Lochiometra
- Malignancy
- CA of uterine body
- Choriocarcinoma

• **Mons pubis**	• **Pad of subcutaneous adipose connective tissue**
• **Labia majora**	• **Are homologous to scrotum and have hair follicles, sweat glands and sebaceous glands**
• **Labia minora**	• **Do not contain hair follicles**
• **Clitoris**	• **Is analogous to penis in males**
• **Anterior perineal triangle is**	• **Urogenital triangle**
• **Posterior perineal triangle is**	• **Anal triangle**
• **Central point of perineum is**	• **Perineal body**
• **Rectouterine pouch is**	• **Pouch of douglas**

• **Embryonic structure**	• **Female**
• **Genital ridge**	• Ovary
• **Genital swelling**	• L. majora
• **Genital fold**	• L. minora
• **Genital tubercle**	• Clitoris

Fallopian Tube

- **Has 4 parts**
- **Lined by ciliated columnar epithelium**
- **Has peg cells**
- **Measures 10 cms**

Female Urethra

- **4 cms in length**
- **6 mm in diameter**
- **Posterior urethrovesical angle is 100°**
- **Has transitional epithelium**

- **Uterine artery arises from internal iliac artery**
- **Vaginal artery arises from uterine artery**
- **Ovarian artery arises from aorta**

The larche, pubarche and menarche is the order of sexual development in girls.

Estrogen

- Produced by the Syncytiotrophoblast
- Its synthesis depends much on the precursor derived mainly from the fetus
- In late pregnancy, **estriol** is the most important estrogen
- Estrogen increases the **secretion and ciliary beating in fallopian tubes**
- Estrogen changes the **cuboidal lining of vagina to stratified**
- Estrogen changes the **breakdown of glycogen into lactate in vagina**
- Estrogen **initiates breast development**
- Estrogen causes **early epiphyseal closure**
- Estrogen causes **water retention**

Progesterone

- Produced by **Syncytiotrophoblast**
- Chief hormone of **Corpus luteum**
- Precursors from fetal origin are not necessary
- After delivery, its level decreases rapidly and is **not** detectable **after 24 hours**

Corpus Luteum Secretes

- **Progesterone**
- **Estrogen**
- **Inhibin**
- **Relaxin**

Ovulation

- Best predictor of ovulation is preovulatory rise in progesterone
- Source of progesterone in normal menstrual cycle is: Corpus luteum

- **Inhibin is secreted by Graffian follicle**
- **Ovulation coincides with LH surge**
- **LH surge proceeds ovulation by 24 hours**
- **Ovulatory period corresponds to 14 days before menstruation**

• **Proliferative phase**	• **Estrogen stimulation**
• **Secretory phase**	• **Progesterone stimulation**
• **Estrogen**	• **Produced by granulosa cells**
• **Progesterone**	• **Produced by corpus luteum**
• **FSH**	• **Stimulates growth of granulosa cells. Measure of ovarian reserve**
• **LH**	• **Stimulates follicle rupture and ovulation**

Supports of Uterus

- **Perineal body**
- **Pelvic diaphragm**
- **Transcervical ligament**
- **Pubocervical ligament**
- **Uterosacral ligament**
- **Uterine axis**
- **Round ligament of uterus**
- **Broad ligament is not a support of uterus**

Anomalies of Uterus

- **Uterus bicornis bicollis: Two uterine cavities, double cervix**
- **Uterus bicornis unicollis: Two uterine cavities, single cervix**
- **Septate uterus: Septum between two fused mullerian ducts**
- **Retroverted uterus: Long axis of body of uterus and cervix are in line instead of normal anteverted and anteflexed uterus**

Supports of Vagina

- **Perineal body**
- **Pelvic diaphragm**
- **Levator ani muscle**

Important Points about Vagina

- **Vagina lacks mucus secreting glands**
- **pH of normal adult vagina: 4.5-5.5**
- **pH of pregnant vagina: 3.5-4.5**
- **Epithelium of vagina: stratified squamous**

Lymphatic Drainage of Uterus

- From fundus and **upper part of body→Preaortic and Lateral aortic** group of nodes
- Cornu of uterus→**Superficial inguinal** lymph nodes
- Lower part of body →**Internal iliac group** of lymph nodes

- Lymphatic Drainage of Cervix
- **External iliac** nodes and **obturator** lymph nodes either directly or through para-cervical lymph nodes
- **Internal iliac** group of lymph nodes
- **Sacral group**

Lymphatic drainage of fallopian tube

- **Para–aortic** group along the ovarian vessels.

Lymphatic drainage of vagina

- **Upper 1/3→Iliac** group
- **Middle 1/3 up to hymen→Internal iliac** group
- **Below hymen→superficial inguinal** lymph nodes

Lymphatics of clitoris: Superficial inguinal, deep inguinal, Cloquets node

Bartholin's Gland

- Correspondes to **bulbourethral glands of male (B-B)**
- Situated in the **superficial perineal pouch**
- Lies **close** to the **posterior end** of vestibular bulb
- Are **pea** sized
- Lie near the junction of the **anterior 2/3 and posterior 1/3 of labium majus**
- It is a Compound **Racemose** Gland and its duct measures about **2 cm**, lined with **columnar Epithelium**
- Its duct passes forward and inward to open **external to the hymen** on **inner side of Labium minus**
- Infection of these glands or their ducts results in **Bartholinitis**

Acute bartholinitis

- Although Gonococcus is always in mind but more commonly **E.coli, Staphylococcus**

Streptococcus or Chlamydia trachomatis are involved

- The end results of acute bartholinitis are:
  - Complete resolution
  - Recurrence
  - Abscess formation
  - Cyst formation

Recurrent Bartholinitis

- Periodic painful attacks cause annoyance to the patient
- Treatment: **Active Phase**: Hot compress, Analgesics and Antibiotics after proper culture
- **Quiescent Phase:** Excision of the gland along with its duct.

Bartholins Abscess

- It is the **end result** of acute bartholinitis
- Duct is blocked by fibrosis, exudates pent up inside to produce abscess
- Treatment: Same as for bartholinitis. Abscess should be drained at the earliest before. It bursts
- **Marsupialization** not only helps in drainage of pus but prevents recurrence of abscess and future cyst formation
- It should be done under **General Anesthesia**
- Reccurrent Bartholin's abscess **Rx** _____ **Excision in Quiescent Stage**

Bartholin's Cyst

- It commonly involves the **duct** and **not** the gland
- Cyst of the duct or the gland can be **differentiated** by the **lining epithelium**

- Sometimes the cyst becomes large up to the size of **Hens egg**
- The shape of vulval cleft changes to **S-shaped**
- Rx: **Marsupialization**

Advantages of Marsupialization over traditional excision

- **Simple**
- **Can be done even under local Anesthesia**
- **Shorter hospital stay**
- **Postoperative complications almost nil**
- **Gland functions remain intact**

Gartners Duct

- Remnant of **wolfian duct**
- Runs below but **parallel** to the fallopian tube in the **mesosalpinx**
- The tubules of the gartners duct may be **cystic**
- The **outer** ones are **Kobelts tubules**
- The **Middle** set, the **Epoophoron**
- The **proximal** set, the **Paroopohoron**
- Small cyst may arise from any of the tubules
- A cystic swelling from the Gartners duct may appear in the anterolateral wall of the vagina **confusing** with cystocele. Cystic swelling is present at the **junction of lower 1/3 and upper 2/3 of vaginal wall**

Gartners Cyst	Cystocele
• Situated **anteriorly** or **anterolateral**	• Situated **anteriorly**
• Size is **variable**	• Size **increases** on straining
• Rugosities of the overlying vaginal. Mucosa is **lost.** Vaginal mucosa over it becomes **Tense and shiny**	• Mucosa over the bulge has **Transverse rugosity** • **No such** thing is seen
• Margins are **well defined**	• Margins are **diffuse**
• **Not** reducible	• Reducible
• **No** impulse on coughing	• Impulse on coughing is present

- **Length of female urethra:** 40 mm
- **Uterine cervix ratio up to 10 years:** 1:2
- Uterine cervix ratio in **adult:** 3:1
- **Normal Urethrovesical angle:** 100°
- **Size of Graffian follicle:** 2 mm

Important Facts about Vulva

- Leukoplakia of vulva is treated by **simple vulvectomy**
- Lymphatics of vulva go to **inguinal lymph nodes**
- Vulval carcinoma metastasizes to **superficial inguinal lymph nodes**
- **Sentinel biopsy is used in vulval cancer**

Important Facts about Vagina

- **Strawberry vagina: Trichomoniasis vaginalis**
- **Clue cells in vagina, fishy odoue, positive whiff test: hemophilus vaginalis**
- **pH of vagina is lowest in pregnancy**

- **Senile vaginitis is due to estrogen deficiency**
- **Vagina has no mucus secreting glands**
- **Lactobacillus is the protective bacterium in normal vagina**

Kartagener's Syndrome

Infertility is common, due to **defective ciliary action in the fallopian tube** in affected females or diminished sperm motility in affected males

In Kartagener's syndrome (KS), primary defects of the ciliary axoneme cause dyskinetic ciliary motion. Because ciliary motion is an important factor in normal ovum transport, ciliary dyskinesia may cause infertility. In active regions, beat frequency ranged from 5 to 10 Hz, approximately 30% of normal

- Electron microscopy shows morphological **defects in** tubal mucosa
- The number of cilia per cell is ↓
- The major ultrastructural abnormality was an absence of the central microtubules
- Electron microscopy demonstrated that the majority of cilia **lack dynein arms** and radial spokes and that various defects of microorgans existed in the sperm

PELVIC INFLAMMATORY DISEASES (PID)

Vaginal Discharge

• Yellow, pH > 5, clue cells, amine odor	• **Bacterial vaginosis**
• Cottage cheese discharge, pruritis	• **Candida**
• Frothy, Foamy discharge and motile trophozites seen	• **Trichomonas vaginalis**

PID

• **Gram-negative diplococcic** in PMNs in urethral Exudate	• **Nisseria gonorrhea**
• **Culture negative** specimen with inclusion bodies	• **Chlamydiae trachomatis**
• Organisms **without cell wall** and **urease positive**	• **Ureaplasma urealyticum**
• **Flagellate protozoa** with motility	• **Trichomonas vaginalis**

Chancroid

- **Hemophilus ducreyi**
  - **Painful ulcer, genital ulceration and inguinal adenitis**
  - **Painful lymphadenopathy seen**
  - Associated with **infection with HIV**
- **School of fish appearance**
- H. ducreyi is a highly fastidious coccobacillary gram-negative bacterium **whose growth requires X factor (hemin)**
- **Chancroid** can be treated effectively with several regimens, including (1) **ceftriaxone**, 250 mg intramuscularly as a single dose; (2) azithromycin, 1 g orally as a single dose; (3) erythromycin, 500 mg orally four times daily for 7 days; and (4) ciprofloxacin, 500 mg orally twice daily for 3 days.

Candida

- Caused by **candida albicans**
- **Recurrent vulvovaginalis: 4 or more episodes per year**
- It is a **gram-positive fungus**
- Common in **pregnancy, diabetes mellitus**
- Commonly seen in **pregnancy, diabetes, antibiotics, OCP use, Corticosteroids**

- **Profuse curdy white curdy** discharge or **cottage cheese appearance**
- Dyspareunia
- Burning sensation
- Intense pruritis

Trichomoniasis

- **Most common vaginal infection**
- **Caused by flagellate parasite 'trichomonas vaginalis'**
  - **Profuse, thin, greeny discharge which is malodorous**
  - **Strawberry vagina/colpitis macularis appearance**
- **Best test: Culture**
- **Metronidazole is DOC**
- **Treat sexual partener concurrently**

Bacterial Vaginosis

Poly microbial caused by:

- **Gardenella vaginalis**
- **Hemophilus vaginalis**
- **Mobilincus**
- **Ureaplasma urealyticum**
- **Mycoplasma hominis**

- **↓Lactobacilli**
- **↓Leucocytes**
- **ALKALINE pH**

- **'Clue cells'** are epithelial cells with bacteria adhering to their surface and sometimes obscuring their borders. Clue cells indicate bacterial vaginosis
- Clue cells were first described by **Gardner and Dukes** in 1955 and were so named **as these cells give an important 'clue' to the diagnosis of bacterial vaginosis (BV)**
- Clue cells are vaginal squamous epithelial cells coated with anaerobic Gram-variable coccobacilli Gardnerella vaginalis.

Pathogenesis:

The detection of clue cells is the most useful single procedure for the diagnosis of BV. Presence of more than 20% clue cells in vaginal discharge is included in Amsel's criteria for the diagnosis of BV. Other criteria for the diagnosis of BV include:

Milky, homogeneous, adherent discharge

vaginal pH greater than 4.5

Positive Whiff test, i.e. typical fishy odor on addition of one or two drops of 10% KOH to vaginal discharge and

Few or no lactobacilli

Metronidazole (DOC) or clindamycin is used in treatment

Metronidazole is used in pregnancy.

LGV

- **Chlamydia trachomatis L type**
  - **Painless ulcer**
  - **Esthiomine seen in LGV**
  - **Groove sign. (Double genitocrural fold)**
  - **Genital elephantiasis is seen**

- Incubation period = 3 days to 3 weeks. **Painless,** vesicle, often transient, followed by **suppurative LAP**
- **Sign of Groove +** (LAP present both above and below inguinal ligament)
- **Elephantiasis** of vulva + Vaginal and rectal strictures seen
- **Frei's** intadermal test +
- **Doxycycline is DOC**

Donovaniosis (Granuloma inguinale)

- **Calymatobacterium granulomaosis**
- **Painless ulcer**
- **Painless beffy red ulcer with fresh granulation tissue**

Herpes Genitalis

- **HSV II virus usual**
- **Painful vesicular lesions**

Condyloma Acuminata

- **Most common** viral STD
- Caused by HPV: **6, 16, 18**
- Immunosuppression, diabetes, pregnancy are predisposing factors
- **Cauliflower like masses**, pedunculated

Treated by:

- **Podophyllin, podophox**
- **Trichloroacetic acid**
- **Imiquimoid**
- **Cryo**
- **LASER**
- **Surgical excision**

Condyloma lata are seen in secondary syphilis

Chlamydia

- Purulent discharge, urethritis, arthritis, conjuctivitis
- **Infertility** associated with fallopian-tube scarring. It appears that subclinical tubal infection **('silent salpingitis')** may produce scarring
- **Ectopic pregnancy**
- **Perihepatitis, or the Fitz-Hugh-Curtis syndrome**, this syndrome should be suspected whenever a young, sexually active woman presents with an illness resembling cholecystitis (fever and right-upper-quadrant pain of subacute or acute onset). Symptoms and signs of salpingitis may be minimal. High titers of antibodies to C. trachomatis are generally present
- **PCR is gold standard for diagnosis**
- **Azithromycin is DOC for uncomplicated chlamydiae**
- **Azithromycin is DOC for chlamydiae in pregnancy**
- **Erythromycin is safe in pregnancy**
- **Azithromycin and contact tracing is the most effective for chlamydiae infections**

Genital Tuberculosis

- Genital TB is almost always **secondary** to focus elsewhere
- Primary focus is in **lungs (50%)**, lymph nodes (40%) cases
- **Hematogeneous spread** is the commonest mode followed by direct spread and ascending route
- **Major forms:**
  - **Tuberculous endosalpingitis**
  - **Tuberculous exosalpingitis**
  - **Interstitial salpingitis**
- Only about 10% of genital TB cases have children
- First site of affection are the **fallopian tubes**
- Commonest site of affection are the **fallopian tubes**
- **'Tobacco pouch appearance'** of fallopian tubes is a feature
- **'Salpingitis isthmica nodosa'** is nodular thickening of tubes in genital TB
- **Endometrium** of uterus is **involved in 60% cases**
- **Cervix** is involved in **10–15% of cases**
- Infertility is due to blockage of fallopian tubes. In the form of TB endosalpingitis
- The first line of treatment is **ATT** (Antitubercular therapy)

USMLE Case Scenario

An 18-year-old girl complains of malodorous vaginal discharge. She is sexually active and uses condoms for sexual intercourse. On examination, a thin, grayish-white discharge is seen. A musty odor is produced when KOH is added to the discharge. The vaginal fluid has a pH of 5. Which of the following is the most likely finding on a microscopic examination of the vaginal fluid?

1. Bacterial vaginosis (BV)
2. Viral inclusions
3. Gram-negative diplococci
4. Lactobacilli
5. Pseudohyphae
6. Motile, flagellated organisms

Ans. 1. Bacterial vaginosis (BV)

Endometriosis

- **Commonest site: ovary**
- Followed by: **pouch of Douglas, uterosacral ligaments, rectovaginal septum**
- Peak age: 30–40 years
- **Common innullipara**
- Chocolate cysts
- Tenderness and nodularity of uterosacral ligaments
- **Sampson's theory of retrograde menstruation. (Most accepted)**
- **Meyer and ivanoffs coelomic metaplasia theory**
- **Direct implantation theory**
- **Halbans lymphatic theory**
- Rare in negroes
- **Pelvic pain** (commonest manifestation)
- **Painful periods** Dysmenorrhea
- **Painful intercourse** Dyspareunia
- **Painful bowel movements** Dyschezia

- Menorrhagia
- Polymenorrhea
- Infertility

Treatment:
- **Progesterone**
- **OCP**
- **CLOMIPHENE (in infertile women)**
- **Danazol**
- **GnRH analogues (leuprolide)**
- **Ovarian cystectomy/oopherectomy/Wedge resection**
- **Paratubal lysis by laproscopy**
- **Total hysterectomy: For diffuse endometriosis interna**

Endometriosis: Atypical Sites

- Abdominal scars
- Bladder/ureter
- Cervix/vagina
- Umbilicus
- Gut
- Lungs

Naked Eye Appearances

- Powder burns
- Red flame shaped areas
- Yellow brown patches
- White areas and circular peritoneal defects

Pseudoxanthoma cells: Adjacent to lining of endometriosis, presence of polyhedral, phagocytic, pigmented cells with hemosiderin

A female of 34 years complain of dysmenorrheal, dyspareunia and dyschezia with fixed retroverted uterus and nodularity of uterosacral ligaments

Adenomyosis

- Endometrial glands without Myometrium of uterine wall
- Secondary dysmenorrhea and menorrhagia are common
- **Uterus is enlarged and tender**
- Treatment: Hysterectomy

A female 36-year-old with dysmenorrhea, **menorrhagia, chronic pelvic pain and symmetrically, enlarged smooth uterus** tender to palpation

CONTRACEPTION

Gossypol

- **Male contraceptive**
- **Direct suppression of semineferous tubules causing azoospermia**
- **Suppresses LH**

IUCD

Act by ovulation inhibition, causing aseptic endometritis
Act by prevention of fertilization
Act by interfering with implantation
Contraindications:
- **PID**
- **Diabetes mellitus**
- **Congenital uterine anomalies**
- **Heart disease**
- **Pelvic TB**
- **HIV Positives**
- **Suspected pregnancy**
- **Previous ectopic**
- **Menorrhagia**

Commonest side effect is bleeding

Nova T has a silver core but contains both copper and silver

- **In CuT_{200}, 200 mean 200 mm^2 of copper**
- **CuT_{200} is inserted postnatally after 8 weeks**
- **If CuT_{200} is implanted in Myometrium treatment is hysteroscopic removal**
- **CuT_{200} should be replaced after every 10 years**

Contraceptive TODAY

Contraceptive TODAY
- **Contains 9 NON OXYNOL**
- **It is a barrier contraceptive**
- **Effective for 24 hours after insertion**
- **Spermicidal in nature**

- **NORPLANT contains levonorgesterol**
- **Centrochroman is antiestrogenic, antiprogestogenic nonteratogenic, long acting pill**
- **Mifeprestone is an antiprogestogen**
- **MINERA is Progesterone IUCD**

Uses of OCP

- **Contraception, emergency postcoital (prophylaxis)** A combination of levonorgestrel 50 or norgestrel with ethinyl estradiolis used as emergency contraception (also called intraception, morning-after treatment, or postcoital contraception) for postcoital birth control, after pregnancy has been ruled out. **The dosing method using high doses of estrogen-progestin hormones is commonly called the Yuzpe method**
- **Acne vulgaris**
- **Amenorrhea**
- **Dysfunctional uterine bleeding (DUB)**
- **Dysmenorrhea**
  - **Hypermenorrhea**
  - **Endometriosis (Prophylaxis and Treatment)**

- **Hirsutism, female**
- **Hyper and rogenism, ovarian**
- **Polycystic ovary syndrome**

WHO Categories Contraindications for Estrogens/OCPS

- Age > 40 years
- Smoker < 35 years
- History of Jaundice
- Mild Hypertension
- Gallbladder disease
- Diabetes
- Sickle Cell anemia
- Headache
- CINor Ca Cervix

- Unexplained Vaginal bleeding
- Hyperlipidemia
- Past Breast Cancer
- Benign Liver tumors
- Heavy smoker
- Breastfeeding

- OCPS protect against **endometrial cancer, Ovarian cancer**
- **OCP of choice in Lactating females is Mini Pill**
- **Fertility returns 6 months after OCP use**

Drugs Decreasing Effectiveness of OCP

- **Barbiturates**
- **Carbamazepine**
- **Phenytoin**
- **Rifampicin**

Levonorgestrel

- Levonorgestrel is a **synthetic progestogen** used as an active ingredient in hormonal contraception
- **Makes endometrium unreceptive**
- **Makes cervical** mucus thick
- It is used effectively in emergency contraception both in **combined form with estrogens as well as levonorgestrel only method**
- Levonorgestrel only method uses **'1500 µgm single dose'** or **'750 µgm' doses twelve hours** apart within 3 days of unprotected sexual activity

Progestasert

- Third generation IUCD containing progesterone
- Decreases blood loss
- Decreases dysmenorrhea
- BUT ↑ risk of ectopics

Third Generation OCP

Contain 3rd generation progesterone
- Desogestrel
- Norgestimate
- Gestodene
  - Lower risk of arterial thrombosis
  - Higher risk of venous thrombosis
  - Lipid friendly

Infertility

- Failure to conceive within one or more years of regular unprotected sex
- Male responsible for 30% cases
- Female responsible for 30% cases

INTRAUTERINE INSEMINATION

Indications

- Hostile cervical mucus
- Cervical stenosis
- Oligospermia
- Immune factors
- Unexplained fertility

INTRACERVICAL INSEMINATION

Indications

- Hypospadias
- Retrograde ejaculation
- Impotence
- Third degree retroversion of uterus

IN VITRO FERTILIZATION

Indications

- Tubal disease
- Unexplained infertility
- Cervical hostility
- Failed ovulation induction
- Endometriosis
- Male factor infertility

Other Assisted Reproduction Techniques

GIFT: Gamete intrafallopian transfer
ZIFT: Zygote intrafallopian transfer
MIST: Microinsemination sperm transfer

- **Aspiration of sperms is done in TESA**
- **In Post-testicular azospermia technique used is PESA/MESA**

- **Ferning pattern of cervical mucus is because of: Estrogen**
- **Palm leaf pattern cervix is due to estrogen**
- **Spinbarkiet phenomenon is maximum in ovulatory phase**
- **Postcoital test determines cervical factor**

Prolapse

- **Cystocele**: Prolapse of upper 2/3 of **anterior** vaginal wall. Formed by **base** of bladder
- **Urethrocele**: Prolapse of lower 1/3 of **anterior** vaginal wall
- **Enterocele**: Prolapse of upper 1/3 of **posterior** vaginal wall
- **Rectocele**: Prolapse of lower 2/3 of **posterior** vaginal wall
- **Uterine prolapse**: Abnormal descent of uterus through vagina
- **Procedentia**: Complete uterine prolapse outside vulva

- Prolapse in pregnant women in **1st Trimester: Pessary**
- Prolapse in pregnant women in **2nd Trimester: Resolves itself**
- Prolapse in young women: **Sling operation, Perineal exercise**
- Prolapse in Women < **40 years with family complete wanting to retain** menstrual function: **Fother gills operation**
- Prolapse in **Women > 40 years with family complete**

Not wanting to retain menstrual function: **Vaginal Hysterectomy**

- Prolapse in **old Women who cannot sustain surgery: Le Fortes surgery**

Complications

- **Elongation of cervix**
- **Cystocele**
- **Decubitus ulcer**
- **Decubitus ulcer is because of venous congestion**

Fistula

- **MC urinary fistula: Vesicovaginal**
- **MC cause of VVF in India: obstructed labor (DOC cystoscopy)**
- **MC cause of Uretrovaginal fistula: injury to ureter in Hysterectomy**
- **MC cause of vesicouterine fistula: cesarean section**
- **MC cause of Rectovaginal fistula: complete perineal tear**

Menstrual Disorders

- **'Menarche'** (First Menstruation) occurs between **11 and 15 years**
- Normal duration of menstrual period is **4–5 days**
- Peak Secretory activity is seen on **Day 22** of menstrual cycle
- Amount of blood loss is **20–80 ml**
- **AVERAGE** blood loss in normal periods is **50 ml**
- **Precocious menstruation** occurs in females aged **less than 10 years**

- **'Menopause'** means permanent cessation of menstruation at an average age of 50 years
- **'Premature menopause'** is when menstruation stops at or below 40 years of age
- **'Delayed Menopause'** is when menopause fails to occur even beyond 55 years

- **Polymenorrhea** is cyclic bleeding **where cycle length is reduced to less than 21 days** and remains constant at that frequency
- **Metorrhagia** is **irregular, acyclic bleeding**
- **Menometorrhagia** is irregular and excessive bleeding to the extent that **menstrual period is not recognized at all**
- **Hypomenorrhea** is scant bleeding lasting for less than 2 days

- **Most common cause of postmenopausal bleeding in India is ca cervix**
- **Most common cause of secondary amenorrhea in India is: endometrial tuberculosis**

Amenorrhea means absence of periods for 6 months or more

Causes of cryptomenorrhea:

- Imperforate hymen
- Transverse septum in vagina
- Noncanalization of cervix
- Cervical canal stenosis

Primary Amenorrhea

Failure of onset of menses in a girl by 16 years of age
Causes:

- **Aplasia/hypoplasia of uterus**
- **Turner's syndrome**
- **Pseudohermaphroditism**
- **Cretinism**

Syndromes Causing Amenorrhea

- **Kallaman's syndrome**
- **Prader willi syndrome**
- **Laurence-Moon-Biedl syndrome**
- **Frohlich's syndrome**
- **Turner's syndrome**
- **Sheehan's syndrome**
- **Sweyer's syndrome**
- **Asherman's syndrome**

Dysfunctional Uterine Bleeding

Menorrhagia without extragenital cause and normal pelvic examination
Associated with metropathia hemorrhagica
Endometrium can be:

- **Normal**
- **Hyperplastic (commonest)**
- **Irregular shedding, irregular ripening**
- **Tubercular endometritis**
- **Chronic endometritis**
- **Progesterone is usually deficient. ↑Estrogen**
- **Estrogen, OCP, progesterone, danazol are used for treatment**

Premenstrual Syndrome: PMS

- **Depression**
- **Irritability**
- **Anxiety**
- **Breast tenderness**
- **Lethargy**
- **Insomnia/Hypersomnia, swelling, weight gains on monthly basis and disappearing with menses**
- **More severe form is premenstrual dysmorphic disorder**
- **Symptoms should occur for 3 consecutive cycles**
- **Must interfere with normal functioning**
- **Must resolve with onset of menses**

Mittelschmerz

- **Lower abdominal pain cyclically 2 weeks before menstruation**
- **In mid menstrual period**
- **Nausea and constipation invariably absent**
- **May be associated with mucoid discharge**

PCOD (Polycystic Ovarian Disease)

Associations:

- **Hirusitism**
- **Obesity**
- **Acne**
- **Acanthosis Nigricans**
- **Infertility**
- **Associated with endometrial hyperplasia and endometrial cancer**
- **↑Testosterone**
- **↑LH/FSH**

Bilaterally enlarged ovaries

- OCPS
- Metformin
- Clomiphene citrate
- Spironolactones are used in treatment

A 20-year-old **obese** female with **irregular menstrual periods, acne, insulin resistance and elevated LH: FSH ratio**

Meyer Rokintansky Hauser Syndrome	Testicular Feminization Syndrome
• 46 XX • Phenotype: Female • Aplasia/hypoplasia of vagina • Ovary present • Female Secondary sexual characters normally developed	• 46 XY • Phenotype: Female • Blind vaginal pouch with absent uterus

Mullerian Agenesis

- Mullerian agenesis **(The Mayer-Rokitansky-Kuster-Hauser syndrome)** second in frequency only to gonadal dysgenesis as a cause of primary amenorrhea
- Caused by mutations in the genes encoding **anti-mullerian hormone (AMH) or its receptor (AMHR)**
- **Women** with this syndrome have a
  - **46, XX karyotype**
  - **Female secondary sex characteristics**
  - **Normal ovarian function,** including cyclic ovulation
  - **Absence or hypoplasia of the vagina**
- **The uterus** usually consists of only rudimentary bicornuate cords, but if the uterus contains endometrium, cyclic abdominal pain and accumulation of blood may occur, as in other forms of outlet obstruction
- One-third of women with this syndrome have **abnormalities of the urogenital tract** and one-tenth has **skeletal anomalies,** usually involving the spine
- **Demonstration of a 46, XX karyotype the biphasic basal body temperature curve characteristic of ovulation and elevated levels of progesterone during the luteal phase establish the diagnosis of mullerian agenesis**

Testicular Feminization Syndrome

- The major diagnostic problem is distinguishing mullerian agenesis from complete testicular feminization
- **46, XY genetic males with testes** differentiate as phenotypic women but with a **blind vaginal pouch and no uterus**
- Women with testicular feminization have **feminized breasts but a paucity of pubic and axillary hair.** The disorder is X-linked and is caused by mutations in the androgen receptor that result in profound **resistance to the action of testosterone**
- Testicular feminization can be diagnosed by demonstrating a
  - **Male level of serum testosterone**
  - **46, XY Karyotype**

- **Doderleins bacillus** is protective bacterium in normal vagina
- **Nabothian follicles** are seen in cervical erosion
- **Lipshutz ulcer effects**: Vagina

Cancer Cervix

Predisposing factors:

- **Early age of coitus**
- **Multiple sex partners**
- **Multiparity**
- **Poor hygiene**
- **Poor socioeconomic status**
- **Smoking, alcohol, drug abuse**
- **Associated STDS**
- **Immunosupression**

- **Most common virus associated with squamous cell carcinoma: HPV 16**
- **Most common virus associated with Adenocarcinoma: HPV 18**
- **Most common virus associated with Verrucous carcinoma: HPV 6**

- Commonest Presenting symptom: **Bleeding pv**
- Arises from **squamo columnar junction**
- Earliest symptom is **postcoital bleeding**
- **MC site is ectocervix**
- Caused By HPV **Virus**
- Mc agent HPV 16
- Types associated with **cervical** carcinoma are **16, 18,** 31, 45 and 51 to 53
- Predisposing factors are: **HSV, HIV, HPV infections**
- **Obturator, hypogastric and external iliac lymph nodes** are affected

Time taken for conversion of CINTO INVASIVE CANCER: 10 YEARS

- Uncomplicated HPV lower genital tract infection and condylomatous atypia of the cervix can progress to CIN. This lesion precedes invasive **cervical** carcinoma and is classified as low-grade squamous intraepithelial lesion (SIL), high-grade SIL and carcinoma in situ
- Approximately 80% of invasive cervix carcinomas are **squamous cell tumors**
- 10 to 15% are adenocarcinomas, 2 to 5% are adenosquamous with epithelial and glandular structures, and 1 to 2% is clear cell mesonephric tumors
- Patients with cervix **cancer** generally present with **abnormal bleeding or postcoital spotting** that may increase to intermenstrual or prominent menstrual bleeding. Yellowish vaginal discharge, lumbosacral back pain and urinary symptoms can also be seen

The staging of **cervical** carcinoma is clinical and generally completed with a pelvic examination under anesthesia with cystoscopy and proctoscopy. **Chest X-rays, intravenous pyelograms and computed tomography are generally required and magnetic resonance imaging (MRI) may be used to assess extracervical extension**

- **Stage 0** is **carcinoma in situ**
- **Stage I** is disease **confined to the cervix**
- **Stage II** disease invades **beyond the cervix but not to the pelvic wall** or lower third of the vagina
- **Stage III** disease **extends to the pelvic wall or lower third of the vagina** or causes hydronephrosis
- **Stage IV** is present when the **tumor invades the mucosa of bladder or rectum or extends beyond the true pelvis**

- Cervical biopsy is the **best method of diagnosing** cervical cancer
- Pap smear is the **best method of screening**
- Renal failure is the **commonest cause of death**
- **100% cure rates** are seen in carcinoma situ

- Treatment of stage II is: Extended hysterectomy, chemotherapy and intracavitary brachytherapy
- Treatment of stage III B is: Radiotherapy and chemotherapy

Cone Biopsy

Indications:

- Cervical lesion cannot be visualized by coloposcope
- Squamo columnar junction is not seen by coloposcope
- Endocervical curettage demonstrates findings positive for CIN II,CIN III
- Lack of correlation between biopsy and coloposcopy
- Microinvasive carcinoma or adenocarcinoma in situ on coloposcopy
- Therapeutic in case of CIN III (Best approach in elderly is hysterectomy)
- Done under general anesthesia ideally

Complications:

- Hemorrhage
- Infection
- Cervical stenosis
- In case of visible mass: Punch biopsy
- In case of no mass: Coloposcopic directed biopsy

Fibroid (Uterine Leiomyoma)

- They are **proliferative, well-circumscribed, pseudoencapsulated, benign Tumors** composed of smooth muscle and fibrous connective tissue
- They are the **most common** uterine mass found in the **female pelvis**
- Most common **neoplasm** found in the female pelvis
- Most common **benign solid tumor** in females
- They are present in **15–20%** of women especially after **30–35 years** of age
- They vary in diameter from **1 mm** to more than **20 cm**
- They are **more** common in **nulliparous**
- The prevalence is highest between **35 and 45 years**

Etiology

- Fibroids are **monoclonal Tumors resulting from somatic mutation**. They arise from
- Single neoplastic smooth muscle cell
- Abnormalities in **chromosomes 6, 7, 12 and 14** have been identified
- Disruption or Dysregulation of the high mobility group genes on **chromosome 12** contribute to fibroid development

Role of Hormones:

- Estrogen is a promoter of fibroid growth **and not** its causal factor
- Fibroids rarely found **before puberty**
- They stop growing **after menopause**
- New fibroids rarely appear **after menopause**
- They often grow rapidly during **pregnancy and amongst Pill Users**
- **GnRH agonists** create a hypoestrogenic environment that results in a reduction of the size of fibroid
- Some **Peptide growth factors** play a role in etiology
- Epidermal Growth Factor **(EGF)** induces DNA synthesis in fibroids and myometrial cells
- Estrogen exerts its effect through **EGF**

PIRFENIDONE, an antifibrotic agent suppresses fibroid growth as it inhibits fibrogenic cytokines including basic **FGF, PDGF, TGF-beta and EGF.**

Intramural or Interstitial Fibroid:

- **Most common** variety
- Occur within the walls of uterus as isolated, encapsulated nodules of varying size
- When they grow they distort uterine cavity or external surface and are pushed inwards or outwards
- They cause **symmetrical enlargement** of the uterus when they occur singly **(Solitary)**

Submucous Fibroid

- Located beneath the endometrium and can grow into the uterine cavity
- Least common **(about 5%) BUT maximum** symptoms

Fate of Submucous fibroid

- Surface necrosis (abnormal bleeding and anemia)
- Polypoid change following pedicle formation
- Infection
- Degenerations including Sarcomatous change

Subserous Fibroid (Subperitoneal)

- Located just **beneath the serosal surface** and grow out towards the peritoneal cavity, causing bulging of the peritoneal surface of the uterus
- They may develop a pedicle, become pedunculated and reach a large size within the peritoneal cavity without producing symptoms

Other Types of Fibroid

- **Wandering fibroid**: In **Subserous** variety, on rare occasion, the pedicle may be torn through; the fibroid gets its nourishment from the **omentum, mesentery** or **bowel** and develop a secondary blood supply. The resulting structure is known as **Wandering fibroid** or **Parasitic fibroid**
- **Intraligamentary fibroid (false or pseudofibroid)**: The **Intramural** fibroid may be pushed out in between the layers of Broad Ligament and is called **Intraligamentary fibroid** or **Broad ligament fibroid**

Cervical Fibroid:

- **Rare** (1–2%)
- **SITE:** Supravaginal part of cervix
- **INTERSTITIAL** variety may displace the cervix or expand it so much that **external os** is difficult to recognize
- All these disturb the pelvic anatomy, specially the **ureter**. In the vaginal cervix, the fibroid is usually **pedunculated** and rarely sessile

Pseudocervical fibroid: A Fibroid polyp arising from the uterine body when occupies and distends the cervical canal, it is called **Pseudocervical Fibroid**

Pathological Changes

1. Fibroids are **pseudoencapsulated** solid Tumors
2. **Well demarcated** from surrounding myometrium
3. The **false capsule** has more parallel arrangement while the tumor has whorled appearance
4. The capsule is pinkish in color in contrast to whitish appearance of the tumor
5. The capsule is separated from the tumor by **A THIN LOOSE AREOLAR TISSUE**
6. The blood vessels run through this plane to supply the tumor
7. The tumor is shelled out during Myomectomy through this plane
8. The periphery of tumor is more vascular and has more growth potentiality
9. The center of the tumor is least vascular and likely to degenerate

CELLULAR LEIOMYOMAS: Are Tumors with mitotic counts of **five to ten per 10** consecutive **high power fields** that **lack** cytological atypia

LEIOMYOSARCOMAS: **Previously** diagnosed on the basis of mitotic count of 10 mitotic figures per 10 high-power fields. The new factors recently recognized are **CELLULAR ATYPIA** and **COAGULATIVE NECROSIS** of tumor cells.

Secondary Changes in Fibroids

1. Degeneration
2. Atrophy
3. Necrosis
4. Infection
5. Vascular changes
6. Sarcomatous changes

Red Degeneration of Fibroid

- Occurs mainly in **large** fibroids
  - **Tumor is red/purple in color**
  - **It is due to thrombosis of large veins in the tumor**
  - **It has apeculiar fishy odor**
- Occurs during **Second half** of pregnancy or **puerperium**
- Most **frequent complication** of myoma during pregnancy

- The tumor assumes a peculiar **purple-red color**
- Cause is **vascular** in nature (Thrombosis of large veins in the tumor)
- Infection has **no** role and the process is an **aseptic** one
- Presentation as a case of an **acute abdomen**
- It produces **pain and tenderness** (hyaline degeneration **does not**)
- Clinical features include **fever**, moderate **leucocytosis** and **increased ESR**
- It has a peculiar **fishy odor**
- **Management is conservative and include:**
  - Bedrest
  - Analgesics and Sedatives
  - The symptoms usually clear off within 10 days
  - **Laparotomy** if done with **mistaken diagnosis,** the abdomen is to be **closed** immediately

Sarcomatous Change in Fibroid

- **Rarest** among all other secondary changes in the fibroid (**0.5%** of all myomas)
- Seen in **women** > **40 years** age
- **Postmenopausal**
- **Intramural and submucous fibroid** > **Subserous (least common)**
- Treatment is total hysterectomy and bilateral salping oophorectomy followed by radiotherapy

Guidelines for the Management of Myomas

- **ASYMPTOMATIC**: **No** treatment required
- **Symptomatic**
  - **Young**
  - **Old And Family Complete**
- Medical Treatment
- Hysterectomy
  - Ru 486 (Mifepristone)
  - GnRH analogues

Surgical (Myomectomy)

Myomectomy

- **Indications**
  - **Infertile Women** in her reproductive period desirous of having a baby
  - **Recurrent pregnancy wastage** due to fibroid
- **Prerequisites Prior to Myomectomy**
  - Examination of **Husband** (From fertility point of view)
  - **Hysterosalpingography** (to detect a fibroid encroaching the uterine cavity OR polyp OR tube)
  - **Diagnostic D+C** (in cases of irregular cycles to exclude endometrial carcinoma)
- **Facts to be in Mind Prior to Consideration of Myomectomy**
- It should be done mainly to **preserve** the reproductive function
- The wish to preserve the menstrual function in parous women should be judiciously complied
- More **risky** operation when the fibroid **is too big** and **too many**
- Chance of **recurrence (5–10%)**
- Chance of **persistence** of menorrhagia **(1–5%)**
- Increased rate of **relaparotomy** to the extent of **20–25%**
- Pregnancy rate is about **40–50%**
- Pregnancy following myomectomy should have a **mandatory hospital delivery**, although the chance of scar rupture is rare.

Contraindications

- Husband proved **infertile**. In the face of advent of ART, counseling is imperative
- Associated **bilateral infective tubo-ovarian** mass
- **Infected** fibroid

Technically Difficult Cases with Poor Reproductive Outcome

- **Big** broad ligament fibroid
- Too many fibroids

Advantages of Hysterectomy Over Myomectomy

- There is no chance of recurrence
- Adnexal pathology and the unhealthy cervix can also be removed

Role of Vaginal Hysterectomy in Fibroid Surgery

- Fibroids with size of **10-12 weeks** of pregnancy and **associated with uterine prolapse** are better dealt by **Vaginal Hysterectomy** with repair of pelvic floor

Indications of Surgery in Asymptomatic Fibroid

- **Size > 12 weeks** of pregnancy
- Diagnosis is **not** certain
- Fibroid **grows during** follow-up
- **Subserous pedunculated fibroid**
- **Unexplained infertility** with distortion of the uterine cavity
- **Unexplained recurrent abortion**
- Situated in the **lower part of uterus** and likely to complicate delivery

Indications of Emergency Surgery in Fibroid

- **Torsion of subserous pedunculated fibroid**
- **Massive intraperitoneal hemorrhage following rupture of veins over subserous fibroid**
- **Uncontrolled infected fibroid**
- **Uncontrolled bleeding fibroid**

- Fibroids are the **commonest benign solid tumors in females**
- Most common variety of fibroid is **intramural/interstitial**
- They are estrogen dependent
- **Most common type of degeneration** is the **'Hyaline Type'** which starts from the center
- **Red degeneration** of fibroid is seen with pregnancy
- **Sarcomatous change** or malignant change is rare (0.5%)
- **Malignant potential** is most in **intramural fibroids**
- **Calcerous degeneration** is most with **sub serous fibroid**
- Most fibroids start as **Interstitial fibroids**
- **Uterine fibroids are associated with endometriosis**
- **Wandering or parasitic fibroid issue serious fibroid**
- **MC symptom is menorrhagia**

Fibroids are associated with

- **Follicular ovarian cysts**
- **Endometriosis**
- **Endometrial Hyperplasia**
- **Endometrial Ca**

Endometrial Carcinoma

Occurs most often in the **sixth and seventh decades of life**

Symptoms often include

- **Abnormal vaginal discharge**
- **Abnormal bleeding which is usually postmenopausal**
- **Leukorrhea**

Between **75 and 80%** of all endometrial carcinomas are **adenocarcinomas**

Adenocarcinoma with squamous differentiation is seen in 10% of patients; the most differentiated form is known as adenoacanthoma and the poorly differentiated form is called **adenosquamous carcinoma**

Most Malignant: Clear Cell carcinoma

Other less common pathologies include:

- **Carcinoma (5%) and papillary serous carcinoma**
- **Secretory (2%)**
- **Ciliated, clear cell**
- **Undifferentiated carcinomas**

Lymph nodes involved are:

- **Para-aortic**
- **Presacral**
- **Inguinal**

Predisposing Factors for Endometrial Cancer

- ***Family History***
- ***Hypertension***
- ***Obesity***
- ***Late Menopause***
- ***Diabetes***
- ***Atypical Endometrial Hyperplasia***
- ***Unopposed Estrogen***
- ***Nulliparity***
- ***Tamoxifen therapy***
- ***PCOD***

The prognosis of endometrial ca depends on:

- **Age at diagnosis (old age: worse prognosis)**
- **Stage of disease**
- **Histological subtype**

Histological Grade

- Myometrial invasion
- Lymph node metastasis
- **Cervical extension** (Cervical involvement is associated with increased risk of extrauterine disease and Lymph node metastasis)
- Tumor size
- **Hormone receptor status** (Receptor positive-better prognosis)
- **Ploidy status** (Aneuploid tumors have better prognosis than diploid tumors)
- **Oncogene expression/mutation** (HER 2/neu, k ras: poor prognosis)

Risk factors for endometrial Hyperplasia are:
- Obesity
- Anovulation
- Low fertility index

'The Lynch syndrome' occurs in families with an autosomal dominant mutation of mismatch repair genes MLH1, MSH2, MSH6, and PMS2, which predispose to nonpolyposis colon cancer as well as endometrial and ovarian cancer

Abdominal Hysterectomy (Indications)

Total abdominal hysterectomy
- DUB
- Uterine fibroid
- Tubo-ovarian mass (T.O. MASS)
- Endometriosis

Subtotal hysterectomy
- Difficult TO mass
- Endometriosis (Rectovaginal septum)
- Obstetric causes

Panhysterectomy
- Indications for total hysterectomy in perimenopausal age

Extended hysterectomy
- Carcinoma Endometrium

Radical hysterectomy
- Carcinoma **cervix I and II**

Adjuvant Radiotherapy in Cancer Endometrium is given in Case of

- Cervical enlargement
- Lymph node involvement
- Carcinoma in situ
- Poor differentiation
- Deep myometrial involvement

- **Commonest cause of Ca endometrium: Unopposed estrogen**
- **Ca endometrium is associated with PCOD**
- **Most malignant endometrial cancer is: clear cell cancer**
- **Atypical endometrial hyperplasia is treated by hysterectomy**
- **Treatment of choice in elderly female with endometrial hyperplasia is Pan hysterectomy**

Important Points about Endometrial Ca

- Combination of Hypertension, Diabetes and Obesity in association with endometrial Ca is called **'Corpus Cancer Syndrome.'**
- Most common type of endometrial Ca is **'Adenocarcinoma/Endometroid'** Ca
- **'Postmenopausal bleeding'** is the most common clinical feature
- **'Simpsons sign'** in endometrial Ca is Referred pain in Hypogastrium or iliac fossa
- **Endometrial aspiration biopsy** is the investigation of choice for **'screening'** 'endometrial Ca

OVARIAN TUMORS

Benign Ovarian Tumors

Serous Cystadenoma

- **Most common benign** tumor of ovary
- **Most common benign** ovarian tumor which **turns** into malignancy
- **Psammoma body** is present in fast growing tumor
- **Intracystic hemorrhage** and **Malignancy (ADENOCARCINOMA)** are highest in **papillary variety of serous cystadenoma**
- Epithelium **resembles** Epithelium of Endosalpinx (Fallopian tube)

REMEMBER 30%

- **Accounts for 30% of ovarian tumor**
- **Bilateral in 30% of cases**
- **Chance of malignancy is 30%**

Mucinous Cystadenoma

- **Largest benign** ovarian tumor
- **Most common ovarian tumor** which can lead to **Pseudomyxoma peritoni**
- Usually **unilateral**
- Epithelium **resembles** Epithelium of Endocervix
- Occasionally, **associated** with **dermoid cysts or Brenner's tumor**
- **Torsion is most frequently** seen with this tumor

Dermoid Cysts (Benign Cystic Teratoma)

- **Most common Germ** cell tumor of Ovary
- **Most common** ovarian tumor found **during pregnancy**
- Chance of malignancy is **lowest** in this type of Benign ovarian tumor (Usually Squamous cell carcinoma)
- **Rokitansky's Protruberance** is seen
- **Most common type** of cyst lying anterior to uterus
- **Most common complication** is Torsion
- Frequently in **association** with **Mucinous Cystadenoma** to form a combined tumor
- The inner surface of the cyst is always irregular and contains **Embryonic Node** from which the hairs project and in which the teeth and bone are usually found
- **Malignancy** which may develop in Dermoid cyst are:
  - **Squamous cell carcinoma**
  - **Mammary cancer**
  - **Malignant thyroid Tumors**

USMLE Case Scenario

A 42-year-old female on account of abdominal discomfort of 6 months duration reports to her obs/gyne physician. On pelvic examination, there is a right adnexal mass. An abdominal USG Followed by a CT scan demonstrates a 5.5 cm cystic mass involving the right ovary. Grossly, the mass on sectioning is filled with abundant hair and sebum. Microscopically, the mass has glandular spaces lined by columnar epithelium, Teeth, squamous epithelium with hair follicles, cartilage and dense connective tissue.

Fibroma

- Most common **benign** ovarian tumor of **connective tissue origin**
- Most common ovarian tumor **associated** with **Meigs' Syndrome**
- They resemble **histologically** with **Brenner Tumor**

Meigs' Syndrome

- Ascites
- Hydrothorax (Right Sided)
- **Benign** tumor of ovary (FIBROMA)

Pseudo-Meigs Syndrome

- Ascites
- Hydrothorax (Right Sided)
- **Malignant** ovarian tumor of ovary

Remember other Points about Benign Ovarian Tumors

- **Struma Ovarii** is a highly specialized, containing Thyroid tissue, which often leads to Thyrotoxicosis
- **Thecomas** (Pure The Ca Cell Tumors) are benign but those with Granulosa cell element may be malignant

MALIGNANT OVARIAN TUMORS

Remember

- **Among** Gynecological cancers it **Ranks 3rd**
- **Among all** Gynecological cancers in India it accounts for **5%**
- **Among all** deaths due to Gynecologic cancers, **most common** cause is due to **ovarian cancer**
- **Most common Ovarian cancer** is **Papillary Serous Cystadenocarcinoma**
- **Second most common** ovarian cancer is **Endometroid Carcinoma**
- **Most common** in women **< 20 years** of age is **Dysgerminoma**
- **Most common hormonally active** ovarian tumor is **Granulosa-Theca cell Tumors**

Epithelial Cancers

Remember

- Constitute about **80%** of all Primary ovarian Carcinomas
- Bilateral **50%** cases
- **Cystic type** is more common than Solid type
- **Most common histological type is Papillary Serous Cystadenocarcinoma**
- Median age **60 years**
- The **single most important risk factor** for Epithelial ovarian cancer is **Age > 40** years

Ovarian Functional and Neoplastic Tumors

Tumor	Features
Follicle Cysts	• Rare in childhood • Frequent in menstrual years • Never in postmenopausal years • Size < **6 cm**, often bilateral • Occasional anovulation with persistently proliferative endometrium
Corpus luteum cysts	• Occur in menstrual years • Size: **4-6 cm**, unilateral
Theca luteincysts	• Occurs with **H.mole, Chorio Carcinoma, Gonado-Trophin or clomiphene therapy** • **4-5 cm**, multiple, bilaterally • (Ovaries may be >**20 cm** in diameter) • Tense consistency, amenorrhea • HCG elevated as a result of Trophoblastic proliferation

Krukenbergs Tumor

- Are Secondary tumor of the ovary
- They are invariably bilateral solid Tumors
- The primary of these Tumors are: Carcinoma of stomach (70%) **(Most Common Site)**, Carcinoma of large bowel (15%), Carcinoma breast (6%)

Gross Features

- **SURFACE:** Smooth with no tendency to form adhesions; No infiltration of capsule
- **SHAPE:** Retains the shape of normal ovary
- **CONSISTANCY:** Solid waxy; Cystic spaces may be seen due to degeneration.
- **MOBILITY:** Freely movable in the pelvis

Microscopy

- Cellular or myxomatous stroma with Scattered **SIGNET RING CELLS.** (Mucin Secreting cells)
- Involvement of Ovary is by Retrograde Lymphatics
- The first halt of tumor cells between **Stomach and Ovary is Superior Gastric Lymph Nodes**

Primary Ovarian Cancers

- **Epithelial ovarian cancer (80%)**
- **Nonepithelial ovarian (10%)**
  - Epithelial Ovarian Cancer: arise from the epithelial surface of the ovary
  - Nonepithelial Ovarian Cancer: arise from
- **Ovarian germ cells**
- **Sex cord cells**
- **Stromal cells**

Malignant Ovarian Tumors

- In Menopausal, Postmenopausal woman **(> 50 yrs)** the chance of malignancy > **50%** (In premenopausal it is 15%)
- Tumors in childhood are usually malignant
- In **Nulliparous**, more commonly seen. Multiparity, to some extent, protects a woman against ovarian malignancy
- Pain (pressure pain can occur with any tumor; but referred pain suggests malignant involvement of N.root
- **Abnormal** uterine bleeding
- **Rapidly growing** tumor
- **Unilateral** edema
- **Cachexia, loss of apetite and loss of weight** (late stage)

Clinical Findings of Malignant Ovarian Tumor

- Bilateral **(About 50%) Solid tumor** except Fibroma, Brenner tumor and few Feminizing Tumors like Thecoma and Granulosa cell tumor
- **Fixed** tumor
- **Presence of Ascites** (Meigs' Syndrome)
- **Hepatomegaly** due to metastasis
- **Unilateral nonpitting edema of leg or vulva. (characteristic of malignancy)**
- The **nodules in Pouch of Douglas** associated to a pelvic mass is highly suggestive of ovarian malignancy

Primary Epithelial Tumors 80%	Nonepithelial Tumors	Hormone-Producing Tumors
• **Mucinous Cystadenoma** or Cystadenocarcinoma • **Serous Cystadenoma** or Cystadenocarcinoma	• Fibroma Dysgerminoma • Teratoma	• **Estrogen-producing** – Granulosa cell tumor – Thecoma
• **Endometrioma** or Endometrioid Carcinoma • **Clear cell carcinoma** • **Brenner Tumor**	• Gonadoblastoma • Yolk-sac tumor	• **Androgen-producing** – Sertoli-Leydig cell tumor – (Arrhenoblastoma) – Hilar cell tumor
		– Lipoid cell tumor (Ovoblastoma Musculinovoblastoma) – Adrenal-like tumor • **OTHERS** – Carcinoid (Seratonin-producing) – Thyroid tumor (Struma Ovarii) – Choriocarcinoma of the ovary

Complications of Ovarian Tumor

- **Torsion of Pedicle**
- **Intracysic hemorrhage**
- **Infection**
- **Rupture**
- **Psedomyxoma peritonei**
- **Malignancy**

TORSION: Torsion of the Pedicle **(Axial Rotation)** is very common during pregnancy (12%) cases.

Structures Forming the Ovarian Pedicle

Laterally: Infundibulopelvic ligament containing structures there in, i.e. Ovarian vessels, nerves and lymphatics

Medially:
- Ovarian ligament
- Medial end of fallopian tube
- Mesosalpinx containing utero-ovarian anastomotic vessels

Middle:-Broad ligament

Torsion is common in tumors having:
- Moderate Size, preferably with round contor
- Free mobility
- Long pedicle

Predisposing factors for torsion
- Trauma
- Violent physical movement
- Contractions of pregnant uterus

Summary of Torsion of Ovarian Pedicle

- Common in **Dermoid or Simple Serous Cystadenoma**
- Partial axial rotation followed by complete torsion is explained by **hemodynamic theory**
- Symptoms of **acute pain** lower abdomen **with a lump**
- General condition remains **unaffected**
- Abdominal examination reveals a **tense cystic tender mass** in the **hypogastrium** arising from the pelvis
- Pelvic examination reveals the **mass separated** from the uterus
- Treatment is **Laparotomy** and **Ovariotomy**

Staging of Ovarian Tumor

STAGE I Lesion confined to Ovaries

- **Ia**____________(One Ovary; No Ascites)
- **Ib**____________(Both Ovary; No Ascites)
- **Ic**____________ (One or two Ovaries with Ascites)
- **STAGE II** One or two ovaries with extension to Pelvis
- **STAGE III** Widespread intraperitoneal metastases (Omentum commonly involved)
- **STAGE IV** Distant Metastases

Treatment

- Surgically Debulk **all Stages** of Tumor that involves:

Total Abdominal Hysterectomy **(TAH) + BSO+ Omentectomy + any other tumor > 2 cm diameter size**

- In Stage III and Stage IV Debulking Surgery is done or **at least** biopsy of the tumor is obtained

ADJUVANT THERAPY

- Radiotherapy _________**STAGE Ib and Ic**
- Chemotherapy ________**STAGE II, III, IV**

Other Facts about Ovarian Cancer

- Accounts for **5%** of all Gynecological cancers in India
- **Most common cause of death** due to Gynecological cancers is **Ovarian Carcinoma**
- **Most common Cancer** is **Papillary Serous Cystadenocarcinoma**
- **Second most common** Ovarian cancer is **Endometrioid Carcinoma**

Clinical Associations of Malignant Ovarian Tumors

- **Nulliparity**
- **Infertility**
- Most common ovarian cancer in women **under the age of 20** is Dysgerminoma
- Most common **hormonally active ovarian tumor is Granulosa-Theca cell Tumors**
- Incidence is **higher** amongst women from the affluent classes (due to high fat content in their diet)
- An enlargement of the ovary in women of **menopausal or postmenopausal** age should be regarded as **malignant until proved Otherwise**

Masculinizing Ovarian Tumors

- Arrhenoblastoma/Androblastoma
- Sertoli Leyding cell tumor
- Sertoli cell tumor
- Leyding cell tumor
- Hilus cell tumor
- Adrenocortical tumor
- Gynandroblastoma

Feminizing Tumors

- Granulosa cell tumor
- Theca cell tumor
- Fibromas

• **Call Exner Bodies**	• **Granulosa cell tumor**
• **Renkies Crystals**	• **Hilus cell tumor**
• **Signet ring cells**	• **Krukenberg's tumor**
• **Schiller Duval bodies**	• **Endodermal sinus tumor**
• **Psommoma bodies**	• **Serous tumors**
• **Meigs' syndrome**	• **Fibroma ovary**
• **Pseudomeigs syndrome**	• **Brenner cell tumor**
• **Walthard cell nest**	• **Brenner tumor**
• **Rokintansky bodies**	• **Teratoma**

Increased Risk Associated	Decreased Risk Associated
• **Early menarche**	• **Pregnancy**
• **Nulliparity**	• **Lactation**
• **Late menopause**	• **OCPs**

Guideline for the management of ovarian tumor in pregnancy

During Pregnancy

Uncomplicated	Complicated
Principle: To remove the tumor as soon as the diagnosis is made **Best Time**: For Elective Operation is **14-18th** week • **If** the diagnosis is made **before** this time the patient should be kept **under observation** • **If** the diagnosis is made in **3rd trimester** **Immediate removal** is done • **If** the diagnosis is made **beyond 36 weeks** The operation is **withheld till delivery** and the tumor is **removed as early in puerperium** as possible	The tumor is **removed irrespective of the period of Gestation**

During Labor

• **If the tumor is well above the presenting part**	• **If the tumor is impacted in the pelvis causing obstruction**
A Watchful Expectancy hoping for Vaginal delivery	Cesarean Section followed by removal of tumor in the same sitting

During Puerperium

On Occasion, the diagnosis is made following delivery. The tumor should be removals early in puerperium as possible.

Remember Risk of Malignancy Index (RMI)

RMI = U × M × CA125

U = USG Score determined by:

- **Multilocular cyst**
- **Solid area**
- **Metastasis**
- **Ascites**
- **b/l lesions**

1 point for each

- M = 3 for postmenopausal women
- CA125 level in units/ml
  - **Low risk: RMI < 25**
  - **Moderate risk: RMI 25–250**
  - **High-risk: RMI > 250**

Regarding Ovarian Tumors

Most common (overall) ovarian tumor	**Epithelial cell tumor**
Most common in less than 20 years of age	**Dysgerminoma**
Most common Benign tumor of ovary	**Dermoid Cyst**
Most common tumor in **young women**	**Germ cell tumor**
Most common Malignant tumor	**Serous Cystadenoma**
Most common tumor diagnosed in pregnancy	**Dermoid Cyst**
Most common tumor to undergo torsion	**Dermoid Cyst**
Most radio sensitive ovarian tumor	**Dysgerminoma**

- Marker for ovarian cancer: **CA 125**
- Marker for granulosa cell tumor: **Inhibin**
- Marker for dysgerminoma: **Serum LDH**
- Marker for dysgerminoma: **Placental alkaline phosphatase**

Pseudomyxoma Peritonei

This is a rare condition resulting from

- **Rupture of a mucocele of the appendix**
- **A mucinous ovarian cyst or**
- **Mucin-secreting intestinal or ovarian adenocarcinoma**
  - The abdomen becomes filled with masses of jelly-like mucus
  - Colloid carcinoma arising from the stomach or colon with peritoneal implants may resemble pseudomyxoma at laparotomy
  - The course of this type of highly malignant tumor is one of rapid cachexia and early death
  - The diagnosis usually can be made by the appearance of many **highly malignant cells in the peritoneal implants**

OHSS (Ovarian Hyperstimulation Syndrome)

It is **enlargement of ovary with multiple follicles after stimulation**

'Necklace sign' of ovaries is seen on USG

- Common with FSH/LH therapy
- Clomiphene therapy
- Pulsatile Gn RH therapy
  - **Ascites, hydrothorax**
  - **Cerebrovascular events, DVT, thromboembolism**
  - **Abdominal pain**
  - **Renal failure**
  - **Torsion of ovarian cysts**
  - **Liver dysfunction**
  - **Coagulopathy**

Ovarian Remanent Syndrome

Persistence of ovarian function even after B/L Oopherectomy presenting with Chronic pelvic pain and dyspareunia due to remaining ovarian tissue.

Trapped Residual Ovarian Syndrome

Presenting with Chronic pelvic pain and dyspareunia due to tension within developing follicles with periovarian adhesions or because of perioophritis.

• MC Type of **vulval carcinoma**	**Squamous cell carcinoma**
• MC Type of **vaginal carcinoma**	**Squamous cell carcinoma**
• MC Type of **cervical carcinoma**	**Squamous cell carcinoma**
• MC Type of **endometrial carcinoma**	**Adenocarcinoma**

Differentiate

Vaginismus	Dyspareunia	Desire Disorder	Arousal Disorder	Anorgasmia
Painful reflex spasm of paravaginal thigh adductors Diagnosed by **physical examination** Almost always **psychogenic** Vaginal dilators useful as therapy	Pain **related to sexual intercourse**	**Apathy for and lack of enjoyment of sex**	**Failure of vaginal lubrication and lack of pelvic engorgement**	Women **never has had organism by any means**

Remember

- **Hirsutism**: Male pattern hair growth in females
- **Virilization**: Male pattern hair growth in females + **Clitoromegaly/Baldness/Loss of female body contours/Lowering of voice/↑Muscle mass**
- **↑DHEA: Adrenal tumor**
- **↑Testosterone: PCOD**
- **↑↑↑Testosterone: Ovarian Tumor (Sertoli leyding, Hilus cell tumor)**
- **↑Serum 17 OH Progesterone levels: Congenital Adrenal Hyperplasia**
- **Maternal virilizing tumor of pregnancy** is called **luteoma of pregnancy** can result in masculinization of female fetus

Clomiphene

- **Antiestrogen with weak agonistic activity as well**
- **Enclomiphene has antiestrogenic effect**
- It is indicated in the **treatment of anovulation or oligo-ovulation** in patients desiring pregnancy, whose sexual partners have adequate sperm, and who have potentially functional hypothalamic-hypophyseal-ovarian systems and adequate endogenous estrogen
- **Chances of pregnancy** are 3 fold as compared to placebo
- Risk of **multiple pregnancy** is 6-10 fold
- It may be used to treat **corpus luteum dysfunction**
- It is used to detect **abnormalities of the hypothalamic-pituitary-gonadal axis in males**
- Used in **Stein Levinthal syndrome**
- It is used to **treat infertility in males with oligospermia**
- It is sometimes given as a **test dose to aid in predicting whether an ovulatory response might occur**

Tamoxifen

- **Nonsteroidal antiestrogenic**
- It is indicated for adjuvant treatment of **axillary node-negative breast cancer** in women following total mastectomy or segmental mastectomy, axillary dissection, and breast irradiation
- Indicated for adjuvant treatment of **axillary node-positive breast cancer in postmenopausal women following total mastectomy or segmental mastectomy, axillary dissection, and breast irradiation**
- That women whose tumors **are estrogen receptor-positive** are more likely to benefit from tamoxifen therapy
- It is indicated to **reduce the risk of developing breast cancer in women who have been determined to be at high-risk for developing this cancer**

Danazol

- Androgen derivative
- Gonadotropin inhibitor

Indications

- **Endometriosis treatment**
- Fibrocystic Breast disease
- **Cyclic mastalgia, noncyclic mastalgia**
- Angioedema, hereditary (prophylaxis)
- **Menorrhagia, primary**
- Gynecomastia
- **Puberty precocious**

GnRH Analogues

- **Goserelin**
- **Buserelin**
- **Nafarelin**
- **Histrelin**
- **Triptorelin**

Used for

- **Precocious puberty**
- **Infertility**
- **Ca breast**
- **DUB**
- **Endometriosis**
- **Fibromyoma uterus**
- **Hirsutism**

Important Syndromes

• **Sheehan's syndrome**	• **Postpartum pituitary necrosis**
• **Asherman's syndrome**	• **Overzealous curettage resulting in endometrial synechia**
• **Stein levinthal syndrome**	• **PCOD**
• **Kallaman's syndrome**	• **Primary amenorrhea, hyposmia, failure of secondary sexual features**

Sheehan Syndrome

- **It is a condition affecting women who experience life-threatening blood loss during or after childbirth**

In Sheehan's syndrome, the damage occurs to the pituitary gland

- **The result is the permanent underproduction of essential pituitary hormones (hypopituitarism)**
- For some women, Sheehan's syndrome seems to cause few, if any, symptoms. For others, Sheehan's syndrome can lead to an adrenal crisis—a life-threatening shortage of the hormone cortisol. Treatment of Sheehan's syndrome involves hormone replacement therapy.

Symptoms:

In most cases, the signs and symptoms of Sheehan's syndrome appear slowly, after a period of months or even years

Signs and symptoms of Sheehan's syndrome include:

- **Slowed mental function, weight gain and difficulty staying warm, as a result of an underactive thyroid (hypothyroidism)**
- **Difficulty breastfeeding or an inability to breastfeed**
- **No menstrual periods (amenorrhea) or infrequent menstruation (oligomenorrhea)**
- **Loss of pubic or underarm hair**
- **Low blood pressure**
- **Fatigue**
- **Weight loss**

Remember

• Donovaniosis	• Calymmatobacter granulomatosis
• LGV	• Chlamydia trachomatis
• Chancroid	• H. ducreyi, Herpes hominis
• Condyloma acuminate	• HPV 6, 11, 16, 18
• Yaws	• T. pertune
• Pinta	• T. carateum

'Clinical Scenarios' of USMLE

• **A** 20-year-old **obese** female with **irregular menstrual periods, acne, insulin resistance and elevated LH: FSH ratio**	• **PCOD**
• A 30-year-old female with **foul smelling, frothy, light green colored vaginal discharge with vaginal erythema and strawberry cervix**	• **Trichomonas vaginalis**
• A female of 25 years with **paresthesias, burning pain in perineal area and vesicles showing Cowdry inclusions. Painful inguinal Lymphadenopathy is also noticed**	• **Herpes Simplex II (Herpes Genitalis)**
• A 30-year-old female with **profuse watery, dirty grey discharge giving positive whiff test**	• **Bacterial vaginosis**
• A 55-year-old female with **constipation, abdominal and pelvic swelling increased CA 125 levels**	• **Ovarian Ca**
• **A 22-year-**old female with **irritability, breast tenderness, fatigue, headache and bloating week before menstrual cycles**	• **Premenstrual dysmorphic disorder**
• A female of **35 years** complain of **dysmenorrheal, dyspareunia and dyschezia with fixed retroverted uterus and nodularity of uterosacral ligaments.**	• **Endometriosis**
• A female 36 years old with **dysmenorrhea, menorrhagia, chronic pelvic pain and symmetrically, enlarged smooth uterus** tender to palpation	• **Adenomyosis**
• **A 16-year-old girl with missing periods, failure to gain weight, emaciated with low LH, FSH and Estrogens.**	• **Anorexia Nervosa**
• A female **with fever, diarrhea, skin rash, headache with hypotension** and altered mental status who **used vaginal tampon.**	• **Toxic shock syndrome**
• A 30-year-old female with **soft, pinkish, cauliflower like lesions** with **multiple sex partners responding to Imiquimod**	• **HPV (Condyloma acuminata)**
• A 25-years female **2 weeks after normal delivery inability to breastfeed her child, nausea, weakness and fatigue with low ACTH, LH, FSH**	• **Sheehans syndrome**
• A 33-year-old who is **38 weeks pregnant with rupture membranes** comes in emergency with **respiratory distress, hypotension with ↓platelets and ↑FDD with fetal cells in maternal blood sample**	• **Amniotic fluid embolism**
• A 57-year-old **obese, hypertensive and diabetic female with vaginal bleeding**	• **Endometrial cancer**
• A 16-year-old **female with amnorrhea, webbed neck, low hair line and widely spaced nipples.** USG shows **streak ovaries**	• **Turner's Syndrome**
• A 24-year-old **female with abdominal pain and adnexal mass.** Pelvic USG showing **heterogenous well circumscribed mass with solid and cystic components with dense calcification.**	• **Teratoma**

USMLE Case Scenario

A woman presents with leakage of fluid per vaginum and meconium stained liquor at 34 weeks of gestation. The most likely organism causing infection would be:

1. Listeria monocytogenes
2. Toxoplasmosis
3. CMV
4. Herpes
5. Trichomonas
6. Candida

Ans. 1. Listeria monocytogenes

USMLE Case Scenario

A painless, discrete, sharply circumscribed, unilateral, rubbery, mobile. Mass:

1. It is the most common benign tumor of the female breast
2. It is the most common malignant tumor of the female breast
3. It is the least common benign tumor of the female breast
4. It is the least common malignant tumor of the female breast

Ans. 1. It is the most common benign tumor of the female breast

USMLE Case Scenario

PCOS is an endocrine imbalance characterized by:

1. Estrogen excess and a ratio of leutinizing hormone (LH) to follicle-stimulating hormone (FSH) greater than 2:1
2. Androgen excess and a ratio of leutinizing hormone (LH) to follicle-stimulating hormone (FSH) greater than 2:1
3. Estrogen excess and a ratio of leutinizing hormone (LH) to follicle-stimulating hormone (FSH) equal to 1:1
4. Androgen deficiency and a ratio of leutinizing hormone (LH) to follicle-stimulating hormone (FSH) greater than 2:1

Ans. 2. Androgen excess and a ratio of leutinizing hormone (LH) to follicle-stimulating hormone (FSH) greater than 2:1

USMLE Case Scenario

An episiotomy tear involving rectal sphincter but not rectal mucosa is:

1. A first-degree tear
2. A second-degree tear
3. A third-degree tear
4. A fourth-degree tear

Ans. 3. A third-degree tear

- A first-degree tear involves the vaginal mucosa or perineal skin, but not the underlying tissue.
- In a second-degree episiotomy, the underlying subcutaneous tissue is also involved, but not the rectal sphincter or rectal mucosa.
- In a third-degree tear, the rectal sphincter is affected.
- A fourth-degree episiotomy involves a tear that extends into the rectal mucosa.

USMLE Case Scenario

Epidemics of puerperal sepsis may be caused by:

1. HSV
2. Cytomegalovirus
3. Group A BETA hemolytic streptococci
4. Group B BETA hemolytic streptococci
5. Toxoplasma gondii

Ans. 3. Group A BETA hemolytic streptococci

USMLE Case Scenario

A 22-year-old primigravida at 31 weeks of gestation has a blood pressure of 162/112 mm Hg, serum total bilirubin level (2.8 mg/dL), serum alanine amino transferase level of 155U/L and platelet count of 72,000/mm^3. All other investigations are normal. She is hospitalized for observation and electronic fetal heart rate monitoring of the following the MOST ominous sign of fetal distress during monitoring would be:

1. Early decelerations
2. Increased beat-to-beat variability
3. Late decelerations
4. Spontaneous accelerations
5. Variable decelerations

Ans. 3. Late decelerations

USMLE Case Scenario

A 17-year-old college student presents in emergency with acute onset right-sided abdominal pain. Her last menstrual period was 2 weeks ago. Her temperature is 38.7 °C blood pressure is 122/70 mm Hg, pulse is 82/min and respirations are 17/min. Examination of the throat reveals mild pharyngitis. Her abdomen is diffusely tender, especially the lower abdomen. Rectal examination reveals tenderness anteriorly on the right side. Stool guaiac is negative. A pelvic examination is performed and there is evidence of cervical tenderness. The most likely diagnosis is:

1. Cholecystitis
2. Ovarian cyst
3. Pyelonephritis
4. Pelvic inflammatory disease
5. Endometriosis
6. Peritonitis

Ans. 4. Pelvic inflammatory disease (PID)

Most patients with PID have signs of abdominal pain, lower abdominal tenderness, and the pelvic examination reveals cervical motion tenderness. In addition, the pelvic examination may reveal purulent cervical discharge and an adnexal mass or tenderness may be present.

USMLE Case Scenario

Relation of the long-axis of the fetus to that of the mother is called:

1. Lie
2. Maternal attitude
3. Fetal attitude
4. Presentation

Ans. 1. Lie

Lie of the fetus refers to the relation of the long-axis of the fetus to that of the mother and is classified as longitudinal, transverse, or oblique. Fetal attitude refers to the fetal posture—either flexed or extended. Presentation refers to the portion of the baby that is foremost in the birth canal.

USMLE Case Scenario

The Bishop score is a way to determine the favor ability of the cervix to Induction. The elements of the Bishop score include:

1. Effacement, contraction, station, consistency and position of the cervix
2. Enhancement, dilation, station, consistency and position of the cervix
3. Effacement, dilation, station, consistency and portion of the cervix
4. Effacement, dilation, station, consistency and position of the cervix

Ans. 4. Effacement, dilation, station, consistency and position of the cervix

USMLE Case Scenario

A 66-year-old female present with white lesions, pruritus in her vulval region which have well defined borders. The histological appearance includes loss of the rete pegs within the dermis, chronic inflammatory infiltrate below the dermis, the development of a homogenous subepithelial layer in the dermis, a decrease in the number of cellular layers. The most likely diagnosis is:

1. Lichen planus
2. Lichen sclerosus
3. Vulval carcinoma
4. Leukoplakia

Ans. 2. Lichen sclerosus

USMLE Case Scenario

A female presents with pseudoprecocious puberty, bleeding or menorrhagia. Most likely diagnosis of a tumor that can be the cause is:

1. Granulosa cell tumor
2. Leydig cell tumor
3. Choriocarcinoma
4. Krukenberg's tumor

Ans. 1. Granulosa Cell Tumor

USMLE Case Scenario

Diethylstilbestrol exposure has been associated with an increased incidence of:

1. Clear cell carcinoma of kidney and endometrial carcinomas
2. Endometrial carcinoma and uterine clear cell carcinoma
3. Vaginal and cervical clear cell carcinomas
4. Uterine Sarcoma and endometrial carcinoma

Ans. 3. Vaginal and cervical clear cell carcinomas

USMLE Case Scenario

Factor believed NOT to decrease the risk of developing ovarian cancer:

1. Oral contraceptive use
2. Multiparity
3. Breastfeeding
4. Late menopause

Ans. 4. Late menopause

USMLE Case Scenario

A 60-year-old woman from South Texas comes to the physician 2 months after her husband died in a vehicular accident. She gets easily fatigued. She has had frequent crying spells at night especially when she is alone associated with thoughts of her husband and feels uninvolved in daily activities. Which of the following is the most likely diagnosis?

1. Conversion disorder
2. Generalized anxiety disorder
3. Major depressive disorder
4. Normal grief
5. Pathologic grief

Ans. 4. Normal grief

USMLE Case Scenario

A 34-year-old G1P0 at 34 weeks gestation presents to a maternity clinic with chief complaints of complaining of a four day history of generalized malaise, anorexia and vomiting. She has also complains of abdominal discomfort, a poor appetite. On physical exam, she has mild jaundice. Her vital signs indicate a temperature of 101 °F, pulse of 74, and BP of 100/70. She has no significant edema, and in fact appears very dehydrated.

Blood results are obtained:

- WBC : 22,000
- HCT : 41.0
- Platelets: 45,000
- SGOT/PT: 292/334
- Glucose: 45
- Creatinine: 2.0
- Fibrinogen : 125
- PT/PTT : 12/50s
- Serum ammonia level: 80 mol/L (n 11–35)
- Urinalysis is positive for 3++protein and ketones

The patient's most likely diagnosis is:

1. Hepatitis A
2. Hepatitis B
3. Acute fatty liver of pregnancy
4. Intrahepatic cholestasis of pregnancy
5. Severe preeclampsia
6. Hyperemesis gravidarum
7. Eclampsia

Ans. 3. Acute fatty liver of pregnancy

USMLE Case Scenario

A 66-year-old woman reports to a physician because of troublesome aches and stiffness in her neck, shoulders, and hips for 2 and half months. Her symptoms are more in the morning hours. She has had chronic fatigue and low-grade fevers during this period. On examination:

- **Range of motion of the neck, shoulders, and hips is normal**
- **The muscles are minimally tender to palpation**
- **Muscle strength, sensation, and deep tendon reflexes are normal**
- **Erythrocyte sedimentation rate is 88 mm/h**

Serum rheumatoid factor and antinuclear antibody assays are negative. Which of the following is the most likely diagnosis?

1. SLE
2. Rheumatoid arthritis
3. Fibromyositis
4. Osteoarthritis
5. Polymyalgia rheumatica
6. Polymyositis
7. Polyarteritis Nodosa
8. Wegner's granulomatosis
9. Seronegative rheumatoid arthritis

Ans. 5. Polymyalgia Rheumatica

USMLE Case Scenario

A 26-year-old woman, gravida 2, para 1, comes to the physician because of vaginal discharge and vulvar pruritus for 8 days. She is allergic to penicillin. Her last menstrual period was 1 week ago. There is a thin, bubbly, pale green discharge. A wet mount preparation shows a mobile, pear-shaped, flagellated organism. Most effective treatment is by:

1. Miconazole
2. Penicillin
3. Spectinomycin
4. Spiramycin
5. Tetracycline
6. Metronidazole

Ans. 6. Metronidazole

USMLE Case Scenario

A 27-year-old woman, gravida 2, para 2, comes to the physician because of vaginal discharge, vulvar pruritus and burning and dyspareunia for 2 days. She has no drug allergies. The vagina is tender and erythematous. A KOH wet mount preparation shows spores and hyphae. Most effective treatment is by:

1. Cefazolin
2. Ceftriaxone
3. Erythromycin
4. Gentamicin
5. Griseofulvin
6. Metronidazole
7. Miconazole
8. Penicillin

Ans. 7. Miconazole

USMLE Case Scenario

A 26-year-old young mother comes to the emergency department with her 5-day-old son. She explains that he has been feeding poorly over the last 2 days and has been very irritable, crying all the time and jittery during the day. She has also noticed that his breathing had become irregular over the last few hours and his hands and feet have turned blue in between. On physical examination, the infant has a temperature of 35.6 °C pulse is 99/min and respirations are 38/min. He is irritable and restless during the exam. The pregnancy was uneventful but labor was prolonged and the membranes had ruptured 12 hours before the baby was delivered. The anterior fontanelle is bulging and there is peripheral cyanosis. Which of the following is the most likely diagnosis?

1. Congenital rubella
2. Congenital syphilis
3. Congenital toxoplasmosis
4. Neonatal herpes simplex virus infection
5. Neonatal sepsis

Ans. 5. Neonatal sepsis

USMLE Case Scenario

A female has amenorrhea with absence of a vagina. Most likely cause is:

1. Wolfian agenesis
2. Mesonephric duct agenesis
3. Hypothyroidism
4. Turner's syndrome
5. Mullerian agenesis

Ans. 5. Mullerian agenesis

Also known as Mayer-Rokitansky-Kuster-Hauser syndrome, presents as amenorrhea with absence of a vagina. The incidence is approximately 1 in 10,000 female births. The karyotype is 46, XX. There is normal development of breasts, sexual hair, ovaries, tubes and external genitalia. There are associated skeletal (12%) and urinary tract (33%) anomalies.

USMLE Case Scenario

During pregnancy:

1. There is an increase in the glomerular filtration rate and a increase in tubular reabsorption of filtered glucose
2. There is an decrease in the glomerular filtration rate and a decrease in tubular reabsorption of filtered glucose
3. There is an decrease in the glomerular filtration rate and a increase in tubular reabsorption of filtered glucose
4. There is an increase in the glomerular filtration rate and a decrease in tubular reabsorption of filtered glucose

Ans. 4. There is an increase in the glomerular filtration rate and a decrease in tubular reabsorption of filtered glucose

The finding of glucosuria is common during pregnancy and usually is not indicative of any pathology. During pregnancy, there is an increase in the glomerular filtration rate and a decrease in tubular reabsorption of filtered glucose. In fact, one of six women will spill glucose in the urine during pregnancy.

USMLE Case Scenario

A female presents with amenorrhea, infantile sexual development, low gonadotropins, normal female karyotype, and inability to perceive odors. Most likely cause is:

1. Mullerian agenesis
2. PCOD
3. Noonan's syndrome
4. McCune-Albright syndrome
5. Kallmann's syndrome
6. Turner's syndrome

Ans. 5. Kallmann's Syndrome

USMLE Case Scenario

A 38-year-old female from Ilinos complains of dysmenorrhea and menorrhagia, examination findings include a tender, symmetrically enlarged uterus without adnexal tenderness. Most likely cause is:

1. Endometriosis
2. Adenomyosis
3. Hypothyroidism
4. Prolactinoma
5. Uterine sarcoma

Ans. 2. Adenomyosis

USMLE Case Scenario

A 28-year-old patient with five months of secondary amenorrhea, A doctor orders serum prolactin. The pregnancy test is positive and the prolactin comes back at 110 ng/mL (normal: 25 ng/mL in this assay). This patient requires

1. No active intervention
2. Bromocriptine to suppress prolactin
3. Evaluation for possible hypothyroidism
4. MRI scan of her sella turcica to rule out pituitary adenoma
5. Repeat measurements of serum prolactin to ensure that values do not increase over 300 ng/mL

Ans. 1. No active intervention

Serum prolactin levels can be elevated in pregnancy

USMLE Case Scenario

A female in her third trimester comes to maternity clinic with pustular eruption along the margins of erythematous patches at points of flexure and extend peripherally with involvement of mucous membrane of oral cavity. Patients has only mild pruritus, but had nausea, vomiting, diarrhea, chills and fever. Most likely cause is:

1. Impetigo by streptococcus
2. Impetigo by staphylococcus
3. Impetigo herpetiformis
4. Herpes gestationis
5. Intrahepatic cholestasis

Ans. 3. Impetigo herpetiformis

USMLE Case Scenario

A CT Scan of a 44-year-old female reveals bilateral, solid masses of the ovary that represent metastases from stomach. They contain large numbers of signet ring adenocarcinoma cells within a cellular hyperplastic but non-neoplastic ovarian stroma. Most likely tumor is:

1. Dermoid cyst
2. Liposarcoma
3. Krukenberg's tumor
4. Gynandroblastoma

Ans. 3. Krukenberg's tumor

USMLE Case Scenario

A 22-year-old female from ilinos G1P0 presents to maternity unit for a routine return visit at 30 weeks. The patient has a number of bruises on the abdomen and chest. After being asked by the doctor what happened and she tells him that the bruises are due to fall from stairs in her apartment. The patient comes again to the clinic twelve days after later for another routine visit, and the doctor notes that she has a black eye. All investigations and psychiatric check-up are normal. Most likely cause is:

1. Sexual abuse
2. Machunsen's syndrome by proxy
3. Domestic violence
4. Coagulopathy

Ans. 3. Domestic violence

USMLE Case Scenario

A 54-year-old postmenopausal female attends to her Gynecologist. She is gravida 3, para 3 and is having trouble some urinary leakage 4–5 weeks in duration. The first step in her evaluation would be:

1. Ultrasound
2. Urinalysis
3. Intravenous pyelogram (IVP)
4. Cystourethrogram
5. Urethrocystoscopy
6. Hysteriosalpingogram

Ans. 2. Urinalysis

USMLE Case Scenario

A 43-year-old female from New Orleans had a baby with Down syndrome 10 years ago. She is Anxious to know the chromosome status of her fetus in a current pregnancy. The test that has the fastest lab processing time for karyotype is:

1. Amniocentesis
2. Cordocentesis
3. Chorionic villus sampling (CVS)
4. Doppler flow ultrasound
5. Cystic hygroma aspiration

Ans. 3. Chorionic villus sampling (CVS) has many theoretical and practical advantages over amniocentesis, including its earlier performance and quicker results.

USMLE Case Scenario

Vaccines are contraindicated in pregnancy, even following maternal exposure, for which of the following diseases?

1. Rabies
2. Tetanus
3. Typhoid
4. Hepatitis B
5. Measles

Ans. 5. Measles

USMLE Case Scenario

A syndrome of multiple congenital anomalies including microcephaly, cardiac anomalies and growth retardation has been described in children of women who are heavy users of:

1. Amphetamines
2. Barbiturates
3. Heroin
4. Methadone
5. Ethyl alcohol

Ans. 5. Ethyl alcohol

Which can cause liver disease, folate deficiency, and many other disorders in a pregnant woman, also can lead to the development of congenital abnormalities in the child.

The chief abnormalities associated with the fetal alcohol syndrome are microcephaly, growth retardation and cardiac anomalies. Chronic abuse of alcohol may also be associated with an increased incidence of mental retardation in the children of affected women.

USMLE Case Scenario

True statement is:

1. Down syndrome is associated with increased levels of maternal serum AFP levels and an elevated maternal serum AFP is associated with abdominal wall defect
2. Down syndrome is associated with decreased levels of maternal serum AFP levels and a decreased maternal serum AFP is associated with abdominal wall defect
3. Down syndrome is associated with increased levels of maternal serum AFP levels and a decreased maternal serum AFP is associated with abdominal wall defect
4. Down syndrome is associated with decreased levels of maternal serum AFP levels and an elevated maternal serum AFP is associated with abdominal wall defect

Ans. 4. Down syndrome is associated with decreased levels of maternal serum AFP levels and an elevated maternal serum AFP is associated with abdominal wall defect.

USMLE Case Scenario

Alcohol is a potent teratogen. Fetal alcohol syndrome is the most common cause of mental retardation in the United States and consists of a constellation of fetal defects including all except:

1. Craniofacial anomalies
2. Growth restriction
3. Behavioral disturbances
4. Brain defects
5. Cardiac defects
6. Spinal defects
7. Aneurysms

Ans. 7. Aneurysms

USMLE Case Scenario

Smoking has been shown to cause Fetal Growth Restriction and is not related to:

1. Increased incidences of subfertility
2. Spontaneous abortions
3. Placenta previa
4. Abruption
5. Post-term delivery
6. Reduced uteroplacental blood flow
7. Fetal hypoxia

Ans. 5. Post-term delivery

USMLE Case Scenario

A 14-year-old girl with amenorrhea, short stature, neck webbing and sexual infantilism is found to have coarctation of the aorta. A chromosomal analysis likely would demonstrate which of the following?

1. Mutation at 21
2. Trisomy 21
3. XO karyotype
4. XXY karyotype

Ans. 3. XO karyotype

Short stature, neck webbing, sexual infantilism and a shield like chest with widely spaced nipples are Features of Turner syndrome, which is usually associated with an XO karyotype.

USMLE Case Scenario

A female in her first trimester meets a doctor and asks for herbal medications. She is taking good diet and examination is normal. In addition to taking her own diet she persistently feels need for something else as a supplement. Recently from her friend she has come to know about herbal medications. She is pretty much impressed about these medications without side effects and says she wants to have them for the well-being of her baby. As a doctor in Maternity unit you would:

1. Recommend to her the use of herbal remedies because such products are classified as dietary supplements and are FDA-regulated for purity, safety, and efficacy and there is no significant data regarding the teratogenic potential of herbal medications in humans
2. Recommend to her the use of herbal remedies because such products are not classified as dietary supplements and are not FDA-regulated for purity, safety and efficacy and there is no significant data regarding the teratogenic potential of herbal medications in humans

3. Not recommend to her the use of herbal remedies because such products are classified as dietary supplements and are not FDA-regulated for purity, safety, and efficacy and there is significant data regarding then on teratogenic potential of herbal medications in humans
4. Not recommend to her the use of herbal remedies because such products are classified as dietary supplements and are not FDA-regulated for purity, safety, and efficacy and there is no significant data regarding the teratogenic potential of herbal medications in humans

Ans. 4. Not recommend to her the use of herbal remedies because such products are classified as dietary supplements and are not FDA-regulated for purity, safety and efficacy and there is no significant data regarding the teratogenic potential of herbal medications in humans.

USMLE Case Scenario

Use of the following drug has been associated with an increased incidence of placental abruption and skull defects, disruptions in urinary tract development, limb defects and cardiac anomalies:

1. LSD
2. Marijuana
3. Prilocaine
4. Cocaine

Ans. 4. Cocaine

USMLE Case Scenario

Amniocentesis performed in the second trimester has been associated with:

1. 1 to 2% risk of amniotic fluid leakage, a fetal loss rate of less than 0.5%
2. 3 to 4% risk of amniotic fluid leakage, a fetal loss rate of less than 5 but more than 2
3. 4 to 5% risk of amniotic fluid leakage, a fetal loss rate of less than 0.5%
4. 1 to 2% risk of amniotic fluid leakage, a fetal loss rate of less than 5 but more than 2

Ans. 1. 1 to 2% risk of amniotic fluid leakage, a fetal loss rate of less than 0.5%

USMLE Case Scenario

A 28-year-old G2P1 is undergoing an elective repeat cesarean section at term. The infant is delivered without any difficulties, but the placenta cannot be removed easily because a clear plane between the placenta and uterine wall cannot be identified. The placenta is removed in pieces. This is followed by uterine atony and hemorrhage. Most likely she is having:

1. Fenestrated placenta
2. Succenturiate placenta
3. Vasa previa
4. Placenta previa
5. Membranaceous placenta
6. Placenta accreta

Ans. 6. Placenta accreta

USMLE Case Scenario

A 30-year-old female from Washington G2P1 presents at 28 weeks gestational age complaining of the sudden onset of profuse red vaginal bleeding. The patient denies any abdominal pain or uterine contractions. Her history is significant for a previous cesarean section at term for fetal breech presentation. She admits to smoking several cigarettes a day, but denies any drug or alcohol use. Most likely she is having:

1. Fenestrated placenta
2. Succenturiate placenta
3. Vasa previa

4. Placenta previa
5. Membranaceous placenta
6. Placenta accreta

Ans. 4. Placenta previa

USMLE Case Scenario

A 39-year-old female on account of abdominal discomfort of 6 months duration reports to her obs/gyne physician. On pelvic examination, there is a right adnexal mass. An abdominal CT scan demonstrates a 5.5 cm cystic mass involving the right ovary. Grossly, the mass on sectioning is filled with abundant, teeth, hair and sebum. Microscopically, the mass has glandular spaces lined by columnar epithelium, squamous epithelium with hair follicles, cartilage and dense connective tissue. True statement about this mass would be:

1. It indicates highly malignant neoplasm
2. It lies within the uterus mostly
3. It is a derived from all three germ layers
4. It is derived from Neural crest

Ans. 3. It is a derived from all three germ layers

The cystic nature and circumscribed appearance of the mass are consistent with a mature cystic teratoma, which contains tissues representing all germ layers of the embryo.

USMLE Case Scenario

A 32-year-old female Late in pregnancy complains of dizziness, light-headedness and syncope after she assumes the supine position. The doctor recommended to her that she should not remain in the supine position for any prolonged period of time in the latter part of pregnancy. It is because:

1. The gravid uterus compresses the aorta and decreases venous return to the heart which results in decreased cardiac output
2. The gravid uterus compresses the inferior vena cava and decreases venous return to the heart which results in decreased cardiac output
3. The gravid uterus compresses the superior vena cava and decreases venous return to the heart which results in decreased cardiac output
4. The gravid uterus compresses the celiac ganglion and decreases venous return to the heart which results in decreased cardiac output

Ans. 2. The gravid uterus compresses the inferior vena cava and decreases venous return to the heart which results in decreased cardiac output

USMLE Case Scenario

True statement is:

1. Bilateral hydronephrosis and hydroureter is a normal finding during pregnancy and does not require any additional workup or concern
2. Bilateral hydronephrosis and hydroureter is an abnormal finding during pregnancy and does require additional workup or concern
3. Bilateral hydronephrosis and hydroureter is a surgical emergency during pregnancy and does require immediate additional workup
4. Bilateral hydronephrosis and hydroureter is a surgical emergency finding during pregnancy and does not require any additional workup or concern

Ans. 1. Bilateral hydronephrosis and hydroureter is a normal finding during pregnancy and does not require any additional workup or concern

USMLE Case Scenario

A 36-year-old female has abdominal tenderness, cervical motion tenderness and adnexal tenderness. She also has a fever, a mucopurulent cervical discharge and an elevated white blood cell count. Most likely diagnosis is:

1. Adenomyosis
2. Endometriosis
3. PCOD
4. PID

Ans. 4. PID

USMLE Case Scenario

The expected date of delivery can be estimated by using Naegele's rule. To do this, a doctor has to:

1. Count back 3 months and then add 7 days to the date of the first day of the last normal menstrual period
2. Count back 4 months and then add 7 days to the date of the first day of the last normal menstrual period
3. Count back 5 months and then add 7 days to the date of the first day of the last normal menstrual period
4. Count back 6 months and then add 7 days to the date of the first day of the last normal menstrual period

Ans. 1. Count back 3 months and then add 7 days to the date of the first day of the last normal menstrual period

USMLE Case Scenario

A 23-year-old pregnant female from Chicago has a history of the onset of an involuntary movement disorder from three weeks that involves rapid and fluid, but not rhythmic, limb and trunk movements. She has no drooling of saliva or intention tremor. There is no family history suggestive of any neurological disorder. She does not suffer from any other disease. Which of the following is the most likely diagnosis?

1. Parkinsonism
2. Lewy Body disease
3. Prion disease
4. Chorea gravidarum
5. Huntington's chorea
6. Alzheimer's disease
7. Multiple sclerosis
8. Amyotrophic lateral sclerosis

Ans. 4. Chorea gravidarum

USMLE Case Scenario

In the Twin-to-Twin transfusion syndrome

1. Hydramnios does not occur
2. Hydramnios can develop in either twin but is more frequent in the recipient because of circulatory overload
3. Hydramnios can develop in either twin but is more frequent in the donor because of circulatory overload
4. Hydramnios can develop in either twin but is equally frequent in both twins

Ans. 2. Hydramnios can develop in either twin but is more frequent in the recipient because of circulatory overload

USMLE Case Scenario

A woman over 45 years of age from North America has hypertension, proteinuria and features suggestive of hyperthyroidism. She hasan enlarged-for-dates uterus and has had intermittent bleeding in the first two trimesters. Grossly her lesions appear as small, clear clusters of grape like vesicles, the passage of which confirms the diagnosis of H. mole A tissue sample would show:

1. No villi
2. Villi without hydropic changes and no vessels

3. Villi with hydropic changes and no vessels
4. Villi with hydropic changes and plenty of vessels

Ans. 3. Villi with hydropic changes and no vessels

USMLE Case Scenario

Fetal hydrops occurs as a result of excessive and prolonged hemolysis due to isoimmunization. Characteristics of fetal hydrops include abnormal fluid in two or more sites such as the thorax, abdomen and skin. The placenta in fetal hydropsis:

1. Pale, enlarged and boggy
2. Pale, smaller and shrunken
3. Erythematous, enlarged and boggy
4. Erythematous, small and shrunken

Ans. 3. Erythematous, enlarged and boggy

USMLE Case Scenario

The therapeutic range of serum magnesium to prevent seizures is:

1. 4 to 7 mg/dL
2. 10 to 12 mg/dL
3. 15 to 20 mg/dL
4. 25-30 mg/Dl

Ans. 1. 4 to 7 mg/dL

At levels between 8 and 12 mg/dL, patellar reflexes are lost. At 10 to 12 mg/dL, somnolence and slurred speech commonly occur. Muscle paralysis and respiratory difficulty occur at 15 to 17 mg/dL and cardiac arrest occurs at levels greater than 30 mg/dL.

USMLE Case Scenario

True statement about appendicitis in pregnancy is:

1. Appendicitis in pregnancy is easy to diagnose and has lesser mortality
2. Appendicitis in pregnancy is easy to diagnose but has more mortality
3. Appendicitis in pregnancy is difficult to diagnose but has lesser mortality
4. Appendicitis in pregnancy is difficult to diagnose and has more mortality

Ans. 4. Appendicitis in pregnancy is difficult to diagnose and has more mortality

The diagnosis is very difficult in pregnancy because leukocytosis, nausea and vomiting are common in pregnancy and the upward displacement of the appendix by the uterus may cause appendicitis to simulate cholecystitis, pyelonephritis and gastritis. Surgery is necessary even if the diagnosis is not certain. Delays in surgery due to difficulty in diagnosis as the appendix moves up are probably the cause of increasing maternal mortality with increasing gestational age.

USMLE Case Scenario

A 26-year-old previously healthy primigravida from New York City is in the first trimester of pregnancy. During two successive prenatal visits, she has fasting serum glucose levels of 129 and 135 mg/dL. Prior to this pregnancy, her fasting serum glucose was 81 mg/dL. A hemoglobin A1C level is 8.1% at the last visit, at 18 weeks gestation. She feels well and has no major health problems. In the latter part of her pregnancy she is likely to have?

1. Agenesis of corpus callosum
2. Ketoacidosis
3. Chondrodysplasia
4. Hyperosmolar coma
5. Teratology of Fallot
6. Placental insufficiency

Ans. 6. Placental Insufficiency

The problem in gestational diabetes is eventual placental malfunction in the third trimester with potential fetal demise.

USMLE Case Scenario

HELLP syndrome is:

1. Hepatitis, elevated liver enzymes, low plasma albumin
2. Hepatitis, elevated liver enzymes, low platelets
3. Hemolysis, elevated liver enzymes, low platelets
4. Hemolysis, elevated liver enzymes, low plasma albumin

Ans. 3. Hemolysis, elevated liver enzymes, low platelets

USMLE Case Scenario

A placenta is seen to be located at the edge of the cervical. It signifies:

1. Complete placenta previa
2. Partial placenta previa
3. Marginal placenta previa
4. Placenta accrete

Ans. 3. Marginal placenta previa

Complete previa describes a placenta that completely covers the cervical os. Partial previa is a placenta that covers some of the cervical os, with the remainder of the os uncovered by the placenta

USMLE Case Scenario

Eyrthroplasia of Querat is:

1. Carcinoma in situ on vulva
2. Carcinoma in situ on lip
3. Carcinoma in situ on scrotum
4. Carcinoma in situ on glans penis

Ans. 4. Carcinoma in situ on glans penis

NOTES

NOTES

NOTES